RECENT ADVANCES IN OBESITY RESEARCH: II

RECENT ADVANCES IN OBESITY RESEARCH: II

Proceedings of the 2nd International Congress on Obesity

23-26 October 1977
Washington DC

Edited by
GEORGE A BRAY
University of California
at Los Angeles

NEWMAN PUBLISHING

British Library Cataloguing in Publication Data:

Recent advances in obesity research.
2: Proceedings of the 2nd International Congress on Obesity, 23-26 October, 1977, Washington DC.
1. Obesity - Congresses
I. Title II. International Congress on Obesity, 2nd, Washington, 1977
III. Bray, George A
616.3'98 RC628

ISBN: 0 7079 6602 7
ISSN: 0306-7548

Published in the UK by
NEWMAN PUBLISHING LTD
48 Poland Street
London W1V 4PP

Printed in Great Britain by
Biddles Ltd, Guildford, Surrey

Preface

The Second International Congress on Obesity met in Washington D.C. on October 23-26, 1977, for the exchange of ideas and information about a problem of major scientific and public interest. The papers from the six lectures and 11 symposia which were presented at this meeting were assembled in this volume to provide the interested reader with an up-to-date review of new vistas in the study of obesity.

The First International Congress on Obesity was held in London in October, 1974, and a third one is planned for Rome in 1980. The initial kernel of an idea for the International Congress as well as the 'International Journal of Obesity' germinated one afternoon along the River Rhine when Dr Alan Howard and I were discussing some of our mutual problems in the field of obesity. Dr Howard took these ideas back to the Association for the Study of Obesity. With their support, and the leadership of Dr Trevor Silverstone and his able committee, the First International Congress on Obesity was organized and held. The Proceedings were duly published under the editorship of Dr Alan Howard. Between the First and Second Congress on Obesity, the 'International Journal of Obesity' was born with Alan Howard and myself as editors. With publication of the Proceedings from the Second International Congress on Obesity, our dreams born by the River Rhine in 1972 have come to life.

Several important areas in the field of obesity are worthy of special comment. The study of the fat cell has provided new insights into basic biology and into the clinical importance of changes in fat tissue. Of particular clinical interest is the observation that success in the treatment of the overweight individual may be related to the size of his fat cells. This suggests that studies evaluating treatment should include measurements of the size and number of fat cells.

Energy expenditure has also received continuing study. There is now convincing evidence that after overeating of a sufficiently large number of calories the metabolic rate may rise up to 15 per cent. Conversely, with starvation, there is a compensatory reduction in metabolic rate. These small but real variations in 'efficiency' of energy utilization may play a role in the differences between lean and obese subjects.

Application of basic information obtained from the study of obese animals and applied to the problem of human obesity may be expected to yield new ways of treating overweight individuals. There are several different models of obesity which have been widely studied. A new enzymatic defect has been proposed which could account for many, if not all, of the biochemical changes in some of these animals. Such a finding may have important therapeutic implications. The importance of the autonomic nervous system as the connection between the central nervous system and the control of insulin secretion has also received emphasis. Insulin, the pancreatic hormone which is central for the storage and utilization of body fuels, is increased in all forms of obesity. Recent studies suggest that this hormone may account for many of the changes which are described in obesity. Finally, the 'supermarket diet' of tidbits from the grocery store will result in obesity when fed to experimental animals. This finding provides an important basis for obesity in experimental animals and may be the best model for human obesity.

The psychological components of obesity and their use in treatment were the focus of several panels. During the past decade there has been a widespread adaptation of techniques of behavioral modification to help overweight people control eating situations. Since the initial flurry of enthusiasm for this approach, there have been a number of well-designed studies aimed at analyzing the successful components of this technique. Although much new information about the behavioral aspects of eating have been generated from these studies, there has been little improvement in the overall success. Indeed, all available evidence indicates that there has been a steady increase in the percentage of overweight people in the population in spite of these technical advances.

Starvation and protein-supplemented starvation have been popularized recently and in the form of liquid protein diets have been widely marketed. The Center for Disease Control in the United States has reported on a number of deaths associated with this form of dietary treatment. Because of this interest surfacing at the time of the Second International Congress on Obesity, the panel on dietary control and protein-supplemented starvation was of particular interest. Although there is some good, sound investigation presented in the accompanying papers, there is still a wide gulf between the theoretical understanding of the way in which the body responds to such a program of treatment and the application of this technique for the widespread treatment of overweight people.

Although millions of people have reportedly participated in the commercial and non-profit self-help groups, there is only a small amount of useful information available for analysis. One study from Europe has found that there are some differences between the outcomes, but that by and large the effectiveness of all the commercial self-help groups are similar. Addition of techniques for behavioral modification may improve the results, but the application of these techniques on a wider basis to commercial groups has not yet been reported.

Government, industry, and the academic community combined forces in the final symposium to present information on the way in which each of these groups might help with the problems of obesity in society. It is now evident that the problem of obesity extends beyond the medical and academic community and that the involvement of commercial enterprises such as food processors and food distributors is essential, if the problem is to be dealt with effectively. This latter area holds major promise for future development.

In 1977/8, the study of obesity is alive and thriving. The chapters in this volume attest to this fact and promise a bright and rewarding future for research in this area. In addition to the papers published in this volume, the abstracts are published in the *International Journal of Obesity* (1978: issues No. 3 and 4 of Vol. 2). In these abstracts are the seeds for many of tomorrow's major advances.

The planning and organization for the Second International Congress on Obesity required the help of many people and organizations whose aid I wish to acknowledge. The sponsoring organizations including the American Medical Association, the American Society of Bariatric Physicians, American Society for Clinical Nutrition, the Association for the Study of Obesity, the National Council on Obesity, and the Nutrition Foundation were most helpful for the people and ideas they contributed. A number of organizations provided financial support including Boehringer Ingelheim Ltd., General Foods Corporation, Hoffmann-LaRoche, the Kroc Foundation, Merck Sharp and Dohme Research Laboratories, Merrell-National Laboratories, Pennwalt Corporation, Proctor and Gamble Co., Riker Laboratories, the A.H. Robins Co., Ross Laboratories, Stokeley-Van Camp, Inc., the Upjohn Company, and Weight Watchers Foundation. Finally, the organizing committee and international liason committee deserve especial thanks for their help with the planning and execution of the program. This committee was composed of Drs George Cahill, Johanna Dwyer, M.R.C. Greenwood, Jules Hirsch, John Garrow, Henry A. Jordan, Judith Rodin, Lester B. Salans, Trevor Silverstone, Ethan A.H. Sims, Albert J. Stunkard, Theodore B. Van Itallie, and Philip L. White. The rapid preparation of this book is a credit to the prompt submission of manuscripts and the enthusiasm of the publishers, in particular Mr Eldred Smith-Gordon. Finally, I am especially indebted to Ms B. Fisher, conference co-ordinator, and to my secretaries Ms J. Martinez and Ms N. deLeon.

Harbor General Hospital
Torrance, California,
December, 1977

George A. Bray, Editor

CONTENTS

1
OBESITY: A PERSPECTIVE

J. HIRSCH
The Rockefeller University, 1230 York Avenue, New York, NY10021, USA.

I find it very difficult to view obesity in perspective. Any discussion of etiology or of treatment, at the present time, must involve social and psychological considerations as well as the input from neurophysiology, biochemistry, pharmacology and other disciplines of biology and medicine. Thus, it is with trepidation that one attempts the evaluation of where we now stand. My views are very subjective, yet I hope you may find them useful. Let me begin with a few facts and a definition of what I consider to be the chief, unsolved problem of obesity.

Obesity has a remarkably high incidence, at least in the Western world. Many efforts have been made to quantify the exact incidence of obesity. But, there is always the problem of how body fat is to be measured and also what cut off point to use to separate the obese from the non-obese. I must say that I have not found such studies to be particularly edifying. It is not unreasonable to state that at least 10 per cent of Americans are obese by almost any standard.

I think we can also agree that the presence of obesity is either a cause or is correlated with a variety of hazards to health, among which diabetes, hypertension and coronary artery disease are particularly noteworthy. The exact level of hazard and the meaning of such co-correlates as hyperlipidemia are difficult to assess. Yet, there is broad agreement that a reduction in the incidence of obesity would advance public health.

The technique for achieving weight reduction is clearly some mixture of reducing food intake and increasing energy use through programs of exercise and physical fitness.

The true problem of obesity is nothing that I have said so far, but rather the sad fact that treatment is in general unsuccessful. It is most discouraging to have such non-toxic and simple treatment as a reduction in food intake and yet have so little treatment success. This, to me, is the central problem of obesity. I find it hard to believe that this problem is due to a lack of nutritional information or to some unusual lack of motivation found in the obese. Indeed, the obese are extremely well motivated to try each new or fad diet that is popularized. New diets and 'how to do it' books periodically become favorite topics of conversation at cocktail parties.

The persistence of obesity in the face of well-publicized information on the health hazard of obesity and readily available, simple means for safely eating less, suggest to me that there is a more subtle problem of obesity that many of us have been led to believe.

I would like to formulate the problem in this way. Every organism is continuously adapting and responding to the signals it receives from within and without. At any moment there is an equilibrium which is the result of the stresses or deformations placed on the system. The state of the system is determined by its genetic endowment and the forces that have acted on it. This is surely as inflexible a law of biology as the principle of rising entropy is to the physicist. The state of health or of disease, whether it be hypertension or diabetes or obesity, is a state of adaptation and equilibrium between the organism and its environment.

The obese individual involved in weight reduction or attempting to live at a new, lower body weight is changing an adaptation and this is experienced as a dysphoric or unpleasant experience. I have no doubt that the adaptation which we call obesity is an unfortunate and risky adaptation, but to call obesity anything other than an adaptation is to believe that obese individuals are in some way capricious. I am unwilling to believe this to be the case.

My colleagues and I have shown that severely obese individuals with childhood-onset disease find that weight reduction leads to disturbances in body image perception, in timing behavior and in affective state. These changes are reminiscent of the response of normal weight individuals to starvation. Such adverse sequelae of weight reduction disappear when the obese state is resumed. It seems almost a tautology to say that all obese who fail to maintain lower body weights experience some adverse consequences of weight loss that exceeds the obvious benefits of being slimmer and healthier. Thus, the former adaptation of obesity is again restored.

Although what I am saying may seem obvious and reasonable, I must point out that this approach to the problem of obesity makes one realize there is no reason for discriminating against the obese or increasing their feelings of guilt and inadequacy. It also leads us to realize how primitive some of our treatments are. It is not my purpose to condemn any currently advocated, radical or 'adventurous' treatments, since I know that obesity can kill and sometimes radical treatment must be used in despair, yet conceptually some suggested means of treatment seem to me to be the modern day equivalent of beating the insane to keep them quiet.

The problem then is why the obese find normal body weight and normal, non-obese patterns of food intake and exercise to be so disequilibrating and so difficult to achieve. What can this be due to?

The simplest answer is direct and mechanistic. They must have some biochemical or cellular defect. In other words, there is either a constitutional or environmentally produced single defect which is ameliorated or adapted to only by the assumption of greater fat storage in adipose tissues. One of my distinguished colleagues has whimsically suggested that there may be some as yet undiscovered enzyme: alpha-corpulase inhibitor. A defect in the production of such an enzyme would be the root cause of all obesity. Given an environment with abundant food, the organism is impelled to react to this deficiency by becoming obese.

This would seem to be an utterly naive answer to the problem, since the obese state is so involved with psychologic and social factors which must differ from one person to another. Yet, it is remarkable how ornate and misleading ignorance can be.

Consider with me, for a moment, a medical fable. I assure you this is purely a fictional tale, but hopefully it illustrates a point.

Many years ago there was a nomadic desert tribe that gave up its wanderings and settled into a very isolated valley. There was a limited water supply - from a single mountain spring. The viability of the group depended on the spring. The tribe could not increase in size and always had to exercise great care in conserving water and drinking as little as possible. Their culture, with its art and symbols, was heavily conditioned by the existence of the mountain spring which was their link to survival.

The isolation of the tribe created the need for consanguineous marriages and this led to many genetic aberrations. The most cruel of all was a disorder of the pituitary - a form of diabetes insipidus. The symptoms were exclusively the need to drink a lot of water and produce a urine of low specific gravity. Since the severity of the disorder varied there were types of over-drinkers - some over-drank a little and some a lot - some began to do so in childhood and others as adults. The combined over-drinkers of childhood and adult-onset were roughly 10 per cent of the population. They were most unhappy unless they could over-drink, although everyone was always a little thirsty in that hot environment. Over-drinkers felt guilty and were the object of discrimination. The theories as to why over-drinking occurred were numerous. Some felt it might be due to over-drinking in childhood - perhaps at some critical time - since childhood over-drinkers became the most severe type of adult over-drinkers. Since water was purchased, there were strong socio-economic correlates of over-drinking. With the coming of a semi-socialistic approach to the distribution of water, the socio-economic factors were difficult to evaluate. Consider this, for example: although, in general, the children of over-drinkers were also over-drinkers - there was less over-drinking on the shady side of the valley in the lower socio-economic groups. But, on the hot and sunny side of the valley, there was a clearer, yet inverse, correlation between social class and the incidence of over-drinking.

Research workers found a way to count the number of water-logged cells in the body. The findings were interpreted as showing that early water-logging of cells might lead to a perpetual thirst from cells formed in childhood.

There were clinics for the behavior modification of drinking and some experimented with an ingenious surgical treatment whereby recently ingested water trickled from the esophagus through a tube, then through a filter and finally, back to the spring. At the recent Second All-Tribe Congress on Over-Drinking, it was suggested that the problem might be biochemical and a lively discussion ensued. This brings us up-to-date on the vexing problem of over-drinking in that desert tribe.

The moral of the fable is obvious. A small amount of pitressin and a little more knowledge would have helped immensely. Are we in the same situation? It is surely possible that all of our deliberations at this Congress would be rendered archaic, even quaint, by a single discovery of basic science. How I wish it would happen and yet my hunch is that this will never be. I do not believe we will ever find a single magic bullet for all cases of obesity. Let me explain.

The biggest segment of man's history is covered by times when food was scarce and was acquired in unpredictable amounts and by dint of tremendous caloric expenditure. Our ontogenesis is, of necessity, a recapitulation of this history. We have developed the capacity to store food as triglyceride in adipose tissue and thus we can, if we wish, eat only periodically and withstand long periods of starvation. The long history of food scarcity and its persistence in much of the world could not have gone unnoticed by such an adaptive organism as man. Hoarding and caloric miserliness are built into our fabric.

To me, it would be most unthinkable if we did not have a complex, integrated system to assure that a fraction of what we eat is put aside and stored. That hepatic, intestinal, hypothalamic and psychologic factors are involved in the operation of this system is no surprise. This is the way that salt and water intake are regulated. All such systems are complex and have many redundancies to assure that the system will continue to operate when one component fails. The system operates to assure a certain level of fat deposition, but with considerable variance. Components can fail and thus one finds anorexic states, lipodystrophies and obesity.

For millenia, the system has been under pressure to operate well in the face of a scarcity of food. Now, food is abundantly available in part of the world. The hedonic aspect of food intake, our delight in eating sweet and savoury dishes which is a behavioral adaptation from the lean years, now has a full opportunity to be expressed. Sweet foods and food of high caloric density are available in machines, in quick over-the-counter restaurants and best of all, in our own pantries. Filling our adipose depots is most pleasant - it leads to a full and gratified feeling that must be the reciprocal affect that our anxious, semi-starved ancestors so often felt. To add to this pleasant feeling, the industrial revolution has provided us with labor-saving devices to assure that each stored calorie is securely locked in its resting place, not to be disturbed by excess energy expenditure.

As our industries produce food and labor-saving devices, they urge us to be avid consumers. It is hard to blame them, for they are fulfilling our wishes. But the result is that our regulation of fat stores is pushed to one extreme. Some of us, for reasons we wish we knew, adapt with extreme obesity. Some lucky ones remain on the lean side, but most of us just go up a bit higher on the scale of weight.

The new environment exerts its effects from earliest infancy. Perhaps at this time further adaptations or tissue changes are set in motion. Certainly we can make fatter or leaner rats more easily by an early nutritional change than by what we do to the adult animal. Although, with a bit of cleverness, we can make rats overeat at almost any age.

And then, in all this cornucopia of plenty, the epidemiologists point out that all this good may be too much good. But it is not easy to change - our bodies were built for other environments. We can no more change our biology of fat storage than we can over night learn to develop all the enzymes needed to inactivate environmental pollutants or to selectively rid ourselves of radioactive contaminants.

One wonders whether behavior modification cannot be successful. It surely can! We have been modified by our environment and by our history to become and stay just as fat as possible. Fortunately, behavior modification is not omnipotent. The supremacy of some biologic systems over behavior modification is shown by the fact that not all of us are immensely obese. Had behavior modification worked better, we all would be!

What then should be our objectives and our priorities? Now I will be even more subjective than I have been already - and thus more liable to error.

One approach is to develop what might be called the 'technologic fix.' Can we find a drug, a device or a dietary gimmick that will give us the best of all possible worlds? Eat all you want, be as inactive as you will and remain slender and healthy. To this end, we should investigate every aspect of food intake regulation and fat storage. When more information is available, perhaps there will be an agent which can be used. None is at hand as yet.

But would such an agent be the best answer? We are built and organized to live in a certain way. Our environment has pushed us to certain limits which are not healthy, so we wish to develop an agent which permits a better adjustment. This is reminiscent of the problem of having very noisy neighbors who interfere with our sleep. The technological and pharmaceutical answer is to take a sleeping pill. Perhaps the neighbors should be given the sleeping pill, or better yet, we should come to some *modus vivendi* that does not involve yet another pill or device.

Yet, every frequency distribution has its extremes. Some will become obese under any reasonable circumstances - perhaps there is a major error in regulation. For these the 'technologic fix' is important and, for such individuals alone as well as for the advancement of knowledge, basic research into caloric storage must have a high priority.

But for the average, obese American, the pills and gimmicks should not be the answer. To some degree we can learn to eat differently and to be more active. There are many efforts in this direction already. The Stanford group have shown that the behavior of entire communities can be reshaped at least to some extent. Not all is venal and ugly in the commercial ventures to aid the obese. The Weight Watchers Organization, for example, is cognizant of the fact that good nutritional advice and some type of behavioral re-organization are central features of bucking the tide which drives us to overweight. With the help of Dr Henry Sebrell and Dr Richard Stuart, they have introduced sound practices into their program and their early results are encouraging. Other individuals and organizations are working in the same direction.

But one must ask whether all efforts should be beamed exclusively at the obese adult. It seems to me that our children may be the ones who are yet plastic enough to develop those better practices that will prevent the usual, mild obesity that holds us in its grip in epidemic proportions. But, most important of all, can't we begin to direct our efforts in an even broader direction? If our problem is the problem of having a biologic system which adapts and an environment which forces us into maladaption - then perhaps we should not ask ourselves to quickly adapt faster and further. It does not seem to work that well - our rate of change is perhaps too slow. Is it unfair to direct our behavior modification at the environment and not ourselves?

Can we not work to create a pattern of living in which there is abundant hedonic return from more physical activity? Is it inconceivable that we re-structure the way we eat, so that mealtime brings conviviality and human warmth, so that our pleasures are not from the amount of food consumed but rather from where and with whom it was eaten? The job of medicine and science should not be only to change the human body to fit the environment. It is our task to examine the environment as well. This is a tall order and the approaches are not well delineated.

Yet, if we can begin to do this in connection with the problem of obesity, we will make a major contribution to our well-being. Sometimes, I feel as though working with the problem of obesity is in some way a lesser activity than probing the intricacies of biochemical genetics or molecular interactions. But, I believe that the solutions to the problem of human obesity can have wider impact than any advance of a more traditional scientific type. Indeed, what we do at this Congress could point the way to solutions of other problems that lie at the interface of man and his environment. For these reasons, I wish you all godspeed and a productive meeting.

2
The role of central catecholamine-containing neurons in food intake

J.F. MARSHALL
Department of Psychobiology, University of California, Irvine, California 92717, USA.

An adequate account of the neural mechanisms controlling food intake would have to explain at least three separate processes. First, such a theory should account for how the central nervous system is informed about bodily nutrient repletion or depletion. Second, it would have to explain the organism's ability to integrate the information concerning its nutrient state with, for instance, its prior experience in consuming certain foods or the other needs which impinge upon it at a given time. Finally, this model would account for how a decision to eat is then translated into an appropriate series of motor patterns, adapted to the animal's immediate environment.

Unfortunately, such a complete account is far from being realized. For instance, it is still unclear how the brain senses nutrient availability. One long-standing hypothesis is that the brain directly samples nutrients such as glucose within the cerebral circulation (Mayer, 1953). Alternatively, it may sense humoral agents which are released peripherally when a meal is eaten (Smith, Gibbs & Young, 1974). Or, it may receive such information indirectly, by sensing the nutrient flux within peripheral organs such as the liver (Russek, Rodriguez-Zidejas & Pina, 1968). While one or all of the above routes may well be used in the control of food intake, a definite resolution to this complex issue is still lacking.

In view of these deficiencies in our understanding of the neural controls over food intake, one may justifiably ask what the study of brain catecholamine-containing neurons can offer to this field. The answer, it seems to me, is that such investigations give us windows into the function of the nervous system. As will be reviewed, experimentally-induced exaggerations or deficiencies in the function of central catacholamine-containing neurons have dramatic effects on the food intake of laboratory animals. Although the mechanisms by which these profound influences are exerted is only gradually becoming clear, these phenomena remain among the most powerful tools we have for gaining insight into how the CNS controls feeding. Thus, while we are still far from developing a complete model of the neural control of feeding, an understanding of the effects of brain catecholamine-containing neurons on this behavior is likely to be one of the most important means available to us for building such an understanding.

Neural control of feeding: a brief history

The recognition that discrete regions of the brain are critical to the control of feeding predates our appreciation that cerebral catecholamines (norepinephrine and dopamine) play an important role in this behavior. The development of the first stereotaxic neurosurgical instrument by Horsley and Clark made possible the localization of particular brain regions, especially with the hypothalamus, important in the control of feeding. Hetherington & Ranson (1940) found that rats ate voraciously, and demonstrated that their obesity was largely a result of excessive food intake.

When a region of the hypothalamus 1.5 to 2.0 mm dorsolateral to the VMH was destroyed bilaterally, quite an opposite behavioral syndrome resulted. Rats, cats, and monkeys, with damage to neural tissue in and around the lateral hypothalamus became totally aphagic (Anand & Brobeck, 1951; Anand, Dua & Shoenberg, 1955; Ranson, 1939) and adipsic (Teitelbaum & Stellar, 1954). Such animals would typically die of inanition unless force-fed. When given adequate intragastric feeding, however, such rats recovered their capacity to eat and drink, and the restoration of ingestive functions occurred in a predictable sequence of stages (Teitelbaum & Epstein, 1962).

More recent investigations have suggested that these syndromes of hyperphagia and aphagia are due not so much to the destruction of hypothalamic cells *per se* as to the transection of fiber systems coursing through the medial (Gold, 1973) and lateral (Morgane, 1961; Ungerstedt, 1970) hypothalami respectively. In addition, it has become clear that these lesions produce multiple behavioral changes in addition to altering food intake. For example, rats with damage to the VMH are hyperaggressive, overreactive to sensory stimuli, and display alterations in the performance of learned behaviors, while rats with destruction of the lateral hypothalamus are hypoaggressive and display profound sensorimotor disturbances (for review, see Marshall & Teitelbaum, 1977). Despite these recent complexities in their anatomical and behavioral interpretation (see last section), the ventromedial and lateral hypothalamic syndromes have served as important reference points in instigating and guiding much of the research concerning the relationship between brain catecholamine-containing neurons and feeding. The purpose of the current chapter is to review the current state of this latter research, and to place it within the framework of the classical syndromes.

Brain norepinephrine (NE) and feeding

NE injections

Vogt (1954) in her classic work on the distribution of NE within the central nervous system determined that the highest brain concentration of this substance occurs in the hypothalamus. In retrospect, it is no mere coincidence that manipulations of this brain region produce marked effects on feeding. Rather, hypothalamic norepinephrine appears to be an important determinant of the feeding behavior of animals. Grossman, in his seminal work of 1960, found that when 1 to 5 μg of NE was administered *via* an indwelling cannula directly into the lateral hypothalamus of sated rats, these animals would eat on the average 3 to 4 grams of food during the subsequent 40 minutes. A substantial, though lesser, eating followed the intrahypothalamic adminstration of epinephrine into the same brain region. Particularly dramatic was Grossman's finding that when cholinergic agents (carbachol, acetylcholine) were delivered into the same region, the rats would drink but not eat. Thus, the stimulation of food intake appeared to be associated specifically with noradrenergic stimulation of the hypothalamus.

Grossman (1960) suggested that his injections of NE into the lateral hypothalamus induced feeding by activating 'feeding-related' neurons within the area. As lateral hypothalamic lesions produced aphagia, and because electrical stimulation of this site had long been known to produce overeating (Brügger, 1943), this interpretation seemed parsimonious. In subsequent work, however, it was found that hypothalamic injections of NE produce feeding more consistently when the cannula tips were located anteromedially to the lateral hypothalamic nucleus (Booth, 1967), particularly within the medial anterior hypothalamus or paraventricular nucleus (Davis & Keesey, 1971; Herberg & Franklin, 1972). Thus, Grossman's NE applications may have been effective in inducing eating because of diffusion of the amine to more anteromedial structures.

The phenomenon of NE-induced eating deserves special consideration from a pharmacological standpoint. This experimental procedure has been criticized because of the quantity and concentration of NE needed to evoke food intake. For example, the threshold dose reported by Leibowitz (1975) for the rat is 0.04 μg in 0.5 μl of solution. This represents a quantity of

NE approximately equal to the total endogenous NE content of the rat's hypothalamus. Furthermore, this concentration (3.8×10^{-4}) of NE is approximately 10^3 times the K_m for physiological processes (uptake of NE into cells, stimulation of NE-sensitive adenylate cyclase).

While these facts raise significant questions regarding the physiological significance of NE-induced eating, several findings support the view that this eating may in fact be due to the action of NE on NE-sensitive hypothalamic receptors. First, several investigators (Booth, 1968; Slangen & Miller, 1969; Leibowitz, 1975) have shown that the effect of applied NE on feeding can be blocked by α-adrenergic blocking agents (phentolamine, phenoxybenzamine) but not by β-adrenergic blocking agents (propranolol). Other work has shown that the order of drug potency for elicitation of eating (clonidine > NE > epinephrine) is suggestive of an α-adrenergic receptor (Grossman, 1960; Ritter, Wise & Stein, 1975). Also, the hypothalamic sites where NE injection is most effective in inducing eating are those which receive extensive innervation by the ascending NE-containing bundles (Fuxe, 1965 and see Fig. 1). Finally, the work of Evetts, Fitzsimons & Setler (1971) suggests that enhanced eating can occur following the release of *endogenous* stores of brain NE. In the four hours following the injection of 6-hydroxydopamine (a compound which exerts a neurotoxic action on catecholamine containing cells) into the preoptic region, rats overeat substantially. This food intake is seen

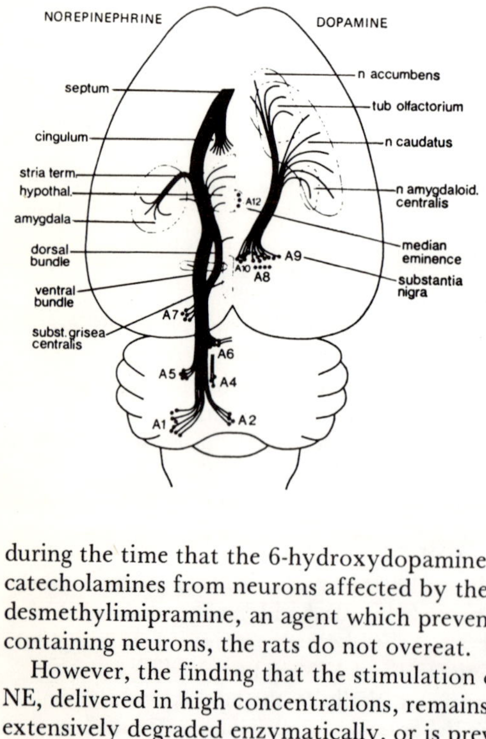

Fig. 1. Horizontal projection of the ascending catecholamine- (norepinephrine- and dopamine-) containing axons in rat brain. This distribution provides the neuroanatomic substrate by which cerebral catecholaminergic influences over feeding are exerted (from Ungerstedt, 1971)

during the time that the 6-hydroxydopamine causes a degeneration-related release of catecholamines from neurons affected by the neurotoxin. When rats are pretreated with desmethylimipramine, an agent which prevents the 6-hydroxydopamine from destroying NE-containing neurons, the rats do not overeat.

However, the finding that the stimulation of food intake requires such large quantities of NE, delivered in high concentrations, remains perplexing. Possibly, the NE is rapidly and extensively degraded enzymatically, or is prevented from having a postsynaptic effect because it is rapidly taken up by CA-containing neurons. In this regard, Booth (1968) and Slangen & Miller (1969) found that NE-induced eating is potentiated by pretreating rats with desmethylimipramine, a drug which prevents the NE from entering nerve terminals of NE-containing cells, thereby presumably increasing its extracellular concentration. A battery of such pharmacological treatments might well be employed in a systematic manner to determine the feasibility of eliciting feeding following the intrahypothalamic administration of more physiological concentrations of NE.

Damage to NE-containing neurons
The role of hypothalamic NE in food intake has become increasingly complex. While intra-hypothalamic NE injections can induce feeding, it has also become apparent that brain lesions, which destroy the NE-containing neurons innervating the hypothalamus, can produce over-eating and increased weight gain (Ahlskog, 1974; Ahlskog & Hoebel, 1973). Rats with damage to the ventral NE-containing bundle, incurred either by electrolytic lesions or 6-hydroxy-dopamine injections along the course of this fiber system, will overeat starting 1 to 4 days post-operatively. This overeating and enhanced weight gain, while modest in comparison with the voracious food consumption of the rat with electrolytic lesions of the ventromedial hypothalamus, is associated with the loss of fluorescent varicosities within the hypothalamus. Furthermore, 6-hydroxydopamine injections along the course of the ventral NE-containing bundle fail to produce overeating if such rats are pretreated with desmethylimipramine which blocks the entry of the neurotoxin into NE-containing cells thereby preventing their destruction (Ahlskog & Hoebel, 1973).

The paradox that both excesses and deficiencies of NE transmission can lead to enhanced food intake has been a formidable obstacle to understanding the role of NE in eating behavior. One suggested resolution is that hypothalamic NE has a biphasic effect on feeding, ie it may stimulate food intake during the day and suppress it at night (Margules *et al.*, 1972).

According to this interpretation, the loss of hypothalamic NE terminals might be expected to suppress daytime feeding and to enhance nightime feeding. Since rats are nocturnal animals and take relatively little food during the day, the net result of NE depletion would be likely to increase 24-hour food intake. Indeed, it has been found that rats with destruction of hypothalamic NE terminals increase their food intake during the night. However, during the day their intake equals controls' (ie there appears to be no suppression of feeding – Ahlskog, Randall & Hoebel, 1975).

An alternative resolution to this paradox is that there are two independent NE-sensitive receptor sites in the hypothalamus which are involved in feeding, such that stimulation of one leads to eating while stimulation of the other suppresses feeding. Support for such a view comes from the recent work of Brown & Leibowitz (1977) in which it was found that dorsal midbrain electrolytic lesions which led to a loss of fluorescent varicosities in the paraventricular and dorsomedial hypothalamic nuclei resulted in aphagia, while ventral midbrain lesions which produced a loss of fluorescent terminals in the perifornical hypothalamus led to hyperphagia. While these results need to be confirmed using injections of 6-hydroxydopamine in order to selectively deplete discrete hypothalamic areas of NE, they suggest that the paraventricular and perifornical NE innervations may exert reciprocal controls over food intake.

Measuring hypothalamic NE content, turnover, and release
While the preceding experiments show that extreme fluctuations in the NE content of hypothalamic areas can influence feeding, they do not tell us directly whether food intake is related to physiologically-meaningful variations of hypothalamic NE. Evidence pertaining to the latter issue comes from two sources: the correlation of hypothalamic NE content with obesity in nerologically intact animals, and the measurement of the hypothalamic efflux of NE in freely-moving animals. Glick & Stanley (1975) found that in a group of female rats weighing between 230 and 350 grams at the time of sacrifice, body weight correlated highly ($r = +0.73$) with the ratio of striatal dopamine content to hypothalamic NE content. In another experiment utilizing genetically obese rats of the Zucker strain, phenotypically obese rats had paraventricular nuclear levels of NE which were lower than those of non-obese littermate controls (Cruce, Thoa & Jacobowitz, 1976). Other workers (Lorden, Oltmans & Margules, 1975), using genetically obese mice (*dbdb* and *obob*) have found higher hypothalamic contents of NE in such animals than among non-obese littermate controls. Finally, van der Gugten & co-workers (in press) reported that male rats have a higher content and higher turnover rate of NE within the perifornical and dorsomedial hypothalamic areas at times of day when the rate

of feeding is high. While these investigations open an exciting new area of research, there are at present many questions regarding their interpretation. Hypothalamic NE levels are not clearly indicative of the rate of release of this neurotransmitter, so that the functional activity of these neurons is uncertain. Also, the analysis of NE in the whole hypothalamus may obscure important regional differences. Finally, circadian variations in feeding are accompanied by similar variations in a plethora of other physiological, endocrine, and behavioral functions, any of which might influence hypothalamic NE.

A second line of evidence relating physiological variations in hypothalamic NE with eating behavior comes from experiments in which push-pull cannulae are used to perfuse the hypothalamus of behaving rats. In this manner, moment-to-moment variations in the extracellular hypothalamic concentration of NE can be correlated with the consumatory behavior of the rat. For example, Slangen & van der Gugten (1977) measured the efflux of NE and dopamine (DA) in the dorsomedial, perifornical, subfornical, and anterolateral hypothalamic regions of freely feeding rats. During feeding, NE (but not DA) release from the dorsomedial and perifornical regions was significantly elevated when compared with pre- or post-feeding values (Fig. 2). An increase of catecholamine release was not observed during

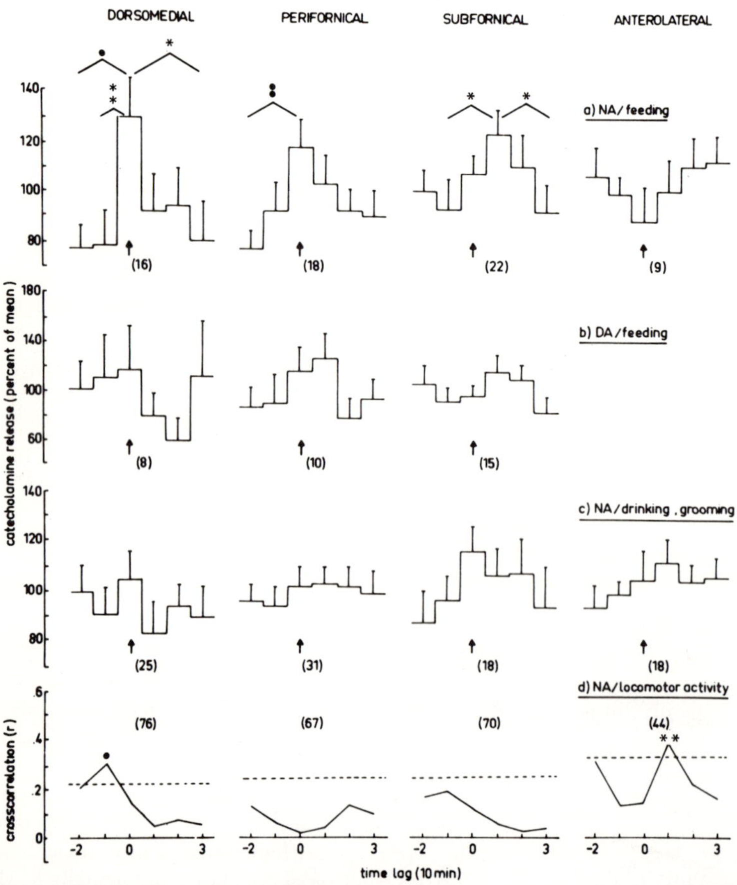

Fig. 2. Relation between catecholamines released from four hypothalamic regions and behaviors observed in rats. Time 0 indicates 10-minute perfusion period during which the behavior of interest occurred. (a) NE and (b) DA release over 10-minute periods before, during, and after occurrence of feeding (c) NE release before, during, and after occurrence of drinking/grooming. (d) Cross correlation between NE release and locomotor activity. $^*P<0.05$; $^{**}P<0.025$; $^{\bullet}P<0.01$; $^{\bullet\bullet}P<0.005$ Van der Gugten *et al.,* 1977)

drinking or grooming. Furthermore, when rats were deprived of food for 16 hours and then fed, these workers found that the rate of NE release from the medial hypothalamus was higher before food presentation than during satiety. This latter finding is important, since it suggests that the hypothalamic release of NE is related to the hunger state, and is not simply attributable to the act of food consumption.

NE-induced eating and the VMH syndrome

I previously stated that the study of the syndromes induced by damage to the ventromedial and lateral hypothalamic regions have served as important guides in the study of how brain catecholaminergic systems influence feeding. One intriguing observation is the similarity between the eating behavior of rats following intrahypothalamic NE injections and that of the rat given VMH lesions. Both procedures, while producing overeating, appear to induce a motivational depression for food (see Herberg & Franklin, 1972). That is, the eating behavior of such rats depends upon the taste qualities of the food and the work demands to obtain food. In contrast to food-deprived rats or rats given electrical stimulation of the LH, rats with VMH lesions or intrahypothalamic NE administration are not hyperphagic if given a bitter-tasting diet or if required to press a bar on a variable-interval schedule for access to food. In addition, the eating due to intrahypothalamic NE injection can be blocked by destruction of the ventromedial hypothalamus (Herberg & Franklin, 1972). One explanation for these findings is that the VMH lesions induce hyperphagia at least in part by interrupting fibers from the paraventricular nucleus and medial anterior hypothalamic sites where NE is effective in inducing feeding. If NE is an inhibitory neurotransmitter in these brain regions, as it appears to be elsewhere in the brain, then VMH lesions should mimic the application of NE to medial anterior hypothalamic areas, since both procedures would depress the activity of efferent fibers. The existence of a fiber system coming from medial anterior hypothalamus to the posterior VMH has been identified (Chi, 1970).

The possible implications of this similarity have yet to be explored. For instance, rats with VMH lesions are known to have important metabolic and endocrine dysfunctions (eg, Hustvedt & Løvø, 1972), which are thought by many workers to make an important contribution to the overeating and weight gain of these rats (Friedman & Stricker, 1976). It would be intriguing to investigate whether similar endocrine changes accompany the intrahypothalamic injection of NE.

Brain dopamine (DA)-containing neurons and feeding

Damage to DA-containing neurons and the lateral hypothalamic syndrome

Whereas the intrahypothalamic administration of NE reliably produces increased food intake, the injection of DA at these same sites (Booth, 1968; Slangen & Miller, 1969) or into the cerebral ventricles (Kruk, 1973) was found to have little or no effect in promoting food intake, and even reduced eating.

Ungerstedt (1971), in the course of his anatomical mapping of the brain dopamine (DA) pathways, noted that one of the major ascending dopaminergic tracts, the nigrostriatal bundle, passes through the far-lateral hypothalamus before terminating in the caudate-putamen. This is the same region of the lateral hypothalamus where electrolytic lesions had previously been shown to produce the most prolonged aphagia and adipsia (Morgane, 1961; Gold, 1967). Ungerstedt hypothesized that the dramatic effects of lateral hypothalamic lesions on food and water intake might be attributable to the transection of these ascending DA-containing fibers. By using intracerebral injections of the neurotoxin 6-hydroxydopamine, Ungerstedt (1970, 1971) showed that rats with preferential destruction of the nigrostriatal DA neurons became completely aphagic and adipsic. Furthermore, if kept alive by force-feeding, such rats would eventually recover the capacity to eat and drink, as do animals with lateral hypothalamic electrolytic lesions.

The behavioral parallels between the rat with 6-hydroxydopamine-induced nigrostriatal

DA depletion and the lateral hypothalamic rat have since been extended by a number of investigators. The 6-hydroxydopamine-treated rat goes through the same four stages of recovery as do rats with lateral hypothalamic lesions. Even when they recover the ability to maintain themselves on dry chow and water, both types of animals show marked impairments in the ability to respond to regulatory challenges. For example, these rats fail to drink normally when given an osmotic load or when the blood volume is reduced. Similarly, they do not eat normally in response to the glucoprivation induced by insulin or 2-deoxy-D-glucose (see reviews by Marshall & Teitelbaum, 1977; Stricker & Zigmond, 1976).

Many lines of evidence now suggest that these behavioral impairments are specifically associated with a loss of brain dopamine. The syndrome of ingestional impairments is seen after administration of 6-OH-DA into many structures eg, the cerebral ventricles, lateral hypothalamus, substantia nigra, or globus pallidus, provided that extensive forebrain DA loss occurs. When rats are given injections of desmethylimipramine before the injections of 6-OH-DA, the DA depletion occurs without substantial loss of brain NE, but the aphagia and adipsia still occur (see reviews by Marshall & Teitelbaum, 1977; Stricker & Zigmond, 1976). Also, several workers using divergent techniques (electrolytic lesions, knife cuts, 6-hydroxydopamine injections) have consistently noted that the duration of aphagia is highly correlated with the reduction of striatal DA levels. Finally, it is possible to restore the feeding and drinking capacities of rats with 6-hydroxydopamine-induced forebrain depletion of DA by supplying the animals with an 'exogenous source of DA'. When aphagic and adipsic rats are given a systemic injection of an agent like apomorphine which stimulates DA receptors, they begin to eat (Ljungberg & Ungerstedt, 1976*a*), and will even drink if made thirsty by injections of hypertonic saline or isoproterenol (Marshall & Ungerstedt, 1976).

Role of brain DA-containing neurons in sensorimotor integration

The preceding findings raise an important issue: what is the nature of the behavioral impairment in rats with dopamine-depleting lesions in the brain? In order to answer this question, we must first review briefly the history of thinking about the lateral hypothalamic syndrome. Earlier research concerning the effects of lateral hypothalamic damage on feeding and drinking emphasized that these rats appeared to be suffering from a motivational impairment. For example, in recovering from the aphagia, the first foods that such rats accept are moist, palatable diets such as a slurry of Pablum or cookie, ie those foods which are highly preferred by an intact rat (Teitelbaum & Epstein, 1962). Even later in recovery, when the rats are maintaining themselves by eating dry chow and water, if their food is made even slightly bitter with quinine, they can become totally aphagic and adipsic once again (Teitelbaum & Epstein, 1962). While not denying the importance of taste, it now appears that many of the symptoms of the rat with lateral hypothalamic damage have a simpler neurological basis. Marshall, Turner & Teitelbaum (1971) found that rats with such bilateral lesions showed a profound sensory neglect for tactile, visual and olfactory stimuli arising on either side of the body. When the damage was unilateral, the neglect was restricted to stimuli on the side of the animal opposite to the damage. Thus, it appears that the rat with bilateral lateral hypothalamic lesions is not simply uninterested in eating or drinking. Rather, such rats have a profound impairment in sensorimotor functions, which affect their ability to localize and ingest food and water. More recent work has shown that rats with intracerebral 6-OH-DA injections, which have suffered extensive damage to the ascending DA-containing neurons, have quite similar sensorimotor impairments (Marshall *et al.*, 1974; Ljunberg & Ungerstedt, 1976*b*).

These findings may help to explain why rats with lateral hypothalamic lesions show a multifaceted syndrome of behavioral impairments. Not only are such rats aphagic and adipsic, they also show impaired performance of learned responses, disturbances of male sexual behavior, and diminished aggressive behavior (see review by Marshall & Teitelbaum, 1977). Thus, the integrity of the ascending DA-containing neurons is important for the expression of a variety of behaviors, not simply for feeding and drinking. These neurons likely play such a wide-ranging role in behavior because they modulate the animal's responsiveness to external stimuli.

Role of brain dopamine-containing neurons in experimentally-induced hyperphagias
(1) VMH lesion hyperphagia
Ungerstedt's (1970, 1971) demonstration of the importance of brain DA-containing neurons to the spontaneous feeding of rats has raised the issue whether these same cells play any role in the feeding behavior induced by several experimental procedures. It would be intriguing, for instance, to attempt to bring together the lateral and ventromedial hypothalamic syndromes by seeing whether the ascending dopaminergic fibers play an important role in the expression of the hyperphagia brought about by damage to the VMH.

The rationale for this investigation came from the work of Marshall (1975), who found that rats with unilateral VMH damage show an exaggerated orientational response to stimuli, particularly touch, on the contralateral side of the body. These findings, as well as others (see Marshall, 1975), are precisely the opposite of what is seen following damage to brain DA-containing neurons, and raised the possibility that following VMH lesions there may be enhanced neurotransmission within ascending dopaminergic fibers.

We reasoned that if brain DA-containing neurons are involved in an important way in the expression of VMH lesion-induced hyperphagia, then the rat which has suffered prior damage to these catecholaminergic pathways should show little or no overeating or obesity. This is precisely what we have found (Fig. 3). Rats which were given intranigral injections of 6-OH-DA, which depleted striatal DA by 90 per cent, and which were allowed to recover from the initial aphagia and adipsia, showed no tendency to overeat or to become obese when given VMH lesions. As a group, they ate no more food or water than rats that had recovered from

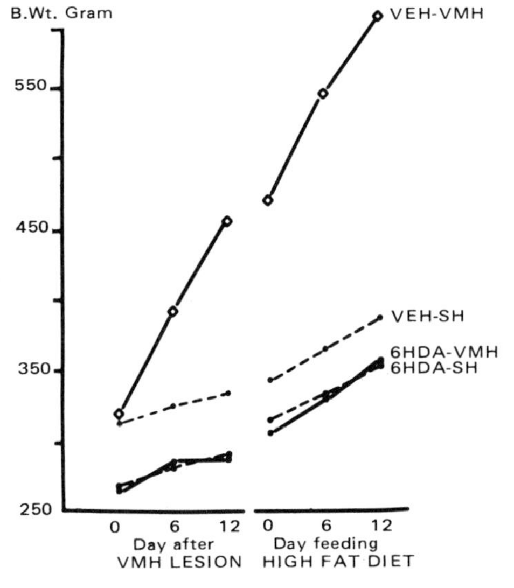

Fig. 3. Body weight (B.Wt.) of rats given DA-depleting 6-hydroxydopamine injections followed by VMH lesions (6 HDA-VMH), 6-hydroxydopamine injections followed by sham lesions (6 HDA-SH), vehicle injections followed by VMH lesions (VEH-VMH), or vehicle injections followed by sham lesions (VEH-SH). Note that DA-depleting 6-hydroxydopamine injections totally blocked the excessive weight gain normally seen after VMH lesions, whether the rats were eating dry pellets or a high fat diet

the 6-OH-DA injections but had not been given VMH lesions. These rats were not hyperphagic when offered dry chow (Purina pellets) or a preferred high-fat diet. These results stand in contrast to the findings of Coscina *et al.* (1973) who found that rats given 6-OH-DA injections and subsequent VMH lesions were just as hyperphagic as were VMH rats with intact DA-containing neurons. However, there appears to be a critical difference between our two experiments. Whereas the 6-OH-DA treatement employed by Coscina *et al.* resulted in 65 to 80 per cent decrease in forebrain DA, our regimen produced an average 90 per cent drop in striatal content of DA. This difference appears crucial. One animal in our experiment which received 6-OH-DA injections followed by VMH lesions did become moderately hyperphagic. The depletion of striatal DA achieved in this rat was the least extensive of the group, only 73 per cent. In other work as well, the extent of striatal DA depletion has been found to be an important determinant of the duration of the behavioral impairments seen after 6-OH-DA injections (Zigmond & Stricker, 1972).

While these findings suggest that the occurrence of hyperphagia after VMH lesions depends upon the integrity of at least a small portion of the ascending dopaminergic fibers, the reason for this dependency remains to be clarified. One possible explanation for these findings is that VMH damage in an otherwise intact rat leads to enhanced DA neurotransmission. If this elevated DA release contributed to the appearance of hyperphagia, then rats with substantial depletions of DA would show little overeating following VMH lesions. This interpretation receives support from our work (Marshall *et al.,* 1977) showing that VMH damage in rats does enhance the striatal release of DA immediately after the lesion. We found that striatal content of homovanillic acid (HVA, a major metabolite of DA, the level of which is frequently used as an index of DA release) was elevated two hours after either direct current or radiofrequency VMH lesions, while striatal DA content was unaffected. However, striatal HVA levels were increased only significantly at two days postoperatively, a finding which casts doubt on the possibility that an enhanced DA neurotransmission contributes to the long-term hyperphagia and weight gain of these animals.

An alternative explanation of our results is that brain DA-containing neurons play a permissive role in the expression of hyperphagia. For instance, the VMH lesion induces metabolic alterations (eg, Hustvedt & Løvø, 1972), which many workers believe are largely responsible for the overeating of these rats (eg, Friedman & Stricker, 1976). Since rats with extensive damage to DA-containing neurons do not eat normally in response to glucoregulatory challenges such as insulin or 2-deoxy-D-glucose (Epstein & Teitelbaum, 1967; Zigmond & Stricker, 1972; Marshall *et al.,* 1974), one might expect that such rats would be unable to eat in order to compensate for the metabolic derangements induced by the VMH damage. From this perspective then, the integrity of the dopaminergic neurons is necessary so that the animal can respond behaviorally to the homeostatic imbalances created by the VMH lesion.

In conclusion, the hyperphagia of the VMH rat depends upon the integrity of brain DA-containing neurons. These findings in no way deny the likely importance of metabolic and endocrine factors to the VMH syndrome. However, since the enhanced food intake of the rat with VMH damage can be lateralized to the sensory field contralateral to the injury (Marshall, 1975), factors other than metabolic must be guiding the food intake of the VMH rat. Clearly, any 'final theory' of the VMH lesion syndrome must take account of both the metabolic abnormalities and hyperreactivity to stimuli of such rats (Powley, 1977), and we suggest that brain DA neurons may figure importantly in such an interpretation.

(2) Electrical brain stimulation and tail pinch

Two additional feeding phenomena have within recent years been linked to brain DA-containing neurons. When rats are given mild electrical stimulation through an indwelling intracranial electrode at particular brain sites, they begin to eat (Brügger, 1954; Valenstein, Cox & Kakolewski, 1970). Similarly, when a rat's tail is mildly pinched, it will begin to consume food (Antelman & Szechtman, 1975).

Both types of eating have been shown to depend upon brain DA neurotransmission. For instance, while the localization of brain sites effective in eliciting 'stimulation-bound' feeding is not precise, electrodes in the vicinity of the lateral hypothalamus are among the most effective (Roberts, 1969). These sites lie in close proximity to the ascending DA-containing fibers, and electrical stimulation of the lateral hypothalamus can increase the release of DA in the ipsilateral forebrain. Also, drugs such as spiroperidol or pimozide, which are potent and selective DA receptor blocking agents, attentuate stimulation-bound feeding (Phillips &.

Nikaido, 1975). Administration of 6-OH-DA also reduced stimulation-bound feeding to the extent that forebrain DA is depleted (Phillips & Fibiger, 1973).

The evidence which links DA neurotransmission with tail pinch-induced eating is quite similar. When rats are given low doses of drugs which block dopamine receptors, tail pinch-induced feeding is largely prevented (Antelman *et al.*, 1975). Injections of 6-OH-DA along the course of ascending dopaminergic fibers, which result in substantial reductions in striatal DA, are similarly effective in attenuating this eating. However, noradrenergic receptor blockers, such as phentolamine or sotalol, are ineffective even at high doses.

From this discussion, it is apparent that there are several similarities between tail pinch and electrical brain stimulation. Perhaps the most striking similarity is the behavioral plasticity encountered in each phenomenon. For instance, the particular behavior elicited by the electrical stimulation largely depends upon the animal's environment during the test. Thus, rats which had been stimulation-bound eaters could be switched to drinkers or gnawers when a water tube or block of wood were presented in lieu of food (Valenstein *et al.*, 1970). Similarly, rats given tail pinch will gnaw wood if a wooden block is presented instead of food. Interestingly, however, it has not been possible so far to induce drinking with tail pinch.

The intriguing similarities between tail pinch and electrical brain stimulation as elicitors of feeding raise the possibility that the electrical current to the brain does not excite a neural substrate specific to hunger, any more than would a pinch of the tail (Antelman, Rowland & Fisher, 1976). Instead both events may enhance the posibility that the animal will respond to environmental cues, thereby engaging in any of a variety of relatively preprogrammed behaviors (eg, eating, gnawing, licking). This formulation of tail pinch and electrical stimulation-induced behaviors, while speculative, is consistent with our previous interpretation of the function of brain DA-containing neurons, based upon the behavior of animals with degeneration of these cells.

References

Ahlskog, J.E. (1974): *Brain Res.* **82**, 211.
Ahlskog, J.E. & Hoebel, B.G. (1973): *Science* **182**, 166.
Ahlskog, J.E., Randall, P.K. & Hoebel, B.G. (1975): *Science* **190**, 399.
Anand, B.K. & Brobeck, J.R. (1951): *Yale J. Biol. Med.* **24**, 123.
Anand, B.K., Dua, S. & Shoenberg, K. (1955): *J. Physiol.* (Lond.) **127**, 143.
Antelman, S.M., Rowland, N.E. & Fisher, A.E. (1976): *Physiol. Behav.* **17**, 743.
Antelman, S.M. & Szechtman, H. (1975): *Science* **119**, 731.
Antelman, S.M., Szechtman, H., Chin, P. & Fisher, A.E. (1975): *Brain Res.* **99**, 319.
Booth, D.A. (1967): *Science* **158**, 515.
Booth, D.A. (1968): *J. Pharm. Exp. Ther.* **160**, 336.
Brown, L.L. & Leibowitz, S.F. (1977): Lesions of catecholamine pathways in the midbrain associated with changes in feeding behavior and hypothalamic catecholamine innervation. *Sixth International Conference on the Physiology of Food and Fluid Intake*, Jouy-en-Josas.
Brügger, M.V. (1943): *Helv. Physiol. Pharmacol. Acta* **1**, 183.
Chi, C.C. (1970): *Brain Res.* **17**, 439.
Coscina, D.V., Rosenblum-Blinick, C., Godse, D.D. & Stancer, H.C. (1973): *Pharmacol. Biochem. Behav.* **1**, 629.
Cruce, J.A.F., Thoa, N.B. & Jacobowitz, D.M. (1976): *Brain Res.* **101**, 165.
Davis, J.R. & Keesey, R.E. (1971): *J. Comp. Physiol. Psychol.* **77**, 394.
Epstein, A.N. & Teitelbaum, P. (1967): *Am. J. Physiol.* **213**, 1159.
Evetts, K.D., Fitzsimons, J.T. & Setler, P.E. (1971): *J. Physiol.* **216**, 68P.
Friedman, M.I. & Stricker, E.M. (1976): *Psychol. Rev.* **83**, 409.
Fuxe, K. (1965): *Acta Physiol. Scand.*, Suppl. 247, **64**, 37.
Glick, S.D. & Stanley, M.D. (1975): *Brain Res.* **96**, 153.
Gold, R.M. (1967): *Physiol. Behav.* **2**, 211.
Gold, R.M. (1973): *Science* **182**, 488.
Grossman, S.P. (1960): *Science* **132**, 301.
Herberg, L.J. & Franklin, K.B.J. (1972): *Physiol. Behav.* **8**, 1029.
Hetherington, A.W. & Ranson, S.W. (1940): *Anat. Rec.* **78**, 149.

Hustvedt, B.E. & Løvø, A. (1972): *Acta Physiol. Scand.* **84**, 29.
Kruk, Z.L. (1973): *Nature* **150**, 52.
Leibowitz, S.F. (1975): *Physiol. Behav.* **14**, 743.
Ljungberg, T. & Ungerstedt, U. (1976*a*): *Physiol. Behav.* **16**, 277.
Ljungberg, T. & Ungerstedt, U. (1976*b*): *Exp. Neurol.* **53**, 585.
Lorden, J.F., Oltmans, G.A. & Margules, D.L. (1975): *Brain Res.* **96**, 390.
Margules, D.L., Lewis, M.J., Dragovich, J.A. & Margules, A.S. (1972): *Science* **178**, 640.
Marshall, J.F. (1975): *Brain Res.* **86**, 373.
Marshall, J.F., Antelman, S.M., Rowland, N.E. & Edwards, D.J. (1977): *Life Sci.* **20**, 1377.
Marshall, J.F., Richardson, J.S. & Teitelbaum, P. (1974): *J. Comp. Physiol. Psychol.* **87**, 808.
Marshall, J.F. & Teitelbaum, P. (1977): New considerations in the neuropsychology of motivated behaviors. In *Handbook of psychopharmacology*, Vol. 7, eds L.L. Iversen, S.D. Iversen & S.H. Snyder, p. 201, New York: Plenum.
Marshall, J.F., Turner, B.H. & Teitelbaum, P. (1971): *Science* **174**, 523.
Marshall, J.F. & Ungerstedt, U. (1976): *Physiol. Behav.* **17**, 817.
Mayer, J. (1953): *New Engl. J. Med.* **249**, 13.
Morgane, P.J. (1961): *Am. J. Physiol.* **201**, 420.
Phillips, A.G. & Fibiger, H.C. (1973): *Behav. Biol.* **9**, 749.
Phillips, A.G. & Nikaido, R.S. (1975): *Nature* **258**, 750.
Powley, T. (1977): *Psychol. Rev.* **84**, 89.
Ranson, S.W. (1939): *Archs Neurol. Psychiat.* **41**, 1.
Ritter, S., Wise, C.D. & Stein, L. (1975): *J. Comp. Physiol. Psychol.* **88**, 778.
Roberts, W.W. (1969): *Brain Behav. Evol.* **2**, 317.
Russek, M., Rodriguez-Zidejas, A.M. & Pina, S. (1968): *Physiol. Behav.* **3**, 249.
Slangen, J.L. & Miller, N.E. (1969): *Physiol. Behav.* **4**, 543.
Slangen, J.L. & Van der Gugten, J. (1977): Release of endogenous catecholamines from rat hypothalamus *in vivo* related to feeding and other behaviors. *Sixth International Conference of the Physiology of Food and Fluid Intake*, Jouy-en-Josas.
Smith, G.P., Gibbs, J. & Young, R.C. (1974): *Fed. Proc.* **33**, 1146.
Stricker, E.M. & Zigmond, M.J. (1976): Recovery of function after damage to central catecholamine-containing neurons: A neurochemical model for the lateral hypothalamic syndrome. In *Progress in psychobiology and physiological psychology*, Vol. 6, eds. J.M. Sprague & A.N. Epstein, p. 121. New York: Plenum.
Teitelbaum, P. & Epstein, A.N. (1962): *Psychol. Rev.* **69**, 74.
Teitelbaum, P. & Stellar, E. (1954): *Science* **120**, 894.
Ungerstedt, U. (1970): *Acta Physiol. Scand.* **80**, 35A.
Ungerstedt, U. (1971): *Acta Physiol. Scand.*, Suppl. **367**, 95.
Valenstein, E., Cox, V.C. & Kakolewski, J.W. (1970): *Psychol. Rev.* **71**, 16.
Van der Gugten, J., De Kloet, E.R., Versteeg, D.H.G. & Slangen, J.L. (1977): *Brain Res.* (in press).
Vogt, M. (1954): *J. Physiol.* **123**, 451.
Zigmond, M.J. & Stricker, E.M. (1972): *Science* **177**, 1211.

3
Activity of chemosensitive neurons related to the neurophysiological mechanism of feeding

Y. OOMURA, M. OHTA, S. ISHIBASHI, H. KITA, T. OKAJIMA and T. ONO*
Department of Physiology, Faculty of Medicine, Kyushu University, Fukuoka, 812 Japan. *Department of Physiology, Faculty of Medicine, Toyama Medical Pharmaceutical University, Toyama, 930-01 Japan.

Glucose, insulin and free fatty acid effects

Glucose-sensitive neurons in the lateral hypothalamus (LH) and glucoreceptor neurons in the ventromedial hypothalamus (VMH) of the rat are well known (Anand *et al.*, 1964; Oomura *et al.*, 1975*b*). Glucose tends to increase the discharge frequency of approximately one-third of the VMH neurons in a dose-response manner with a threshold value of 2 mmol/l and to decrease the discharge frequency of glucose-sensitive neurons in the LH. Insulin alone tends to inhibit VMH neuronal discharge, but it enhances the effects of glucose when both are applied simultaneously (Fig. 1*a*). In the LH, only glucose-sensitive neurons are affected by insulin and they are excited in a dose-response manner which indicates a reaction of one molecule

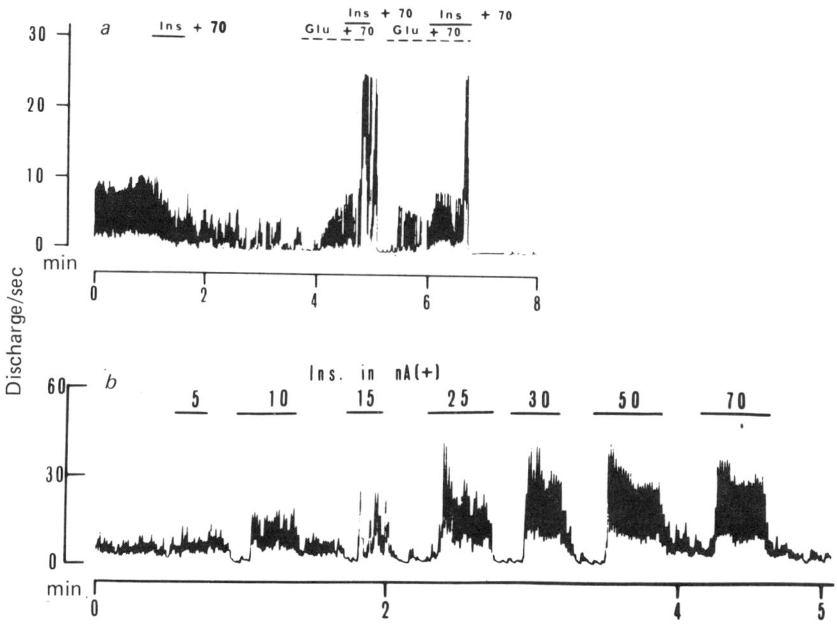

Fig. 1. Single neuron activity showing the effect of insulin. *a:* Glucoreceptor in rat VMH neuron. Insulin application decreased frequency, glucose slightly increased frequency, and glucose plus insulin strongly facilitated the unit (Oomura, 1973). *b:* Glucose-sensitive rat LH neuron activity at various concentrations of insulin application (indicated by nA). Insulin effect is saturated at currents greater than 40nA. Strength of application expressed in nA. Stimulation time is indicated by horizontal lines (Oomura *et al.*, 1975*b*).

per receptor site (Fig. 1*b*). The threshold level for insulin effect is approximately 5 x 10^{-9} i.u. Each chemical factor discussed in this report is applied electroosmotically through one barrel of a multibarrel pipette, unless otherwise indicated.

The effects of glucose, insulin, and glucose plus insulin are summarized in Fig. 2*a* (Oomura, 1976). Membrane hyperpolarization might explain inhibition by insulin. Insulin is known to cause hyperpolarization in muscle membrane by increasing electrogenic sodium-pump activity combined with intracellular K^+ accumulation (Creese & Jenden, 1968; Zierler, 1966). This would explain inhibition by insulin, but not stimulation by glucose or enhancement by glucose plus insulin. It is possible that insulin may increase neuron uptake of glucose at the specific neuronal glucoreceptive membrane site as it does in the fat cell membrane. Among the glucose analogues 3-OMG (3-O-methyl-glucose) clearly shows an inhibitory effect on VMH neurons. Figure 2 shows the inhibitory effect of 3-OMG alone, and its suppression of glucose-induced activity.

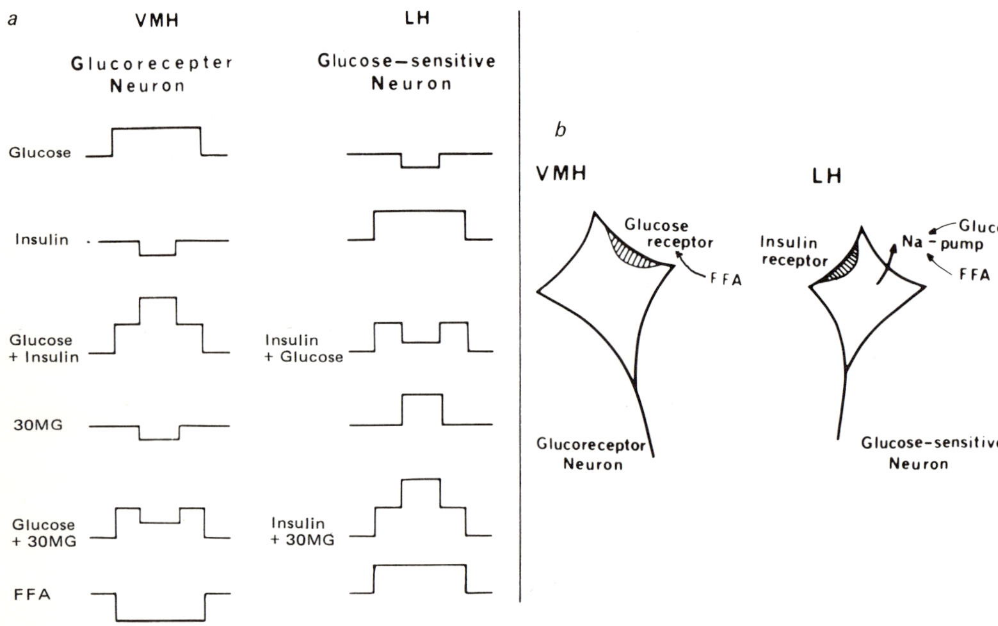

Fig. 2. a: Schematic representation of the effects of glucose, insulin, glucose analogue, FFA, and their combined effects on rat neuronal discharge frequency. Left: Glucoreceptor VMH neuron. Right: Glucose-sensitive LH neuron. Upward deflection, discharge frequency increase. **b: Schematic illustration of glucoreceptor neuron in the VMH and glucose-sensitive neuron in the LH.** Left: Glucoreceptor neuron has glucose receptor sites. FFA inhibits firing of this neuron by interposing between the glucose molecules and the receptor site, hence inhibiting binding or uptake of glucose by the neuron. Right: Glucose-sensitive neuron has insulin receptor sites. Na-pump action is accelerated by glucose but slowed by FFA (Oomura, 1976)

There are few, if any, glucoreceptors in the LH, but about one-third of the neurons in the LH are glucose-sensitive. Intracellular recording of neuronal activity shows approximately 5 mV hyperpolarization of the membrane during glucose inhibition (Oomura *et al.*, 1974); at this time, change in membrane conductance cannot be seen. Since this glucose sensitivity can be diminished by cardiac glycosides or antimetabolites, which inhibit extrusion of intracellular sodium by the sodium-pump, it is apparent that the glucose effect is caused by activation of the energy-dependent sodium-pump and its resultant hyperpolarization, not by a change in permeability.

Insulin functions through insulin receptors on the glucose-sensitive neurons (Oomura *et al.*, 1975*b*). The decrease of the insulin effect by glucose is probably caused by the hyperpolarization mentioned above, and the enhancement of the insulin effect by glucose analogues is probably due to depolarization caused by slowing of the sodium-pump, perhaps from partial interruption of cellular metabolism.

FFA extracted from deprived or sated rats (Oomura *et al.*, 1975*a)* is a powerful excitant of glucose-sensitive neurons in the LH regardless of its source. Figure 3 *b* and *c* illustrates typical results of application of FFA to glucose-sensitive neurons in the LH. In the beginning, the spontaneous activity was near zero, and FFA increased the discharge rate with a few seconds latency. The first application was from a fasted rat, the second from a sated rat. The effect

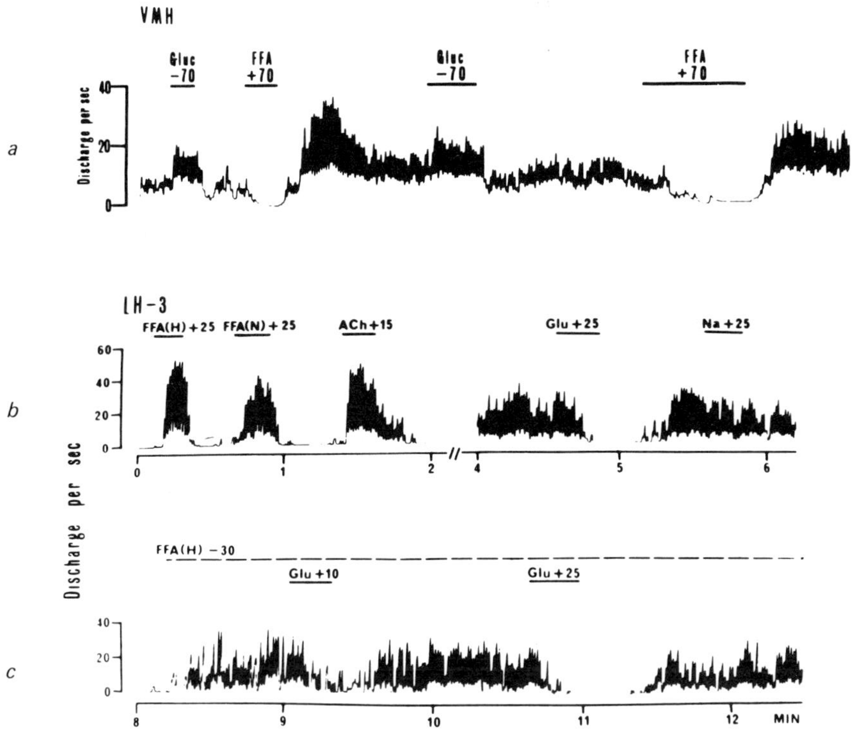

Fig. 3. a: Effect of FFA on rat glucoreceptor neurons. Glucose applied at -70 nA during period under bar increased discharge frequency and FFA applied at +70 nA almost completely inhibited the neuronal activity (Oomura, 1976). **b: Effect of FFA on glucose-sensitive rat LH neurons.** FFA (H)+25 (FFA extracted from blood of deprived rats applied at +25 nA for period indicated by underscore) increased discharge from almost zero level. FFA (N)+25 (FFA extracted from sated rat, otherwise as above) had similar but slightly less effect than FFA (H). ACh applied at +15 nA caused nearly instantaneous discharge increase. Glucose applied at +25 nA inhibited discharge. Na had no effect. **c: Interaction between glucose and FFA effects.** Continuous application of FFA (H) at -30 nA gradually increased firing. FFA activity facilitation partially inhibited by glucose at 10 nA, completely with 25 nA (Oomura et al., 1975b)

usually persisted for several seconds after termination of the current. The discharge frequency of this cell was increased by application c acetylcholine (ACh). After increasing the frequency with several applications of L-glutamic acid, glucose caused complete suppression of activity. The absence of response to sodium application indicates that this neuron was not osmosensitive. When glucose was applied during FFA excitation, a small dose diminished the excitation and a large dose, as shown in Fig. 3*b* and *c*, completely supressed the activity. The threshold for FFA application was approximately 1 mEq/l, which is comparable to the normal FFA level of about 0.75 mEq/l in rat blood. The difference in effect of FFA on glucose-sensitive and nonglucose-sensitive neurons is significant. To determine the relative effectiveness of the components of FFA, palmitic and oleic acids (which together comprise approximately 70 per cent of the FFA in rat blood) were tested separately. Both showed effects on glucose-sensitive neurons that were similar to the effects of complete FFA.

In the VMH, glucose and FFA reverse their relative functional roles from those exhibited in the LH (Oomura, 1976). Figure 3*a* shows glucose stimulation, and FFA suppression of a VMH neuron. After FFA suppression, the neuron was again facilitated by glucose, allowed to recover to normal, and again inhibited by application of FFA. Since growth hormone, as well as FFA, increases in the blood during hunger, growth hormone was tested for its effect on glucoreceptor neurons in the VMH. It had no effect, either excitatory or inhibitory on a glucoreceptor neuron. The FFA effect is shown schematically in Fig. 2*a*.

FFA, when it affects VMH neurons, is mostly suppressive in its effect on glucoreceptors and it has no effect on non-glucoreceptors. In the LH, FFA functions by affecting the uptake of glucose by the neuron (Bornstein & Park, 1953). In the VMH, it appears, from data in this report, that the glucoreceptor neurons are normally excited by glucose binding at a receptor site followed by incorporation and subsequent metabolism. Since FFA prevents all glucose uptake, it stops the activity which depends on glucose and thus causes decreased activity.

Figure 2*b* illustrates schematically the one difference between the glucoreceptor neurons of the VMH, and the glucose-sensitive neurons in the LH. The glucoreceptor neuron has glucose receptor sites, whereas the gluco-sensitive neuron has insulin receptor sites.

Food intake and body weight in mammals are closely correlated with lipogenesis and lipolysis. It has been proposed that the VMH functions as a deterrent to addition of excess fat (Kennedy, 1966) while the LH acts to conserve fat (Nisbett, 1972). The roles of FFA and other metabolic substances in the regulation of food intake have been emphasized (Kennedy, 1966). Furthermore, it is supposed that: (1) neurons that control appetite and maintain body weight will also detect the concentration of metabolic substances, (2) as a result of constantly monitoring the level of FFA, glucose, insulin, growth hormone, adrenalin, and other blood chemicals, they will immediately be aware of changes, and (3) these neurons will be located in the LH and/or in the VMH. The remarkable sensitivity of the LH glucose-sensitive neuron and the VMH glucoreceptor neuron to FFA is shown in Fig. 3. Efficient feeding behavior requires increased activity of glucose-sensitive neurons that respond to FFA, decreased activity of neurons that would inhibit effective behavior or instigate counter-behavior, and animation of neuronal networks which are controlled by chemosensitive neurons. The effective functioning of FFA in the LH to accomplish the first and third of these requirements, and its equally effective functioning in the VMH to meet the second and third, has been demonstrated.

Glucose and insulin in the blood varies as a function of hunger and satiation, but the concentrations remain low from a relatively long time prior to, until just after, initiation of eating (Steffens, 1970). Consequently, the explanation of hunger or the onset of eating under *ad lib.* conditions is difficult in terms of these substances alone. On the other hand, the FFA level falls shortly after the onset of eating and recovers as glucose and insulin decrease (Steffens, 1970). During hunger, this level increases along with the decrease of glucose and insulin, but at a much higher relative rate. Simultaneously, growth hormone (Himsworth, 1972), ACTH, cortisol and epinephrine increase (McNew *et al.,* 1972). Liberation of FFA by these substances is well known (Goodman, 1970; Goodner *et al.,* 1973). Thus glucose and insulin are both closely related to FFA, as are epinephrine and growth hormone, during the hunger stage. It has been demonstrated that glucose-sensitive neurons in the LH, and glucoreceptor neurons in the VMH, both have, in reality, complex chemosensitivy to FFA as well as to glucose and insulin.

Obese subjects have high FFA levels (Nisbett, 1972). Diabetics, who are usually hyperphagic, have a high FFA blood level. Obesity is produced by VMH lesions which result in disinhibition of the LH. At that time, the levels of FFA and insulin in the blood increase (Hongslo, 1974), as does gastric acid secretion (Ridley & Brooks, 1965). All these factors together may lead to feeding. Repetitive stimulation of the LH which leads to feeding also leads to increased levels of glucose (Kokka & George, 1970), FFA, and growth hormone (Barkai & Allweis, 1972). Growth hormone in turn stimulates further production of FFA. This large increase in FFA will overcome the glucose effect on glucoreceptor neurons and inhibit the VMH. A cold environment facilitates feeding more than a warm environment. This can also be explained by increased FFA, which again inhibits the VMH even in the presence of glucose (Gross & Migliorini, 1977). Amino acid injections may cause anorexia by lowering FFA level (Nisbett, 1972). These facts explain relationships by which FFA level controls hunger-connected behavior.

Glucose mechanism in VMH

The glucose-sensitive neurons in the LH have been studied extensively and their glucose induced decrease in activity is understood (Oomura *et al.*, 1974). The mechanism by which glucose excites VMH neurons has been unknown until now. The investigation discussed here was initiated to determine whether or not receptor binding was sufficient for generation of the observed excitation, and/or if cellular incorporation was necessary. In the light of recent results, the response of these neurons to gastrointestinal polypeptides, and to thyrotropin releasing hormone (TRH) was also probed. King Wister rats were used under urethan anesthesia.

*The glucose analogues, 1-deoxy-*D*-glucose (poligalitol) and 2-deoxy-*D*-glucose (2-DG)* have no effect on VMH glucoreceptor neurons when used alone, but both suppress glucose stimulation of VMH glucoreceptors. Figure 4 illustrates the effect of glucose, the lack of effect of poligalitol alone, and poligalitol suppression of glucose stimulation. The effects of 2-DG and of 2-DG plus glucose mimic those shown in Fig. 4. These results indicate that the mechanism, whatever its nature, is peculiar to glucoreceptor neurons.

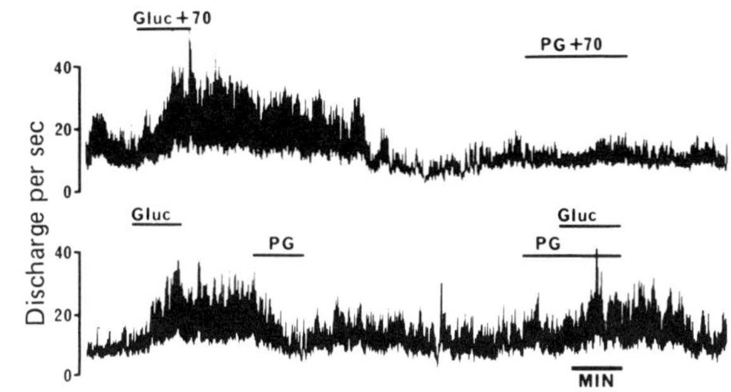

Fig. 4. Effects of glucose (top and bottom), poligalitol(PG) alone (top), and poligalitol(PG) plus glucose (bottom) on VMH glucoreceptor neuron. Note that effect of glucose endures after application (Oomura *et al.*, 1978)

α and β D*-glucose* stimulation of insulin secretion indicates that β cells in the rat pancreas can differentiate the molecular configuration of anomers and thus respond more to α than to β D-glucose (Niki *et al.*, 1974). This differentiation is indicative of a binding site function since the metabolic process should not discriminate between the α and β configurations (Niki *et al.*, 1974). The effects of α-methyl-glucose (αMG) and β-methyl-glucose (βMG), which were used because they remain stable and do not mutarotate, were assessed on VMH neurons. Figure 5 shows the dose relations for two different glucoreceptor neurons. Beta-methyl-glucose is more effective at lower doses, whereas the difference between αMG and βMG

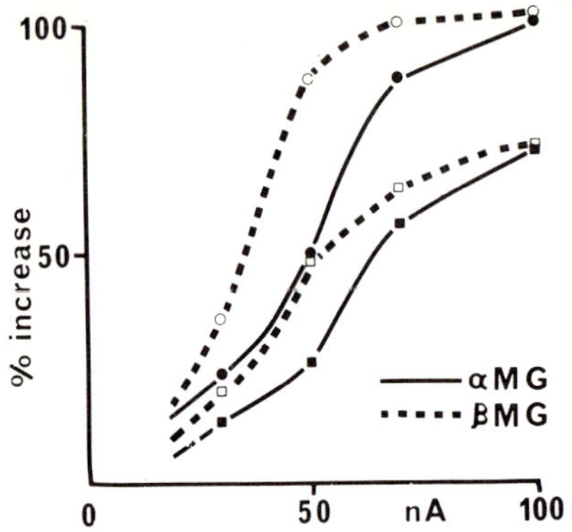

Fig. 5. Dose relations of two different VMH glucoreceptor neurons. Ordinate: discharge rate; abscissa: electroosmotically ejected α or β methyl glucose (MG) expressed as nA. One neuron did not reach saturation for the dose shown (Oomura *et al.*, 1978)

decreases as concentration increases. Approximately 30 per cent of the VMH cells tested were glucoreceptors most of which responded in this manner to αMG and βMG. Non-glucoreceptors were completely non-responsive. The differentiation at low concentration is assumed to indicate binding site activity, while the similarity at high concentration inducates that at high concentrations the metabolic effect may mask the binding site effect (Oomura *et al.*, 1978). Although the glucoreceptor membrane appears from these results to be able to recognize the difference between αMG and βMG, it is still impossible to determine conclusively if simple receptor binding of the glucose molecule is adequate, or if assimiliation and metabolism by the neuron is necessary to produce the results observed in Fig. 4.

Phlorizin blocks the glucose effect and inhibits glucose induced electrical activity of pancreatic β cells. Phlorizin also has a depolarizing effect *per se* on the β cell membrane and initially stimulates insulin release (Dean, Matthews & Sakamoto, 1975). These effects could be due to the binding of the glucose part of the phlorizin molecule to the cell membrane, insofar as the molecule might be too large to penetrate the cell membrane. Electro-osmotic application of these two materials to the same neuron demonstrated the enhancing effects of glucose and of phlorizin on VMH glucoreceptor neurons. Only glucoreceptor neurons are affected in this way by phlorizin, while non-glucoreceptors are not.

One receptor site reacts to two molecules of either glucose or phlorizin according to the Beidler taste equation (Beidler, 1971; Oomura *et al.*, 1975*b*) which was used to evaluate their dose effectiveness. The α MG and βMG data also showed that two of these molecules combine with one membrane receptor site.

Antigen-antibody reactions were considered in order to furnish incontrovertible proof of the presence of specific receptor sites on VMH cell membranes. Rat VMH antibody and caudate antibody were prepared in rabbit serum and their potencies verified. Figure 6 *a* illustrates the test for antibody potency and specificity. The photograph, as explained by the schema beneath it, shows each precipitation line resulting from both VMH and caudate homogenate reactions with the crude, non-specific antibody produced in rabbit serum. After treatment with caudate homogenate to adsorb the general rat serum antibody and the common neuronal tissue antibody, the serum reacted to only VMH homogenate as shown by the single precipitation line. Rat VMH antibody specifically decreased neuron activity when applied electroosmotically to rat VMH glucoreceptors. Fresh antibody produced a large transient increase followed by irreversible cessation of neuronal activity. With old antibody, due to probable deterioration of unstable portions, the activity depression was less pronounced and was reversible. Figure 6*b* shows (above) the response of a VMH glucoreceptor neuron to electroosmotic application of glucose for 30 seconds at 80 nA, and (below), the response of the same neuron to the same measure of VMH antibody application.

Table 1 summarizes the antibody reactions of 126 glucoreceptive and non-glucoreceptive

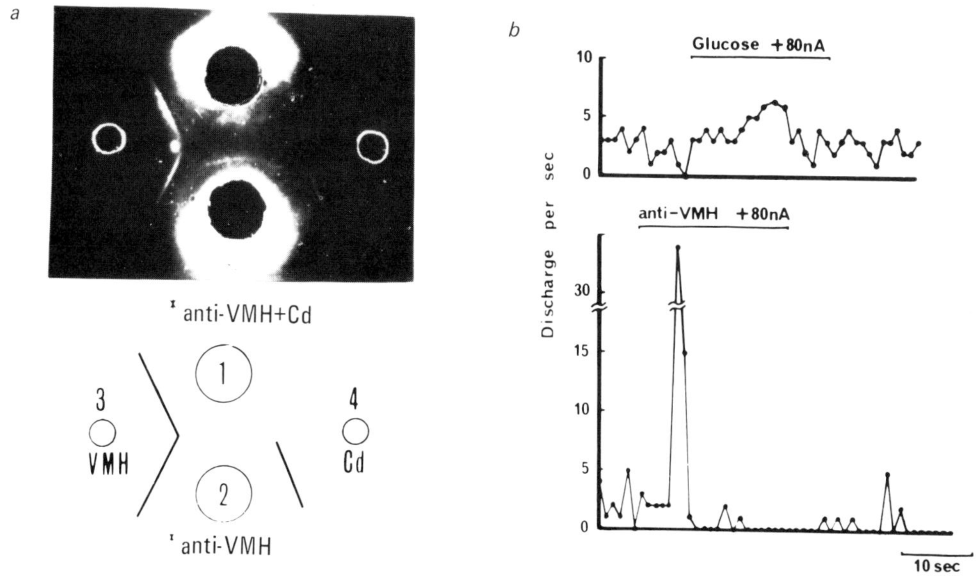

Fig. 6. Identification of glucoreceptor site in VMH glucoreceptor neuron. a: Crude VMH antibody produced in rabbit serum (anti-VMH) reacts with both VMH and caudate nucleus (Cd) homogenates. After absorbing nonspecific common antibodies of rat serum and Cd (anti–VMH+Cd), VMH antibody makes one precipitation line with VMH homogenate. b: Anti-VMH specifically suppresses rat glucoreceptor neuron. Above, response of glucoreceptor neuron to electroosmotic application of glucose. Below, response of same neuron to anti-VMH antibody shows injury discharges followed by cessation of firing.

VMH neurons. Normal rabbit serum (NRS) and antibody for rat caudate nucleus (anti Cd) had no effect on VMH neurons, but the latter did inhibit unit activity in caudate neurons (Oomura *et al.*, 1971). Specific membrane receptor binding sites are thus shown to exist on glucoreceptor neurons in the VMH, and these sites offer one route for producing the excitatory effect that glucose has on VMH neurons.

Table 1. Effects of VMH antibody on rat VMH neurons. ↑: increase, ↑→: injury discharge and stop, ↓: decrease, nc: no change

a: **VMH neurons not classified for glucoreceptivity.***

	anti-VMH		anti-Cd ↑	anti-Cd ↓	anti-Cd nc	NRS ↑	NRS ↓	NRS nc
VMH	↑	4	1	0	0	1	0	2
unit	↑→	8	0	0	1	0	0	2
(80)	↓	32	0	2	15	3	0	18
	nc	36	3	1	21	3	0	28

b: **VMH neurons classified for glucoreceptivity.****

	Glucose		anti-VMH ↑	anti-VMH ↑→	anti-VMH ↓	anti-VMH nc	anti-Cd ↑	anti-Cd ↓	anti-Cd nc	NRS ↑	NRS ↓	NRS nc
VMH	↑	19	0	1	11	5	2	2	8	6	0	9
unit	↓	0										
(46)	nc	27	1	1	1	22	2	0	19	2	0	19

* Correlation of anti-VMH antibody specificity to VMH neurons (McNemar test) : $P<0.005$
** Correlation of anti-VMH antibody specificity to VMH glucoreceptor neurons (Fisher exact method) : $P<0.001$

The results produced by this line of investigation indicate that the increase in discharge rate could be due to a simple binding of glucose to the receptor membrane, so that binding alone can be considered to be sufficient to achieve the effects which glucose has on glucoreceptors. However, the prolonged after-effect of glucose, which is evident in Fig. 4, indicates that assimilation and metabolism are probably also involved. Further investigation is necessary to ascertain the true mechanism of this post-injection activity.

A preliminary appraisal of putative satiety agents

Extracts of gastrointestinal mucosa were related to appetite as early as 1960 and 1968. Since then materials have been refined and experiments have proliferated (Gibbs, Young & Smith 1973; Gibbs, Falasco, & McHugh, 1976; Stern, Cudillo, & Kruper, 1976), but many questions still remain to be answered (Sturdevant & Goetz, 1976). Behavioral experiments have been reported which show cholecystokinin (CCK) to be a potent appetite depressant, and gastrin to be effective but somewhat less potent, following intraduodenal, intraperitoneal, intravenous, or intraventricular injection. Behavioral experiments indicate the potential efficacy of these hormones as appetite depressors, but do not disclose the mechanism, or site, or sites of their action. A third gastrointestinal hormone, secretin, has been shown to be ineffective in appetite suppression. Three hypothalamic related hormones, somatostatin (SRIF), TRH, and luteinizing hormone-releasing hormone (LHRH) have been shown, when injected into the third ventricle, to inhibit intake of food or water or both (Vijayan & McCann, 1977), with TRH being the most potent of the three. Experiments were performed to examine the direct effects of cholecystokinin (CCK), gastrin, secretin, and TRH on neurons in the VMH, LH, and parietal cortex. The results of these tests are summarized in Table 2.

Table 2. Effects of CCK, tetragastrin (GAST), secretin, and TRH on rat VMH and LH neurons

Effects	CCK	GAST	Secretin	TRH
Cortex				
Stimulated	20% (17)	8% (4)	(0)	x
Inhibited	3% (3)	2% (1)	(0)	x
No effect	77% (67)	90% (43)	(6)	x
Total	(87)	(48)	(6)	x
LH				
Stimulated	(0)	(0)	(0)	21% (28)
Inhibited	1% (1)	(0)	2% (1)	7% (8)
No effect	99% (81)	(40)	98% (57)	72% (84)
Total	(82)	(40)	(58)	(116)
VMH				
Stimulated	4% (2)	6% (1)	6% (1)	11% (5)
Inhibited	2% (1)	(0)	(0)	11% (5)
No effect	94% (49)	94% (16)	94% (15)	78% (34)
Total	(52)	(17)	(16)	(44)

CCK and gastrin are effective in stimulating cortical neurons, with CCK being about 2.5 times as effective as gastrin. The inhibitory effects in the cortex, and all effects in the LH and VMH, are either negligible or non-existent for both factors. Secretin is completely ineffective in all three regions. The few results seen in the LH and VMH were consistent with the glucose response of the neurons recorded. The one unit which was inhibited in the VMH was not a glucoreceptor (Oomura *et al.*, 1978). TRH was not tested in the cortex; it was most effective in stimulating the LH, but one-third of the stimulated neurons were glucose-sensitive, while half of the inhibited neurons were. Likewise, in the VMH, the inhibited neurons were not glucoreceptors, but 60 per cent of the stimulated neurons were. TRH appeared to have the same kind of reactions as those observed from noradrenalin (NA) when applied to the same neuron. However, phentolamine which blocked the NA effect was only partially effective in blocking the TRH effect. This indicates that the TRH effect is direct and is not mediated by NA.

Summary

FFA has strong effects on the glucose-sensitive neurons in the LH and the glucoreceptor neurons in the VMH which function to induce hunger, reduce starvation, and generate feeding behavior. FFA level is controlled by insulin, growth hormone, adrenalin, and other hormones which affect lipogenesis and lipolysis. The effect of FFA in the LH can be deeply suppressed by the presence of glucose.

Glucose strongly stimulates the VMH and mildly inhibits the LH. Both effects tend to depress hunger, enhance satiation, and reduce or terminate feeding behavior. Glucose is removed from the circulatory system by insulin which enhances glucose uptake by cells and adipose tissue. The glucose effect in the VMH is strongly enhanced by insulin, and suppressed by FFA. The presence of glucose in the LH tends to decrease the stimulating effect in the LH and mildly inhibits the VMH in the absence of glucose, however, it strongly enhances glucose stimulation of the VMH. Insulin stimulation of the LH is diminished by glucose. Insulin secretion is induced by orogastric stimulation, by glucose, and by other hormones. Its presence in the absence of glucose and FFA is a pathologic condition, although it acts to remove both of these factors from the circulatory system, and to modify their effects on CNS control of hunger sensation and feeding behavior. Initial VMH glucoreceptor reaction to glucose is through membrane receptor sites which are immunologically specific to protein, but evidence suggests that assimilation and metabolism also contribute to the effect.

Preliminary results indicate that the gastrointestinal hormones: cholecystokinin, gastrin and secretin are ineffective in glucoreceptors and glucose-sensitive neurons of the VMH and LH, although CCK affects the parietal cortex. TRH affects glucose-sensitive and glucoreceptor neurons in the LH and VMH in ways which are consistent with its observed effect on feeding behavior.

Acknowledgements – We thank Professor A. Simpson, Showa University, for help in preparation of this manuscript. This work was partly supported by grants 844023, 948272, 044067, 087099, 187015, 139017, and 157033 from the Ministry of Education.

References

Anand, B.K., Chhina, G.S., Sharma, K.W., Dua, S. & Singh, B. (1964): *Am. J. Physiol.* 207, 1146.
Barkai, A. & Allweis, C. (1972): *J. Lipid Res.* 13, 725.
Beidley, L.M. (1971): Taste receptor stimulation with salts and acids. In *Handbook of sensory physiology,* ed L.M. Beidler, p. 200. Berlin: Springer.
Bornstein, J. & Park, C.R. (1953): *J. Biol. Chem.* 205, 503.
Creese, R. & Jenden, D.J. (1968): *J. Physiol.* 197, 255.
Dean, P.M., Matthews, E.K. & Sakamoto, Y. (1975): *J. Physiol.* 246, 459.
Gibbs, J., Young, R.C., & Smith, G.P. (1973): *J. Comp. Physiol. Psychol.* 84, 488.
Gibbs, J., Falasco, J.D. & McHugh, P.R. (1976): *Am. J. Physiol.* 230, 15.
Goodman, H.M. (1970): *Physiologist* 13, 75.
Goodner, C.J., Koerker, D.J., Werrbach, J.H., Toivola, P. & Gale, C.C. (1973): *Am. J. Physiol.* 224, 534.
Gross, J.L., Migliorini, R.H. (1977): *Am. J. Physiol.* 232, E165.
Himsworth, R.L., Carmel, P.W. & Frantz, A.G. (1972): *Endocrinol.* 91, 217.
Hongslo, C.F., Hustvedt, B.E. & Løvø, A. (1974): *Acta Physiol. Scand.* 90, 757.
Kennedy, G.C. (1966): *Br. Med. Bull.* 22, 216.
Kokka, N. & George, R. (1970): *Neuroendocrinol.* 6, 1.
McNew, J.J., Sabbot, I.M., Hoshigaki, J., Mandell, A.J., Spooner, C.E., Marcus, I. & Adey, W.R. (1972): *Am. J. Physiol.* 222, 640.

Niki, A., Niki, H., Miwa, J. & Okuda, J. (1974): *Science* **186**, 150.
Nisbett, R.E. (1972): *Psychol. Rev.* 79, 433.
Oomura, Y., Ono, T., Sugimori, M., Nakamura, T. & Ooyama, H. (1971): Antigen-antibody reaction in the satiety center of the rat hypothalamus. In *Proc. XXV Int. Cong. Physiol. Sci.* **9**, 4.
Oomura, Y. (1973): Central mechanisms of feeding. In *Advance in biophysics,* ed M. Kotani, p. 65. Tokyo: Tokyo University Press.
Oomura, Y., Ooyama, H., Sugimori, M., Makamura, T. & Yamada, K. (1974): *Nature* 247, 284.
Oomura, Y., Nakamura, T., Sugimori, M. & Yamada, Y. (1975*a*): *Physiol. Behav.* **14**, 483.
Oomura, Y., Sugimori, M., Nakamura, T. & Yamada, Y. (1975*b*): Contribution of electrophysiological techniques to the understanding of central control systems. In *Neural integration of physiological mechanisms and behavior,* eds G.J. Mogenson & F.R. Calaresu, p. 375. Toronto: University of Toronto Press.
Oomura, Y. (1976): Significance of glucose, insulin, and free fatty acid on the hypothalamic feeding and satiety neurons. In *Hunger, basic mechanisms and clinical implications,* ed D. Novin, W. Wyrwicka & G. Bray, p. 145. New York: Raven Press.
Oomura, Y., Ohta, M., Kita, H. & Ishibashi, S. (1978): Hypothalamic neuron response to glucose, phlorizin, and cholecystokinin. In *Proc. XXVII Int. Cong. Physiol. Sci. Sat. Symp:* Iontophoresis and transmitter mechanisms in the mammalian central nervous system, eds R.W. Ryall & J.S. Kelly. Amsterdam: Elsevier.
Ridley, P.T. & Brooks, F.P. (1965): *Am. J. Physiol.* **209**, 319.
Steffens, A.B. (1970): *Physiol. Behav.* **5**, 147.
Stern, J.J., Cudillo, C.A. & Kruper, J. (1976): *J. Comp. Physiol. Psychol.* **90**, 484.
Sturdevant, R.A.L. & Goetz, H. (1976): *Nature* **261**, 713.
Vijayan, E. & McCann, S.M. (1977): *Endocrinol.* **100**, 1729.
Zierler, K.L. (1966): *Am. J. Med.* **40**, 735.

4
Some expected and unexpected effects of glucose on food intake

D. NOVIN
Psychology Department and Brain Research Institute, University of California, Los Angeles, CA 90024, USA.

The effect of a glucose infusion on hunger ought to be simple and well known. By any current theory of hunger, giving glucose to man or animal should result in decreased hunger for some period after that infusion. The extent and time course of the effect presumably depends upon the amount given. This would be predicted by a glucoreceptor, glucose utilization, energy flow, lipostatic, or any theory, whereby hunger and metabolism are linked.

In the last few years workers in my laboratory have looked intensely at the question of the effects of glucose (and to some extent other sugars) on appetite. For the most part this review will be restricted to our own work. The reason is not vanity but the difficulty of interlaboratory comparisons when seemingly even minor variations in procedure may have profound effects on the way in which sugars affect feeding. Depending upon a complex interaction of factors such as nutritional state, route of infusion, time of day and amount given, glucose can depress, enhance or have no effect on subsequent food intake. In addition, some denervations and lesions profoundly influence the effect glucose has on feeding. Are these effects random, or is there a mechanism or mechanisms that could account for expected as well as seemingly paradoxical results following what would appear to be simple experiments? I believe it an important question because glucose is an important source of energy and an understanding of these mechanisms would be essential for any complete understanding of the psychophysiology of food intake. In addition, these findings might well have implications for dietary treatment of obesity, particularly the ongoing controversy about the effectiveness of low carbohydrate diets.

Initial studies

Based upon a wide variety of studies Russek (1971) concluded that the liver was the primary locus of nutrient receptors controlling feeding. In an attempt to test this hypothesis we did a simple experiment in which duodenal and hepatic-portal glucose infusions were compared for their effects on short-term feeding in undeprived rabbits. In both hepatic-portal and duodenal infusions the glucose solution was 5 per cent (w/v), given at a rate of 1 ml/min for 10 min. The results suggested that the gut, rather than the liver, might be more important in suppressing food intake to a glucose load (VanderWeele *et al.*, 1974). These data for the first hour are given in Fig. 1. There were, however, enough discrepant results in the literature (see Novin, 1976 and Novin & VanderWeele, in press) for me to believe that these results should be investigated further.

Locus of infusion interacts with nutritional status

We then compared the effectiveness of duodenal and hepatic-portal glucose infusions in 22-hour deprived rabbits (Novin, Sanderson & VanderWeele, 1974). We hypothesized that the effectiveness of these procedures would be reversed when compared to results in free-

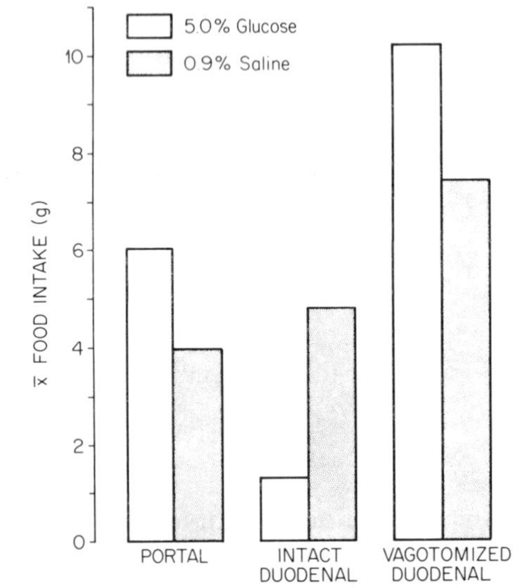

Fig. 1. Food intake in the first hour following the administration of 5 per cent glucose solution or 0.9 per cent saline either through the hepatic-portal system ('portal'), the duodenum, or the duodenum of the sub-diaphragmatically vagotomised rabbit. The rate was 1.0 ml/minute and volume was 10 ml. There was no prior food deprivation. (Reprinted with permission of Brain Research Publications, Inc.)

feeding animals. The predicted results were in fact obtained. These are illustrated in Fig. 2. The reasoning behind this prediction was that the suppression of feeding by glucose in the duodenum depended upon the presence of liver glycogen. Moreover, it was proposed that hepatic-portal glucose infusions would only suppress feeding when glycogen and perhaps intracellular glucose levels in the hepatocytes were low.

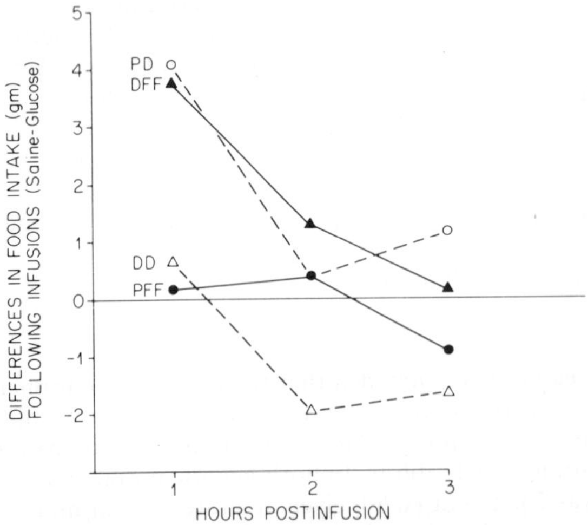

Fig. 2. Differences in feeding after 0.9 per cent saline minus feeding after 5 per cent glucose. PD refers to hepatic-portal infusions in 22-hr deprived rabbits. DFF refers to duodenal infusions in free-feeding rabbits. DD refers to duodenal infusions in deprived rabbits and PFF refers to hepatic-portal infusions in free-feeding rabbits. The rate was 1.0 ml/min and volume 10 ml

The relationship of food deprivation to liver glycogen had been examined by Forsgren (1928). He showed that in the rabbit, liver glycogen was significantly depleted within hours after a meal. We replicated this finding showing that after 4 to 6 hours there is a significant drop in liver glycogen in the rabbit. If our prediction were true that the effective locus of the suppression of glucose-induced feeding and glycogen were related then the crossover point where duodenal infusions fall and hepatic-portal infusions become effective should come quite early in the deprivation period. This prediction was confirmed (VanderWeele, Skoog & Novin, 1976).

Amount and concentration of glucose

In the previous experiments infusions of isotonic glucose were used. If small amounts suppress food intake moderately then one might expect that larger quantities would suppress feeding to a greater extent. In one study in the rabbit (Rezek, Havlicek & Novin, 1975) we found the typical suppression of feeding with 10 ml of 5 per cent glucose solution when duodenally administered. However, when 30 ml of the same solution was given feeding was increased in the immediate postinfusion period when compared to a control saline infusion.

In another study (Martin & Novin, unpublished results) we varied not only volume but concentration and found an inverted V-shaped function. Again 10 ml of 5 per cent glucose solution suppressed food intake, while a 10 per cent solution did not. When a 20 per cent solution was administered suppression was also seen. This latter result, however, is not a response to glucose *per se* but is probably a non-specific effect. High concentrations are making the animal sick; since pairing this concentration with a distinctive flavor creates a taste aversion indicative of non-specific malaise.

When rabbits are allowed to drink glucose solutions, other sugars, and possibly non-nutritive sweet substances we have noted that the most typical response is to increase the subsequent intake of their pelleted laboratory chow (Geiselman, G. Rogers & Novin, unpublished results).

Effects of other hexoses

We have only just begun to look at the effects of duodenal infusion of other hexoses besides glucose on feeding. Fructose in equiosmotic concentrations was at least as effective and possibly more so than glucose when given during the daylight. Galactose, in contrast, showed no effect in suppressing food intake. When these same experiments were done during the dark period galactose was effective in suppressing food intake, and in the first half-hour, was the only hexose of the three to yield significant feeding suppression. All the hexoses have significant effects on feeding one hour after the infusion and the effects begin to fade by 90 minutes.

Denervation and lesion effects

Russek (1971) has proposed that important metabolic information might reach the brain via the vagus nerves. This was in part based upon the work of Niijima (1969) who showed in the isolated guinea pig liver a linear decreasing relation between glucose concentration and rate of firing on the vagus nerve. For this reason many of the experiments outlined above were done not only in cannulated animals but also in animals following recovery from subdiaphragmatic vagotomy. Details of this procedure and the verification of vagotomy are given in VanderWeele *et al.* (1974). Vagotomy eliminated the suppressive effects of glucose on feeding (Novin *et al.*, 1974; VanderWeele *et al.*, 1974). In fact, glucose enhanced subsequent food intake when compared to a control infusion. In one situation where drinking 35 ml of 5 per cent (w/v) glucose solution enhanced subsequent feeding the effect was apparently greater in vagotomized rabbits (Novin, 1976).

Because of the many similarities between the effects of vagotomy and lateral hypothalamic lesions (Novin, 1976), we tested the effects of glucose on feeding in rats with lateral hypothalamic (LH) lesions. The LH is the classic feeding center, so called because lesions decrease feeding. Rats can recover from LH lesions and after sufficient time will eat nearly normal amounts of food (Teitelbaum & Epstein, 1962). Based upon a notion of an LH 'feeding center' one might predict that conditions which reduce food intake (ie cause satiety) might be more effective in these lesioned animals since the 'satiety center' is intact. However, we have proposed a model in which the LH subserves many of the same functions as the vagus nerves in the control of food intake and thus predicted that LH lesions should eliminate glucose-induced satiety. The results supported our prediction rather than the classic view (Novin, Gonzalez & Sanderson, 1976).

Conclusions

These results suggest the importance of visceral receptors in the short-term control of food intake. While gut and liver receptors, under appropriate conditions (see VanderWeele *et al.*, 1976), respond to glucose by limiting subsequent food intake, central nervous system (Epstein, 1960) and systemic intravenous infusions (Novin, unpublished observations) are largely without immediate effect.

The effectiveness of visceral administration of glucose depends upon an intact neural circuit involving both vagus nerves and lateral hypothalamic area. This had led us to the hypothesis that the vagus carries information to the lateral hypothalamic area from visceral receptors sensitive to glucose or glucose-related events (metabolite, enzyme or hormone). At this stage of our work we cannot say with certainty whether other nutrients also activate this system. Some work from our laboratory (Gonzalez, Sanderson & Novin, unpublished observations) suggests that an amino acid solution (FreAmine, McGaw Laboratories), but not fat, is dependent upon an intact vagus to suppress feeding in rats. However, in another study (Rezek & Novin, 1976) casein hydrolysate was effective in suppressing feeding in vagotomized rabbits. Fat, however, was independent of the vagus in its ability to suppress feeding. Thus, glucose depends upon vagal innervations while fat does not. The means by which proteins and protein metabolites affect hunger remains uncertain until we can unconfound the form in which protein is given with the species which receives it.

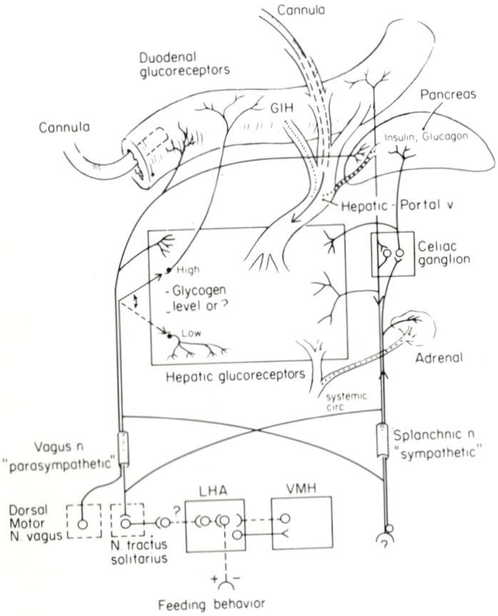

Fig.3. A schematic representation of the way in which glucose, and possibly other hexoses and nutrients, might affect food intake. Visceral receptors innervated by the autonomic nervous system with connections to the lateral hypothalamic area forms the key neural substrate. Liver glycogen level is thought critical in determining the locus of satiety signals. Gastrointestinal hormones (GIH) and the output of the system to endocrine glands are recognized as important but not emphasized in this model. (Reprinted by permission of Academic Press.)

Focusing on glucose, we have represented diagrammatically a general scheme by which glucose is presumed to affect food intake in the short term (Fig. 3). Thus vagotomy and LH lesions are readily explained as eliminating afferent input and integration from the viscera. However, this scheme fails to explain why after vagotomy glucose no longer suppresses feeding but causes increased food intake. Moreover, it cannot account for why small volumes and low concentrations are more effective than greater amounts of glucose; nor, more startling, why relatively large amounts of glucose may actually enhance eating. It appears as if glucose can make experimental animals hungry under certain circumstances, rather than cause satiety as one would expect. We have no explanations, only speculation. One possibility might be that we are seeing reactive hypoglycemia caused by excessive insulin secretion. In the case of vagotomy, where small glucose loads invariably increase feeding, that explanation would appear at first unlikely. The reason is that most studies find that vagal stimulation increases insulin output and vagotomy has either little effect or decreases insulin levels (Woods & Porte, 1974). However, more recently Louis-Sylvestre

(1977) has reported that, following vagotomy, oral glucose loads yield greater insulin secretion overall, despite the absence of the initial peak ('cephalic phase') seen in intact rats. What the result of LH lesions might be on the dynamics of insulin secretion is unknown.

In response to large loads of glucose one could speculate that excessive insulin secretion could lead to a subsequent hypoglycemia. Insulin is more involved in the uptake of glucose by muscle and fat and less important for liver and brain. Most theories for regulation of food intake invoke receptors in liver and/or brain. Excessive insulin might then result in lowered glucose uptake in those organs which contain receptors designed to signal satiety.

Additional effects of insulin are to promote lipogenesis and depress lipolysis. Excessive insulin secretion could increase lipid synthesis at the expense of other metabolic pathways such as glycogenesis or the tri-carboxylic acid cycle that are more likely to provide satiety signals. In experiments using (-)-hydroxycitrate the possibility that glycogen levels were more important than lipids in satiety has been proposed (Sullivan & Triscari, 1976). Many other explanations are possible. We have focused on insulin because of the obvious role of insulin in energy metabolism. It is clear that insulin secretion is finely tuned to feeding, as either excessive insulin secretion, as in obesity, or decreased insulin secretion, as in severe diabetes, are both associated with increased food intake. We are now beginning experiments designed to look simultaneously at insulin and food intake following glucose infusions, especially in those situations where glucose increases food intake.

Our frequent observations that glucose can stimulate eating in animals may have some parallels in humans. Most people eat a relatively high carbohydrate diet in which 50 per cent or more of the calories are typically from starches and sugars. Such a distribution of calories may not be as satiating as equicaloric diets where fats or proteins comprise a larger proportion of the diet. This lack of satiating potency may be particularly apparent when balanced but calorically restricted diets are used. Moreover, if our animal results could be extended to the human case the carbohydrates in such a diet may increase sensations of hunger.

Is then the widespread popularity of the low carbohydrate diets based upon real consequences in that they are easier to follow? In any case, our observations suggest that there are animal models of dietary restriction that are worth pursuing. First, because one can exert absolute control over activity and diet. Second, one can measure 'hunger' in the psychological sense accurately and objectively in the rat or rabbit. Finally, a resolution of the very controversial question of the efficacy of low carbohydrate diets has great practical and theoretical significance.

Acknowledgements — The work on which this paper is based was supported by NINCDS # NS 7687. All of this work represents a collaborative effort with many present and past members of my laboratory. Especial thanks to Ms Paula Geiselman who suggested some interesting connections between our animal data and human clinical results.

References

Epstein, A.N. (1960): *Am. J. Physiol.* 199, 969.
Forsgren, E. (1928): *Scand. Archs Physiol.* 53, 137.
Louis-Sylvestre, J. (1977): Sixth International Conference on the Physiology of Food and Water Intake, Jouy-en Josas.
Niijima, A. (1969): *Ann. N.Y. Acad. Sci.* 157, 690.
Novin, D. (1976): *Hunger: basic mechanisms and clinical implications,* ed D. Novin, W. Wyrwicka & G. Bray, p. 357. New York: Raven Press.
Novin, D., Gonzalez, M.F. & Sanderson, J.D. (1976): *Am. J. Physiol.* 230, 1084.
Novin, D., Sanderson, J.D. & VanderWeele, D.A. (1974): *Physiol. Behav.* 13, 3.
Novin, D. & VanderWeele, D.A. (in press): *Progress in psychobiology and physiological psychology,* Vol. 7, ed J.M. Sprague & A.N. Epstein, p. 193. New York: Academic Press.

Rezek, M., Havlicek, V. & Novin, D. (1975): *Am. J. Physiol.* 229, 545.
Rezek, M. & Novin, D. (1976): *J. Nutr.* **106**, 812.
Russek, M. (1971): In *Neurosciences research,* Vol. 4, ed S. Ehrenpreis, p. 213. New York: Academic Press.
Sullivan, A.C. & Triscari, J. (1976): *Hunger: basic mechanisms and clinical implications,* ed D. Novin, W. Wyrwicka & G. Bray, p. 115. New York: Raven Press.
Teitelbaum, P. & Epstein, A.N. (1962): *Psychol. Rev.* **69**, 74.
VanderWeele, D.A., Novin, D., Rezek, M. & Sanderson, J.D. (1974): *Physiol. Behav.* 12, 467.
VanderWeele, D.A., Skoog, D.R. & Novin, D. (1976): *Am. J. Physiol.* 231, 1655.
Woods, D.C. & Porte, D. (1974): *Physiol. Rev.* 54, 596.

5
The intestinal control of food intake

H.S. KOOPMANS
Dept. of Psychology, Columbia University, 116th St. and Broadway, New York, N.Y. 10027, USA.

The small intestine is the major site for the absorption of nutrients into the bloodstream. Since almost all absorbed nutrients must pass through its mucosa, the intestine could relay neural or hormonal messages to the brain that estimate the amount of absorbed food and provide a control over food intake. Several investigators have tried to assess the importance of the gut to feeding behavior by infusing substances directly into the intestine and the results have been contradictory. Some investigators report a dose-dependent reduction of food intake when glucose or other simple nutrient solutions are infused into the duodenum. (Campbell & Davis, 1974; Novin, Sanderson & VanderWeele, 1974; Snowdon, 1975). Others report that the infusion of nutrients is no more effective in reducing food intake than an equiosmotic control solution (Ethman, Albert & Jamieson, 1971; Yin & Tsai, 1973; Stephans & Baldwin, 1974; Houpt, 1977). All find some reduction of food intake.

The common technique of these studies is the continuous infusion of a laboratory-prepared, chemical solution through a tube that terminates at one site in the duodenum. A more effective technique for investigating the role of the intestine in the inhibition of food intake is the delivery of normal food mixed with digestive enzymes by a physiological control system. This paper describes how this physiological delivery of food to the intestine can be accomplished.

Surgical procedure

Twelve pairs of parabiotic rats were created by sewing together the skin and muscle of the flanks of two inbred Lewis rats. A 3 cm circular opening was made in the peritoneal muscle of each rat and was sewn together by a continuous 2-0 gut suture producing a common peritoneal cavity. Six of these rat pairs underwent a second operation. After a midline incision, the intestines were carefully mobilized and transected 5 cm below the stomach and 35 cm further down in the lower jejunum. The isolated segment was sewn back into an equivalent position in the digestive tract of its partner with continuous 7-0 Connell sutures (see Fig. 1). The rats were closed and allowed to recover for two to three weeks. After the crossed intestines operation, the food eaten by one rat of a pair arrives in its own stomach, travels through 5 cm of its own duodenum and, then, crosses over into the lower duodenum of its partner. After moving through 30 cm of its partner's small intestine, the unabsorbed food crosses back into the intestine of the rat that fed. The crossed intestines preparation does not require the transection of any major blood vessels or gastrointestinal nerves. It is particularly useful in determining whether intestinal signals reduce food intake. The food that moves into the partner rat's intestine is mixed with saliva, gastric secretions and biliary and pancreatic secretions. The bile duct enters the intestines 1 to 2 cm above the first crossover, and food moving into the cross segment should be mildly basic and nearly isotonic. The rate of delivery of food to the intestinal segment is controlled by motility of the partner's stomach and duodenal bulb.

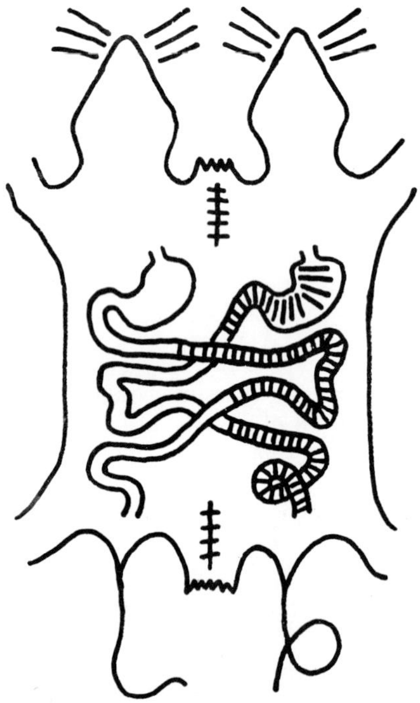

Fig. 1. A diagram of the crossed intestines rats. The striped digestive tract belongs to the rat on the right. No major intestinal blood vessels or nerves need to be transected to alter the flow of ingested food

Behavioral study 1

Four pairs of each type of rat were placed on a ten hour deprivation schedule. They were fed the liquid diet, Nutrament (1 kcal per ml), at 7 p.m. at night and were returned to their home cage the next morning at 9 a.m. where only water was available. The two rats of each pair were fed together within a few minutes of being put in a modified Bollman restraining cage or after a 30 or 60 minute delay. Food intake was measured for 30 minutes. In the experimental conditions, one rat of each pair was fed immediately upon being put back in the restraining cage and its partner was fed either 30 or 60 minutes later. Since either rat of a pair could be fed first, each data point represents an average over eight rats. Three repeated measurements were made on each rat for each condition and the seven conditions were run in random order.

There are two special aspects of the experimental design. If the intestine is important for controlling food intake, then feeding behavior is expected to both increase and decrease. Physical discomfort is unlikely to produce both changes. In addition, the parabiotic rats serve as psychological controls. Psychologically induced changes in food intake that do not depend upon the crossing of the intestines will occur in both types of rat pairs.

The data in Table 1 show that there are strong psychological effects of feeding rats by themselves or together regardless of the type of rat preparation. When one rat is fed by itself immediately after being put into the restraining cage it eats more than when it is fed with its partner. This result is surprising because the rats can not see each other: a black Plexiglass barrier separates them. The smell of food is an unlikely cue since it is present whether the rat has been allowed to feed or not. Apparently, the rats are aware of their partners feeding

Table 1. The 30 minute food intake (ml±s.e.m.) of rat pairs when they are fed at their normal hour or after a delay. Each table entry represents 24 observations. (Three repeated measures on eight rats)

	Delay (min.)		
	0	30	60
Crossed intestines rats			
Fed together	6.6 ± 1.2	8.9 ± 1.8	12.2 ± 1.7
Fed alone with 30 min delay	9.5 ± 1.7	11.2 ± 1.8	
Fed alone with 60 min delay	9.9 ± 1.4		12.7 ± 2.3
Control parabiotic rats			
Fed together	6.3 ± 1.2	8.4 ± 1.1	10.1 ± 1.1
Fed alone with 30 min delay	8.6 ± 1.1	10.5 ± 1.0	
Fed alone with 60 min delay	8.1 ± 1.1		10.1 ± 1.5

condition by noticing body movements or by hearing sounds. When some rats are not allowed to feed, they go to sleep or wait anxiously; other rats move around restlessly and gnash their teeth against the bars of the cage. In any case, the rat that feeds alone in either type of rat pair increases its food intake. This phenomenon also occurs when the rats are fed 30 minutes after being put in the restraining cage. The rat feeding alone eats more than when it eats with its partner ($F=10.8$, $P<0.05$). Of course, this rat is now eating alone after its partner has completely satiated itself and is usually still and dozing. After a 60 minute delay, this psychological effect seems to disappear ($F=0.27$, $P>>0.05$).

There is also a significant increase in food intake when the rat's feeding is delayed whether it eats with its partner or not. The rats eat more after a 30 minute delay and still more after a 60 minute delay ($F=45.4$, $P<0.01$). This significant increase could be interpreted as a physiological compensation for the food not eaten and absorbed during the delay or as a psychological reaction to the frustration of not being fed.

All of these significant changes in food intake occur in both types of rat pair and are not dependent upon the crossing of the intestine. If the intestines were important in reducing food intake, one could expect a significant interaction between the type of rat pair and the amount eaten by the rats fed alone. For example, the crossed intestines rat fed alone lacks signals coming back from its 12 inch crossed intestinal segment because that segment is connected to its partner. If those intestinal signals were important in reducing food intake, the crossed intestines rat fed first should eat more than its parabiotic control to compensate for the lost signals. In contrast, the crossed intestines rat fed 30 or 60 minutes after its partner should have received all of the intestinal signals during that 30 or 60 minute period and it should eat less than the control. In short, if the crossed intestinal segment is important in controlling food intake, there sould be a significant interaction between the type of rat pair and the time of feeding. Figure 2 presents the relevant data for the 30 minute delay (also

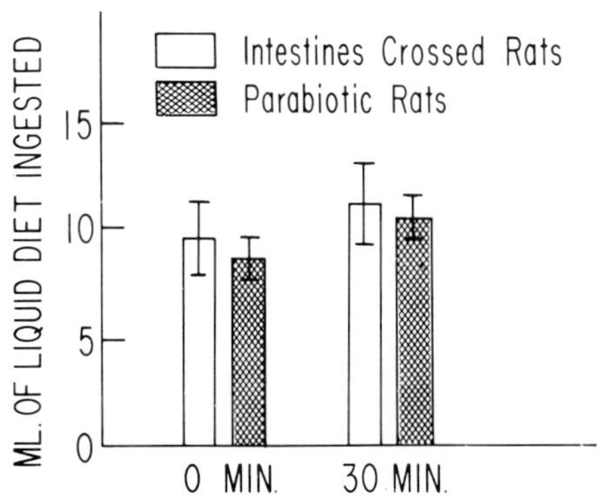

Fig. 2. The 30 minute food intake of each type of rat pair, when one rat in each pair is fed immediately after being put in the restraining cage (0 min), or after a 30 minute delay (30 min). Brackets indicate s.e.m.

presented in lines 2 and 5 of Table 1). The two bars above the 0 minute label show food intake for each type of rat pair when one rat is fed alone immediately after being put in the rat cage. The two bars above the 30 minute label show the food intake when the second rat of a pair is fed alone 30 minutes after its partner begins eating. As can be clearly visualized, there is no significant interaction ($F=0.11$, $P>>0.05$). A 60 minute delay also produces no significant interaction ($F=0.72$, $P>>0.05$).

Absorption study

The results of the feeding behavior studies are important only if food enters the crossed intestinal segment and is absorbed by this segment during the time period when the rat's feeding behavior was measured. To determine how much food was absorbed into each rat, I added small amounts of tritium labelled glucose or amino acids into the normal liquid diet of six pairs of each type of rat. Eight ml of these diets were injected through a chronically implanted stomach tube into the stomach on one rat of each pair at a rate that approximated the normal feeding behavior (1.5 ml per minute for the first 2 minutes and 1.0 ml per minute for the next 5 minutes. A one-tenth ml sample of blood was drawn from the tail of each rat before the stomach injection and every 10 minutes for the next hour. These samples were precipitated in Bray's solution, centrifuged, transferred to counting vials and counted in a Beckman scintillation counter. The number of disintegrations per minute for each of these blood samples is presented in Fig. 3.

Tritiated glucose is rapidly absorbed into the parabiotic rat that was fed. Only a small amount of radioactive label crosses through the capillaries of the skin and muscle into the rat that was not fed. In contrast, the labelled glucose was rapidly absorbed into both of the crossed intestines rats. In fact, in the first 10 minutes more glucose was absorbed into the rat that was not fed and remained hungry than into its fed partner. This difference rapidly disappeared and after 30 and 60 minutes the blood level of glucose -^{3}H was approximately the same in the two rats. These absorption curves establish two facts: that food does arrive in the crossed intestinal segment during the behavioral study and is absorbed through it. Unfortunately, the blood levels of free glucose do not tell us how much food was absorbed into each rat. First, the labelled glucose was added to a complex diet that contained large starch molecules. These starches require digestion and may be absorbed in different regions

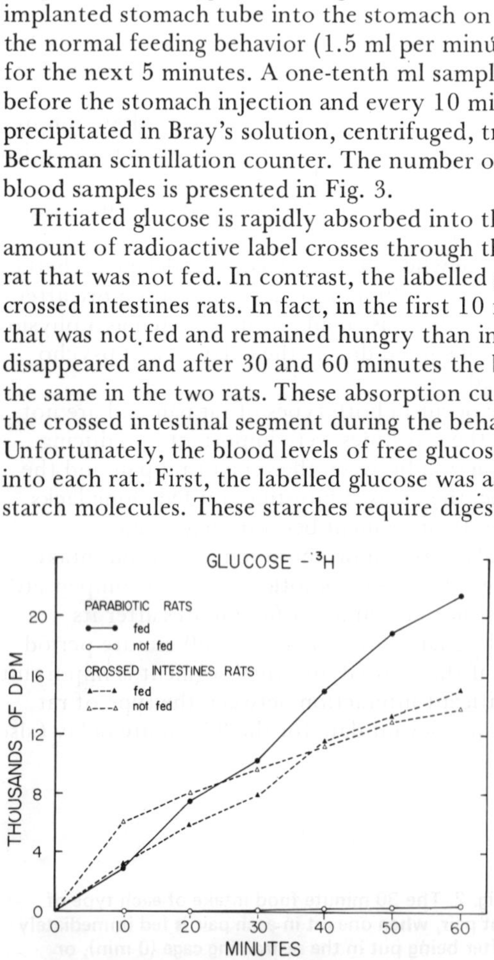

Fig. 3. The number of disintegrations per minute in a 0.1 ml blood sample taken from the tail of each rat every ten minutes after one rat of each pair was fed 8 ml of its normal liquid diet thoroughly mixed with small amounts of glucose ^{3}H

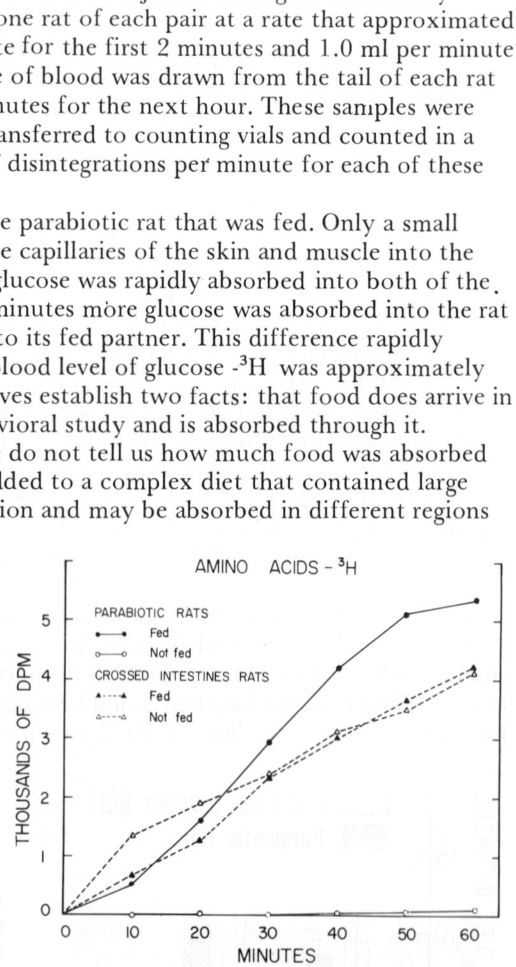

Fig. 4. The number of disintegrations per minute in a 0.1 ml blood sample taken from the tail of each rat every ten minutes after one rat of each pair was fed 8 ml of its normal liquid diet thoroughly mixed with small amounts of amino acid - ^{3}H mix

of the digestive tract than free glucose. Furthermore, the blood level of the labelled glucose is the result of two dynamic processes: the absorption of labelled glucose from the digestive tract and its removal from the blood. If the level of glucose in the blood is different in the two rats, then the rate of removal is likely to be different and blood level will not provide an accurate estimate of the amount of absorption. Fortunately, the blood levels of the two crossed intestines rats are approximately the same and it is reasonable to conclude that free glucose is absorbed about equally in the two rats (at 30 minutes $F=0.61$, $P>>0.05$).

Figure 4 presents similar data for the absorption of a labelled amino acid mix when these free amino acids are added to the 8 ml of liquid diet injected into the stomach. The results are essentially the same: the blood level of tritiated amino acid is approximately the same in both rats of a crossed intestines pair. Hence, free amino acid is absorbed about equally into the two rats (at 30 minutes, $F=0.04$, $P>>0.05$).

These two studies establish that food is present in the crossed intestinal segment within a few minutes after the rat begins feeding and that this food is continually being absorbed from the segment during the 30 or 60 minute delay between the feeding of the first rat of a pair and the feeding of its partner. The absorption studies also show that free glucose and amino acids are absorbed equally into the two rats of a crossed intestines pair. A substantial portion of the more complex nutrients are likely to be absorbed by the crossed intestinal segment. The crossed segment measures 30 cm in length and comprises more than one quarter of the total length of the small intestine which averages 110 cm. Gastrointestinal physiologists (Davenport, 1971) have repeatedly established that 80 to 90 per cent of the ingested food is absorbed in the first half of the small intestine, comprising the duodenum and jejunum. The second half of the small intestine, the ileum, is largely responsible for the absorption of salts, water and bile acids. A small amount of poorly digested food will be absorbed in the ileum. The crossed segment of the intestines is located proximally, beginning only 5 cm below the stomach, and the total length of the segment is more than half the length of the first half of the small bowel. Assuming that the crossed segment is fairly normal in its activity, it is reasonable to assume that 40 to 45 per cent of the ingested food is absorbed through the crossed segment. This conclusion is supported by the results of the absorption study on free glucose and amino acids where about half of the labelled nutrients were absorbed into each rat. Despite the considerable loss of nutrients from the intestine of one rat and the absorption of sizable amounts of food into the bloodstream of the partner, there were no changes in the short-term feeding behavior of the two crossed intestines rats when their feeding was compared to control parabiotic rats. Apparently, the signals that control short-term feeding behavior do not arise in the crossed intestinal segment and do not appear to be related to the amount of food absorbed. Instead, these internal physiological signals must arise in the stomach, proximal duodenum or the lower jejunum and ileum. The signals that are effective in reducing food intake are either neural or hormonal signals because the amount of absorbed food does not seem to be involved in inhibiting food intake.

Behavioral study 2

The first behavioral study established that the crossing of the intestines has no effect on the feeding behavior of rats in the first 90 minutes when one rat of the pair is deprived. The loss of nutrients from one rat to the other might begin to change the rat's feeding behavior after the first or second meal and cause an increase in the total food intake of this rat. To test this possibility, one rat of each type of rat pair was deprived of food for five days while its partner was allowed to feed freely. Total daily food intake was measured for six pairs of each type of rat. The average total food intake and average pair body weight are presented in Fig. 5.

There were three periods of measurement of baseline food intake and body weight: days 1 to 5, 9 to 11 and 17 to 21. On days 6 to 8, the rats' normal liquid diet, Nutrament, was diluted with an equal volume of water. The rats compensated for the diet dilution by eating 1.7 times the volume of food or 0.85 times the calories on the average. They did not quite

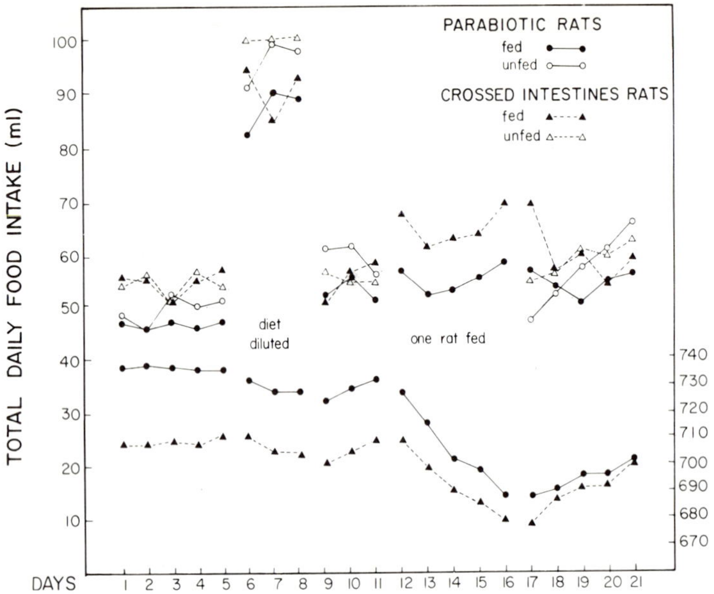

Fig. 5. The daily food intake and body weight of crossed intestines and parabiotic rat pairs. On days 6 to 8, the diet was diluted with an equal volume of water. On days 12 to 16, only one rat of each pair was allowed to feed

compensate for the caloric dilution and lost some body weight. After returning to baseline food intake for three days, one rat of each pair was deprived of food for five days. The free food intake of the partner rat is recorded on days 12 to 16. The fed parabiotic rat should not be expected to increase its food intake since the fed rat experiences the normal satiety signals and loses very little food to its partner. The small amount of nutrient lost in the blood travelling through the capillaries of the parabiotic union is largely returned as mobilized nutrient in the blood arriving from the partner. The net loss of nutrient is small and the fed parabiotic rat does not increase its food intake. In contrast, the fed crossed intestines rat might be expected to increase its food intake because of the loss of substantial amounts of food into the intestines and bloodstream of its partner. The fed rat does show a small increase in average food intake when its feeding behavior is compared to its own intake during the three baseline periods, but the increase is not significant ($F=1.32$, $P>0.25$). Although the feeding rat is losing a substantial portion of its ingested food into its partner, the fed rat does not significantly increase its food intake during the five day period and shows no greater average intake four or five days after its partner is deprived than on the first day. In contrast, when the rat's diet is diluted with an equal volume of water, the increase in intake is immediate and highly significant ($F=40.1$, $P<0.01$). The rat appears to be able to detect and adjust to dilution of the diet when it occurs at the level of the mouth, but does not detect the loss of a substantial amount of nutrient from the duodenum.

Discussion

The short-term experiment shows that signals that arise in the crossed intestinal segment have no effect on feeding behavior in a single meal. This observation is particularly important because the crossed intestines preparation provides a unique method of testing what factors control satiety. The food delivered to the crossed segment arrives in a highly physiological manner. It has been mixed with salivary secretions during feeding and has been partially digested by stomach acid and enzymes before moving into the duodenum. Two cm above the cross-over point, the partially digested food is neutralized by bicarbonate and mixed with pancreatic enzymes and bile salts. It arrives in the crossed intesinal segment in a form very similar to that arriving in the same segment of an intact single rat. The glucose absorption data suggest that food empties more rapidly from the stomachs of crossed intestines rats and enters the crossed intestinal segment more quickly during the first ten minutes of feeding. This physiologically rapid rate of stomach emptying more critically tests the importance of the crossed intestines segment in changing food intake. After ten minutes, the rate of stomach emptying declines as signals from the upper duodenum, lower jejunum and ileum inhibit stomach motility.

The most striking conclusion from the short-term study is that the regulation of meal size does not seem to depend upon the amount of ingested food absorbed. The blood level of labelled glucose is the same in the fed and unfed crossed intestines rats, yet one rat is hungry, as indicated by willingness to eat more than 10 ml of diet if allowed to feed, and the other rat is satiated and does not eat even though it has food freely available. In addition, the unfed crossed intestines rat eats just as much as the unfed parabiotic rat even though its blood level of absorbed free glucose and amino acids is high and the blood level of the unfed parabiotic rat is very low. If one further assumption is made, that the absorbed glucose provokes the release of insulin, the results of these experiments provide evidence counter to the glucostatic theory (Mayer, 1955).

It is critically important to know the approximate amount of food absorbed into each crossed intestines rat to interpret the feeding data. If very little ingested food is lost to the intestine of the partner rat, then the failure to find changes in food intake is not very interesting. The radioactive absorption studies show that about equal amounts of free glucose and amino acids are absorbed into each of these rats, but the measurements of absorbed radioactive glucose and amino acids give only a rough estimate of the amount of food absorbed into each rat. These radioactive nutrients were added to the rat's normal liquid diet, Nutrament, which contained complex carbohydrates, proteins and fats. Complex nutrients require further digestion by secreted enzymes and might be absorbed further down in the digestive tract. An accurate estimate of the amount of food absorbed into each crossed intestines rat would seem to require uniform labelling of the entire liquid diet and whole body radiography at the end of the absorptive period. Fortunately, a probable estimate can be made from well-established observations of gastrointestinal physiologists. It has long been known that between 80 and 90 per cent of the ingested food is absorbed in the first half of the digestive tracts of several different species (Davenport, 1971). The crossed segment of the intestines comprises 30 cm of the 55 cm length of the first half of the small intestine of the rat or, approximately, 55 per cent. If we accept the conservative estimate of 80 per cent of the food absorbed in the first half of the small intestine and, again, conservatively ignore the fact that the crossed segment is in the upper half of the first half, we estimate that 44 per cent of the ingested food is absorbed through the crossed segment, a remarkably close correspondence to the observed proportion of free glucose and amino acids absorbed through the crossed segment. On the other hand, if we completely ignore the results of the gastrointestinal physiologists and assume that every portion of the small intestine absorbs food equally, then an estimated 27 per cent of the ingested food would still be lost through the crossed intestinal segment.

The results of the crossed intestines experiment show that absorbed food and the related metabolic changes in the crossed segment do not control the size of a single meal. Rats eat the same size meals whether these signals are present or not. Several other possible satiety signals can be ruled out by this experiment. Any neural or hormonal signal arising in the crossed intestinal segment also does not produce satiety. Iggo (1957) has recorded from the intestinal nerves of the crossed segment in the normal cat and found individual neurons that responded to stretching of the intestine by saline infusion. The most sensitive neurons responded to a pressure increase of as little as 2 mm of mercury. Sharma & Nasset (1962) have recorded from similar nerves and found units that changed their firing rate after perfusion of the intestine with dilute sugar solutions and other units that responded to perfusion with amino acid solutions. Finally, Youmans (1968) has reviewed the substantial literature showing that nerves in this region of the small intestine are involved in regulating gastrointestinal motility. None of these neural signals could be critically important in producing satiety. Fed crossed intestines rats that lack these neural messages are fully satiated and unfed rats that could process these neural signals remain hungry.

The crossed intestinal segment contains several hormones that could serve as satiety signals and the results of the crossed intestines experiment can be used to evaluate the importance of these hormones in producing satiety. The role of cholecystokinin (CCK) as a satiety signal has recently been in dispute. Glick & co-workers (1971) found that intravenous injections of physiological doses of CCK did not inhibit feeding behavior in rats. Koopmans, Deutsch & Branson (1972) showed that i.p. injected CCK could reduce food intake in mice, but any dose that reduced food intake also reduced water intake. They believed that CCK had non-specific effects on feeding behavior. However, Gibbs & co-workers (1973) showed that high doses of CCK could inhibit feeding behavior in rats and they did not find a reduction of water intake or a conditioned aversion to the injection of the same dose of CCK. More recently, Kraly (1977) has used a more sensitive behavioral test and discovered that the doses of CCK that inhibit food intake also produce a mild conditioned aversion. He does not conclude that CCK fails to produce satiety through physiological means, but considers the results ambiguous.

The crossed intestines preparation allows us to determine whether the physiological release of CCK provoked by the presence of food in the gut can inhibit feeding behavior. Bloom (1974) has measured the amount of cholecystokinin present in different regions of the rat's gastrointestinal tract by reacting a crude extract from each region with an antibody for CCK. Although the technique has limitations, he found that about half of the CCK was located in the crossed segment of the crossed intestines preparation. Koopmans & Heird (1977) did a study in which they measured the total enzyme flow from the pancreas of each rat of a crossed intestines pair under the same conditions as the feeding and glucose absorption studies. They found that enzyme flow was much higher in the unfed and hungry rat than in its fed partner. If pancreatic flow is largely controlled by the level of cholecystokinin in the blood, as is widely believed (Grossman, 1977), then cholecystokinin was present in higher concentration in the blood of a rat that remained hungry than in its satiated partner. In this light, cholecystokinin does not seem to be an effective satiety agent. Two other hormones, gastric inhibitory polypeptide and motilin, are present in higher concentrations in the crossed intestines segment than in other regions of the gut (Bloom, 1975). By comparison with the results on cholecystokinin, these hormones should also not be capable of producing normal satiety.

The results of the crossed intestines experiment also have implications for the role of the liver in the control of food intake. Russek (1971) has argued that the presence of glucose in the portal vein causes glucoreceptors in the liver (Niijima, 1969) to decrease their firing rate and produces satiety. He found that intraportal injection of glucose was much more effective than intravenous injection in reducing food intake. Novin & co-workers (1974) found that intraportal injections of glucose were effective in inhibiting food intake in a 24-hour deprived rabbit, but not in a free-feeding rabbit. Recently, he has discovered that some infusions of glucose into the portal vein enhance feeding (Novin, this volume). In the crossed intestines rats, digested carbohydrate and protein absorbed through the crossed intestinal segment enters the portal vein and goes directly to the liver. The absorption studies have shown that about equal amounts of free glucose and amino acids enter the bloodstream of the two crossed intestines rats. Since these nutrients enter the general circulation through the liver, glucose and amino acids have made contact with hepatocytes and have probably entered the cells and decreased the firing rate of the hepatic glucoreceptors (Niijima, 1969). Despite the absorption of large amounts of nutrient into both rats and changes in hepatic metabolism, one rat remains hungry and the other rat is satiated. The apparent contradiction between these results and those of Russek (1971) and Novin *et al.* (1974) where glucose injections into the portal vein inhibited food intake, may possibly be caused by a non-physiological consequence of direct injection of nutrients into the portal vein. Control injections of substances such as hypertonic sodium chloride or urea do not provide exact controls for glucose injection because sodium chloride, urea and glucose have different cell membrane permeabilities. In addition, the absorption of glucose through the crossed intestines causes the release of hormones and probably stimulates neural reflex circuits that may help the liver process the blood nutrients. The combination of absorbed nutrients and concurrent physiological signals does not inhibit food intake in the unfed crossed intestines rat.

The importance of the liver in controlling feeding behavior is also called into question by several studies using portacaval shunts (Assal *et al.*, 1971; Herz *et al.*, 1972). These experimenters have shown that portacaval shunt in the rat produces a small reduction in food intake and a 5 to 10 per cent loss of body weight. In the shunt preparation, absorbed food bypasses the liver and enters directly into the general circulation. Much of the absorbed food will pass from the gastrointestinal tract to the body's tissues without ever passing through the liver which receives blood only from the hepatic artery. If the liver were involved in assessing the total amount of absorbed food and inhibiting feeding behavior to compensate, then animals with portacaval shunts would have a liver that has less absorbed nutrient passing through it and the animal ought to overeat. The exact opposite result is reported in the literature: animals show a small reduction of food intake. To investigate whether the reduction might be due to the toxicity of absorbed substances not cleared by the liver, we did an unpublished study of feeding behavior on a highly refined food, Nutrament, in cages that prevented coprophagia. We found a minimal 4 per cent decrease in body weight resulting from a recovery from surgery that was prolonged by two days. At no time did we see a significant increase in meal size or in total food intake. The diminished hepatic satiety signals did not increase feeding behavior in a portacaval shunt study specifically designed to observe food intake changes.

Both the crossed intestines studies and the portacaval shunt studies suggest that the liver can not be an important site for the regulation of feeding behavior under normal conditions. Unfed crossed intestines rats that are receiving strong hepatic signals do not diminish food intake and portacaval shunted rats that have fewer hepatic signals do not increase feeding behavior. The liver probably has some role in controlling food intake under unusual conditions such as the intraportal injection of 2-DG (Novin, VanderWeele & Rezek, 1973) or systemic injection of insulin (Stricker *et al.*, 1977).

The rather sweeping negative conclusions of the crossed intestines experiment raise the legitimate question of the validity of the results. In a previous study (Koopmans, 1975), I crossed a somewhat shorter and more distal 25 cm segment of the intestine and found essentially the same behavioral results with 30 and 60 minute delays. A second experiment in which a large (14 ml) injection was made into the stomach just minutes before the crossed intestines partner was fed also had no effect on feeding behavior. Moreover, the behavioral studies reported here are internally consistent. Both the short-term feeding study and the five day deprivation study show that rats ignore signals arising in the crossed intestinal segment. If the rats do not adjust to loss of nutrients from the intestines in five days, then surely they will not adjust in a single meal.

The negative conclusions of the crossed intestines experiment fail to establish that there is no role in the control of food intake for any of the signals present in the unfed crossed intestines rat. Any of these signals could act in conjunction with signals that are present in the fed and fully satiated crossed intestines partner. The experiments do establish that none of these signals produce satiety by themselves or in conjunction with other signals from the crossed segment.

The results of the crossed intestines experiment allow only a few, rather general positive conclusions. The signals that inhibit feeding behavior in crossed intestines rats must arise in the mouth, throat, stomach, upper duodenum, lower jejunum or ileum. These signals apparently do not arise in the crossed segment comprising lower duodenum and upper jejunum. The signals could be either neural or hormonal, but are not produced by nutrients absorbed into the blood. The signals that terminate feeding behavior are unlikely to arise in the mouth and throat. Studies with esophageal fistulae on dogs (Hull *et al.,* 1951; Janowitz & Grossman, 1949) and with gastric fistulae with rats (Smith, Gibbs & Young, 1974) show that oropharyngeal signals by themselves are relatively unimportant in the control of food intake and that other signals further down in the digestive tract must play some role in inhibiting feeding behavior. These other signals from the stomach, upper duodenum and lower small intestine may inhibit feeding behavior alone or may interact with oropharyngeal cues to terminate feeding.

Another possible explanation for the results of the current experiment is that in the two to three weeks of recovery from the intestinal surgery, the crossed intestines rats learned the nature of the satiety signals that they could expect after a meal and adjusted by paying attention only to those self-generated signals. They learned to ignore signals produced in the crossed intestinal segment. This interpretation is possible, but it implies that the rats can make distinctions about the origin of gastrointestinal signals and that they choose to pay attention to those internal signals that were not directly connected to the amount of absorbed food. They attended to cues arising in the stomach, upper duodenum and lower small intestine where only a portion of the ingested food was absorbed.

The results of the five day deprivation study show that learning is an unlikely explanation of the internal control of feeding behavior. During the five days when one rat was completely deprived of food, the other rat did not learn that it was losing a substantial portion of its ingested food into its partner. During these five days, the rat could have become aware of the different types of internal cues because they were more consistently and clearly defined, but it failed to significantly increase food intake.

In theory, learning must be based upon some fundamental unconditioned stimulus as a reference point to guide changes in behavior and if the rat can chose any internal cue to pay attention to, it is difficult to imagine what the unconditioned stimulus is. The crossed intestines preparation shows that the unconditioned stimulus is not the amount of food absorbed, the expected unconditioned stimulus for controlling food intake. The unconditioned stimulus must be one of the other physiological stimuli arising in the gut and if it is, then, by definition, it is not one of the stimuli that the rat can choose to pay attention to. A more likely explanation of the crossed intestines results is that the rat is unaware of its nutritional state, but further experiments have to be done to clarify these issues.

The possibility that either learning or habit explains the results of the crossed intestines preparation could modify some of the positive conclusions. The feeding behavior of the rat might not depend upon the signals arising in the stomach or lower intestine but would depend on learned experience. The negative conclusions of the experiment remain unchanged. All signals from the crossed intestinal segment including absorbed food do not affect food intake regardless of whether food intake is controlled by other physiological signals or by learned responses and habitual behavior.

The five day deprivation experiment produces the most striking results. While it is plausible to believe that the physiological signals that control feeding behavior act without reference to the amount of nutrient absorbed into the bloodstream during a single meal, it is much more difficult to accept that the rats do not show a significant increase in food intake during the 40 or 50 meals that would normally be eaten throughout the five day deprivation period. Since the rats show a small but non-significant increase and the results are so unusual, it is reasonable to wonder whether a substantial amount of food has been lost from the crossed segment. The amount of ingested food lost from one crossed intestines rat to its partner can not be determined from body weight loss because in these experiments we weigh the pair and not the individual rat. The individual weights but not the weight loss could be determined at sacrifice. In the present experiments, we choose to measure post-deprivation food intake rather than sacrifice weight. As a result, the argument about lost ingested food must be more indirect. The absorption data for free glucose and amino acids show that about half of these nutrients are absorbed into each of the crossed intestines rats. These measurements may not reflect the total amount of food lost since the diet that the rats ate contained carbohydrates, proteins and fats that were more complex than the free glucose and amino acids. As argued above, these complex nutrients require digestion and might be absorbed in different regions of the gut. To gain perspective on the labelled glucose and amino acid absorption study, let us make the minimal assumption that each section of the small intestine is equally important in absorbing food. Then, as argued above, 27 per cent of the food ingested by one rat will be absorbed into its partner. If the feeding rat were to compensate for the food lost during deprivation of its partner than it should eat 77.4 ml per day, which is 12.7 ml more than its observed average intake of 64.7 ml. The small observed increase in food intake during the five day deprivation period was not significant, but if 12.7 ml were added to each rat's intake per day and the observed variability was retained, the hypothetical increase would be highly significant ($F=8.57$, $P<0.01$). In short, the rats do not seem to be compensating for lost nutrients even when the amount lost is calculated on the basis of small intestinal length alone.

If we accept the estimate of gastrointestinal physiologists that 80 to 90 per cent of ingested food is absorbed by the first half of the small intestine (Davenport, 1971) then, as argued above, 44 per cent of this food should be lost through the crossed intestinal segment. In order to compensate, the fed rat should increase its food intake to an average of 85.6 ml per day, This estimated quantity of food intake approaches the 88.5 ml average daily food intake of these same rats during the diet dilution period. The rats can process this volume of food at least in the upper regions of the digestive tract before water is removed by intestinal absorption.

There is little reason to reject either of the estimates made above. The crossed intestinal segment looks normal to gross inspection at sacrifice and the crossed intestines rats can live for more than a year in a healthy state. If even the minimal estimate is accepted, then a substantial amount of food has been lost to the crossed intestines partner and signals from the crossed intestinal segment do not significantly alter food intake over a five day period.

The long-term behavioral study shows that rats can adjust almost immediately to a dilution of their diet that occurs at the level of the mouth. They compensate for the diminished number of calories per unit volume by nearly doubling their food intake. However, if they lose a substantial amount of their ingested food at mid-duodenum, they do not make significant adjustments in food intake within five days and show no tendency to increase their intake during these five days. Clearly, physiological signals from mouth, throat, stomach, upper duodenum, lower jejunum and ileum can respond appropriately to dilution of the diet, but not to duodenal loss of ingested food.

During the five day deprivation period, the crossed intestines pairs lost 4 per cent of their body weight, and their combined decrease in food intake was 47.8 ml per day. These lost calories would have been largely replaced by mobilized free fatty acids. The shift to a lipolytic state or the loss of triglyceride stores in adipose tissue does not lead to a significant increase in food intake during the five day deprivation period.

In conclusion, the many signals arising in the crossed intestinal segment after the ingestion of food do not as a group affect food intake. The most important result is that the absorbed food and several metabolic changes that follow the absorption of food do not alter feeding behavior. Instead, physiological signals from the stomach, upper duodenum and lower small intestine control food intake. These signals predominate not only during a single meal but over a period of five days.

Summary

The importance of the intestine in controlling food intake was investigated with a surgical preparation that allows the delivery of normal food mixed with digestive enzymes into the upper duodenum at a near physiological rate. Parabiotic pairs of rats had a 30 cm segment of the lower duodenum and upper jejunum exchanged with the same segment of their partner's intestine. When food was eaten by either rat of this crossed intestines pair, it arrived in the stomach of the feeding rat, travelled through 5 cm of its upper duodenum and crossed into the intestine of its partner. After passing through 30 cm of the partner's intestine, the undigested food returned to the lower jejunum of the rat that fed. The importance of the crossed intestinal segment in reducing food intake was investigated by feeding one rat first so that it lacked signals from the crossed intestines and feeding the second rat 30 or 60 minutes later after it had experienced the intestinal signals during the delay. There was no change in the feeding behavior of either rat when compared to control parabiotic rats. Apparently, signals arising in the crossed intestines do not alter food intake during a single meal. The many signals that do not change food intake in this physiological preparation include neural and hormonal signals from the crossed intestinal segment, absorbed food and signals from the liver and adipose tissue that indicate a change in metabolism. The importance of the intestine and of absorbed food in altering food intake was further explored by depriving one rat of each crossed intestines pair of food for five days. Despite the loss of a considerable portion of the ingested food to its partner, the feeding rat did not significantly increase its food intake. The food intake of these rats appears to be controlled by signals arising in the stomach, upper duodenum and lower small intestine.

Acknowledgements – This research was supported by Career Development Award AM 00198 and NIH Research Grant AM 17926.

References

Assal, J.P., Levrat, R., Cahn, T. & Renold, A.E. (1971): *Z. Ges. Exp. Med.* **154**, 87.

Bloom, S.R. (1974): *Br. Med. Bull.* **30**, 62.

Bloom, S.R. (1975): In *Proc. 5th Internat. Symp. on Gastrointestinal Motility,* ed M.D. Vantrappen & H.O. Agg. Belgium: Typoff Press.

Campbell, C.S. & Davis J.D. (1974): *Physiol. Behav.* **12**, 377.

Davenport, H.W. (1971): *Physiology of the digestive tract,* p.183. Chicago: Yearbook Medical Publ.

Ethman, G.K., Albert, D.J. & Jamieson, J.L. (1971): *Canad. J. Psych.* **25**, 147.

Gibbs, J., Young, R.C. & Smith, G.P. (1973): *J. Comp. Physiol. Psych.* **84**, 488.

Glick, A., Thomas, D.W. & Mayer, J. (1971): *Physiol. Behav.* **6**, 5.

Grossman, M.I. (1977): *Fed. Proc.* **36**, 1930.

Herz, R., Sautter, V., Robert, F. & Bircher, J. (1972): *Europ. J. Clin. Inv.* **2**, 390.

Houpt, K.A. (1977): Sixth International Conference on the Physiology of Food and Fluid Intake, Paris.

Hull, C.L., Livingston, J.R., Rouse, R.O. & Barker, A.N. (1951): *J. Comp. Physiol. Psych.* **44**, 236.

Iggo, A. (1957): *Q. Jl Exp. Physiol.* **42**, 130.

Janowitz, H.D. & Grossman, M.I. (1949): *Am. J. Physiol.* **159**, 143.

Koopmans, H.S. (1975): *Behav. Biol.* **14**, 309.

Koopmans, H.S., Deutsch, J.A. & Branson, P.J. (1972): *Behav. Biol.* **7**, 441.

Koopmans, H.S. & Heird, W.C. (1977): Sixth International Conference on the Physiology of Food and Fluid Intake, Paris.

Kraly, F.S. (1977): Sixth International Conference on the Physiology of Food and Fluid Intake, Paris.

Mayer, J. (1955): *Ann. N.Y. Acad. Sci.* **63**, 15.

Niijima, A. (1969): *Ann. N.Y. Acad. Sci.* **157**, 690.

Novin, D., Sanderson, J.D. & VanderWeele, D.A. (1974): *Physiol. Behav.* **13**, 3.

Novin, D., VanderWeele, D. & Rezek, M. (1973): *Science*, **181**, 858.

Russek, M. (1971): In *Neurosciences Research,* eds S. Ehrenpreis & O.C. Solnitzky, New York: Academic Press.

Sharma, K.N. & Nasset, E.S. (1962): *Am. J. Physiol.* **202**, 725.

Smith, G.P., Gibbs, J. & Young, R.C. (1974): *Fed. Proc.* **33**, 1146.

Snowdon, C.T. (1975): *J. Comp. Physiol. Psych.* **88**, 231.

Stephans, D.B. & Baldwin, B.A. (1974): *Physiol. Behav.* **12**, 923.

Stricker, E.M., Rowland, N., Saller, C.F., & Friedman, M.I. (1977): *Science* **196**, 79.

Yin, T.H. & Tsai, C.T. (1973): *J. Comp. Physiol. Psych.* **85**, 258.

Youmans, W.B. (1968): In *Handbook of physiology,* Vol. 4, ed C.F. Code, p. 1655, section 6. Washington DC: American Physiological Society.

6
Metabolically driven and learned feeding responses in man

J. LE MAGNEN
Laboratoire de Neurophysiologie Sensorielle et Comportementale, C.N.R.S., Collège de France, 11, place Marcelin Berthelot, 75231 - Paris Cedex 05, France.

Regulatory behaviours are motor patterns from the central nervous system, by which an animal 'anticipates', by reaction to, or actions upon, its environment, the later consequences of these reactions and actions on its life. The permanent recording of past experience, through learning and memory modulates all regulatory and anticipatory behaviours by negative and positive feedback mechanisms. Learning is a basic property of the nervous system and thereby of a living animal system. Throughout the individual's life, positively reinforced responses are selected and maintained, whereas negatively reinforced or non-reinforced responses are eliminated. This selection through learning of the response which is most likely to be effective is not merely the result of each individual's own experience. The selection is also a continuation of the process of natural selection. Evolution of species is produced through the survival value of regulatory behaviours which are most successful. Ineffective regulatory behaviours are eliminated. Thus, learning of regulatory behavioural responses occurs over a background of phylogenetically preadjusted reactions with its corresponding neuronal organization. Man is man because he has added to this genetic transmission of experiences a recording of past experience through language and education.

Food habits and feeding behaviour in man will thus be the result of three different processes of learning: (1) the phylogenetically inherited responses, (2) the automatically reinforced or non-reinforced responses and, (3) the knowledge and beliefs of sociocultural origin. From the interplay of these three, there results either the regulatory nature of human feeding behaviour or its non-regulatory achievement leading to nutritional diseases such as obesity.

Basic mechanisms of feeding behaviour

Sensory and neuroendocrine systems which drive feeding behaviour are the behavioural aspect of the overall process of regulation of body energy balance and the requirements for specific nutrients. Although body energy losses and the corresponding utilization of metabolites fluctuate widely over time, they are nevertheless continuous. Since both body weight and body composition are maintained, these losses must be matched by eating. However, caloric input is essentially discontinuous in nature. Man, together with every other animal, does not eat continuously. He exhibits a 'feeding pattern' made of eating episodes, or 'meals' of various sizes, separated by periods of no-feeding. Since it is difficult to eat and to sleep simultaneously, man eats almost exclusively during the active part of the day. With various materials available as foods, man and animals are either stimulated, or not, to eat these foods and to eat various amounts of each of them until the termination of the meal.

A hunger-satiety system appears to be involved in the temporal pattern for the onset of successive meals. Much evidence has been provided showing that the onset of eating results from a combination of internal and external signals. A fall below a given value for glucose

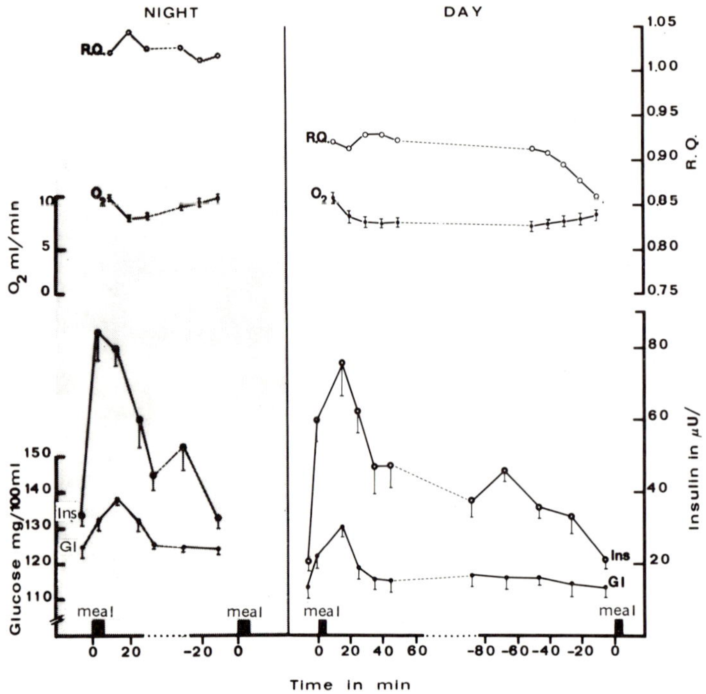

Fig. 1. Metabolic events from meal to meal in rats fed *ad lib.* at night compared to daytime. In the day, contrary to the night, meals start at a low level of the respiratory quotient and at a lower blood glucose and IRI levels. At night as well as in the daytime, meals start after an increase of oxygen consumption

oxidation, and presumably for glucose uptake, may give rise to 'hunger arousal' (Fig. 1). This state, in turn, gives rise to seeking, which is followed by food-taking, chewing and swallowing. The duration of the post-meal period of no-feeding before the onset of a new meal, is dependent on the meal-to-meal balance between the amount of food eaten in the meal and the rate of metabolic food utilization during the post-prandial period. We, and others, have shown that in rats, there is a positive nocturnal correlation between the amount of energy taken in a meal and the time elapsed until the onset of a new meal (Ardisson *et al.*, 1974; Balagura & Coscina, 1968; De Castro, 1975; Duncan, 1960; Le Magnen & Tallon, 1963; Le Magnen & Tallon, 1966; Natelson, 1977 unpublished; Sanderson & VanderWeele, 1975; Snowdon, 1969; Thomas & Mayer, 1968). In addition to a short-term glucoregulatory mechanism involved in this meal-to-meal balance, there are long-term liporegulatory mechanisms (Le Magnen & Devos, 1970; Le Magnen *et al.*, 1973). In rats, a part of the food utilized for fat synthesis accounts both for a shortening of the duration of satiety after each meal and for the general increase of meal frequency. In the daytime and eventually from day-to-day, the utilization of mobilized fats as an endogenous source of calories acts to delay the onset of eating. A defect in this lipo-regulatory mechanism and its effect on the feeding pattern increasingly appears to be responsible for the disruption of the body energy balance, which leads to leanness or obesity (Fig. 2).

Meal-to-meal regulation is operative only during *ad lib.* feeding. It is upset in man, who is constrained by social habits to a feeding schedule of three regularly spaced meals. We shall see below how learning by conditioned hunger and satiety partially compensates for this limitation of the regulatory mechanism.

A distinct mechanism obviously determines meal size and the nature and amount of foods

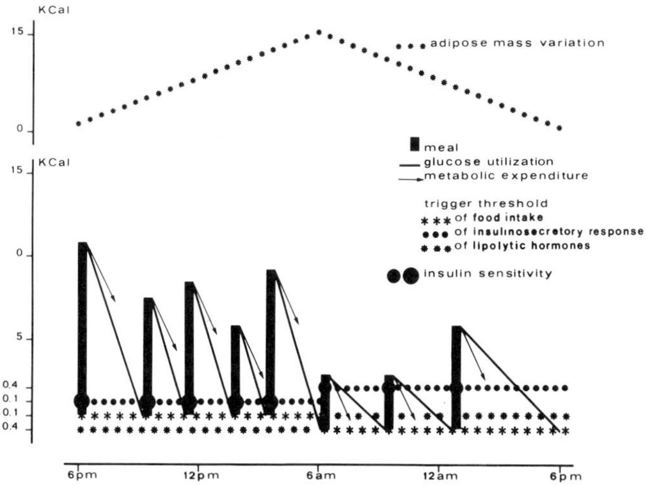

Fig. 2. In ordinate: glucose availability postulated to be, by its action on specific brain or peripheral targets, a signal both of feeding and lipogenic or lipolytic hormone secretions. In abscissae: time from the beginning of dark until the end of light periods. At night, the start of each meal is stimulated at a threshold of lowered glucose availability higher than the threshold of lipolysis. A low threshold of insulinosecretory responsiveness brings about from meal to meal a sharing of the utilization of ingested foods between glucose utilization for cell oxidations and fat synthesis. This results in accelerating the meal frequency (high onset ratios) and in a cumulated increase of body fats (top). In daytime, as an effect of the liporegulatory mechanism, lipolysis occurs at a lower, and the start of meals at a higher, threshold of glucose uptake of target tissues while the insulinosecretory responsiveness and the insulin sensitivity (Randle's effect) are reduced. This results in a fat mobilization which accounts for the prolongation of meal-to-meal intervals. Thus, feeding would be the behavioural component of an overall short-term glucoregulatory and long-term liporegulatory mechanism of body energy balance

eaten. Following the initial stimulation to eat in response to hunger or other cues, what factors lead to the termination of eating? It is, of course, the act of having eaten by mouth, and having swallowed, a given amount of food. Thus, the question may be reformulated as follows: what action or combination of actions of the food along the alimentary canal during the meal acts to satiate the initial stimulation to eat? Despite a tremendous amount of experimental investigation, the answer to this question is not clear. However, much experimental evidence indicates that the sensory effect of food in the mouth, and perhaps its effect on neural afferents from the stomach and intestine, acts as a conditioned stimulus to eat and to terminate eating. This could account for the anticipatory nature of the learned eating response to a particular food. It has also been clearly demonstrated that post-ingestional metabolic repletion acts not only as a direct factor in the immediate satiation but also as an unconditioned stimulus or reinforcer of the conditioned components of this response. The so-called 'palatability' of a food, its ability to stimulate an eating response as an oral-sensory cue and to contribute to satiation, is a learned response. On a background of inherited preferences and aversions such as the preference for sweet and aversion for bitter substances, the learning of palatability makes the anticipatory response to various foods possible in as much as these responses are positively or negatively reinforced by the post-ingestional metabolic effects of the food. The demonstration that oral effects of food are involved in determining the meal-size in rats was provided in the 1950s. The basic experiments may be recalled here. The intake of the same diet with two different flavoured forms, one of which is associated with post-prandial administration of a glucose solution (or insulin) which makes it more metabolically satiating, leads to a lower intake of the diet labelled with the flavour associated with administration of glucose (Le Magnen, 1955; 1957; 1969). The same conditioning is manifested when rats are alternatively offered a calorically dense and a diluted diet (Booth, 1972). 'Conditioned taste aversion', already known 40 years ago, is a particular case of the condiitioned response to palatability. Several characteristics of physiological learning (Le Magnen, 1952) have been studied in greater detail (Rozin & Kalat, 1971). It is learned very rapidly (one trial) and is 'long delay' learning. Post-ingestional reinforcement with a poison, for example, may act to induce taste aversion ten hours or more after the oral intake (Nachman & Jones, 1974). During normal feeding, not only the immediate effect of ingested food, but delayed post-absorptive effects as well, may act as an unconditioned stimulus for the palatability of food.

In the regulation of the eating pattern and meal size, both metabolic depletion and repletion act either directly or indirectly as reinforcers of learned responses. Depending on the feeding schedule, the part due for metabolically driven and learned responses will be different. Because man is man, his feeding condition is a very particular case where learning is predominant.

Conditioned hunger and the hunger arousal of palatability

Balagura, Harrell & Roy (1975) and Woods & co-workers (1977) have demonstrated that rats placed on one or two meals per day offered at the same hour, learned to be hungry at the time of feeding. The time and/or the flavour repeatedly associated with the subsequent presentation of food rapidly becomes a conditioned stimulus for a neuroendocrine state, of a low blood glucose level, and insulin release which reproduces the blood pattern giving rise to arousal of hunger. This release of insulin conditioned by the usual meal-time or by external stimulation from foods has not been demonstrated in man. But it is likely that such a conditioned hunger plays a major role in stimulation of eating at the time of the meal. In addition to metabolic depletion, external stimuli associated with the regular meal such as the room, the table setting and the ambient food odours, obviously stimulate a conditioned hunger and 'appetite'.

This conditioned insulin release and the induced increase in hunger prior to a regular meal

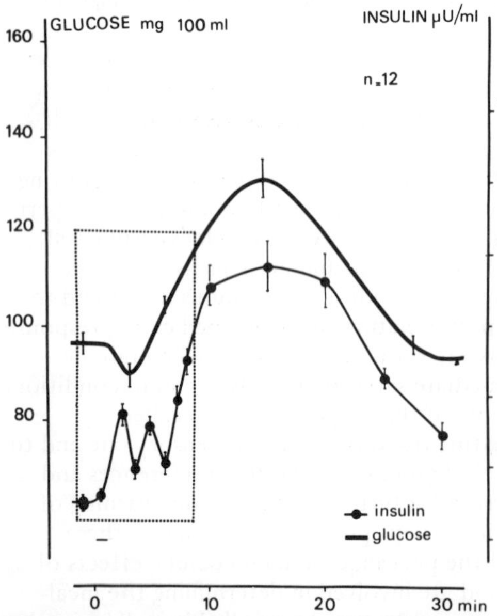

Fig. 3. Pre and post-absorptive plasma IRI and BG levels obtained in normal rats after a free oral intake of 1 ml of a 50 per cent glucose solution. Values are means ± s.e.m. Horizontal bar represents the minute of intake

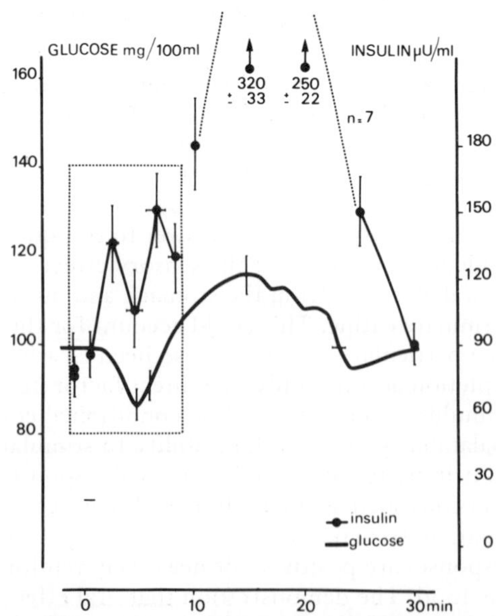

Fig. 4. Pre and post-absorptive plasma IRI and BG levels obtained in hyperphagic rats after a free oral intake of 1 ml of a 50 per cent glucose solution. Values are means ± s.e.m. Horizontal bar represents the minute of intake

are not different from a recently studied and very important component of the neuroendocrine basis for feeding (Louis-Sylvestre, 1976; Louis-Sylvestre, unpublished).

Rats offered a drink of a glucose solution exhibit, within the first minute of oral intake, an increase of the plasma insulin concentration immediately followed by a transient fall of the blood glucose level (Fig. 3). A second peak of insulin occurs some minutes later, preceding the sustained rise of both blood glucose level and insulin concentration resulting from the absorption of ingested glucose. The oral intake of a saccharine solution only induces the two initial peaks of insulin release. Either glucose or saccharine solutions elicit only the second peak, when given directly into the stomach. In vagotomized rats the initial peak is eliminated. It is considerably exaggerated in hyperphagic rats with ventromedial hypothalamic lesions (Fig. 4). Thus a palatable food reflexly induces a vagally mediated release of insulin at the beginning of the meal. The release of insulin will increase the metabolic conditions of hunger, and in turn the hunger-dependent palatability of the food at the beginning of the meal. Thus, a sensory-endocrine type of feedback amplifies the palatability of the food. The well known hyper-reactivity of hyperphagic hypothalamic rats to the sensory aspect of their foods, ie finickiness, could be the result of the observed exaggeration in such rats of the oro-pancreatic loop and, through this mechanism, the direct cause of hyperphagia. This orally elicited insulin release is a 'conditioned' response. In rats repeatedly offered a non-nutritive saccharine solution, the insulin-secretory response rapidly undergoes extinction (Deutsch, 1974). Thus it was suggested that the post-ingestive repleting effects of a food acts as an unconditioned stimulus for the conditioned secretion of insulin in response to taste. This suggestion was supported by the results of another experiment (Le Magnen, 1975; Le Magnen *et al.*, unpublished). By repeated association of an i.v. glucose load (0.5 g/kg) with the odour of amylacetate, this substance becomes a conditioned stimulus for the rise of plasma insulin concentration and a consequent fall of blood glucose level. When amylacetate is added as a flavour to the familiar food it transitorily enhances the palatability of this food (Fig. 5). It is likely that the unconditioned stimulus, or reinforcer, represented by the post-ingestional repletion of food, conditions both the level of activity of the food as an oral stimulant to feeding and its amplification by the release of insulin. Through this suggested mechanism, highly palatable foods would be a direct cause of hyperinsulinemia, which would further enhance the palatability and the amount eaten. The overstimulation of this positive feedback may be a cause of the hyperphagia and obesity as seems to be the case after the VMH lesion in rats. Various experimental results are explained by and support this hypothesis (Powley, 1977). It has been shown that the succes-

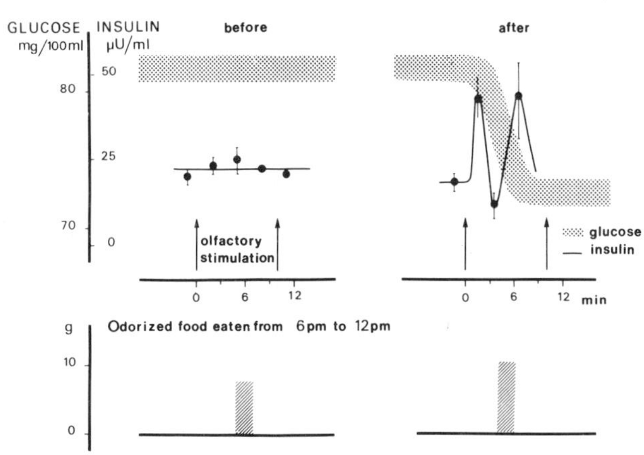

Fig. 5. Effect of the olfactory stimulation by amylacetate on the blood glucose and plasma IRI levels and effect of amylacetate added as flavour of the familiar food upon food intake. On the left: control. On the right: after a conditioning of amylacetate as a conditioned stimulus of insulin release by repeated association with i.v. glucose load as unconditioned stimulus

sive or simultaneous presentation of differently flavoured forms of a diet induces a considerable increase in the size of the meal (Le Magnen, 1959; 1960). In addition to a flavour-specific satiation, the cumulated insulin release stimulated by each successive flavour may explain the retardation of the onset of satiety. It has recently been shown by various investigators (Panksepp, 1974; Rowe & Rolls, 1977 unpublished; Sclafani, 1972) that rats offered simultaneous access to highly palatable foods (supermarket foods) were hyperphagic and rapidly became obese. The obesity related to a highly palatable diet may be associated with overstimulation of insulin secretion.

This so-called supermarket obesity in rats represents the best and most plausible model of human obesity. The reflexly-induced insulin release elicited by the sight, taste and smell of palatable foods has recently been shown to be present in man (Rodin, 1977 unpublished). In human meals, the succession of various courses and the refined variety of flavours represent the optimal condition for a high degree of prandial insulin secretion. In addition, psychological and sociocultural factors which lead to the acquisition of highly palatable foods will give rise to the vicious circle of hyperinsulinemia, and to both primary and secondary chronic hyperphagia.

Primary and secondary or acute and chronic feeding

On the basis of experimental investigations regarding 'food associated drinking', Fitzsimons & Le Magnen (1969) distinguished between primary and secondary modes of drinking. During acute water deprivation, the onset and termination of the drinking is primarily driven by metabolic stimuli and their suppression. In the steady and chronic state, a conditioned thirst and its conditioned relief associated with feeding anticipate the later requirements of body water balance. Likewise primary and secondary feeding are observed. They are distinguishable by the respective role of metabolically driven and learned responses in determining the quantity and quality of foods eaten. In the acute condition produced either by food deprivation, or by a sudden change in the metabolic rate (exercise, cold exposure), or by the change of food, a primary feeding is observed in which the metabolic pattern of hunger and its post-feeding suppression directly governs the sizes and patterns of meals. In rats, the size of a meal during *ad lib.* feeding was not correlated with the inter-meal interval, but became so after a fast (Le Magnen, 1977 unpublished). Similarly, the size of the first meal after administration of insulin exhibited a dose-response relation (Corriol & Le Magnen, unpublished). When eating 'familiar foods', metabolically driven responses are replaced by learned and anticipatory responses. Under chronic conditions, rats were observed to learn to eat in a meal and to be satiated by the amount of food needed to match the metabolic expenses during the time allowed after the meal (Le Magnen, 1957).

The regular time of a meal may condition the start of a meal, whereas the time without food after a meal acts as an unconditioned stimulus for a conditioned satiation by a given food. We have recently re-examined eating patterns after four to eight hours of chronic food deprivation, and compared the results with the same response after acute deprivation. Chronically, the rats tended to increase the size of the meal prior to the regular withdrawal of the food, while they decreased the size of the first meal after food deprivation. The effect decreased with increasing time of food deprivation (Le Magnen & Tallon, unpublished). Some evidence exists that the same process is operative in *ad lib.* fed rats offered their familiar food calorically diluted by the addition of inert material. At first, rats compensated for the loss of calories per volume by shortening the post-meal interval. Then they rapidly compensated by regulating meal size (Le Magnen, 1969). This relearning of the palatability and 'satiation power' of food is analogous to that demonstrated by Booth (1972).

In man, conditioning of satiation is evident in various experiments. Change of the caloric density of the diet taken orally, or the addition of an intragastric feeding to the oral intake, did not acutely elicit a regulatory increase or decrease in oral intake (Jordan, 1969; Spiegel, 1973; Wooley, 1971). Slowly, and only in a part of the subjects studied, did the adjustment occur with a particular liquid diet. Such conditioning by the energy content of a meal has been beautifully demonstrated in man by Booth using the procedure of flavoured diets which had previously applied to rats (Booth, Lee & McAleavey, 1976).

It is likely that man learns to eat in each of his three meals enough food to balance his needs. This long-term balance seems to act as a post-ingestional reinforcer with a long delay in learning. Man would, thus, eat in a meal the amount of food required to suppress hunger and to be satiated over a period of time.

Whether or not the subjective correlation of the palatability of various foods, such as flavour preferences and aversions, is anticipatory in nature is disputed. 'Conditioned taste aversion' was demonstrated for the first time in man by the use of emetic drugs in the detoxication of chronic alcoholics. But these alcoholics had previously acquired a strong preference for alcoholic beverages. Many taste and smell preferences and aversions are in agreement with positive or negative post-ingestional reinforcement. Odours associated with foods are obviously pleasant or unpleasant depending on whether they are used as a food flavour. The flavour of methylsalicylate, which is pleasant and makes palatable the rootbeer for an American, is highly aversive in Europe because it is not used as a flavour and is associated with the ambient odour of pharmacies. The change in food preferences correlated to changes in the metabolic requirements has hardly been investigated. However, such a change has been indicated in a study of 60 ex-prisoners in concentration camps in the Second World War. Interviews with these subjects showed that at the time of their recovery from loss of weight and specific nutritive deficiencies, there occurred striking changes in their previous likes and dislikes for various foods. These changes were of the regulatory type (Berger & Le Magnen, 1960).

Specific reinforcers in human feeding behaviour

This area of interest is encompassed by the fields of psychology, anthropology and sociology. Only those problems and concepts which have emerged from a limited number of studies on human food habits and from common knowledge will be outlined.

Eating behaviour of humans is profoundly affected by food habits which are inherited and learned either from science or from traditions of the sociocultural background. In educated populations humans may learn from the science of nutrition about their metabolic needs and the safety and nutritive properties of various foods. With this knowledge, their feeding behaviour may be in part regulated. However, it is misleading to think that such knowledge and conscious control might be a substitute for physiological regulation. No one, for example, is presently able to indicate and prescribe the daily requirement of protein since the exact value of the daily protein turnover is still in question (Young *et al.,* 1975). From sociocultural patrimony, humans inherit and learn as the traditions and beliefs, the prescriptions and prohibitions to the whole social ritual of feeding. Man learns to eat as he learns to speak. The social pressure of reward or punishment represents positive and negative external reinforcers which by far outweigh the metabolic reinforcers. In the animal kingdom, only man is allowed to die or to be severely ill because some foods are socially prohibited. Some forms of juvenile obesity may be the consequence of maternal overfeeding of their children.

Another bias of the physiological feeding behaviour is specific to humans. The feeling of pleasantness associated with eating a food is the subjective priming of learned regulatory responses. However, in man this 'pleasure' of the sensations is in itself a cause of self-reinforcement. Eating becomes a chemosensory self-stimulation which either partially or entirely escapes the control of metabolic feedback. A pathological form of this hedonic eating leads to compulsive eating analogous to drug addiction, in which a paroxistic search for subjective pleasures is induced in compensation for mental distress. The recently discovered overeating induced in rats by repeated tail-pinching (Antelman, Rowland & Fisher, 1976) is a plausibly good model of such pathological human behaviour which may lead to obesity. In rats, the electrical self-stimulation of the lateral hypothalamus and the learning of a pre-prandial self-administration of insulin (Jouhaneau, 1976) are likewise reminiscent of this aspect of human eating behaviour.

The moderate expression of such chemosensory self-stimulation by eating belongs to the aesthetic. The infinite refinement of high cuisine which aims at obtaining highly palatable foods, is an aesthetic of flavours. It is more and more an important part of the cultural repertoire of each country and universally of human civilization. The nature of man is to develop gratuitous behaviours whose physiological risks are assumed and accepted.

In conclusion, it can be said that, contrary to animals, man does not know how to eat and learns to be overfed or underfed by badly selecting and eating his foods.

Summary

Recording of past experience and its selective action upon behaviour are the basis for the necessary anticipatory nature of regulatory behaviours. From a phylogenetic selection of pre-adjusted responses, learning by selective reinforcements modulates sensory guided responses. In addition, in man, habits result from memory and the across-generation experience transmitted by education.

In feeding behaviours, the respective part of metabolically driven and of anticipatory learned responses in sensory mediated stimulations and inhibitions to eat varies depending on acute or chronic conditions of feeding. In man, as in animals placed on a human feeding schedule, conditioned stimulations to eat and not to eat are prevalent. New experimental evidence indicates that an acquired overpalatability of foods by determining a prandial hypersecretion of insulin may introduce a disruption of post-ingestional regulatory reinforcement. In addition to social habits, the development in man of a chemosensory self-reinforced and self-stimulatory behaviour by eating further acts to prevent the direct and, through learning, the indirect metabolic regulation of feeding.

References

Antelman, S.M., Rowland, N.E. & Fisher, A.E. (1976): *Brain Res.* **102**, 346.
Ardisson, J.L. *et al.* (1974): *Archs Sci. Physiol.* **28**, 67.
Balagura, S. & Coscina, D.V. (1968): *Physiol. Behav.* **3**, 641.
Balagura, S., Harrell, L.E. & Roy, E. (1975): *Physiol. Behav.* **15**, 245.
Berger, P. & Le Magnen, J. (1960): *Ann. Nutr. Alim.* **14**, 101.
Booth, D.A. (1972): *J. Comp. Physiol. Psychol.* **81**, 457.
Booth, D.A., Lee, M. & McAleavey, C. (1976): *Br. J. Psychol.* **90**, 137.
De Castro, J.M. (1975): *Physiol. Behav.* **15**, 13.
Deutsch. R. (1974): *J. Comp. Physiol. Psychol.* **86**, 350.
Duncan, C.J. (1960): *Ann. Appl. Biol.* **48**, 409.
Fitzsimons, T.J. & Le Magnen, J. (1969): *J. Comp. Physiol. Psychol.* **67**, 273.
Jordan, H.A, (1969): *J. Comp. Physiol. Psychol.* **68**, 498.
Jouhaneau, J. (1976): *C.R. Acad. Sci., Paris* **282**, 1685.
Le Magnen, J. (1952): *Le Comportement alimentaire et l'appetit,* 11, Commité nationale de recherche scientifique.
Le Magnen, J. (1955): *C.R. Acad. Sci., Paris* **240**, 2436.
Le Magnen, J. (1957): *Archs Sci. Physiol.* **11**, 263.
Le Magnen, J. (1957): *J. Physiol. , Paris* **49**, 274.
Le Magnen, J. (1959): *J. Physiol., Paris* **51**, 987.
Le Magnen, J. (1960): *Archs Sci. Physiol.* **14**, 411.
Le Magnen, J. & Tallon, S. (1963): *J. Physiol., Paris* **55**, 283.
Le Magnen, J. & Tallon, S. (1966): *J. Physiol., Paris* **58**, 323.
Le Magnen, J. (1969): *Ann. N.Y. Acad. Sci.* **157**, 1126.
Le Magnen, J. & Devos, M. (1970): *Physiol. Behav.* **5**, 805.
Le Magnen, J., Devos, M., Gaudillière, J.P., Louis-Sylvestre, J. & Tallon, S. (1973): *J. Comp. Physiol. Psychol.* **84**, 1.
Le Magnen, J. (1975): In *Olfaction and taste, V,* eds D.A. Denton & J.P. Coghlan, p. 381. London: Academic.
Louis-Sylvestre, J. (1976): *Am. J. Physiol.* **230**, 56.
Nachman, M. & Jones, D.R. (1974): *J. Comp. Physiol. Psychol.* **86**, 949.

Panksepp, J. (1974): *Fed. Proc.* 33, 1150.
Powley, T.L. (1977): *Psychol. Rev.* **84**, 89.
Rozin, P. & Kalat, J.W. (1971): *Psychol. Rev.* 78, 459.
Sanderson, J,D. & VanderWeele, D.A. (1975): *Physiol. Behav.* **15**, 357.
Sclafani, A. (1972): *Physiol. Behav.* **8**, 977.
Snowdon, C.T. (1969): *J. Comp. Physiol. Psychol.* 69, 91.
Spiegel, T.A. (1973): *J. Comp. Physiol.* **84**, 24.
Thomas, D.W. & Mayer, J. (1968): *J. Comp. Physiol. Psychol.* **66**, 642.
Woods, S.C., Vasselli, J.R., Kaestner, E., Szakmary, G.A., Milburn, P. & Vitiello, M.V. (1977): *J. Comp. Physiol. Psychol.* 91, 128.
Wooley, O.W, (1971): *Psychosom. Med.* 33, 436.
Young, V.R., Steffee, W.P., Pencharz, P.B., Winterer, J.C. & Scrimshaw, N.S. (1975): *Nature* 253, 192.

7
First steps towards an integrated quantitative approach to human feeding and obesity with some implications for research into treatment

D.A. BOOTH
Department of Psychology, University of Birmingham, P.O. Box 363, Birmingham B15 2TT, England.

Theory and model

Most therapeutic techniques are explicitly or implicitly based on a theory. From a systems theoretical point of view, the considerations which have apparently been behind many treatments of obesity seem unrealistically limited. It appears to have been assumed that a marked reduction in absorptive surface by surgery, or an acute drug-induced reduction in appetite, or a punishment for eating as behavioural therapy, will in each case by itself reduce the amount of fat in the body without any risk of countervailing adjustment in other parts of the system and without worse consequences for other sub-systems in the whole individual, who is after all a person not just an energy-balancing organism. Even if such problems are acknowledged in principle, often the treatment in question is at best developed empirically, with little attention to validation or even valid statement of the purported theoretical under-pinnings. The main question is taken to be whether it works, not whether it should work. That is of course a fallacy. Unless we have a sound theory with which to design and to interpret clinical tests of a treatment, there will be no rational basis for generalising from a clinical test under particular circumstances to a clinical recommendation or condemnation of usefully wide application.

Energy flow in control of appetite

Our feeding model has been 'sarcischystatic' - or, what is probably better Greek and better biochemistry, 'cytischystatic'. The theory is that appetite and its role in energy balance is ultimately controlled by the net flow of utilised energy (*ischys* - strength, power, ie calories per minute, joules per second or watts) in working tissues (*sarx* - flesh; *cytos* - cell). This energy supply theory (Fig. 1) was originally less aptly dubbed 'energostatic' (Booth, 1972*b*).

On occasions, for example perhaps after a large meal, the energy flow becomes excessively positive and tends to accumulate energy in liver and muscle. When that happens the brain reduces the likelihood of such an excessive inflow in future by aversively conditioning the stimuli which predicted it. Whatever aspects of a situation predict excessive inflow - a particular foodstuff, the time of day, developing bodily sensations, or some combination of these and other stimuli - will in future tend to suppress food intake and the interest in feeding. This suppression is conditioned satiety (Booth, 1977*a*). The aversively accumulating energy generates oversatiation. The rise in absorption of glucose as the starch in a meal begins to be digested is probably a major normal satiety cue (Booth & Jarman, 1976; Booth, Toates & Platt, 1976).

Typically towards the end of absorption, energy flow becomes excessively negative.

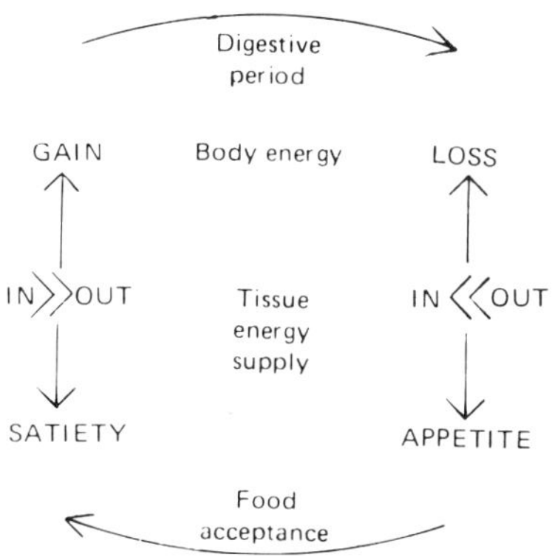

Fig. 1. The energy flow cycle. Changes in state of energy supply to working tissues as time passes during and between meals with food freely available

Energy begins to be lost by liver and muscle, ie non-storage energy begins to be utilised, as well as fat and glycogen stores metabolised. This occurs late in the phase of absorption between meals taken at a normal frequency. That is, energy flow deficiency is occurring as we become hungry in the normal way. Stimuli which predict the removal of this outflow become appetitively conditioned. That is to say, situations which consistently predict the removal of hunger come to elicit interest, approach and consumption. This is conditioned appetite. Feeding situations predict the correction of negative energy flow as the ingested food begins to be absorbed.

Energy is used at 100 kW (about 2 kcal per min) or more, depending on the level of physical activity. Lipolysis, glycogenolysis and gluconeogenesis are unlikely to exceed 40 to 50 kW at best. So when absorption falls well below 50 kW, as it does within an hour or so of a 4 MJ (about 1000 kcal) meal, then increasing negative energy supply develops (50 + 40 - 100 = -10). After a meal, absorption can reach 500 kW. This generates a large positive energy flow, even allowing for much of absorption to go into glycogen and lipid synthesis (¼ x 500 - 100 = +25).

One may suppose that both the deficient flow and the excessive flow are detected by neural elements or adjacent cells affecting them in the liver, the hypothalamus, or elsewhere. These detectors may be sensitive to their own metabolism, like the neuronal units Oomura (1973) has recorded in the lateral hypothalamus of the rat and Niijima (1969) has recorded in vagal afferents from the perfused liver of the guinea pig. In both cases, it is thought that energy supply determines activity of the sodium pump and hence the polarisation and firing rate of the cells. Alternatively or as well, there may be detectors with selective metabolic sensitivities or membrane receptor specialisations, which generate separate influences on appetite of glucose, fatty acids, glycerol, amino acids, or other energy-yielding substrates. In either case, the capacity of the liver to synthesise and/or to spare glucose from most energy substrates will be likely to give this organ a transducer role; it could translate the current supply of energy for utilisation into a locally or centrally detected signal. Although evidence for such signals accumulates for physiological responses like gastric acid secretion and adrenomedullary adrenalin secretion, there is as yet no direct evidence that such cellularly recorded metabolic or chemosensitive detectors contribute to the control of feeding behaviour. Similarly, there is now considerable evidence that systemic delivery of energy substrates inhibits appetite by action on probably more than one type of receptor or transducer but the identity and characteristics of any such neural receptor cell remain to be determined.

Cytischystatic simulations

Put such an energy-flow monitoring system into the context of what really happens in the body and in the external environment. Add the conditioning processes mentioned above, which seem likely to dominate behaviour and sensations in human appetite and satiety. Can realistic meal patterns and changes in body composition be calculated by such a model? In the rat, we had found that they could be (Booth, 1978; Booth & Toates, 1974; Booth *et al.*, 1976; Toates & Booth, 1974).

We were somewhat taken aback to find that our first tentative attempt to extend such a theory to building a model of human appetite and body composition also worked (Booth & Mather, 1978) (Fig. 2). We had expected that social factors would

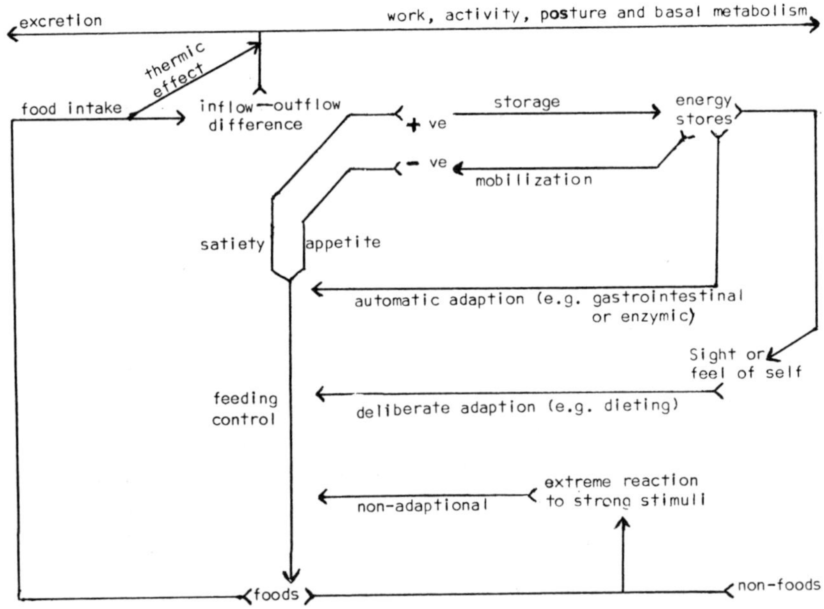

Fig. 2. Some processes likely to affect appetite, satiety and body weight. The computer model discussed in this paper includes explicitly or implicitly a representation of each process indicated in this diagram

dominate the picture so much that the influence of physiological factors would be almost totally obscured. In retrospect, this pessimism was ill-founded in two ways. First, we were modelling only a general case. No doubt social factors can dominate the timing of a meal on particular occasions, and sometimes even strongly influence its composition. In general, however, it could surely be that social conventions and microcultural habits have adapted to the average physiology and the pattern of energy demands for human beings in that culture. Secondly, the conditioning theory provides a specific mechanism by which social and cognitive factors can in fact acquire physiological roles. It is not only flavours, and also gastrointestinal and metabolic stimuli, which can gain anticipatory control of attitudes to specific foodstuffs, when such stimuli are classically conditioned by the hunger-removing or over-satiating consequence of experiencing such cues. Cues like time on the clock, knowledge of how long it has been since the last meal, and expectancy of a vigorous sporting engagement, can also become 'conditioned stimuli' which control feeding for its physiological consequences in such circumstances.

Steps of calculation

Table 1 lists equations used in this preliminary model to calculate major flows of energy within the body and their effects on feeding behaviour. The values of the parameters k_1 to k_7 were chosen to be within the range indicated by the literature, which

Table 1. Main equations of basic feeding model (Booth & Mather, 1978). An example of a set of values for parameters k_1, k_2, k_3, k_5, k_6 and k_7 is given in Table 2; k_4 was -10^{-6} per min

Energy flows

Stomach contents	= stomach contents	+ eating rate	$- k_1 \sqrt{\text{stomach contents}}$
Absorption rate at t	= gastric emptying rate at t-6 min		$= k_1 \sqrt{\text{stomach contents at t-6min}}$
Metabolic rate	= basal mr	+ activity mr	+ 0.1 x absorption rate
Lipogenesis rate	$= - k_2$ [absorption rate	− metabolic rate] when ar > mr	
Lipolysis rate	$= - k_3$ [absorption rate	− metabolic rate] when ar < mr + k_4 fat energy	
Net energy supply rate	= absorption rate	− metabolic rate	+ lipolysis/genesis rate

Energy stores

Fat energy	= fat energy	− lipolysis/genesis rate
Non-fat energy	= non-fat energy	+ net energy supply rate

Feeding controls

Hunger = 1 when net energy supply rate < k_5 = feeding threshold for single diet

Hunger = 0 when net energy supply rate > conditioned satiety value for diet and time

Conditioned satiety = conditioned satiety + target maximum energy supply (k_6) − actual last maximum rate

Eating rate = food availability x food & body acceptability state

= k_7 x hunger for a single diet *ad lib.*

was often very wide. The values were further attuned to give a standard stimulation which kept almost constant body weight and composition and showed limited ability to defend that composition against some displacements. The justifications of the choices of equations used and also the details of the calculations are given by Booth & Mather (1978).

Tests for potential influences on body composition

Booth & Mather (1978) conducted an initial exploration of the characteristics of a system working on the above principles. We varied the value of each of the system's parameters in turn and recorded the effects on the timing and sizes of meals and on the increments of lean and fat mass.

Not surprisingly, the most dramatic effects on body weight and composition were generated by varying the characteristics of modelled lipid metabolism and of modelled sensitivity to the postprandial satiating effects of food (Table 2). As expected from previous experience (Booth, 1976), the stomach emptying pattern is also a major influence. Subtler effects of varying certain other parameters were seen, and these may be no less significant clinically (see below). No systematic effect should be ignored After all, dramatic gains or losses of fat are by no means the phenomena to be concentrated on. On one hand, obesity can be insidious in onset. On the other, programmes of weight loss which were gentler than current therapies could have better long-term success.

Lipid metabolism

There were small but systematic effects on meal timings and sizes resulting from simulated variations in the proportion of the absorption-expenditure mismatch which is covered by lipolysis energy (k_3, Tables 1 and 2) or diverted into lipogenesis energy (k_2). The most substantial effects were increases in sizes of breakfast and supper with increasing proportions of energy supply diverted into fat storage. Body energy gain

Table 2. Sensitivity of a basic feeding model (second version of Booth & Mather, 1978) to variation in parameter values set for constant body composition

Parameter	Symbol*	Basic value	For a 1% increase in parameter value: Conversion to fat increases by (%)	Total body energy increases daily by (%)
Gastric emptying rate factor	k_1	0.192 $kcal^{1/2}$/min	0.089	−0.04
Lipogenesis factor	k_2	0.554	0.343	0.013
Lipolysis factor	k_3	0.407	−0.280	0.0007
Activity metabolic rate	–	1.4 kcal/min	−0.001	0.0001
Hunger threshold	k_5	1.08 kcal/min	0	0.0003
Satiety target	k_6	1.49 kcal/min	0.025	0.011
Eating rate	k_7	47.5 kcal/min	0	−0.001

* Used in Table 1 above

increased under these conditions. Variations in proportional lipolysis, on the other hand, had negligible effect on body energy gain. Nevertheless, as readily foreseen, either more efficient lipogenesis or less efficient lipolysis led to a relatively greater distribution of stored energy into fat rather than lean, whether or not the total energy gain occurred.

The converse simulation might have encouraging implications for attempts to develop drugs for weight control based on interference with synthesis or breakdown of energy stores. Simulations of decreased lipogenesis or increased lipolysis showed the expected diversion of energy away from fat into lean - again without large changes in meal timings or sizes.

Adaptation of lipogenesis Rats trained to feed once a day for only two hours (gorgers or 'meal feeders') show greatly increased postprandial lipogenesis, compared with rats which take their meals *ad lib.* (free feeders or 'nibblers'). In some dieting regimes the slimmer is therefore advised to take at least three or four meals a day of modest size and to avoid taking only one really large meal in a day. Gorgers force-fed with the same amount of energy as free feeders do accumulate more fat (Cohn & Joseph, 1959). However, the biochemically measured lipogenic activation coincides with a marked loss of body fat, which occurs because the rats fail to maintain *ad lib.* daily intake when transferred to the 2 h/day schedule. We are left with little evidence that frequency or size of meals is a primary cause of obesity or a variable worthy of therapeutic attention. Furthermore, as Palmquist, Learn & Baker (1977) emphasise, there are marked species differences even among rodents. In man, although low frequency of meals is associated with obesity (Fabry & Tepperman, 1970) and a frequency as low as one or two meals a day has metabolic effects, it appears not to have a substantial obesity-inducing effect (Young *et al.*, 1971), except when only two meals per day are eaten (Metzner *et al.*, 1977). If lipogenic activation by schedule feeding has any clinical import, it might rather be to raise a further doubt about the efficacy of rapid dieting.

Sensitivity to satiety after meals

In following a simplified form of the conditioned satiety theory, the model seeks an optimum level of energy supply shortly following a meal (k_6, Table 2). The energy supply rate at which the next subsequent meal is stopped is adjusted up or down according to whether postprandial energy supply undershoots or overshoots this predetermined target. Now, an individual may have too high a target for the satiating energy supply. Someone might be generally insensitive to the satiety affects which do the conditioning. He might be poorly conditionable to the potential satiety cues, internal or external, which predict the conditioning after-effects of meals. In all such cases, the effective target will permit the conditioned satiety level to rise. Meals will increase in size, with lunch being the most dramatic in the simulations of Booth & Mather (1978). Even though the larger meals will take longer to clear and release feeding again (unless gastrointestinal or metabolic processing adapts to speedier clearance), lunch and supper are still taken, albeit later in the day. On the present assumptions of the model, the effect of one day's intake on the next day's intake is very small and also can be weak compared with behavioural factors such as immediate satiety control. So total intake rises with raised satiety target. Energy deposition follows. However, these simulations show no differential deposition of energy into fat rather than non-fat mass. In that sense, then, this effect is more like normal growth than it is like becoming obese. Here the simple assumptions of the model must be recalled. No adaptations to increases in meal size are allowed for. Even if there are no hyperlipogenic adaptations to frequent meals, such adaptations may occur with repeated large meals. A simulation on such assumptions would produce an obesifying effect of a raised satiety target.

Thus the therapeutic benefits of improving the control of satiety may be substantial (Booth, 1976).

The benefits of gaining control of hunger are less obvious from the simulations to date. Although Booth & Mather (1978) did not represent appetite conditioning, it seems likely that their unconditioned appetite process would not differ greatly in effect from conditioned appetite processes on a constant diet. The day's meals seemed to compensate amongst themselves for variations in hunger threshold. Little or no effect on energy deposition was simulated (k_5, Table 2).

Gastric emptying

We have been impressed by the importance of the shape and steepness of the curve of emptying from the stomach in simulations of appetite and body weight in rats (Booth & Toates, 1974; Booth *et al.,* 1976). In the preliminary human simulations, variations in the relation between gastric contents and gastric emptying rate also had some effect on the meal pattern and body weight.

Table 2 shows how the deposition of energy in fat increased relative to non-fat energy deposition as the gastric emptying rate factor (k_1) increased (ie with higher rate of emptying or a given gastric contents). A 10 per cent increase in the rate factor yielded a shift towards fat deposition of almost 1 per cent. A related effect of relatively energy-rich diet on gastric emptying may account for the correlation between chubbiness and dietary energy density reported by Hunt, Cash & Newland (1975) and Fomon (1975). On the other hand, such an increase in the rate factor reduced total body energy in that simulation, by reducing the quantities taken at breakfast and lunch.

Conversely, a lower rate factor increased breakfast and lunches sizes. Body weight increased too, until (at only a few per cent lower emptying rate factor) the sizes of breakfast and lunch and the lateness of lunch, because of slow emptying and a large breakfast, combined to delay supper so much that the simulated individual was predicted not to get hungry before bed. Two meals a day produced a precipitate loss of weight.

These effects on food intake and body composition seemed relatively minor compared with some we had seen in rat modelling. However, the simulations of the rat included adaptation of the lipogenesis to speeded gastric emptying to account for hypothalamic obesity (Booth, 1978). This human model does not include adaptations, and these could amplify or bias the consequences of a change in gastric emptying.

Furthermore, the above simulations altered the gastric emptying rate factor at all times. The changed gastric emptying shortly after a meal tended to counteract the same change continued throughout the rest of the period until the next meal, at least in the effects of the change on satiety. A fast stomach soon after a meal decreased meal size, by conditioning satiety. A fast stomach during most of the absorptive period hastened the arrival of hunger and the next meal. Altering gastric emptying at only one phase should have much more marked consequences.

Occasional (Axelsson, Dano & Hylander, 1976) or systematic relations (Johansson & Ekelund, 1976) have been reported between body weight and gastric emptying of liquid test meals. The aetiological significance of unusual gastric emptying characteristics merits closer investigation, using ordinary meals in unoperated individuals with weight problems, whether or not overweight at the time of measurement. The correlations could arise rather from adaptation of the gastroduodenal system to eating style or body composition.

Even if no type of weight control problem involves an extreme of gastric emptying characteristics, the use of biofeedback, drugs or other means to change gastric emptying might still be of considerable therapeutic potential (Booth, 1976). It could prove crucial to time such changes appropriately in relation to meals.

Exercise

Our simulations include a representation only of the direct effects of exercise, within the energy expenditure component. They therefore illustrate with empirical detail the purely thermodynamic principles of a beneficial contribution of exercise to altering the energy balance in overweight.

Intriguingly, the simple thermodynamics interacts with the set of assumptions used by Booth & Mather (1978) to yield a complete breakdown in the feeding system when the rate of exercise gets too low. This breakdown occurs below the lower end of the most sedentary occupations in the model which has been attuned to no weight gain in an average sedentary life. Mayer, Roy & Mitra (1956) suggested that the feeding and bodyweight control system breaks down at low activity rates in man, although their data in support of the idea remain to be replicated. However, some extra assumption(s) will have to be improved to yield a simulated increase in fat in the absence of exercise. The present model simply stops feeding altogether. The stimulating effect of a variety of foodstuffs (Booth, 1976) would be one unmodelled factor preventing this consequence in reality.

A potential snag with dependence on heavy exercise for weight control is indicated by the simulation of energy expenditure rates higher than those at which the Booth & Mather (1978) model was attuned to constant weight. A slight residual increase in body energy was observed (Table 2). More of the gain was in lean mass than in fat mass on the assumptions written in, but fat was increasing along with muscle, etc. The simulated lunches and suppers came earlier and were larger, generating this tendency. The relative roles of expenditure modification and intake modification is a complex issue currently receiving increased attention. In due time, simulation work may be the only way of analysing the problem and constructing systematic or individualised clinical recommendations for experimental trial.

Adaptive thermogenesis In the simulations considered here, components of energy expenditure besides the cost of physical activity are kept constant. In reality people vary considerably in basal metabolic rate, even when calculated relative to body mass or some suitable derivative. Basal metabolic rate and the thermic effect of food may also change at least in some people. Conditions leading to adaptation may include food restriction or overfeeding. If the extent of such changes can be established, equations to represent such adaptations might be estimated and then added to the model. Like elaborations of other adapting relationships between components, such additions are likely to improve the realism of simulations of long-term effects. Furthermore, some of the consequences of such adapting functions for body composition are not readily intuited, especially if the human being is a feedback system in which the consequences of the adaptations affect appetite in turn.

Slow eating

Behaviour modification packages generally include instructions to eat slowly. One rationale for this appears from related aspects of the instructions to be based on the belief that 'savouring' the food will be helpful. The logic here is obscure. If overeating is an emotional reaction to stress or hedonic compensation, 'stretching' the calories involved might be helpful but increasing the duration and salience of food-generated stimulation could further reinforce the maladaptive use of food. More specifically for the present theory of normal feeding control, protraction of the presentation of food cues will change the temporal relations to their postingestional correlates and consequences. The immediate effect and the eventual effect after the new conditioning had been set up would not be simply predictable, as will be seen when we turn to another rationale for slow eating.

A clearer theory behind the attempt to slow the slimmer's eating is that this will give time for the onset of satiety before too much food has been ingested. However, this hypothesis in its simplest form presupposes that the onset of complete satiety, or the rise of intensifying satiety, has a fixed time-course. I know of no evidence for this. If postingestional events have any graded effects, then the time-course is liable to vary when the rate of delivery of nutrients down the throat is varied. Slower eating may delay the satiety it is supposed to be waiting for.

On the assumptions in the Booth & Mather (1978) model, slowing the rate of energy intake (k_7, Table 2) actually proves to have an antitherapeutic short-term effect. Variations in the rate of energy intake had small effects on the timing and sizes of meals which did not appear very systematic over the limited range of conditions tested. However, slower eating was systematically related in the model to increased energy deposition in the body (and speeded eating caused decreased deposition). These effects arise because the change in rate of intake changes the relationship between the amount of intake and the pattern of absorption after a meal, by varying the amount that can accumulate in the stomach during a meal. Larger amounts in the stomach give higher emptying rates and so higher average absorption rates. On the model's assumptions, these encourage more efficient conversion of food to body weight. The normal conditioning of satiety would correct some of the increased average absorption rate, but it appears from this simulation that not all of the increase is counteracted by the type of satiety conditioning assumed. If this is a weakness in the real system also, it could be worse in overweight individuals. They could have difficulty in satiety conditioning because a greater proportion of moderately overweight than other people suffer overstrong unconditioned reactions to external stimuli (Rodin, 1977), including feeding-predictive stimuli which otherwise are readily conditioned. Also, at least some overweight may have learned not to attend to postingestional internal events (Stunkard & Koch, 1964; Bruch, 1973) and it is such events which serve as unconditioned stimuli to condition the satiety reactions to feeding situations.

Some general implications

Support of simulation work

Data on eating patterns, patterns of gastric emptying and the effects of absorption in man are accumulating. A considerable variety of increasingly realistic simulations is becoming practicable. However, simulation takes time. Intelligent simulation takes more time, as it requires close acquaintance with the best available theoretical insights and with the latest available experimental data. Solely on the issue of the effects to be expected from modifying eating patterns, many months of simulation work would currently pay off quite as much as the equivalent time spent in basic or clinical experimentation or observation. Such simulation work should be provided with the necessary financial support, ideally within or in collaboration with laboratories also involved in the relevant experimentation and treatment programmes.

Momentary process, not cause out of context

It seems clear that we will not get far by simply classifying people, foodstuffs, stomachs or fat cells. Attribution of observed variance to this or that causation can be a useful first step in analysing a phenomenon, but the approach is limited even when the causes do not interact statistically as they are liable to do in a mechanistically integrated system. Predictive explanation of the phenomenon requires a mechanistic theory which invokes systematically interconnected processes and their changes in state over whatever time period is significant.

Palatability is a clear case of a concept which needs improvement. Theorists keep returning to the insight that reactions to the sensory qualities of foodstuffs are critical to appetite control (Jacobs & Sharma, 1969; Wyrwicka, 1969; King,1976) and, of course, no amount of nutritional biochemistry or hypothalamic neurophysiology will replace behavioural and phenomenological analysis of the reactions to foodstuffs. A moment's thought about the phenomena of interest should make clear that this must be the case. Eating is an oral sensorimotor reaction or local reflex. The immediate difference between one food and the next is its impact on eyes, nose and mouth. All control of feeding must work through 'palatability' (Booth, 1972*a*) - calories, gastric distension, adipose, if relevant at all, act on the reactions to food-induced stimulation. The force of this insight is not met by looking at the effects of adulteration with quinine or saccharin on feeding. Nor will one create an explanation or prediction of the consumption of a food if one subjects it only to sensory evaluation procedures which depend on a context-free concept of invariant acceptability. The sensory effect of a foodstuff on feeding will depend on the percipient's current state, which will include his concept of the time of the next meal and of the composition of the last meal, his attitudes to foodstuffs of the type presented, and so on.

Similarly, we need to know how stomachs empty all sorts of real meals, not the emptying time for a convenient liquid load. We need metabolic conversion rates, not blood concentrations. And so on. Such measurements are important for valid qualitative theory, not just for quantitative modelling. Some current interpretations of behavioural effects of surgery or infusions could be considerably changed if the effects on gastrointestinal processing or tissue substrate uptakes during such behaviour were adequately measured biochemically.

Flow, not amount

Appetite and satiety are frequently conceptualised in terms of the amount of energy which is taken during a meal or in a day's intake. Weight control is considered in terms of body weight or, at best, amount of body fat.

The amount of body fat, is, of course, the presenting problem but the theoretical and practical issue is what the fat does and what can be done to it. Also, how much an individual says he or she wants is one *prima facie* legitimate measure of appetite, as is the amount taken when an organism is allowed to eat 'to appetite' or until satiation. This mode of thought has become more strongly and widely engrained recently by the not unworthy fashion for analysing feeding patterns into meal size and meal-to-meal intervals. The unfortunate tendency would be to treat such data as a behaviourally exhaustive analysis of feeding.

I would urge that an approach which is more likely to be productive would focus on the processes which are current at any instant during or between meals, or at any state of body composition. Even if we can see the size of a meal and feel something of its bulk abdominally, and even if the quantity of fat in the body is measured somehow, these signals will be processes of some sort. The chances are that most quantities are measured as their effects on local flow rates or concentrations, even before the brain deals with them all as rates of neuronal firing. The proposal that the amount of adipose triglyceride in the body is measured as an average or basal rate of glycerol and/or non-esterified fatty acid release is a case in point. Putting a realistic level of such a signal into the human feeding model generates a slow but precise equilibrating influence on adiposity (Booth & Mather, 1978). Another reason to concentrate on processes rather than objects or bulks is that control signals are likely to depend on several amounts if they relate to any at all (eg, rate of energy expenditure, rate of eating, rate of intestinal absorption, rate of lipid or glycogen synthesis). The total amount in the body seldom matters in a biochemical calculation. Maybe it should not be the main focus of those of us who are trying to understand or control what is going on behaviourally. Even self-perception or body image is unlikely to relate closely to actual body weight or composition. It seems that cues such as the feel of the clothes and the sight of the thighs or belly are likely to be the signals for weight control cognitively, and the name, colour, smell and texture of the food the signals of nutritional quantities. Except for a small minority of users, bathroom scales and calorie charts are likely to be poor calibrators, even when they are consulted.

For similar reasons, hours of food deprivation may not be a very useful variable in appetite studies, and per cent of free-feeding body weight even less so. Such variables seem distant from the processes likely to be influential. Psychologists have found that people are very bad at discriminating levels of 'hunger' (Wooley, 1976). Of course, even without the sight of a clock, people have a good idea how long ago it was they last had a meal. So such experiments have tested for effects after meals with disguised differences in energy content. It does not follow from such results that people are bad at discriminating internal signals at the times they are relevant to normal food intake. One hour after a meal the rate of absorption is changing very slowly and differs little between meals of different sizes, by comparison with the variations during and shortly after meals. A focus on rates of processing, and the timing of changes in such rates, is more likely to encourage the design of experiments which elucidate the behaviourally powerful variables.

Consideration of the roles of conditioning and learning adds an extra twist. To the extent that appetite is acquired behaviour, it will not be current flows, current quantities, or any current signals which dominate behaviour, although currently present signals may often contribute. The interpretation of current events will be critically dependent on past experience of what such events mean. Remembrance of fluxes past will be used to allow for fluxes shortly to come. The cognitive processes in feeding control are acquired concepts and attitudes which are circumstance-dependent in their relevance and application. Concepts of a foodstuff's palatability and satisfying power are, I believe, built up to a great extent from experience of its effects on energy supply following ingestion, and these consequences vary with context. We have indeed found that the pleasantness of eating a foodstuff varies with context and this variation is closely related to variation in behaviour towards the foodstuff - so closely that it is possible to believe that the context-sensitivity of the concept is sufficient to explain the familiar cycle of the food's selection and rejection (Booth, 1977*b*).

The normal human meal pattern is a repletion-depletion cycle of very high amplitide when considered in terms of energy flows. It is beside the point that body weight, body fat content, liver glycogen content, blood glucose concentration, and like, vary so little during a normal meal pattern. It is not critical that the stomach actually becomes empty or that it be filled sufficiently to produce gastric or intestinal bulk effects. What may be the most relevant fact ultimately is that the stomach emptying curve is negatively accelerated. That means that intestinal absorption is substantially faster around the end of a meal than it is an hour or two later. The flows of substrates to tissues switch from prime dependence on intestinal supply to majoring on gluconeogenic, glycogenolytic and lipolytic supply. The energy 'cash flow' swings from abundance to deficit, even though there may be enough energy in the body to sustain life for a month. Positive balance may arise when these large and frequent tides of metabolism are only slightly perturbed, so long as the perturbation is persistent.

Envoi

Sassoon (1973) also emphasised the need to pay close attention to changes in processes over time in obesity. Hopefully, his insights will be put into a quantitative basis fairly soon by extensions of the present line of modelling, or - better still - the combination of these models with others more adequately representing parts of the system.

The fact that a model computes, and even produces a plausible simulation of one general case, does not mean that the theory behind it is correct. We know that every component of the present model is a crude oversimplification of reality. Many important interactions and additional components are obviously missing from the version presented. Nevertheless, the present model is a system synthesised from independently measurable real elements, and the first such which simulates human feeding and body composition changes. It is therefore conceivable that the theory is on the right track, even though clearly inadequate in its detail at present. In such a situation there follows a responsibility to see the model refined. The data which will fill the gaps and rectify the crudities may have to be collected and will certainly have to be evaluated and expressed in programmable form. The improved models must be tested for sensitivity to variations in their parameter values and robustness over varying combinations of conditions. Their implications for treatment of weight problems might then be clear enough to warrant direct clinical trial.

Summary

A prototype quantitative computer simulation of the control of human feeding is presented. It is based on the theory that satiety and appetite are conditioned responses to feeding situations and that these external and internal cues have been conditioned by the consequences that feeding has for the supply of energy-yielding substrates to working tissues. Some simulation results illustrate effects to be expected on the basis of one particular set of such assumptions. Food intake and the deposition of fat are differentially sensitive to variations in different characteristics of the control system. A realistic quantification of such sensitivities is needed by any rational weight control therapy. The immediate implication for research into treatment for obesity is that we need better quantitative data on the most influential controls of normal human feeding, as well as continued efforts to identify distinctive biochemical, physiological and psychological characteristics amongst those disposed to overweight. Only with such data and with work on more sophisticated quantitative system simulation can we expect to develop successful rational treatments for obesity under its varied maintaining conditions.

References

Axelsson, C., Dano, P. & Hylander, E. (1976): *Scand. J. Gastroent.* 11, Suppl. 38, 113.

Booth, D.A. (1972*a*): *Physiol. Behav.* 8, 891.

Booth, D.A. (1972*b*): *Physiol Behav.* 9, 199.

Booth, D.A. (1976): Approaches to feeding control. In *Appetite and food intake*, ed T. Silverstone, p. 417. Berlin: Dahlem Konferenzen, Abakon.

Booth, D.A. (1977*a*): *Psychosom. Med.* 39, 76.

Booth, D.A. (1977*b*): Appetite and satiety as metabolic expectancies. In *Food intake and chemical senses*, ed Y. Katsuki, M. Sato, S. Takagi & Y. Oomura. p. 259. Tokyo: University of Tokyo Press/Baltimore: University Park Press.

Booth, D.A. (1978): Prediction of feeding behaviour from energy flows in the rat. In *Hunger models: computable theory of feeding control*, ed D.A. Booth. London and New York: Academic Press.

Booth, D.A. & Jarman, S.P. (1976): *J. Physiol.* (Lond.) 256, 71.

Booth, D.A. & Mather, P. (1978): Prototype model of human feeding, growth and obesity. In *Hunger models: computable theory of feeding control*, ed. D.A. Booth. London and New York: Academic Press.

Booth, D.A. & Toates, F.M. (1974): *Bull. Psychon. Soc.* 3, 442.

Booth, D.A., Toates, F.M. & Platt, S.V. (1976): Control system for hunger and its implications in animals and man. In *Hunger: basic mechanisms and clinical implications*, ed D. Novin, W. Wyrwicka & G.A. Bray. p. 127. New York: Raven Press.

Bruch, H. (1973): *Eating disorders: obesity, anorexia nervosa and the person within.* New York: Basic Books.

Cohn, C. & Joseph, D. (1959): *Am. J. Physiol.* **196**, 969.
Fabry, P. & Tepperman, J. (1970): *Am. J. Clin. Nutr.* **23**, 1059.
Fomon, S.J. (1975): *Acta Paediat. Scand.* **64**, 172.
Hunt, Cash & Newland (1975): *Lancet* **8**, 905.
Jacobs, H.L. & Sharma, K.N. (1969): *Ann. N.Y. Acad, Sci.* **157**, 1084.
Johansson, C. & Ekelund, K. (1976): *Gut* **17**, 456.
King, K.R. (1976): *Physiol. Psychol.* **4**, 405.
Mayer, J., Roy, P. & Mitra, M.P. (1956): *Am. J. Physiol.* **110**, 329.
Metzner, H.L., Lamphiear, D.E., Wheeler, N.C. & Larkin, F.A. (1977): *Am. J. Clin. Nutr.* **30**, 712.
Niijima, A. (1969): *Ann. N.Y. Acad. Sci.* **157**, 690.
Oomura, Y. (1973): *Adv. Biophys.* **5**, 65.
Palmquist, D.L., Learn, D.B. & Baker, N. (1977): *J. Nutr.* **107**, 502.
Rodin, J. (1977): The effects of stimulus-found behavior on biological self-regulation: feeding, obesity and external control. In *Consciousness and self-regulation,* Vol. 2, ed G. Schwartz & D. Shapiro. New York: Plenum Press.
Sassoon, H.F. (1973): *Am. J. Clin. Nutr.* **26**, 776.
Stunkard, A.J. & Koch, C. (1964): *Arch. Gen. Psychiat.* **11**, 74.
Toates, F.M. & Booth, D.A. (1974): *Nature* **25**, 710.
Wooley, S.C. (1976): Human experimental psychology. In *Appetite and food intake,* ed T. Silverstone, p. 331. Berlin: Dahlem Konferenzen, Abakon.
Wyrwicka, W. (1960): *Physiol. Behav.* **4**, 853.
Young, C.M., Scanlan, S.S., Topping, C.M., Simko, V. & Lutwak, L. (1971): *J. Am. Diet. Ass.* **59**, 466.

8
Human feeding in the laboratory

V.E. PUDEL
Department of Psychiatry, University of Goettingen, von-Siebold-Strasse 5, 3400 Goettingen, F.R.G.

Human eating behavior is often studied in the laboratory even though innumerable opportunities arise every day in which the interested scientist might observe people eating in a variety of situations. Lately, free, systematic observational methods have been employed, much like those developed by child psychologists at the beginning of this century. A comparison of the results of such studies impressively points towards the considerable influence of environmental conditions on human eating habits (Stunkard & Kaplan, 1977). Typical differences between normal and obese persons are difficult to detect by this method, because human eating behavior introduces very large variances in the observational data. Certainly it is necessary to check hypotheses related to the pathogenesis of obesity in natural settings, for it is in these natural settings that obese people have gained weight, not in the laboratory. Methods of free observation are thus a worthwhile supplement offering the possibility to validate laboratory findings.

Yet the complexity of human eating behavior also compels the application of methods used in studies of animal experiments as well. Through planned, controlled experiments, causal relationship may be established, whereas free observation offers only statistical correlations. Laboratory experiments and free observations supplement each other ideally, as exemplified by an observational study conducted in public places by Wooley, Tennenbaum & Wooley (in press). This study concluded that obese persons in a cafeteria serving a large variety of palatable food ate more than normals; in a cafeteria serving mediocre food, they ate less than normals. This finding relied on laboratory controls in which standardized food was offered, so that an interaction between food intake and body weight status could not be detected. The experimenter can determine, from natural observations, which factors should be manipulated as independent variables, so that clinically useful results can be compiled.

Laboratory experiments have attempted to determine, above all, which variables influence the beginning and end of food ingestion. Many possible parameters have been investigated, including the following: caloric density and volume of food (Campbell, Hashim & Van Itallie, 1971; Spiegel, 1973; Wooley, Wooley & Woods, 1975*a*); effects of preloading and food deprivation (Nisbett, 1968; Walike, Jordan & Stellar, 1969; Wooley, Wooley & Dunham, 1972*a*); meal frequency, taste, palatability and availability of food (Cabanac, Duclaux & Spector, 1971; Nisbett, 1969; Price & Grinker, 1973; Wooley, Wooley & Dunham, 1972*a*); appetite suppressants (Pudel, 1975; Wooley, Wooley & Williams, 1976*b*; Wooley, O.W. *et al.*, 1977); effects of anxiety and stress (Abramson & Wunderlich, 1972; Kaplan & Kaplan, 1957; McKenna, 1972; Meyer & Pudel, 1972; Schachter, Goldman & Gordon, 1968); influences of cognitive factors such as time of day (Schachter & Gross, 1968), caloric labelling (Wooley, Wooley & Dunham, 1972*b*; Wooley, S.C., 1972), and false feedback on calorie (Pudel, 1973) and volume intake (Pudel & Oetting, in press).

Of particular interest were the possible interactions between these variables and the body weight of the test subjects. In order to gain insight into the etiology and therapy of obesity, laboratory experiments demand methods which estimate such subjective experiences as appetite, hunger and satiation in a meaningful way. Among these methods are hunger and satiation rating with various scales, as well as hedonic ratings for measuring differences in taste.

In addition to these more subjective methods, the following methods have been applied: determination of volume, weight or caloric content of ingested food which normally is delivered in liquid form from visible or hidden containers by food dispensing machines (Hashim & Van Itallie, 1964; Jordan *et al.*, 1966; Pudel, 1971). Recently, Silverstone & Fincham (in press) developed a food dispensing device for administering a variety of food in solid form. Food was generally orally ingested, but has also been ingested intragastrically or parenterally (Jordan *et al.*, 1974). More recent experimental methods measure reactions that cannot be willingly influenced by the subject, for example, salivation (Wooley & Wooley, 1973) or psychogalvanic skin response (Linton *et al.*, 1972; Pudel & Oetting, in press). These methods have been stimulated by the hypothesis (Schachter, 1971) that normal subjects have a higher responsiveness to short term 'internal cues' than obese subjects do. The concept of 'internal cues' was first made operational by systematically manipulating the caloric density or the volume of test meals, holding constant all sensory properties. Many studies have independently concluded that the caloric content of a meal has little or no influence on food intake or satiation ratings (Jordan, 1969; Wooley, 1971; Wooley, Wooley & Dunham, 1972*b;* Wooley, S.C., 1972). This finding is particularly true of obese subjects, whereas normal subjects were occasionally influenced by variations in caloric content (Spiegel, 1973), particularly under long-term experimental conditions (Campbell, Hashim & Van Itallie, 1971; Hashim & Van Itallie, 1965). However, a complete compensation of caloric variations through changes in the volume of food intake could not be proven.

It should be noted that, in the laboratory, relatively low caloric concentrations were administered, test diets ranging from 2.0 kJ (0.5 kcal) to 7.5 kJ (1.8 kcal) per gram, in contrast to caloric densities normally encountered eg, bread with 10.4 kJ (2.5 kcal) /g; chocolate with 23.1 kJ (5.5 kcal) /g or even bacon with 29.3 kJ (7.0 kcal) /g. For this reason we administered a diet of pudding with caloric densities ranging from 2.9 kJ (0.7 kcal) to 20.5 kJ (4.9 kcal) per gram, to 36 subjects of varying body weight. Pudding portions of either 150 g or 300 g contained either 985 kJ (235 kcal) or 3102 kJ (740 kcal). Directly after a meal, satiation ratings were ascertained, and then hourly thereafter. Contrary to the internal hypothesis, no differences in satiation ratings between the body weight classes could be determined. Even the ratings registered directly after a meal showed a distinct relation to caloric content. A statistically significant influence of food volume on the degree of satiation could not be determined. On the other hand, studies show that upon administering oral and gastric preloads, subsequent intake from food dispensers is depressed as a function of both size and time of preload (Jordan, 1969; Walike, Jordan & Stellar, 1969). But compensation is not complete, so that these subjects ate more than their baseline amounts.

These results agree somewhat with a study that we conducted with a group of 63 subjects comprised of latent (Meyer & Pudel, 1977; Pudel, Metzdorff & Oetting, 1975) and manifest obese and non-obese persons. All subjects received 150 ml or 300 ml of soup as a preload and directly after, or 15 minutes after the preload, they were fed *ad lib.* by a food dispenser. Water preloads were adminstered as a control. Once again the internal hypothesis was refuted, in that no difference was established in the data between weight groups. Preloads, in general, suppressed intake by about 30 per cent, which did not completely compensate for the volume of preloads. Neither the volume of the preloads nor the timing had a statistically significant effect on the subsequent food intake. The caloric content of the soup, varying from 12.6 kJ (3 kcal) to 521.6 kJ (60 kcal) per 100 ml, did not influence food intake. The satiation ratings were similar in all preload situations, with the exception of the water preload which did not

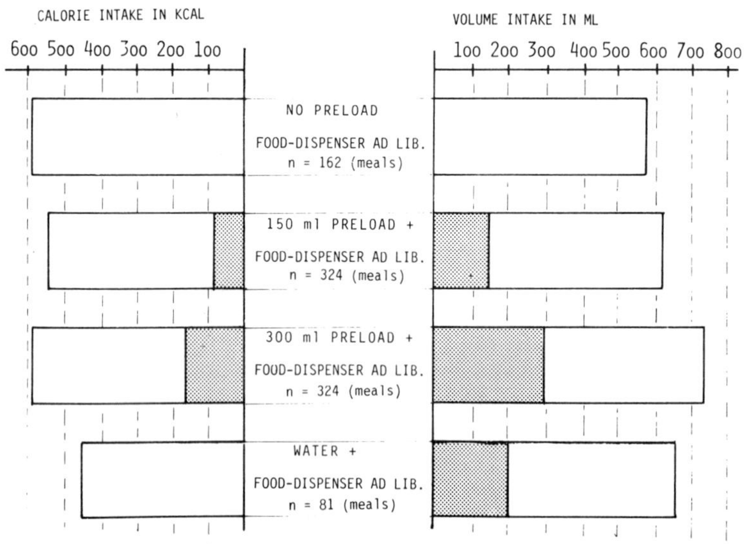

Fig. 1. Comparison between volume and energy intake of 63 subjects following different preload conditions

lead to subjective satiation. This finding is in accordance with an experiment by Wooley, Wooley & Dunham (1972*b*) who showed that a subjective feeling of satiation is more strongly influenced by the putative caloric content of a meal than by its actual caloric content. Water preloads obviously are not considered to have an effect on satiation.

The non-uniformity of many findings are better understood when one considers that calories and volumes were varied to different degrees. For example, a volume variation of 400 ml *vs* 800 ml is an overbearing stimulus compared with caloric variation between 2.1 kJ (0.5 kcal) *vs* 4.2 kJ (1 kcal) per ml in the test diet. We adjusted a large variety in caloric densities with a modest variation in volume. The resultant satiation rating fluctuated accordingly.

With respect to Hunt's thoughts regarding the relationship between nutritive density and gastric emptying (Hunt & Stubbs, 1975; Hunt, Cash & Newland, 1975) the problem could be better solved by considering the mutual interaction of calories and volume, rather than viewing these factors independently of each other. In addition to these two parameters, food intake is influenced by other factors such as, the type of the preload and the circumstances under which the test meal is administered (Shaw, 1973), as well as the interplay between oral and gastric factors as described in studies by Jordan (1969).

Often a rating scale, the method of measurement favored by psychologists, is employed. An interesting phenomenon was revealed in a study undertaken by Kindermann (1976). Unlike many authors who applied a single scale with opposing 'hunger' and 'satiation' poles, Kindermann utilized two scales in which 'hunger' and 'satiation' were graded separately. After administering 200 test meals to 48 subjects, a high negative correlation was established between the two scales ($r = -0.66$) for those subjects of normal weight, but not for overweight subjects ($r = -0.33$, not significant). Valid predictions of food intake for the obese subjects could only be made from the hunger rating, not from the satiation rating. This might give us good reason to reevaluate our own methods. It is interesting to note the finding of an older study on the theory of cognitive dissonance: subjects who voluntarily deprived themselves of food experienced differing degrees of hunger, depending on whether or not they had been paid for this task (Brehm & Cohen, 1962).

Particular attention should be drawn to the method developed and propagated by Wooley & Wooley (1973), namely, measuring the rate of salivation. The authors succeeded in showing that, upon presenting subjects with palatable food, their salivation response was inhibited if a high calorie meal had been administered one hour before; a lower degree of inhibition corresponded to low-calorie meals. Obese subjects generally displayed less inhibition in their salivation responses. Differences in hunger ratings could not be established (Wooley, Wooley & Woods, 1975*a*). The authors were also able to prove that amphetamine, but not fenfluramine, inhibited salivation. Again, differences in hunger ratings were not determined (Wooley *et al.*, 1977). The authors designate their method as an involuntary measure of appetite. It would seem worthwhile to apply these methods in the laboratory more often.

Not only the amount of food, but also the manner in which food is ingested must be considered. Experimental studies and observations indicate that, on average, obese people eat faster than slender people (Gaul, Craighead & Mahoney, 1975; Kindermann, 1976; Nisbett, 1972). For this reason, methods of slowing down the consumption rates are often employed in behavioral therapy programs (Stuart, 1967). The following related laboratory findings are worth mentioning: Wooley, Wooley & Turner (1975*b*) instructed subjects to eat precisely the same meal either hurriedly or slowly. Subjects salivated less while viewing palatable food one hour later when required to eat slowly.

Experiments using food dispensers and liquid diets showed that the cumulative intake curves differ between subjects while within a subject the shape is relatively constant (Meyer & Pudel, 1972; Meyer & Pudel, 1977). Negatively accelerated intake curves were recorded from infants, children between ages four and six and from non-obese adults. Obese subjects, people over 65 years of age and patients suffering from arteriosclerotic dementia tend to display linear intake curves and, in the latter cases, even towards progressively accelerated curves. The negatively accelerated curves (which have similarly been obtained from animals)

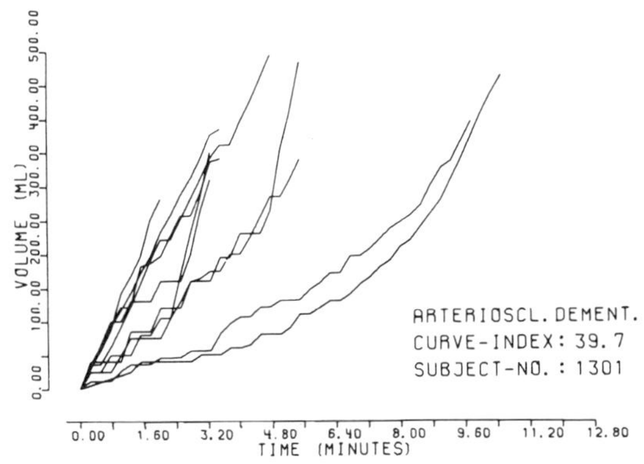

Fig. 2. Cumulative intake curves of a patient suffering from arteriosclerotic dementia. This patient only consumed on average 39 per cent of the total intake in the first half of the mealtime. The curves are in contrast to biological intake curves progressively accelerated

were labelled as 'biological satiation curves'. Recently we have attempted to simultaneously monitor these intake curves along with subjective satiation ratings. Subjects recorded their subjective degree of satiation on a continuous mechanical rating scale every 30 seconds. We have not yet been able to find a mode of evaluation that might detect a correlation or difference between the weight groups. Yet distictly different types of curves can be recognized independent of the weight groups. Many subjective satiation curves display an initial time delay followed by a steep rise, and then gradually level off. It appears that the time function of food intake may influence the feeling of satiation. In a pilot study we examined whether the time function of food intake could possible be modified by external influences. Six obese subjects who initially displayed linear intake curves in à baseline experiment were fed from a food dispenser accompanied by green and red light signals along an electronically synthesized biological satiation curve. After applying this type of feedback during ten meals, spontaneously recorded intake curves became distinctly similar to biological satiation curves directly after testing as well as three weeks thereafter.

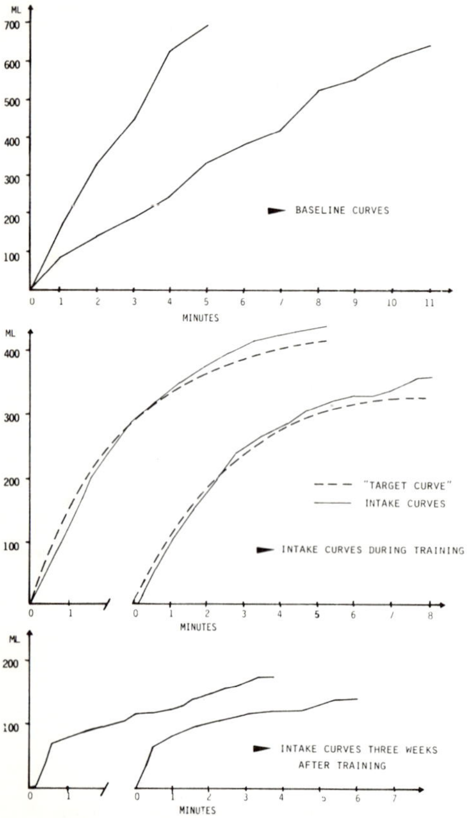

Fig. 3. Cumulative intake curves of one obese subject under three different conditions: (1) spontaneous recorded baseline intake curves when fed from a food dispenser; (2) intake curves during feed back training when the intake is guided by external signals along a synthesized biological target curve; (3) recorded intake curves three weeks after training

Along with the concept of 'internal cues', the complementary concept of 'external cues' (Schachter & Rodin, 1974) has been examined in the laboratory. A review of all the studies involving internal-external hypothesis would present a diversity of contradictory findings (Leon & Roth, 1977; Rodin, 1976). With regard to this topic, I wish to briefly refer to the following paper of J. Rodin, and to certain findings that are necessarily connected to special conditions of laboratory experiments.

Contrary to the internal hypothesis, the external hypothesis claims that obese subjects display a hyper-responsiveness to external cues, while normal individuals remain relatively uninfluenced. This hypothesis would seem to require detailed investigation, particularly in light of its enormous influence in behavioral therapy.

Laboratory results which are not in agreement with the Schachter hypothesis (1971) have arisen mainly from studies which investigate the influence of external cues *per se*. In these experiments normal subjects react just as externally as obese ones. From this observation a parallel can be drawn from those experiments which varied internal cues exclusively (eg, volume, calorie content) in which, likewise, no differences between weight groups could be determined. This seems to contradict the internal-external hypothesis. In contrast, experiments have been developed in which internal and external cues were varied simultaneously, and whose information was mutually contradictory; that is, a discrepancy existed between internal and external cues (Meyer & Pudel, 1977), which could only be accomplished with certain experimental techniques. I wish to briefly mention an experiment (Pudel & Oetting, in press) in which subjects received a liquid diet from a visible receptacle of a food dispenser, which could be electronically manipulated to lower the liquid levels of the container without the knowledge of the subject, thereby misrepresenting the true volume ingested. It could then be determined to what degree the subject was influenced by internal cues (the actual amount filling the stomach) and by external cues (the fluid level of the container).

The analysis of the data led to the following equations which predict behavior:

non-obese subjects: intake $= 0.83 \times R_i + 0.17 \times R_e$

manifest and latent obese subjects: intake $= 0.43 \times R_i + 0.57 \times R_e$

'R_i' (response, intern) represents the amount of food ingested that lead to a constant filling of the stomach under all experimental conditions, that is, the exclusively internally-controlled reaction. 'R_e' (response, extern) represents the food intake were the subject to rely solely on liquid level fluctuations, that is, the exclusively externally-controlled reaction.

Both parameters were accordingly weighted with constants that describe the various reaction tendencies of the subjects under an external-internal stimulus discrepancy. If only the internal or external cues were varied, then comparable reactions should result; this expectation does, in fact, agree with previous experiments.

As an example of this approach, Wooley, Tennenbaum & Wooley (in press) emphasized the importance of high palatability in influencing the food intake of obese individuals. Palatability is a paradigmatic variable which might stimulate a discrepancy outside the laboratory, whereas other external-internal discrepancies are restricted to artificial laboratory procedures. Given the case that a certain degree of food deprivation would lead to consumption of ten crackers, independent of internal cues, eight crackers would be eaten due to palatability alone. The equations would predict a mean intake of 9.7 crackers for non-obese and 8.9 for obese subjects. However, a slight external-internal discrepancy exists. If these crackers were smothered with butter, roastbeef and asparagus, and if subjects, because of the taste alone, theoretically choose to eat as many as 20 pieces, then 11.7 would be consumed by the non-obese subjects, and 15.7 by obese persons. Differences between the groups are connected with the degree of internal-external decrepancy.

Palatability, therefore, is a factor that can introduce a large internal-external discrepancy, and that can stimulate overeating in everyday situations as well. In the light of previous experiments, one might consider whether the selected test diets (most of low palatability) might significantly influence the experimental results. If, for example, in the preload study mentioned earlier we had used a cold buffet rather than a liquid diet from a food dispenser, then it is likely that we would have determined a difference between the weight groups.

An important point that can also lead to non-uniform results is the lack of standardization in random samples. The criterion of body weight alone seems inadequate. Yet this is often the sole criterion considered in experimentation and evaluation of therapy. It is recommended that groups be classified according to age, sex, degree of overweight, onset of obesity and motivational status (Price & Grinker, 1973; Pudel, 1976; Schumacher & Wagner, 1977). Recently the aspect of 'restrained and non-restrained eaters' has been dealt with (Herman & Polivy, 1975; Herman & Mack, 1976). Restrained eaters show similarities to latent obese patients; the latter are slender individuals with personal histories of weight problems which they overcame through self-control and orientation counselling. Only a few studies have employed control groups selected on the basis of 'no history of weight problems' (Price & Grinker, 1973; Wooley *et al.*, 1975*a*).

In experiments involving an external-internal stimulus discrepancy, latent obese subjects reacted quite similarly to manifest obese subjects (Pudel & Oetting, in press). However, the result of a smaller study indicated a large difference in reactions between latent and manifest obese subjects. Test subjects were given food *ad lib.* served as a liquid in a bowl. On the fourth day a self-refilling bowl was installed without their knowledge. The subjects were later informed of the trick device, and were subsequently administered six more meals. In this experimental situation a cognitive control is possible. During the last six meals the non-obese

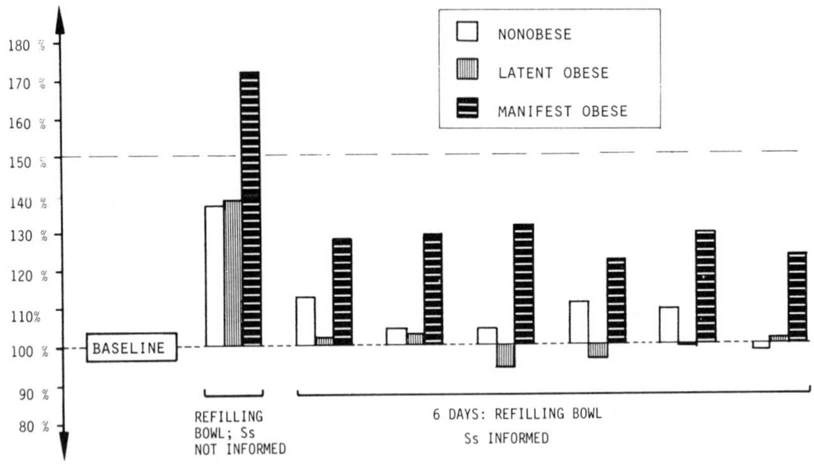

Fig. 4. Percentage deviation from ingested baseline volume in three groups of subjects when normal bowl was replaced by a 'self-refilling bowl'

subjects returned to their baselines, the obese subjects overate, while the latent obese tended to overcompensate by undereating.

Another subject of experimentation was the influence of psychological variables such as anxiety, fear and stress on food intake. Clinical observations have determined that stress can lead to either undereating or overeating depending on the individual. Experimental studies designed to examine hyperphagic reactions have not been able to determine the psychogenesis of overeating. It remains to be seen whether underlying causes involve a compensatory mechanism in the psychoanalytic sense (Abramson & Wunderlich, 1972; Kaplan & Kaplan, 1957; McKenna, 1972), or a reaction due to lack of internal responsiveness according to Schachter's hypothesis (Schachter *et al.,* 1968), and/or conditioned responses acquired during childhood (Jung, 1973; Meyer & Pudel, 1977).

Hyperphagic reactions are often displayed by overweight women. Experimental studies with children show that increased food intake usually does not arise until the early school years (Jung, 1973). The food intake of people over 65 years of age is generally uninfluenced by stress; they are probably neither internally nor externally controlled, but rather display 'automated' food intake (Pudel & Meyer, 1977). Approximately one-fifth to one-third of overweight people react by overeating during and following stress. Meyer & Tuchelt-Gallwitz (1967) showed that this group tends to score high on neuroticism in personality tests compared with other obese individuals. It seems to me that behavioral therapy techniques which have been developed so far are not properly oriented toward this special group of obese individuals.

What can we learn from laboratory experiments? First of all they show us that it is still too early to consider any theory of human eating behavior as being valid in absolute terms, mainly because experimental findings have not been independently replicated with a high degree of certainty (eg, Cabanac, 1971; Wooley *et al.,* 1972*a*). The high variance in laboratory data even acquired under the strictest conditions indicates that the search for more important variables must be intensified. Even differences that are statistically significant in spite of the wide variances are often of minor therapeutic importance, because of their small effect eg, if obese subjects ate 20 grams of crackers more than normals.

Nevertheless, important tendencies reflected by laboratory data have provided the foundation for therapeutic techniques, particularly in behavioral modification programs. It has been found that palatability is a very important determinant. Only when people find themselves in an environment with food of high palatability, differences between the eating behavior of obese and non-obese persons can be determined. Laboratory data indicate that certain dietetic factors should be dealt with more thoroughly in behavioral therapy. Food volume and caloric density are determinants in satiation, provided that interfering factors of palatability are controlled. The following behavioral therapy guidelines have been confirmed in the laboratory: (1) reduction of eating speed, (2) consumption of low calorie preloads some minutes before a meal, (3) arranging fixed food portions at the beginning of a meal, (4) leaving small amounts of leftovers on the plate, and (5) avoiding having good food on hand.

The group of hyperphagic-reacting obese patients cannot be treated effectively under a single, standardized program. Only when obese patients are recategorized according to specific criteria, can we expect to develop therapeutic approaches which are better suited to individual needs in the treatment of obesity. It appears to me that the entire spectrum of behavior therapy is aimed at transforming manifest obese patients into latent obese individuals; this implies that it is not the disposition or deep-rooted disturbances that are treated, but rather the patient learns certain techniques with which he overcomes his habit of overeating.

Acknowledgements – The research for this paper was supported by the German Research Foundation (SFB 33).

References

Abramson, E.E. & Wunderlich, R.A. (1972): *J. Abnorm. Psychol.* **79**, 317.
Brehm, J.W. & Cohen, A.R. (1962): *Explorations in cognitive dissonance.* New York: Wiley.
Cabanac, M. (1971): *Science* **173**, 1103.
Cabanac, M., Duclaux, R. & Spector, N.H. (1971): *Nature* **229**, 125.
Campbell, R.G., Hashim, S.A. & Van Itallie, T.B. (1971): *New Engl. J. Med.* **285**, 1402.
Gaul, D.J., Craighead, E. & Mahoney, M.J. (1975): *J. Consult. Clin. Psychol.* **43**, 123.
Hashim, S.A. & Van Itallie, T.B. (1964): *Fed. Proc.* **23**, 82.
Hashim, S.A. & Van Itallie, T.B. (1965): *Ann. N.Y. Acad. Sci.* **131**, 654.
Herman, C.P. & Polivy, J. (1975): *J. Abnorm. Psychol.* **84**, 661.
Herman, C.P. & Mack, D. (1976): *J. Personality* **43**, 647.
Hunt, J.N. & Stubbs, D.F. (1975): *J. Physiol.* **245**, 209.
Hunt, J.N., Cash, R. & Newland, P. (1975): *Lancet* **8**, 905.
Jordan, H.A. (1969): *J. Comp. Physiol. Psychol.* **68**, 498.
Jordan, H.A., Stellar, E. & Duggan, S.Z. (1968): *Comm. Behav. Biol.* **1**, 65.
Jordan, H.A., Wieland, W.F., Zebley, S.P., Stellar, E. & Stunkard, A.J. (1966): *Psychosom. Med.* **28**, 836.
Jordan, H.A., Hamilton, M., McFayden, B.V. & Dudrick, S.J. (1974): *Psychosom. Med.* **36**, 144.
Jung, F. (1973): *Prax. Kinderpsychol.* **22**, 167.
Kaplan, H.I. & Kaplan, H.S. (1957): *J. Nerv. Ment. Dis.* **125**, 181.
Kindermann, F.W. (1976): Experimentelle Untersuchungen zur kurzfristigen Sättigungskontrolle. Doctoral Dissertation, University of Dusseldorf.
Leon, G.R. & Roth, L. (1977): *Psychol. Bull.* **84**, 117.
Linton, P.H., Conley, M., Kuechenmeister, C. & McClusky, H. (1972): *Am. J. Clin. Nutr.* **25**, 368.
McKenna, R.J. (1972): *J. Pers. Soc. Psychol.* **22**, 311.
Meyer, J.E. & Pudel, V. (1972): *Psychosom. Res.* **16**, 305.
Meyer, J.E. & Pudel, V. (1977): *Psychosom. Med.* **39**, 153.
Meyer, J.E. & Tuchelt-Gallwitz, A. (1969): *Z. Psychosom. Med.* **13**, 73.
Nisbett, R.E. (1968): *Science* **159**, 1254.
Nisbett, R.E. (1969): *J. Pers. Soc. Psychol.* **10**, 107.
Nisbett, R.E. (1972): *Psychol. Rev.* **79**, 433.
Price, J. & Grinker, J. (1973): *J. Comp. Physiol. Psychol.* **85**, 265.
Pudel, V. (1971): *Z. Ernaehrungswiss*, **10**, 382.
Pudel, V. (1973): *Z. Exp. Angew. Psychol.* **20**, 653.
Pudel, V. (1975): Psychological observations on experimental feeding in the obese. In *Recent advances in obesity research:* 1, ed A. Howard, p. 217. London: Newman.

Pudel, V. (1976): Experimental feeding in man. In *Appetite and food intake* ed T. Silverstone, p. 245. Berlin: Dahlem Konferenzen, Abakon.
Pudel, V., Metzdorff, M. & Oetting, M. (1975): *Z. Psychosom. Med.* 21, 345.
Pudel. V. & Oetting, M. (in press): *Int. J. Obesity* 1, 369.
Rodin, J. (1976): The role perception of internal and external signals on the regulation of feeding in overweight and non-obese individuals. In *Appetite and food intake* ed T. Silverstone, p. 265. Berlin: Dahlem Konferenzen, Abakon.
Schachter, S. (1971): *Am. Psychol.* 26, 129.
Schachter, S., Goldman, R. & Gordon, A. (1968): *J. Pers. Soc. Psychol.* 10, 91.
Schachter, S. & Gross, L. (1968): *J. Pers. Soc. Psychol.* 10, 98.
Schachter, S. & Rodin, J. (1974): *Obese humans and rats.* Washington DC: Erlbaum/Halsted.
Schumacher, J.F. & Wagner, M.K. (1977): *J. Am. Diet. Ass.* 70, 275.
Shaw, J.C. (1973): The influence of food type and method of presentation. Doctoral Dissertation, University of Pennsylvania.
Silverstone, T. & Fincham, J. (in press): Measurement of hunger and food intake. In *Central mechanisms of anoretic drugs* ed S. Garattini & R. Samanin. New York: Raven Press.
Spiegel, T.A. (1973): *J. Comp. Physiol. Psychol.* 84, 24.
Stuart, R.B. (1967): *Behav. Res. Ther.* 5, 357.
Stunkard, A. & Kaplan, D. (1977): *Int. J. Obesity.* 1, 89.
Walike, B.C., Jordan, H.A. & Stellar, E. (1969): *J. Comp. Physiol. Psychol.* 68, 327.
Wooley, O.W. (1971): *Psychosom. Med.* 33, 436.
Wooley, O.W., Wooley, S.C. & Dunham, R.B. (1972*a*): *Physiol. Behav.* 9, 765.
Wooley, O.W., Wooley, S.C. & Dunham, R.B. (1972*b*): *J. Comp. Physiol. Psychol.* 80, 250.
Wooley, O.W., Wooley, S.C. & Woods, W.A. (1975*a*): *J. Comp. Physiol. Psychol.* 89, 619.
Wooley, O.W., Wooley, S.C. & Turner, K. (1975b): The effects of rate of consumption on appetite in the obese and nonobese. In *Recent advances in obesity research: I* ed. A. Howard, p. 212. London: Newman.
Wooley, O.W., Wooley, S.C. & Dunham, R.B. (1976*a*): *Physiol Behav.* 17, 187.
Wooley, O.W., Wooley, S.C. & Williams, B.S. (1976*b*): Salivation as a measure of appetite: studies of the anorectic effects of calories and amphetamine. In *Hunger: basic mechanisms and clinical implications,* ed D. Novin, W. Wyrwicka, G. Bray, p. 421. New York: Raven Press.
Wooley, O.W., Wooley, S.C., Williams, B.S. & Nurre, C. (1977): *Int. J. Obesity* 1, 293.
Wooley, S.C. (1972): *Psychosom. Med.* 34, 62.
Wooley, S.C. & Wooley, O.W. (1973): *Psychosom. Med.* 35, 136.
Wooley, S.C. & Tennenbaum, D. & Wooley, O.W. (in press): *Psychosom. Med.*

9
Has the distinction between internal versus external control of feeding outlived its usefulness?

J. RODIN
Department of Psychology, Yale University, Box 11A Yale Station, New Haven, Connecticut 06510, USA.

While, on one front, investigators were trying to understand obesity as a dysfunction in the metabolic and hormonal economy involved in energy storage and regulation, others were looking for more psychological or behavioral explanations. Stimulating this early research was Bruch's (1961) suggestion that the obese may simply confuse a variety of internal arousal states, such as fear or anxiety, with hunger and therefore eat indiscriminately. When Stunkard & Koch (1964) demonstrated that some overweight people were much less likely than the non-obese to correlate their stomach contractions with the conscious experience of hunger, there was increasing interest in the possibility that obesity was caused by defects in the perception of internal signals of hunger and satiety that served as regulatory mechanisms in the non-obese. Schachter and his colleagues (Schachter, 1971; Schachter & Rodin, 1974) systematically studied this hypothesis in a series of studies whose novelty attracted wide attention since they manipulated hunger and presented food to experimental subjects who were unaware that their eating was being measured. These studies suggested a dichotomy between internal and external control of feeding and went further to suggest that the eating behavior of normal weight people was responsive to internal stimuli. They argued that, by contrast, the eating behavior of overweight people was unresponsive to internal stimuli and instead was primarily controlled by external cues.

Schachter and his associates postulated that internal controls were peripheral and central physiological events within the organism that signalled hunger and satiety. External controls were factors outside the individual that affected eating and its cessation. Included among these were environmental cues such as the time of day, the visual prominence and variety of food, and the sight of other people eating. In addition, cultural habits, family eating practices and attitudes, and social factors may all be considered forms of external controls, although these were not studied by Schachter and his co-workers. Also viewed as external stimuli, and here is where the dividing line gets somewhat hazy, were cognitive cues such as thoughts about food or food imagery, and palatability including the taste and smell of food, which are clearly not simply properties of the food itself, but depend on the state of the organism. Although I have questioned whether or not oropharyngeal stimuli can even be considered external cues (Rodin, 1977), there is a far more basic question that I would like to address in this paper, and that is the evidence for the internal versus external construct itself.

The internal-external distinction is a widely held and widely cited framework. It appears, for example, in every introductory textbook published in psychology in the last five years. Yet it now appears that the injunction of extreme discontinuity between internal-physiological and external-environmental stimuli may have been premature, especially for eating behavior. In addition, there are now also many indications that the internal versus external view is far too simple a description of, or explanation for, differences between obese and normal people.

First, let us consider how this dichotomy was developed initially. Schachter was greatly influenced by the studies of Stunkard & Koch (1964) who reported high correlations between hunger and gastric contractions for normals but not for many overweight individuals. On this basis, he argued that the eating behavior of normals was more influenced by internal signals like gastric motility but that motility was not a hunger cue for the obese, However, in reviewing the role of the gastrointestinal tract in the regulation of food intake, Janowitz (1967) concluded that while deficits of nutrients give rise to a complex of sensations which includes the epigastric hunger pang, gastric hunger contractions appear to be a dispensable component since eating proceeds normally in their absence. In fact, Janowitz claimed that 'at present, no published data exist about any species that indicate whether or not *food intake* or other hunger-motivated behavioral parameters are actually correlated with gastric hunger contractions' (p. 220). Thus, relying heavily on gastric motility as an important internal signal that predicts differential feeding behavior in overweight and normal weight persons was to rely on a cue that does not appear to play a crucial role in the initiation of eating.

The second kind of evidence taken as a lack of internal responsiveness in the obese came from studies demonstrating their failure to respond to caloric preloading as accurately as did normals (Nisbett, 1968; Pliner, 1974; Schachter, Goldman & Gordon, 1968). However, it may simply be that the level of preload used in these and other comparable studies was insufficient to be detected by the overweight subjects. For example, it has been suggested (Nisbett, 1972) that many overweight individuals are physiologically deprived due to dieting or at least due to conscious restraint of their eating. If they are literally starving, they would overeat whether they had already received a 200 or 500 calorie preload since neither of these would be sufficient to satisfy their current nutritional needs. Thus, their short-term feeding could actually be seen as highly responsive to their internal physiological state at the moment.

One does not have to accept the Nisbett hypothesis to predict that overweight and normal weight individuals should not be equally responsive to preloading manipulations. The corpulent person demonstrates a number of metabolic and endocrine abnormalities, generally as a result of overeating and adiposity (Sims *et al.*, 1973). Because of these weight-related metabolic differences, overweight people may be responding to different levels or different kinds of internal signals. This in turn could make them responsive to a different amount or concentration of caloric preload than normals, but not unresponsive.

Third, as concluded by the psychology group of the Dahlem Workshop on appetite and food intake (Wooley *et al.*, 1976), there is now a great deal of evidence that normal weight people also show poor regulation based only on internal signals. Despite evidence that experimental animals are able to adapt relatively promptly and accurately to caloric dilution, studies with normal weight humans have shown that only some subjects are able to compensate over several days for changes in the caloric density of liquid diets and in nearly all cases, consumption is sluggish and incomplete (Campbell, Hashim & Van Itallie, 1971; Jordan, 1969; Spiegel, 1973; O. Wooley, 1971). Other studies examining the short term effects of changes in caloric loading have also shown that internal signals do not appropriately guide eating behavior towards stable caloric intake for most people unless cognitive or external cues regarding amount are also present (Spiegel, 1973; S. Wooley, 1972). These results strongly suggest that very few people can ordinarily perceive variations in deprivation within the moderate or physiologic range.

The studies using a preload-test meal paradigm are also difficult to assess because the test meal forces the initiation of eating in a situation in which the natural response might have been to delay eating. Once a meal is begun, there is a tendency to continue eating until satiety. Thus probability of eating cannot be equated with amount consumed in such experimental probes. The temporal features of eating therefore still have to be examined in order to understand the integrated relationship between those internal physiological and external variables that influence both the initiation and the termination of feeding.

Finally, most people are responsive to some external food cues. Moreover, a variety of studies have shown that there are people in all weight categories who are *highly* responsive to these external cues. We have tested several hundred subjects with varying degrees of overweight in our studies and found that degree of overweight was not well correlated with degree of responsiveness to external cues. However, using scores of external responsiveness standardized on the entire sample in each study, we did find that when group averages were compared, moderately overweight subjects were more external than either the normals or the extremely obese. This finding was consistent from study to study and was true for consumption of good-tasting milkshakes (Rodin, 1975); ratings of the palatability of increasingly sweet-tasting glucose solutions (Rodin, Moskowitz & Bray, 1976); ratings of the palatability of milkshakes that differed in sweetness but not in caloric value (Rodin, 1975); responsiveness to preloads of varying caloric density (Rodin *et al.*, 1976); and eating and non-eating responses to manipulations of external cue salience (Rodin, Slochower & Fleming, 1977). Moderately overweight subjects also appeared most willing to work to obtain a highly preferred milkshake when permitted to sample it first. However, the actual ease or difficulty of ingesting the milkshake (manipulated by straw width) once they obtained it, had a greater impact on their preference ratings and level of consumption than it did for either normal weight people or the extremely obese (Rodin, 1975). These results are all based on group means however, and since we have demonstrated that there are some externally responsive individuals in every weight category, I believe it is no longer sufficient to categorize either experimental subjects or clinical patients on the basis of weight alone. This is especially true since we have found that responsiveness to external stimuli among overweight people does not change – either to increase or decrease – as a function of weight gain or loss.

These data, and others that I will present later, lead me to conclude that overeating, in the short term, is controlled to a great extent by external and social factors. Indeed we have demonstrated (Rodin & Slochower, 1976) that high responsiveness leads to overeating and weight gain even among normal weight people placed in a food abundant environment. But whether or not the person becomes overweight, and the degree of obesity attained, is determined by mechanisms for weight regulation that have little or nothing to do with external responsiveness. Let us return to the issue of short-term controls.

To summarise, there are clear difficulties, outlined above, with a view that dichotomizes internal and external controls and then uses this distinction to explain differences between overweight and normal weight people. The extreme separation of these factors is no longer conceptually useful nor empirically supported. Instead internal and external factors depend upon, and should in part be defined by, the state and role of the other rather than as two opposite ends of the same continuum. For example, it is certainly true that external cues always trigger eating against a background of certain physiological conditions. In most studies, overweight individuals have consumed more than normals, but often not everything, suggesting that consumption may influence responsiveness to external stimuli either by changing the perceived palatability of the food stimulus (Cabanac, 1971) or through some other post-absorptive consequence of food. Indeed, internal factors may play an important role in modulating responses to sensory or external signals. An explicit link between these factors has been drawn by Cabanac and his associates (Cabanac, 1971; Cabanac & Duclaux, 1970) who demonstrated that the pleasantness of sweet taste is determined, in part, by the nutritional needs of the organism. Sweet taste appears especially good when the individual is deprived and relatively unpleasant after satiety. There have been several studies examining the effects of body weight and/or deprivation on palatability (Grinker, 1976; Nisbett, 1968, 1972; Rodin, 1975; Rodin *et al.*, 1976) which show that level of acute and chronic energy supply do indeed affect palatability. These relationships are complex, however, and depend in part on the way energy deficit is accomplished, current level of body weight and the type of food being tasted.

Level of deprivation also affects thoughts of food, and extreme hunger, as Keys and his co-workers (1950) have demonstrated, can lead to obsessional food fantasies. Hunger affects how appealing various foods look and how much is purchased in a supermarket (Nisbett & Kanouse, 1969). In addition, the Wooleys and their co-workers have demonstrated that level of deprivation and rate of eating affect the salivary response to highly palatable stimuli. Salivation is greater to palatable food presented one hour after a high calorie meal and when a meal is eaten quickly rather than slowly (Wooley, Wooley & Woods, 1975).

It now seems likely that the opposite direction of influence is true. In other words, external stimuli can directly influence internal physiological states. We pursued this question in our laboratory when we asked whether heightened external responsiveness could lead to overeating by triggering physiological responses. As one example of such a process, Teitelbaum and his co-workers (Wolgin, Cytawa & Teitelbaum, 1976) suggested that external and sensory stimuli (taste, smell, sight of food) have a general activating component which energizes the organism. These are separate from their directing and incentive value, although the degree of arousal may depend, in part, on the hedonic value of the stimuli. They argued that this arousal plays a crucial role in the control of feeding, and that lack of activation may be a contributing factor to the lack of interest in food seen in lateral hypothalamic-lesioned animals.

The view takes on added significance in the light of Marshall's data (1975, 1976) from animals with unilateral ventromedial hypothalamic lesions. Since the neural region on one side of the brain is responsive to the external environment on the contralateral side, Marshall varied the location of food-dispensing dishes for these animals. He first found that 13 of the 14 rats with unilateral damage showed an increase in responsiveness to contralateral sensory stimuli of all kinds; they showed increased orienting, exaggerated response to whisker touch, head turning, increased biting of noxious stimuli, and aggressive responses to attack. Most important, when eating, the unilateral animals began taking a significantly greater proportion of their daily food from the contralateral food dish. This suggests that the lesion itself was enhancing cue responsiveness. In other words, medial damage might produce hyperresponsiveness which influences the animal's reactivity to external stimuli. This in turn influences feeding. Gibson & Gazzaniga (1971) noted a similar finding in split brain monkeys with unilateral hypothalamic damage. Such monkeys overate only when using the eye that projected to the hemisphere with the ventromedial lesion, suggesting that external visual cues were what influenced overeating.

Marshall (1976) suggested that medial damage might produce hyperresponsiveness by increasing activity within catecholamine-containing systems, such as the nigrostriatal bundle, that run through the hypothalamus. In intact animals, arousal appears to increase catecholaminergic activity within these same pathways, and external cues seem to be responsible for insuring the release of appropriate behaviors from the behavioral repertoire in response to this arousal. Certainly one can argue for the biological significance of a mechanism by which an aroused organism would be better off to attend and respond to salient external stimuli. A non-monotonic relationship is expected, however, since at the extreme of arousal such attention would be, by and large, maladaptive. This line of reasoning is further supported by studies with animals, showing that low doses of D-amphetamine (Glick & Muller, 1971) and mild tail pinch (Antelman, Rowland & Fisher, 1975; Rowland & Antelman, 1976) reliably induce eating in sated rats. The eating behavior appears quite normal, proceeds without obvious pain, and if the tail pinch procedures or amphetamine administration continues over days, the animals gain weight.

Pharmacological studies have led to the proposal by Antelman and Fisher and their colleagues that tail pinch-induced eating also involves preferential facilitation of brain catecholaminergic function leading to a heightened sensitivity and responsivity to most survival-oriented and/or pre-potent environmental stimuli. They suggest that the tail pinch induces a consumatory response by heightening the valence of sensory cues from available environmental stimuli and recently have presented data that precisely parallel our human data (Rodin, 1977; Schachter & Rodin, 1974). For example, they show that there is less tail pinch-induced drinking for quinine adulturated milk and greater drinking for sweetened milk than in non-tail pinched animals. Thus the hedonic value of the external stimulus may be a key determining factor for the tail pinch phenomenon. The dopamine-mediated disinhibitory action of the tail pinch could lower sensory motor thresholds and promote heightened sensitivity and responsivity to environmental stimuli that are salient or high in hedonic value.

These converging lines of evidence may be summarized as follows: activation and arousal by external stimuli are related to the return of normal feeding in LH lesioned and dopamine depleted animals, and hyperarousal in response to external stimuli appears to be related to overeating in VMH lesioned animals, in tail pinch-induced animals, and in many overweight people. In each of these groups, heightened responsiveness to external stimuli leads to weight gain over time. The neurochemical pathways involved in these responses are involved in the general arousal of the organism and its specific responsiveness to hedonically valued external stimuli. As Stricker & Zigmond (1976) have suggested, an external stimulus would thus be seen as having two effects — a specific one which activates neurons that are involved in eliciting some appropriate motivational state and a non-specific one that removes a gate and thereby permits such responses actually to occur. Thus an individual could literally be turned on by an external stimulus, and at the same time arousal makes an organism even more responsiveness to external stimuli. The neurochemical link between responsivity, arousal and feeding systems has exciting implications for the study of external responsiveness in human obesity.

At present I am certainly not arguing for the underlying anatomical or neurochemical dysfunction of these responses in humans. However, others have proposed, notably Maddi (1968), and Thayer (1967), that there are large individual differences both with regard to rate of activation change and basal levels of arousal. These individual differences may be especially important for eating. I think that this same line of reasoning can also explain arousal-induced eating in many overweight people without relying on psychodynamic explanations. While there is no good evidence to date that arousal increases hunger or that overeating is anxiety reducing (Leon & Roth, 1977), arousal can lead to overeating even in normal weight organisms, based on the mechanism that I have just outlined.

In addition to general arousal, a second role of external cues on internal processes would arise from the effects of these cues on metabolic events or digestive processes. The Wooleys have demonstrated that salivary response to a food stimulus varies as a function of palatability of the food and beliefs regarding its caloric value and its availability for subsequent ingestion (Wooley & Wooley, 1973). We reasoned that insulin release would be a major candidate for an intervening physiological mechanism that might be responsive to external stimuli. Insulin is involved in promoting increased ingestion and in increased storage of nutrients as fat.

In rats, Nicolaidis (1969) and Steffens (1970) have both demonstrated an early release of insulin in response to gustatory stimuli, and recently Woods and his colleagues (1977) reported that rats develop the tendency to secrete insulin in the presence of stimuli that reliably predict the opportunity to eat. In some instances this was time of day and in others, odor. Most directly relevant, however, was the report of Parra-Covarrubias, Rivera-Rodriguez & Alamaraz-Vgalde (1971) that obese adolescents tended to secrete insulin at the sight and smell of food. In this study, however, no normal weight persons were tested as a control group and the first blood sample was taken after five minutes, thus eliminating the possibility of assessing an early insulin response if it were to occur.

To consider this question, we have followed the same basic procedure in several studies. All subjects are non-diabetic with normal glucose tolerance. Subjects are advised to eat at least 40 per cent of their diets as carbohydrates for three days prior to the study. They come to the laboratory at lunch time, having eaten nothing since dinner at 7 p.m. on the previous evening. In order to minimize stress, an indwelling catheter is placed under local xylocaine anesthesia in an antecubital vein and kept open with a slow i.v. drip of saline solution. After three control bloods are taken, a partly cooked beefsteak is brought in and grilled, crackling in a frying pan in front of the subject, to provide rich visual, auditory and olfactory food cues. Try to picture yourself sitting there, hungry, watching, hearing, and smelling a large juicy steak that the experimenters have promised you will soon be able to eat!

Small continuous blood samples are taken for the first ten minutes and then again at 15 and 20 minutes after the presentation of the steak. At -3, +3, and +20 minutes, subjects rate their hunger and at +3, and +20 minutes they also rate how appetizing the steak looks; in other words, how much they would like to eat it right at that moment.

On the next figure are some pilot data, based on only three overweight (+18 per cent to +60 per cent OW) and four normal weight (-6 per cent to +8 per cent OW) subjects. The mean fasting plasma immunoreactive insulin level was 18.7 μU/ml in the obese compared to 10.4 μU/ml in the normal weight subjects and the data are expressed as change scores from basal. Figure 1 shows a biphasic secretion of insulin: both an early phase that peaks at two to three minutes and a later phase rising again at 15 to 20 minutes after stimulus introduction.

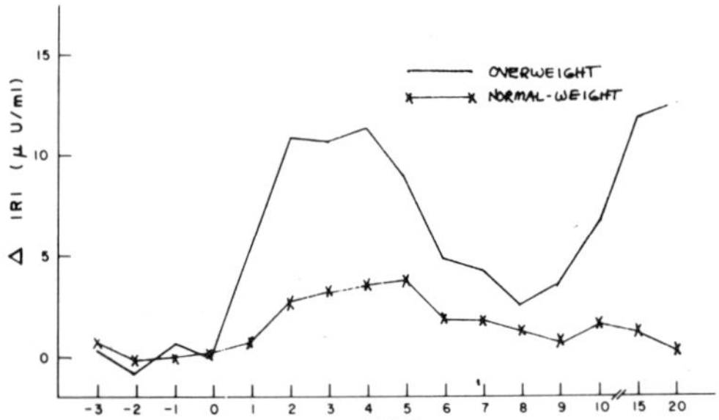

Fig. 1. Mean plasma insulin levels in 18-hour deprived overweight and normal weight subjects. Scores are expressed as a change from basal levels in response to presentation of a grilling steak

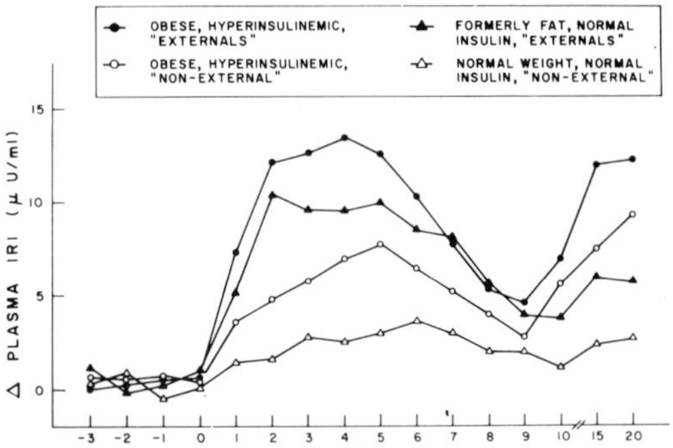

Fig. 2. Mean plasma insulin levels in 18-hour deprived overweight and normal weight subjects grouped according to prior assessments of their degree of responsiveness to external stimuli. Scores are expressed as a change from basal levels in response to presentation of a grilling steak

If this is a real effect, the first possibility is that it is due to the B cell - either because the B cell has been reset by obesity or because the obese are typically hyperinsulinemic. Since insulin release obeys the law of initial values, hyperinsulinemia alone could have made them more responsive. However, we know that a hypocaloric diet and some weight loss leads to a drop in basal insulin to normal levels. Therefore, we replicated the first study using several subject groups including dieted, formerly overweight people.

Eleven stabilized overweight subjects were selected. Five were highly responsive to food-relevant environmental stimuli as assessed by prior ingestion and performance measures used reliably in our laboratory (cf. Rodin *et al.*, 1977), and six were not externally responsive by these measures. Both groups had high basal insulin levels, averaging 20.4 μU/ml and 23.2 μU/ml respectively. There were five non-externally responsive, normal weight subjects with an average basal insulin of 11.6 μU/ml and five formerly overweight subjects who were currently within normal weight range and whose basal insulin levels averaged 12.6 μU/ml—well within the normal range.

Figure 2 shows some contribution of hyperinsulinemia but more from external responsiveness. In other words, regardless of current weight, those individuals whose eating behavior was most responsive to environmental stimuli associated with food, show the greatest insulin response to the sight and smell and sound of the grilling steak.

In the next experiment, we asked whether the magnitude of the hormonal response was correlated with the palatability of the food stimulus. Wooley & Wooley (1973) found that degree of salivation to food stimuli varied directly with their subject-rated appeal, and we expected the same sort of relationship for insulin release. Palatability was determined in advance by presenting a pilot group of subjects with a list of foods and asking them to rate how much they would like to eat each of them at that moment. This time the foods were all carbohydrates. All pilot subjects had been fasted overnight and so were in a state of deprivation identical to that which was to be used in the study itself.

The experimental subjects (n = 10) were then tested on two separate days with presentations of foods at three palatability levels of increasing goodness (1, 5, and 9,), and no food. Two were presented each day, separated by half an hour in counterbalanced order, and in a double blind procedure in which the food stimulus or an empty plate was presented.

Table 1 shows that overweight, externally responsive subjects had an insulin response which was significantly more affected by palatability than the normal weight non-external subjects. If externally responsive people oversecrete insulin in the presence of compelling food cues, they might eat more calories in order to balance this hormonal and metabolic output and they might also store more of the food in fat. Thus appetite is stimulated and overeating may result as a consequence of increased responsiveness to potent, palatable stimuli.

Table 1. Peak change in plasma insulin within five minutes after presentation (μU/ml) of no food or one of three foods varying in palatability

Group		Palatability		
	No food	1	5	9
Overweight externals	3	−2	7	13
Normal weight non-externals	0	1	3	6

Food industries have been attempting to fabricate palatable, low calorie analogs of certain foods rich in energy. However, it is not clear whether this approach would actually help many overweight people to diet and lose weight. If the original internal-external formulation were entirely correct, the obese who are presumably highly external should be just as satisfied by the calorically dilute food analogs as by the calorically concentrated original, so long as each food tasted about the same. Based on the internal versus external framework, their high external responsiveness and minimal perception of internal signals should allow them to meet their hedonic needs at a lower caloric price. By contrast, on the basis of the data that I have just described, we might expect the low calorie, good tasting cues to stimulate metabolic responses and subsequent overeating in the same way as their high calorie counterparts. Indeed, Nicolaidis (1969) reports the same metabolic effect for buccal stimulation with nutritive or non-nutritive sweet solutions. Thus a piece of sweet diet chewing gum or some rich tasting visually compelling low calorie cake may stimulate hunger and food seeking, or lead to greater consumption if food is already available. In fact, the richer looking and tasting the food stimulus, regardless of the food's actual caloric value, the more it might stimulate the appetite. This provides a double bind: it does not provide ample calories to satiate and may actually encourage subsequent seeking and/or ingestion of other, more calorically dense foods.

It is possible that some portion of this insulin response is reflexive and another portion is conditioned as certain salient food stimuli are consistently paired with eating. If so, weight reduction procedures might focus more on explicit extinction techniques for these associative links that are related to the onset of eating rather than, or in addition to, reprogramming the environment with behavior modification (Jordan, 1975; Stuart, 1975).

External and sensory cues may also trigger physiological states relevant to the termination of feeding. Since the energy-relevant physiological consequences of eating may occur too slowly to play a major role in the cessation of intake, it has recently been suggested by Booth (1972, 1976), following the work of LeMagnen (1969), that sensory qualities of food such as taste or texture or environmental stimuli such as time or place (Woods *et al.*, 1977) may participate in the control of intake as conditioned stimuli. Presumably the pairing of these sensory qualities of food with the delayed physiological consequences of ingestion can and do occur and could subsequently guide eating. The specific physiological unconditioned stimuli for this associative process are, as yet, unclear but the notion is intriguing and has important clinical implications if it is correct. Epstein (1967) and Kraly (1976) both suggest that oral sensations are also capable of leading to the behavioral sequence of satiety in animals (termination of feeding, grooming, etc.) even in the absence of ingestion and absorption. However, full satiety requires both that the receptors of the oropharynx be stimulated and that the material reach the stomach and be absorbed (Young *et al.*, 1974).

It is on satiety that there is already the clearest evidence for the possibility of an interaction. Whether this is also true for purely external stimuli needs to be tested. Cabanac and his associates have demonstrated that the pleasantness of the smell or taste of food stimuli diminishes after a meal or a glucose load. Cabanac (personal communication) believes that the internal signal for this phenomenon is concentration of the stimulus. It still has not been empirically validated that this shift in perceived palatability actually plays a role in the termination of feeding but that possibility seems quite likely.

In another demonstration of how internal state might affect responsiveness to sensory cues, we (Rodin *et al.*, 1976) recently reported that patients with intestinal bypass surgery resulting in a greatly shortened intestinal tract showed a preference curve for sweetness intensity that changed dramatically after surgery and in a direction which was identical to the curve obtained for normals. This is demonstrated in Fig. 3. Figure 4 shows that obese people who lost relatively identical amounts of weight by dieting did not show this changed preference curve following weight loss. The bypass patients also spontaneously reduced their food intake. These data suggest local changes in the intestinal tract itself, for example, the

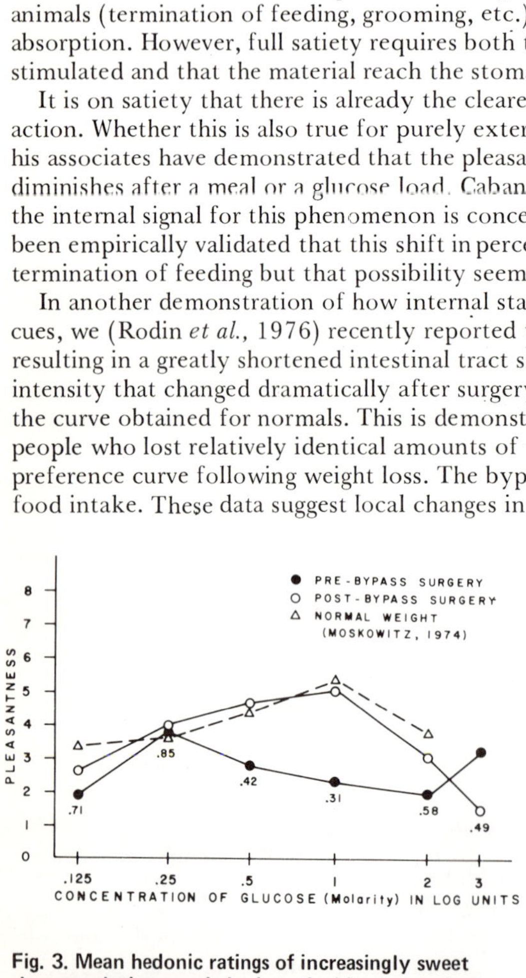

Fig. 3. Mean hedonic ratings of increasingly sweet glucose solutions made by intestinal bypass patients before and after surgery and weight loss. A typical curve for normal weight people from Moskowitz, 1971 is superimposed for comparison. (From Rodin, Moskowitz & Bray, 1976)

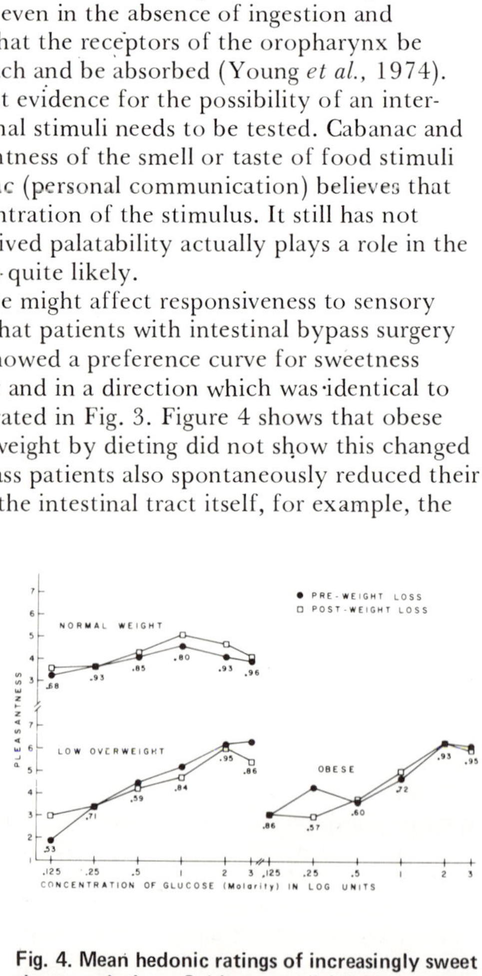

Fig. 4. Mean hedonic ratings of increasingly sweet glucose solutions. Subjects are divided into groups on the basis of their degree of overweight prior to weight loss and tested before and at the conclusion of a two-month weight reduction program

amount of intact absorptive surface remaining or number of local glucoreceptors, might influence sweet taste of perception and amount of food consumed.

Thus we must conclude that eating is regulated by a multiple process governed by interactions among physiological, sensory, cognitive and external factors. The act of eating involves the integration of these systems, even in the disordered state of obesity. I believe that the data no longer support the internal versus external distinction to explain overweight-normal weight differences. At present it should be used mainly as an organizing principle for the human literature of the late 1960s and early 1970s since most work during that period was articulated within that framework. It is my belief that theoretical developments and clinical applications will advance fruitfully from a conceptualization which acknowledges the bidirectional influence of internal and external control factors and then seeks to explain how they can produce overeating and obesity.

Summary

The studies of Schachter and his co-workers suggested a dichotomy between internal and external control of feeding and went further to suggest that the eating behavior of normal weight people was responsive to internal stimuli. They argued that, by contrast, the eating behavior of overweight people was unresponsive to internal stimuli and instead was primarily controlled by external cues. Internal controls were peripheral and central physiological events within the organism that signalled hunger and satiety. External controls were factors outside the individual such as time of day that affected eating and its cessation. It now appears however that the injunction of extreme discontinuity between internal-physiological and external-environmental stimuli may have been premature especially for eating behavior. Further, there are now many indications that the internal versus external view is far too simple a description of, or explanation for differences between obese and normal people. These include evidence that gastric motility is a dispensable component for hunger-motivated behavior including intake, that most people regardless of weight have difficulty adjusting their eating on the basis of disguised variations in caloric dilution alone, and that most people regardless of weight are somewhat responsive to external food cues and some in all weight categories are highly responsive.

Instead of putting internal and external controls against one another, they should be seen as depending upon and influencing one another quite directly. Internal factors may play an important role in modulating responses to sensory or external signals and reciprocally, external stimuli can directly influence internal physiological states. One example of the second process is the general activating property of external and sensory cues which energizes the organism. These are separate from the directing and incentive value of such stimuli although the magnitude of the degree of arousal may depend, in part, on hedonic value of these stimuli. In addition to general arousal, a second role of external cues on internal processes would arise from the effects of these cues on digestive processes or metabolic events. It now appears that insulin, which is involved in hunger and the storage of nutrients as fat, is responsive to variations in external stimuli among certain individuals. Those people whose food consumption is most influenced by manipulations of external food-relevant cues show the greatest increase in insulin levels when shown food which they believe they will soon eat. The magnitude of the response increases with the palatability of the stimulus. Not only onset of eating is affected by these reciprocal processes; it is with regard to satiety that there is already the clearest evidence for the possibility of an interaction of internal state and sensory cues.

References

Antelman, S.M., Rowland, N.E. & Fisher, A.E. (1975): *Physiol. Behav.* **17**, 743.
Booth, D.A. (1972): *J. Comp. Physiol. Psychol.* **81**, 475.

Booth, D.A. (1976): Approaches to feeding control. In *Appetite and food intake*, ed T. Silverstone. Berlin: Dahlem Konferenzen, Abakon.
Bruch, H. (1961): *J. Nerv. Men. Dis.* **133**, 46.
Cabanac, M. & Duclaux, R. (1970): *Science* **168**, 469.
Cabanac, M. (1971): *Science* **173**, 1103.
Campbell, R.G., Hashim, S.A. & Van Itallie, T.B. (1971): *New Engl. J. Med.* **285**, 1402.
Epstein, A.N. (1967): Oropharyngeal factors in feeding and drinking. In *Handbook of physiology: alimentary canal, I*, ed C.F. Code. Washington, DC: American Physiological Society.
Gibson, A.R. & Gazzaniga, M.S. (1971): *Physiologist* **14**, 150.
Glick, S.D. & Muller, R.U. (1971): *Psychopharmacologia* **22**, 396.
Grinker, J. (1976): Taste factors in human and animal obesity. In *Hunger: basic mechanisms and clinical implications*, ed D. Novin, W. Wyrwicka & G. Bray. New York: Raven Press.
Janowitz, H.D. (1967): Role of the gastrointestinal tract in the regulation of food intake. In *Handbook of physiology: alimentary canal*, I, ed C.F. Code. Washington DC: American Physiological Society.
Jordan, H.A. (1969): *J. Comp. Physiol. Psychol.* **68**, 498.
Jordan, H.A. (1975): Physiological control of food intake in man. In *Obesity in perspective*, ed G.A. Bray. Washington DC: US Govt. Ptg. Office.
Keys, A., Brozek, J., Henschel, A., Mickelson, D. & Taylor, H. (1950): *The biology of human starvation.* Minneapolis: University of Minnesota.
Kraly, F.S. (1976): Pre-gastric stimuli are sufficient for short-term satiety in 3-hour food deprived rats. Paper presented at Eastern Psychological Association meeting, New York.
LeMagnen, J. (1969): *Ann. N.Y. Acad. Sci.* **157**, 1126.
Leon, G.R. & Roth, L. (1977): *Psychol. Bull.* **84**, 117.
Maddi, S.R. (1968): *Personality theories: a comparative analysis.* Homewood, Illinois: Dorsey Press.
Marshall, J. (1975): *Brain Res.* **86**, 373.
Marshall, J. (1976): Neurochemistry of central monoamine systems as related to food intake. In *Appetite and food intake*, ed T. Silverstone. Berlin: Dahlem Konferenzen, Abakon.
Nicolaides, S. (1969): *Ann. N.Y. Acad. Sci.* **157**, 1176.
Nisbett, R.E. (1968): *J. Pers. Soc. Psychol.* **10**, 107.
Nisbett, R.E. (1972): *Psychol. Rev.* **79**, 433.
Nisbett, R.E. & Kanouse, D. (1969): *J. Pers. Soc. Psychol.* **12**, 289.
Parra-Covarrubias, A., Rivera-Rodriguez., I. & Almaraz-Vgalde, A. (1971): *Diabetes* **20**, 800.
Pliner, P. (1974): On the generalizability of the externality hypothesis. In *Obese humans and rats*, ed S. Schachter & J. Rodin. Washington, DC: Erlbaum/Halsted.
Rodin, J. (1975): *J. Comp. Physiol. Psychol.* **89**, 100.
Rodin, J. (1977): *Personality Soc. Psychol. Bull.* **3**, 333.
Rodin, J., Moskowitz, H.R. & Bray, G.A. (1976): *Physiol. Behav.* **17**, 591.
Rodin, J. & Slochower, J. (1976): *J. Pers. Soc. Psychol.* **33**, 338.
Rodin, J., Slochower, J. & Fleming, B. (1977): *J. Comp. Physiol. Psychol.* **91**, 586.
Rowland, N. & Antelman, S. (1976): *Science* **191**, 310.
Schachter, S. (1968): *Science* **161**, 751.
Schachter, S. (1971): *Emotion, obesity and crime.* New York: Academic Press.
Schachter, S., Goldman, R. & Gordon, A. (1968): *J. Pers. Soc. Psych.* **10**, 91.
Schachter, S. & Rodin, J. (1974): *Obese humans and rats.* Washington, DC: Erlbaum/Wiley.
Sims, E.A.H., Danforth, E. Jr., Horton, E.S., Bray, G.A., Glennon, J.A., & Salans, L.B. (1973): *Recent progress in hormonal research* **29**, 457.
Spiegel, T. (1973): *J. Comp. Physiol. Psychol.* **83**, 24.
Steffens, A.B. (1975): *Am. J. Physiol.* **228**, 1738.
Stricker, E.M. & Zigmond, M.J. (1976): Brain catecholamines and the lateral hypothalamic syndrome. In *Hunger: basic mechanisms and clinical implications*, ed D. Novin, W. Wyrwicka & G.A. Bray. New York: Raven Press.
Stuart, R.B. (1975): Behavioral control of overeating: a status report. In *Obesity in perspective*, ed G.A. Bray. Washington DC: US Govt. Ptg. Office.
Stunkard, A.J. & Koch, C. (1964): *Archs Gen. Psychiat.* **11**, 74.
Thayer, R.E. (1967): *Psychol. Rep.* **20**, 663.
Wolgin, D.L., Cytawa, J. & Teitelbaum, P. (1976): The role of activation in the regulation of food intake. In *Hunger: basic mechanisms and clinical implications*, ed D. Novin, W. Wyrwicka & G.A. Bray. New York: Raven Press.
Woods, S.C., Vasselli, J.E., Kaestner, E., Szakmary, G.A., Milburn, P., & Vitiello, M.V. (1977): *J. Comp. Physiol. Psychol.* **91**, 128.
Wooley, O.W. (1971): *Psychosom. Med.* **33**, 436.
Wooley, O.W., Wooley, S.C. & Woods, W.A. (1975): *J. Comp. Physiol. Psychol.* **89**, 619.

Wooley, S.C. (1972): *Psychosom. Med.* 34, 62.
Wooley, S.C., & Wooley, O.W. (1973): *Psychosom. Med.* 35, 136.
Wooley, S.C., Wooley, O.W., Bartoshuk, L.M., Cabanac, M.J.C., Feistl, R., Gutezert, G.W.R., McFarland, D.J., Oetting, M., Pudel, V.E., Rodin, J. & Simoons, F.J. (1976): Psychological aspects of feeding group. In *Appetite and food intake,* ed T. Silverstone. Berlin: Dahlem Konferenzen, Abakon.
Young, C.M., Scalan, S.S., Topping, C.M. *et al.* (1971): *J. Am. Diet. Ass.* 59, 466

10
Psychological and behavioural factors in weight loss

P. LEY
Reader in Psychology, University of Queensland, St. Lucia, Queensland, Australia 4067.

The problem of clients' and patients' non-compliance with advice has received increasing attention over the past decade (Davis, 1966; Ley & Spelman, 1967; Stewart & Cluff, 1972; Mitchell, 1974; Sackett & Haynes, 1976). The magnitude of the general problem can be seen in Table 1 (from Ley, 1976).

Table 1. The frequency with which patients fail to follow medical advice

Type of advice	No. of studies	Percentage of patients who did not follow advice		
		Range	Mean	Median
A. Medicine taking				
(1) PAS and other TB drugs	20	8-76	37.5	35
(2) Antibiotics	8	11-92	48.7	50
(3) Psychiatric drugs	9	11-51	38.6	44
(4) Other medicines, e.g. antacids, iron	12	9-87	47.7	57.5
B. Diet	11	20-84	49.4	45
C. Other advice, e.g. child care, ante-natal exercises	8	30-79	54.6	51
D. All advice	68	8-92	44.0	44.35

Ley *et al.* (1974) argued that investigation of the management of obesity, as well as being of intrinsic importance, would provide valuable data on the problem of non-compliance in general. Two of the main advantages of studying the obese are that they are not hard to find and that therefore large-scale experiments are feasible, and that weight loss provides an objective measure of compliance with advice.

The experiments to be described have all been concerned with the instigation and maintenance of short-term weight loss by the manipulation of variables which it was thought would affect compliance with a dietary regimen.

Subjects involved have been women between the ages of 20 and 60, who answered newspaper and television appeals for obese subjects to help in research on the topic. All have been at least 10 per cent over the average weight for their age group as assessed by the norms provided by Montegriffo (1968). The majority of the subjects have been in the age group 30 to 49, and the median per cent overweight has fallen somewhere in the range 30 to 39. A detailed description of these characteristics for one sample of subjects is given by Ley *et al.*

(1974) and the one experiment which does not conform to the above description is that of Ley *et al.* (1977*a*) for which full descriptive details are given by Yorke, Holland & Massey-Lynch (1973). The experiments were all conducted in the United Kingdom, and no charge was made to subjects. The diet used was the Servier low carbohydrate diet, copies of which were kindly provided by the company.

A scheme of the experimental programme is given in Fig. 1.

Fig. 1. The experimental programme

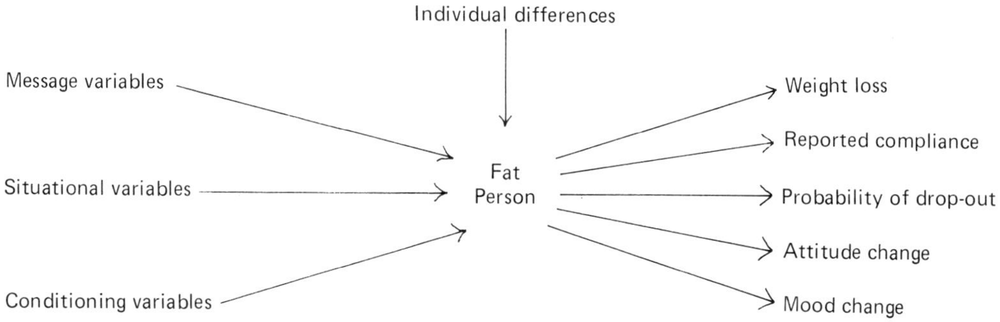

The message variables investigated have been sidedness of communication; comprehensibility and ability to remember; fear arousal; position of fear message; and frequency of fear message. Detailed justification for investigating these variables has been provided by Ley *et al.* (1974), Ley *et al.* (1977*b*), and Skilbeck, Tulips & Ley (1977). Briefly, it would be expected that two-sided communications would lead to greater resistance to counter-propaganda and thus to better long-term compliance; that more understandable and more easily remembered messages would produce better results; and that the use of degree of fear arousal, the position of fear arousal in relation to recommendations and the frequency of such arousal might well exert effects.

The situational variables studied have included the effects of group membership; the channel used to convey the messages, and group cohesiveness. More detailed justification for investigating these variables is given by Ley & Spelman (1967) and Ley *et al.* (1977*b*). The question of whether group situations produce more compliance than individual ones, and whether the degree to which the group is a cohesive one makes any difference are obviously sensible ones to ask in the light of what is known in the field of group dynamics (Shaw, 1971). It is also sensible to investigate the relative effectiveness of messages presented by a person in the flesh as opposed to a person on a videotape or as opposed to leaflet presentation.

Experiments on classical and operant conditioning have also been conducted. The effects of self-control procedures, a system of reinforcement with points and classical aversive and appetitive conditioning have been investigated. Detailed reviews of the literature on conditioning as treatment for obesity are provided by Stuart & Davis (1972); Yates (1975); Stunkard & Mahoney (1976). In the present series, experiments were conducted partly for their own sake and partly to provide some comparative data on the effectiveness of both novel and established conditioning procedures on weight loss in samples such as ours.

The individual differences investigated have included the personality variables of extraversion-introversion; neuroticism; perceived locus of control; attitudinal variables; degree of fear experienced by subjects after hearing frightening messages; and such mundane things as knowledge of the diet, initial starting weights, and initial weight loss. The other variables in the diagram are self-explanatory.

In most of the experiments, designs using factorial analysis or variance have been used and in all experiments subjects have been assigned at random to experimental conditions. The usual sequence of the experiments has been an initial treatment phase followed by follow-up at two, four and eight weeks, with several experiments providing a 16 week follow-up as well. However, in order to standardize the presentation of results, these are given for the eight-week follow-up. In general, 16-week follow-up results have been the same as for eight weeks except that drop-out rates were higher. More detailed accounts of these experiments are given elsewhere (Ley *et al.*, 1974; Ley *et al.*, 1977*a, b;* Skilbeck *et al.*, 1977, and Whitworth *et al.*, 1977). Brief summaries of each experiment are given in the Appendix. Experiments are numbered and numbers in the tables in the Results section refer to the experiments as numbered in the Appendix.

Results

Before turning to the detailed results, it will be useful to summarize the information given to subjects in the experiments with message variables. This consisted of a definition of overweight; statements to the effect that overweight was caused by taking in too many calories; a summary of the dangers of being overweight; and the recommendation that adherence to a diet was the best way to lose weight. Sidedness of communication was manipulated in the sections on the dangers of being overweight and methods of weight loss. In the two-sided version, possible advantages of being overweight were listed and countered, and in the Methods section possible methods of weight loss other than dieting were described and refuted. Fear arousal was manipulated in the section on consequences of being overweight, by the description of the dangers in more or less vivid detail. Differences in level of fear arousal were checked in three ways: (1) ratings by judges, (2) ratings by subjects, (3) post-lecture fear level as assessed by standardized anxiety checklists. In the experiments on fear, the fear-arousing material was placed either at the beginning, or just before the recommendation, or right at the end of the lecture.

Weight losses are reported as mean weight in kilograms lost by the indicated groups of subjects.

The effects of message variables

The prediction made for the effects of sidedness of communication is that while one-sided communications might produce better initial results, two-sided ones will overtake them and produce better results in the long run. Technically, there should be an interaction between sidedness and time. No such interaction has been found nor has sidedness produced any overall differences, as can be seen in Table 2 (Ley *et al.*, 1977*b*; Skilbeck *et al.*, 1977).

The prediction for the ease of understanding and remembering messages was that, the easier the message was to understand and remember, the greater would be the compliance. In the three experiments summarized in Table 3, subjects were told that the main programme was oversubscribed but that to avoid disappointment they could be given the information in leaflet form. The standard leaflet was moderately easy as assessed by the Flesch Formula (Flesch, 1948; Ley 1973), while the experimental leaflet was very easy, contained repetition,

Table 2. Effects of one-sided versus two-sided communications on weight loss

	Weight loss kg		
	2 weeks	4 weeks	8 weeks
Experiment No. 1			
1-sided	2.00	2.27	2.86
2-sided	2.49	2.99	3.90
Experiment No. 4			
1-sided	2.59	4.13	5.40
2-sided	2.81	4.45	5.81

and was explicitly categorized. These features have been shown to affect comprehensibility and ease of memorizing (Ley *et al.*, 1972, 1973; Bradshaw *et al.*, 1975). Both leaflets contained basic information given in the standard two-sided moderate fear lecture. Despite an impressive initial success, it can be seen in Table 3 that two out of three experiments produced negative results (Ley, 1976; Ley *et al.*, 1977*b*).

Table 3. Effects of comprehensibility and memorability on weight loss at eight weeks

		Weight loss kg	
	Expt. No. 7	Expt. No. 9	Expt. No. 10
High comprehensibility and memorability leaflet	5.58	3.40	4.49
Control leaflet	3.49	3.76	4.67
p	(<0.01)	(ns)	(ns)

Predictions as to the effects of fear arousal vary depending on which theorist is preferred. Janis's (1967) theory would in general predict curvilinear relationships between fear and compliance, while Leventhal (1970) would not be surprised to find non-curvilinear ones. In the present experiments, three levels of fear were used with the results shown in Table 4 which also shows the relationship between fear *experienced* by the subjects after hearing the lecture and their subsequent weight loss (Ley *et al.*, 1974; Skilbeck *et al.*, 1977).

Table 4. Effects of fear-arousingness of message and fear aroused by message on weight loss at eight weeks

	Weight loss kg	
	Expt. No. 1	Expt. No. 4
Level of fear-arousingness		
Low	3.08	6.21
Moderate	3.67	4.99
High	3.49	5.44
p	(ns)	(<0.05)
Degree of fear experienced by subjects		
Low	–	5.40
Moderate	–	7.30
High	–	4.81
p	–	(<0.05)

The level of fear aroused by the lecture had no consistent effect. (In the second experiment, the significant effect had disappeared at the 16-weeks follow-up.) However, there is a clear curvilinear relationship between fear *experienced* and weight loss. Subjects who reported themselves as moderately frightened after hearing the lecture lost more weight than those who reported either high or low fear.

No predictions were made about the effects of the position and exposure to fear. The latter was manipulated by presenting subjects with booklets containing one sheet for each day in which to record their food intake. Both groups of subjects heard the initial lecture, but subjects in the multiple-exposure condition had reminders of the fear message printed at the top of each daily sheet. The single-exposure group had no such reminders. Results for the effects of these two variables are shown in Table 5 (Skilbeck *et al.*, 1977).

Table 5. Effects of fear exposure and fear position on weight loss

	Weight loss kg					
	Expt. No. 4			Expt. No. 5		
	Follow-up			Follow-up		
	2w.	4w.	8w.	2w.	4w.	8w
Fear exposure						
Single	2.63	4.31	5.99		–	
Multiple	2.72	4.17	5.03		–	
p	(<0.05)					
Fear position						
At start - well before recommendations		–		1.86	2.68	3.99
In middle - just before recommendations		–		3.18	3.95	5.90
At end - after recommendations		–		2.04	2.95	4.72
p				(<0.05)		

In both cases significant results were obtained. Multiple exposure to the fear message produced less weight loss than the single exposure, and placing the fear arousing message just before the recommendation to that, produced more weight loss than putting it in any other position.

The effects of situational variables

Three experiments have been completed on the effects of group variables. The first compared the effects of listening to a lecture with the effects of the group decision procedures described by Lewin (1954). In these, subjects receive the same information as in the lecture condition, but discuss it and publicly commit themselves to trying to follow the advice. Three group leaders each ran three groups of six subjects, and subjects were randomly assigned to each of the nine groups.

The other two experiments investigated the effects of cohesive group membership. Subjects in cohesive groups were given targets as well as individual ones, had name badges, were seated facing one another and were given plenty of time for social interaction. Subjects in the social group condition all attended at the same time in a group but no effort was made to increase cohesiveness. Subjects in the nominal group were given a wide range of times on which they could attend, and although they would meet people they had met before while waiting, they were essentially not members of a group. The results of these manipulations are shown in Table 6 (Ley *et al.*, 1974; Ley, 1976; Ley *et al.*, 1977*b*).

Table 6. Effects of group factors on weight loss at eight week follow-up

	Weight loss kg		
	Expt. No. 1	Expt. No. 8	Expt. No. 11
Lecture	3.49	–	–
Group decision	4.13	–	–
p	(ns)	–	–
Nominal group	–	4.08	4.67
Social group	–	–	5.26
Cohesive group	–	5.72	5.62
p	–	(<0.001)	(ns)

Only one of the experiments yielded significant results. In Experiment No. 8 cohesiveness produced significantly more weight loss. Post-experimental checks of subjects' ratings of group cohesiveness in Experiment No. 11 showed (a) that the social and cohesive groups did not differ in perceived cohesiveness, and (b) that perceived cohesiveness was correlated with weight loss ($r = +0.48$, $P<0.05$). Thus the negative results of Experiment No. 11 cannot be taken at face value.

No predictions were made about channel factors. The practical importance of investigating them is obvious in that if leaflet or videotape presentation is as effective as personal presentation, a great deal of expert time can be saved. Two experiments were conducted on this topic, and the results are shown in Table 7. Despite the failure to achieve significance in Experiment No. 12, there is a remarkable similarity in absolute weight loss in the video and booklet groups in both experiments (Ley *et al.*, 1977*b*).

Table 7. Effects of channel of communication on weight loss at eight weeks

	Weight loss kg	
	Expt. No. 11	Expt. No. 12
Lecture	5.40	–
Booklet	4.35	4.45
Video	5.76	5.76
p	(<0.05)	(ns)

The effects of conditioning variables

The first experiment on conditioning variables compared the self-control procedures advocated by Ferster, Nurnberger & Levitt (1962) and Stuart (1967, 1971) with diet alone and a willpower placebo treatment. All subjects heard the standard lecture, but subjects in the experimental and placebo groups received a booklet which either outlined the methods suggested by the self-control theorists and provided concrete instructions in what to do, or which recommended the exact opposite of the self-control procedures with the rationale that exposure to temptation leads to the development of resistance to it. The results of this experiment are shown in Table 8. No significant differences were obtained (Ley *et al.*, 1974).

Table 8. Effects of self-control techniques on weight loss in Expt. No. 1

Group	Weight loss kg		
	2 weeks	4 weeks	8 weeks
Control (diet alone)	2.22	2.54	3.08
Placebo (willpower instructions)	1.95	2.77	3.49
Self-control	2.68	3.36	4.49

A second experiment argued on the basis of the Premack Principle (Premack, 1965) that, as eating high carbohydrate foodstuffs was reinforcing to obese subjects, it should be possible to affect compliance by using a reinforcement system of 'points' with a diet holiday as a back-up. It is also well known that fixed and variable schedules differ in their effects (Honig, 1966), so this variable was investigated as well. Results are shown in Table 9, where it can be seen that the experimental manipulations failed to have the desired effect on either the number of days on which subjects complied with their diets or on their weight loss (Ley *et al.*, 1974).

Table 9. Effects of various schedules of contingent and non-contingent reinforcement by diet holiday on (a) weight loss and (b) mean days compliant in Expt. No. 2

Group	Mean weight loss at 7 weeks (kg)	Mean days compliant in 7th week
Control (diet alone)	1.51	4.8
Non-contingent reinforcement		
fixed	2.01	3.5
variable	1.17	0.5
Contingent reinforcement		
fixed	0.38	2.8
variable	1.56	3.5

More success has been obtained in attempts to use classical aversive conditioning to increase weight loss. The aversive unconditioned stimuli used have been (a) sniffs of butyric acid or ammonium sulphide or acetamide, (b) descriptions of and suggestions of nausea and vomiting (covert sensitization procedure), and (c) subjects' own pictures of themselves in scanty underwear or bikinis. Conditioned stimuli have been actual samples of or imagined samples of the subjects' preferred high carbohydrate foods. In attempts to alter subjects' liking for low carbohydrate foods, these have been paired with a positive unconditioned stimulus. The one used in the present series has been the respiratory relief method described by Orwin (1972, 1973). In this, the subjects are instructed to exhale and then hold their breath until it becomes absolutely unbearable. They then inhale and experience an intense feeling of relief. This has been claimed by Orwin to be useful in the rapid treatment of phobias where by pairing the phobic object with the inhalation a counter-conditioning effect can be achieved. It therefore seemed possible that non-preferred foods could be made more attractive by pairing them with respiratory relief. Results of these experiments on classical conditioning are shown in Table 10 (Ley *et al.*, 1974; Maher, 1974).

Table 10. Effects of aversive and appetitive classical conditioning on weight loss

	Mean weight loss (kg) at	
	1 week	5 weeks
Experiment No. 3		
Control (diet alone)	–0.02	–0.02
Overt aversive conditioning	1.09	0.64
Covert sensitization	0.77	0.95
	Mean weight loss (kg) at 8 weeks	
Experiment No. 14		
Control	3.40	
Aversive conditioning	6.08	
Appetitive conditioning	4.67	
Aversive conditioning *plus* appetitive conditioning	6.26	

In both of the experiments involving classical aversive conditioning, this technique has produced a significant effect. In Experiment No. 3 a shortlived one, but in Experiment No. 14 a more substantial one.

Effects of individual differences

The relationships found between personality variables and weight loss are summarized in

Table 11. Rotter's locus of control variable has been reliably associated with weight loss in the present programme but neither extraversion nor neuroticism has had such a consistent relationship (Ley *et al.*, 1974; Kincey, 1976).

Table 11. Relationships between personality variables and weight loss

Personality variables	Correlation with weight loss at eight weeks	
Experiment No. 1	*r*	*p*
Internal-external control	+0.31	<0.05
Neuroticism	−0.08	(ns)
Extraversion	+0.06	(ns)
Experiment No. 4	*r*	*p*
Internal-external control	+0.24	<0.05
Neuroticism	−0.25	<0.05
Extraversion	+0.09	(ns)

Table 12 also shows weight loss achieved by subjects in relation to their perceived locus of control for the two, four and eight-week follow-up sessions. In both experiments, there is an interaction between this variable and time. The only other variable to show a significant correlation with weight loss was knowledge of the diet as measured by a simple test of the content of the diet booklet. The correlation coefficient was + 0.29, $P<0.05$ for the subjects in Experiment No. 1.

Table 12. Weight loss achieved by internally and externally controlled subjects at different follow-up stages

Type of subject	Weight loss (kg) at		
	2 weeks	4 weeks	8 weeks
Experiment No. 1			
Internally controlled	2.41	3.03	4.52
Externally controlled	2.37	2.68	2.95
Experiment No. 4			
Internally controlled	2.87	4.51	5.92
Externally controlled	2.56	4.06	5.29

Following Fishbein's early model (Fishbein & Ajzen, 1975), attempts were made to assess the relationship between attitudes to dieting in specific situations and intentions to diet in these situations and weight loss. Attitudes to dieting assessed in this way shared no relationship to either intention to diet or weight loss. However, relationships emerge when account is taken of all the variables in the early Fishbein model which states that:

$$B \sim BI = \left[A_{act}\right] w_o + \left[NB_p\right] w_1 + \left[(NB_s) + (MC_s)\right] w_2$$

where

B = behaviour
BI = intention to behave
A_{act} = attitude to that behaviour
NB_p = personal normative beliefs about that behaviour
NB_s = social normative beliefs, ie the perceived expectations of others
MC_s = motivation to comply with social normative beliefs
w_0, w_1, w_2 = empirically determined weights.

(The more recent version of this model has dropped the NB_p component on the grounds that it has proved empirically to be very highly correlated with BI. In the present series, however, although NB_p and BI have been significantly correlated the correlations have been low. The NB component has therefore been preserved).

Correlations between measures of A_{act} and BI and between A_{act} and weight loss showed a median of +0.38 and +0.15 respectively, while correlations between combined measures of all the Fishbein components increased these to +0.86 and +0.55 respectively (Ley *et al.*, 1977*b*).

Changes in dependent variables other than weight loss

In every experiment the appropriate analyses have been conducted to look for possible relationships between the experimental variables and drop-out rates. No significant relationships have been found, nor have personality variables been found to be related to drop-out. However, some significant correlations between weight loss, mood and drop-out have emerged. Table 13 shows the correlations between failure to attend a given session and weight loss up to the previous session, and mood as measured at the previous session. These data are taken from Whitworth *et al.* (1977). In the second series of patients, weight loss was consistently correlated with drop-out. The mean differences in weight loss between those who did and did not attend in future being 0.77 kg and 0.73 kg at two and four weeks.

Table 13. Correlations (r)† between drop-out at a given session and (a) weight loss and (b) mood at the previous session

	Follow-up session at which drop-out was observed		
Predictor:	2 weeks	4 weeks	8 weeks
Experiment No. 1			
Anxiety (MAACL)	0.041	0.170	0.201
Depression (MAACL)	0.122	0.168	0.194
Weight loss	–	0.205	0.043
Experiments No. 4, 5			
Anxiety (MAACL)	0.198*	0.281***	0.110
Depression (MAACL)	0.133	0.226**	0.148
Depression (Beck)	0.096	0.243**	0.134
Weight loss	–	0.246**	0.257***

*P<0.05 **P<0.01 ***P<0.001

† All correlations are positive

In the present programme, the effects of conditioning on attitudes to foodstuffs were measured in investigations by Barnes (1973) and Maher (1974). Barnes found that attitudes were changed, while Maher did not. Further, Barnes found that although attitudes changed, reported intake of the foodstuffs did not, and Maher found that although attitudes did not change, her procedures produced weight loss.

Finally, the effects of dieting and weight loss on mood have been examined in two series of subjects (Whitworth *et al.*, 1977). In both of these experiments anxiety and depression were measured by the Multiple Affect Adjective Check List (Zuckerman & Lubin, 1965), and in the second experiment the Beck Depression Inventory was also used. The findings from these studies were: (1) that the more overweight the subject was, the higher tended to be anxiety and depression, and (2) the greater the weight loss, the lower were the anxiety and depression. Correlations at the eight-week follow-up are shown in Table 13. Division of the subjects into poor and good weight losers by a median split show that the correlations between weight loss and mood were due to the poor losers becoming more depressed and anxious and the good losers becoming less so. Mean mood scores for these subjects are also shown in Table 14 (Whitworth *et al.*, 1977).

Table 14. Correlations (r) between degree of overweight weight loss and mood variables at the eight week follow-up

		Expt. No. 1	Expt. No. 4, 5
Correlations between:			
Degree of overweight and:			
MAACL Anxiety		+0.23*	+0.13
MAACL Depression		+0.32**	+0.16*
Beck Depression		—	+0.16*
Weight loss and:			
MAACL Anxiety		−0.37*	−0.21**
MAACL Depression		−0.41*	−0.26**
Beck Depression		—	−0.13
Mean change in mood scores for:			
Good losers	MAACL Anxiety	−2.3	−1.6
	MAACL Depression	−4.3	−1.1
	Beck Depression	—	−6.0
Poor losers	MAACL Anxiety	+0.9	−0.2
	MAACL Depression	+2.6	+2.7
	Beck Depression	—	−3.8

* $P<0.05$ ** $P<0.01$

Discussion and summary

Investigations of the message variables have yielded disappointing results. Sidedness has had no effects, and fear arousal no simple ones. While there is the negative conclusion that high fear has never produced better results than low fear, it is clear from the relationship between experienced fear and weight loss that there must be important interactions between degree of fear arousal and subject characteristics.

Further complications arise from the findings that the position of the fear message matters, and that multiple exposures produce poorer effects than single ones. Future experiments on the effects of fear will have to ask questions like: what level of fear in what position with how many exposures produces the best result with subjects with particular characteristics?

Ley & co-workers (1977*b*) have argued that it is possible that because the subjects in the present series of experiments were volunteers and because fear arousal and sidedness of communication might exert any effects they have through their effects on motivation, there might be a mismatch between the use of these techniques and the subjects' characteristics. Subjects will either be motivated to lose weight or not, and will have the technical skills to do so or they will not. This yields a fourfold classification, into groups, which require a different package of techniques. This is shown in Table 15.

Table 15. Categories of obese persons and the types of communication they need to lose weight

	Own efforts would be	
	Successful	Unsuccessful
Motivated	none	technical advice
Not motivated	persuasive	persuasive plus technical advice

On this analysis the subjects in the present investigations would presumably be motivated to lose weight, but their own techniques would not have been successful. They should therefore only need technical advice.

If this is so, then variables such as sidedness and fear arousal would show no effects with these subjects, but would with less motivated subjects. To test this possibility, Ley *et al.* (1977*a*) randomly assigned 720 subjects from the sample described by Yorke *et al.* (1973), who were known to be overweight, but who had not applied to attend a slimming clinic, to receiving one of six letters and a questionnaire. The letters differed in fear arousal (three levels: low, moderate, high) and sidedness. They contained a summary of the standard lectures used in the experiments with message variables. The questionnaire asked a variety of questions about current weight, health and the like, but contained two items concerning (a) interest in receiving details of a slimming scheme, and (b) interest in participating in such a scheme. While fear arousal had no effect on the way subjects answered these questions, sidedness did. In both instances, the two-sided communication produced greater expressed interest. As this sample of subjects had not volunteered to join in a scheme before being exposed to fear arousal and sidedness, it is plausible to argue that they would be on average less motivated than the subjects in the main series. Other possible explanations for the failure of fear arousal and sidedness to exert effects are discussed by Ley *et al.* (1977*b*).

In view of the evidence implicating poor comprehension and memory as possible determinants of non-compliance (Ley, 1977), it was surprising that the attempts to increase compliance by improving memory and comprehension met with so little success. This mirrors the general lack of consistent results for these variables in other fields such as taking medicine (Colcher & Bass, 1972; Sackett *et al.*, 1975; Ley, Jain & Skilbeck, 1976).

The investigations of situational variables also yielded meagre pickings. It seems probable that placing clients in cohesive groups will lead to greater weight loss, and the videotape presentation is as good as personal presentation and better than mere written information, but our findings are mixed. Certainly there is no reason on the basis of our data for concluding that group treatment in general, regardless of degree of group cohesiveness, produces better results than individual treatment.

Probably the most controversial findings are those on self-control procedures and classical aversive conditioning. Neither the self-control nor the willpower placebo techniques were significantly better than diet alone. It can be argued that one of the ways of classifying placebo treatment is along the dimensions of theoretically strong or weak, and convincing or unconvincing to the subjects. Theoretically, strong ones involve procedures opposite to those recommended by theory, and where it is ethically permissible to use them they can provide convincing negative evidence. Our willpower training seemed to meet these requirements, thus the negative result is of some importance. However, it will be noted that all of the subjects in this experiment were exposed to the standard lecture and all were counting units of carbohydrates ingested and were regularly weighing themselves. These procedures can sometimes be effective in themselves, at least in the short term (Romanczyk, 1974), and may have obscured the effects of self-control. Further, it might be that the advantages of self-control procedures lie more in the maintenance than in the instigation of weight loss.

For classical aversive conditioning, the results of the present series are largely consistent. Aversive conditioning has produced weight loss while appetite conditioning has neither been able to produce weight loss nor add to the effects of aversive conditioning. Unfortunately in these experiments there has been no theoretically strong placebo. An experiment using one in an analogous situation is that of Foreyt & Hagen (1973), who used a pleasant stimulus instead of an aversive one as the unconditioned stimulus in a covert placebo control. The failure of covert sensitization to be superior to their placebo, shows the possible dangers of interpreting the present results as being due to classical conditioning, since a successful outcome for aversive procedures is not always found (Stuart & Davis, 1972; Abramson, 1973; Stunkard & Mahoney, 1976).

The finding that perceived locus of control is correlated with weight loss is discussed in detail by Kincey (1976). Once more there is some conflict between the present findings and those of other investigators. Thus Craddock (1975), Leon (1975), and Rodin & co-workers (1977) have all failed to replicate this finding. While subject differences may be of relevance here, it is important to note that the Rotter Internal-External control questionnaire has been shown to measure a number of factors (eg, Gurin *et al.*, 1969; Mirels, 1970; Collins, 1974). Ley & his co-workers have used the five-item personal control subscale of Gurin *et al.* (1969) on the assumption that it is personal control rather than other aspects of control ideology which is most likely to be related to compliance. Other investigators have used total scores on the Rotter Scale, except for Balch & Ross (1975) who used the Mirels factor scores as well as total scores. It is possible that this difference in measuring instruments accounts for the differences in results.

In a very interesting analysis, Kincey (1976) has shown that what seems to happen is that externally controlled individuals are more likely to stop losing weight, presumably as a result of giving up complying, than internally controlled subjects, but that amongst those with external control who do not give up, weight loss is just as great as amongst those with internal control.

The findings of essentially zero relationships between attitudes and weight loss, and attitude change and weight loss, echo the increasing evidence that there are no necessary relationships between attitudes and behaviour, nor between attitude change and behaviour change (Fishbein & Ajzen, 1975). The results also support the theoretical model of Fishbein and Ajzen, and suggest that it might be valuable to conduct further, and more sophisticated, investigations using this approach.

The correlations between mood and weight loss are also of some interest. Subjects who lost more weight tended to be less anxious and depressed than those who lost less weight. It is not possible on the basis of the present data to say whether it was the weight loss which improved mood, or whether it was mood which prevented weight loss. However the results do prove that weight loss is not generally accompanied by increases in anxiety and depression.

Drop-out rates have not been affected by any of the experimental or personality variables. In the present experiments, drop-out rates have ranged from 23 to 74 per cent with a median of 48 per cent (see Appendix). This seems high in relation to the review provided by Hall & Hall (1974) who report a range from zero to 83 per cent with a median of 10 per cent. Indeed, several of the investigations reviewed by Hall & Hall report zero drop-out rates. Why there should be such differences is not clear, and it is likely that drop-out is controlled by variables different from those controlling weight loss. Within the present programme, there are only two possible leads. First, the experiments on the effects of increasing ease of understanding and ease of remembering showed much higher drop-out rates (53, 68, and 74 per cent) than the average. Secondly, there is some scanty evidence in the present series that weight loss and mood have some effect on drop-out. It is clear that research into variables controlling drop-out is urgently required.

The overall results of the programme are summarized in Table 16 which shows the best results obtained with the different variables and the gain they show over diet alone. The figures for group decision and self-control may be a little on the low side because they were obtained from the first series of experiments in which weight losses were generally lower than in other series, (Ley *et al.*, 1977*b*).

Leaving aside the group decision, the self-control and the individual variables of individual differences, the experimental manipulations produce improvements in weight loss of 65 to 85 per cent over diet alone. An experiment comparing a combination of these best variables with placebo and controls given diet-only needs to be conducted, but it looks as though at their best a number of very different procedures can produce worthwhile gains in weight loss over that achieved by diet alone.

Finally, there is emerging from the conflicting findings within this programme, and the frequent disagreements between other investigators, the obvious conclusion that there remains a great deal of unexplained variance. Much more research will be needed before confident claims can be made that any treatment is (a) effective and (b) works for the reasons stated.

Table 16. The best weight loss obtained at eight weeks by the different methods

	Mean weight loss (kg)	% gain over diet alone
Diet alone	3.4	—
Message variables:		
Two-sided communication	5.8	70
Low fear arousal	6.2	82
Fear just before recommendations	5.9	74
Single exposure to fear	6.0	76
Increased comprehension and memory	5.6	65
Situation variables:		
Group decision	4.1	21
Cohesive group	5.7	68
Video presentation	5.8	70
Conditioning variables:		
Self-control	4.5	32
Aversive conditioning	6.1	79
Individual differences:		
Moderate fear experienced	7.3	115
Internal control	5.9	74

APPENDIX

Expt.		No. of Subjects	Drop-out rate at 8 weeks	Variables investigated
No. 1.	Levy *et al.*, (1974); Kincey (1976); Whitworth *et al.* (1977)	131	48%	(a) Group decisions vs lecture (b) Level of fear arousal (c) Sidedness of communication (d) Self-control procedures (e) Personality variables: extraversion, neuroticism, internal/external control (f) Mood variables
No. 2.	Ley *et al.*, (1974)	68	(44% at 7 weeks)	Points reinforcement schedule
No. 3.	Ley *et al.*, (1974)	28	—	Covert and overt aversive conditioning
No. 4.	Skilbeck *et al.* (1977); Kincey (1976); Whitworth *et al.* (1977)	136	32%	(a) Fear arousal (b) Fear exposure (c) Sidedness of communication (d) Internal-external control (e) Mood variables
No. 5.	Skilbeck *et al.* (1977)	66	30%	Position of fear-arousing material
No. 6.	Ley *et al.* (1977*b*)	64	56%	Difficulty level of lecture
No. 7.	Ley (1976)	44	68%	Comprehension of and memory for material
No. 8.	Ley (1976)	44	41%	Group cohesiveness
No. 9	Ley *et al.* (1977*b*)	47	74%	Comprehension of and memory for material
No. 10.	Ley *et al.*(1977*b*)	75	53%	(a) Comprehension of and memory for material (b) Format of leaflet

No. 11.	Ley *et al.* (1977*b*)	102	44%	(a) Channel of communication (b) Group cohesiveness (c) Fishbeinian attitude variables
No. 12.	Ley *et al.* (1977*b*)	39	59%	(a) Difficulty level of material (b) Channel of communication
No. 13.	Barnes (1973)	32	–	Classical conditioning of attitude to foods
No. 14.	Maher (1974)	52	23%	Classical aversive and appetitive conditioning
No. 15.	Ley *et al.* (1977*a*)	720	–	Effects of sidedness and fear arousal on interest in slimming scheme

Acknowledgements – The experiments described in this paper have been supported in part by the United Kingdom Health Education Council, and in part by the Department of Health and Social Security. Their generous support of this programme is gratefully acknowledged.

References

Abramson, E.E. (1973): *Behav. Res. Therap.* **11**, 547.
Balch, P. & Ross, A.W. (1975): *J. Consult. Clin. Psychol.* 43, 119.
Barnes, W. (1973): Attitude formation in the obese by the covert application of Premack's Principle. Unpublished B. Phil. dissertation: University of Liverpool, England.
Bradshaw, P.W., Ley, P., Kincey, J.A. & Bradshaw, J. (1975): *Br. J. Clin. Soc. Psychol.* **14**, 55.
Colcher, I.S. & Bass, J.W. (1972): *J. Am. Med. Assoc.* 222, 657.
Collins, B.E. (1974): *J. Pers. Soc. Psychol.* 29, 381.
Craddock, D. (1975): Psychological and personality factors associated with successful weight reduction: a ten year follow-up of 134 personal cases. In *Recent advances in obesity research:* I, ed A.N. Howard. London: Newman.
Davis, M.S. (1966): *J. Med. Educ.* **41**, 1037.
Ferster, C.B., Nurnberger, J.I. & Levitt, E.B. (1962): *J. Mathetics* **1**, 87.
Fishbein, M. & Ajzen, I. (1975): *Belief, attitude, intention and behavior.* Massachusetts: Addison-Wesley.
Flesch, R. (1948): *J. Appl. Psychol.* 32, 221.
Foreyt, J.P. & Hagen, R.L. (1973): *J. Abnorm. Psychol.* **82**, 17.
Gurin, P., Gurin, G., Lao, R.C. & Beattie, M. (1969): *J. Soc. Issues* 25, 29.
Hall, S.M. & Hall, R.G. (1974): *Behav. Ther.* 5, 352.
Honig, W.K. (1966): *Operant behavior: areas of research and application.* New York: Appleton-Century-Crofts.
Janis, I.L. (1967): Effects of fear arousal on attitude change. In *Advances in experimental social psychology,* Vol. 3, ed L. Berkowitz. New York: Academic Press.
Kincey, J.A. (1976): The relationship between internal-external control and compliance with a weight loss regime. Unpublished Ph.D. Thesis. University of Liverpool, England.
Leon, G.R. (1975): Personality, body image and eating pattern changes in overweight persons after weight loss. In *Recent advances in obesity research:* I, ed A.N. Howard. London: Newman.
Leventhal, H. (1970): Findings and theory in the study of fear communications. In *Advances in experimental social psychology, Vol. 5,* ed L. Berkowitz. New York: Academic Press.
Lewin, K. (1954): Studies in group decision: In *Group dynamics,* ed D. Cartwright & A. Zander. London: Tavistock Press.
Ley, P. (1973): *J. Inst. Hlth Educ.* **11**, 17.
Ley, P. (1976): Towards better doctor-patient communication: contributions from experimental and social psychology. In *Communications between doctors and patients,* ed A.E. Bennett. London: Oxford University Press for the Nuffield Provincial Hospitals Trust.
Ley, P. (1977): Psychological studies of doctor-patient communication. In *Contributions to medical psychology 1,* ed S.J. Rachman. Oxford: Pergamon Press.
Ley, P. & Spelman, M.S. (1967): *Communicating with the patient.* London: Staples Press.
Ley, P., Goldman, M., Bradshaw, P.W., Kincey, J.A. & Walker, C.M. (1972): *J. Inst. Hlth Educ.* **10**, 47.
Ley, P., Bradshaw, P.W., Eaves, D. & Walker, C.M. (1973): *Psychol. Med.* **3**, 217.
Ley, P., Bradshaw, P.W., Kincey, J.A., Couper-Smartt, J. & Wilson, M. (1974): Psychological variables in

weight control. In *Obesity*, ed W.A. Burland, P. Samuel & J. Yudkin. London: Churchill Livingstone.
Ley, P., Jain, V.K. & Skilbeck, C.E. (1976): *Psychol. Med.* 6, 599.
Ley, P., Whitworth, M.A., Woodward, R. & Yorke, R.A. (1977*a*): *Hlth Educ. J.* to appear.
Ley, P., Whitworth, M.A., Woodward, R., Kincey, J.A., Skilbeck, C.E., Bradshaw, P.W., Tulips, J.G., Barnes, W., Maher, J., Couper-Smartt, J. & Wilson, M. (1977*b*): *Hlth. Educ. J.* to appear.
Maher, J. (1974): Aversive conditioning and respiratory relief in the treatment of obesity. Unpublished M. Psychol. Dissertation. University of Liverpool, England.
Mirels, H.L. (1970): *J. Consult. Clin. Psychol.* 34, 226.
Mitchell, J.H., (1974): *Health Education Monographs* 2, 75.
Montegriffo, V.M.E. (1968): *Ann. Hum. Genet.* 31, 389.
Orwin, A. (1972): *Br. J. Psychiat.* 119, 635.
Orwin, A. (1973): *Br. J. Psychiat.* 122, 171.
Premack, D. (1965): Reinforcement theory. In *Nebraska symposium on motivation,* ed D. Levine. University of Nebraska Press.
Rodin, J., Bray, G.A., Atkinson, R.L., Dahms, W.T., Greenway, F.L., Hamilton, K. & Molitch, M. (1977): *Int. J. Obesity* 1, 79.
Romanczyk, R.G. (1974): *Behav. Ther.* 5, 531.
Sackett, D.L. & Haynes, R.B. (1976): *Compliance with therapeutic regimens.* Baltimore: John Hopkins University Press.
Sackett, D.L., Haynes, R.B., Gibson, E.S., Hackett, B.C., Taylor, D.W., Roberts, R.S. & Johnson, A.L. (1975): *Lancet* 1, 1205.
Shaw, M.E. (1971): *Group dynamics.* New York: McGraw-Hill.
Skilbeck, C.E., Tulips, J.G. & Ley, P. (1977): *Europ. J. Soc. Psychol.* (in press).
Stewart, R.B. & Cluff, L.E. (1972): *Clin. Pharmac. Ther.* 13, 463.
Stuart, R.B. (1967): *Behav. Res. Ther.* 5, 257.
Stuart, R.B. (1971): *Behav. Res. Ther.* 9, 177.
Stuart, R.B. & Davis, B. (1972): *Slim chance in a fat world.* Champaign, Illinois: Research Press.
Stunkard, A.J. & Mahoney, M.J. (1976): Behavioral treatment of eating disorders. In *Handbook of behaviour modification and behaviour therapy,* ed H. Leitenberg. Englewood Cliffs, New Jersey: Prentice Hall.
Whitworth, M.A., Skilbeck, C.E., Woodward, R. & Ley, P. (1977): *Mood change and weight loss in a slimming regime.* Awaiting publication.
Yates, A.J., (1975): *Theory and practice in behavior therapy.* New York: Wiley.
Yorke, R.A., Holland, M.A.J. & Massey-Lynch, M. (1973): *Jl R. Coll. Gen. Pract.* 23, 730.
Zuckerman, M. & Lubin, B. (1965): *Manual for the multiple affect adjective check-list.* San Diego: Educational and Industrial Testing Service.

11
OBESITY AND DIABETES

G. F. CAHILL, Jr.
Joslin Research Laboratory, Joslin Diabetes Foundation, Inc. and Harvard Medical School, and the Department of Medicine, Peter Bent Brigham Hospital, Boston, Mass., USA.

A correlation of diabetes mellitus with obesity has been known for millenia. Ancient descriptions recorded in India and passed along in Ayurvedic medicine (Ajgaonkar, 1972) related diabetes *(Madhumeha)* to corpulence and overnutrition, and, with even more perception, suggested a genetic transmission, as it 'passed through the seed'. The markedly strong genetic input in maturity-onset diabetes, as will be discussed subsequently, is now amply confirmed by the very high concordance in identical twins (Gottlieb & Root, 1968; Tattersall & Pyke, 1972) and its relationship to obesity has been noted repeatedly in innumerable publications. This brief account will try to apply current knowledge to these relationships with some speculation on their phylogenetic etiology.

The correlation of obesity and diabetes is not unique to Homo sapiens and appears to be present in most mammalia, especially those which have become associated with man. One can only speculate whether other species, not maintained easily in captivity or domesticated, would also become diabetic. The common bond may simply be a combination of overnutrition and a confined sedentary environment. Renold and colleagues have reviewed this correlation in a number of publications (Renold & Dulin, 1967; Stauffacher *et al.*, 1971; Cameron, Stauffacher & Renold, 1972; First Brook Lodge Workshop on spontaneous 'diabetes' in animals, 1967; Second Brook Lodge Workshop on spontaneous 'diabetes' in animals, 1970; Third Brook Lodge Workshop on spontaneous diabetes in laboratory animals, 1974; Renold *et al.*, 1977) and have catalogued the species, including the dolphin, hippopotamus, sand rat and a number of other rodents, almost all sub-human primates kept in captivity (old and

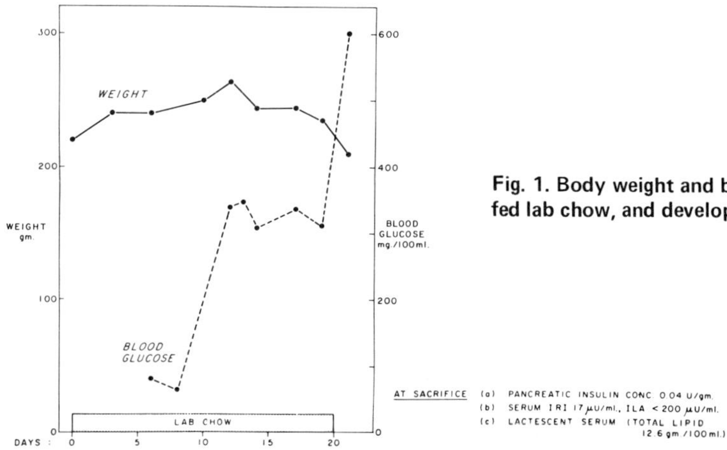

Fig. 1. Body weight and blood glucose in a sand rat fed lab chow, and developing acute diabetes

new world monkeys, chimpanzees, Celebes apes) cattle, pigs, and very frequently, the household cat or dog. The sand rat is a typical example (Fig. 1), living a precarious existence in the desert and eating submarginal roughage, but, when brought to the laboratory and presented with typical commercial rodent feed, it overeats, increases its weight slightly and develops diabetes, eventually succumbing to total beta cell failure and death (Miki *et al.*, 1966). Even the Chinese hamster, elegantly studied by Gerritsen and colleagues at the Upjohn Company, in whom an additive effect of probably four genes predisposes the animal to diabetes (the more of the diabetes genes it has, the more the diabetes), can be spared from developing diabetes by dietary restriction (First Brook Lodge Workshop, 1967; Second Brook Lodge Workshop, 1970; Third Brook Lodge Workshop, 1974; Butler & Gerritsen, 1970).

In a very similar fashion, human populations, long challenged by undernutrition, when exposed to a more sedentary existence and ready access to energy intake, demonstrate a dramatic increase in the prevalence of diabetes, and also, of course, obesity. These observations have been made, to name a few, on Indian populations in South African cities such as Durban (Campbell, 1963), in New Zealand Maoris (Prior & Davidson, 1966) and *in extenso* in North American tribes such as the Seneca (Doeblin *et al.*, 1969), Cherokee (Stein *et al.*, 1965) and especially the Pima (Rushforth *et al.*, 1971; Bennett *et al.*, 1976. In the Pima, the incidence of grossly abnormal tolerance increases with age and is well in excess of 50 per cent in women over 30. Paradoxically, the Eskimo does not appear to be similarly predisposed (Mouratoff & Scott, 1973).

Further support for the additive effects of diet and physical activity, an excess of the former and a deficiency of the latter, is derived from more acute changes in population habits. Himsworth (1949) correlated death rates from diabetes in England and Wales during and after the First and Second World Wars with rationing rather than with the war itself. Similar observations were made during and after the Second World War in Japan (Goto, Nakayma & Yagi, 1958) and in Germany (Schliack, 1954). Bouchardat (1883) commented extensively on the decrease in the prevalence of diabetes during the prolonged and famine-associated siege of Paris at the end of the Franco-Prussian war of 1870. Obviously, during periods of international hostility, environmental changes do not involve diet alone, but also other factors such as increased physical activity and emotional tension. Indeed it is impossible to differentiate between the influence of changes in diet alone and changes in the amount of physical exercise, because data for such a differentiation are not available.

Continuing along the line of thought that diet and diabetes are related, but not merely to energy intake alone, it has been argued that refined dietary sugars (Cohen, Teitelbaum & Saliternik, 1972; Cleave, 1974), removal of fibres from flour and other food (Trowell, 1974), as well as fat (Himsworth, 1935) are diabetogenic. It is even possible that environmental toxins, either exogenously consumed or endogenously produced from food additives or intestinal flora, such as alloxan or streptozotocin (Issenberg, 1976), may contribute to the progressive demise of the beta cells, especially in maturity-onset diabetes. On the other hand, an identifiable role for dietary factors such as sugar has been denied (Booyens *et al.*, 1970; Kahn *et al.*, 1971). On the basis of all the available evidence it appears that the most important dietary factor increasing the risk for diabetes is the total calorie intake and subsequent fat accumulation, irrespective of the source of the calories, as long as they are in excess of need or expenditure.

A few scattered studies (O'Sullivan & Mahan, 1965; Medley, 1965) have shown little direct effect of obesity on diabetes, but many others, in widely different populations, have consistently confirmed this strong relationship Marble *et al.*, 1971; Pyorala, Lehtovirta & Llomaki, 1974; Medalie *et al.*, 1975; Rimm *et al.*, 1975). It has even been suggested that central obesity, which is that which is more frequently found in the middle-aged or hypertrophic type of obesity, has a higher correlation with diabetes (Feldman, Sender & Siegelaub, 1969; Vague, 1956; Boyer *et al.*, 1968; West *et al.*, 1974) than do the peripheral forms, the latter more likely being hyperplastic and developed in youth. A study of 375 middle-aged

Norwegian men followed for 10 years (Westlung & Nicolaysen, 1972) showed a linear correlation of diabetes and obesity, thin men escaping diabetes and massively obese men almost uniformly contracting the disease.

Pathophysiology

Other papers in this volume deal with the etiology of obesity, the controversy of environmental-versus-hereditary factors, the important and elegant studies differentiating hypertrophic and hyperplastic obesities, and the highly complex and as yet unclarified roles of central versus peripheral processes in regulating caloric intake and expenditure, and thereby of caloric balance. Emphasis in this section will be on insulin and its relationship to obesity.

That insulin deficiency, or at least something in the pancreas, was fundamental to diabetes was known and amply documented by the turn of the century, especially after Von Mering & Minkowski (1890) described diabetes in pancreatectomized dogs. With the advent of insulin in 1922, clinicians rapidly realized that fat diabetics needed more insulin (Marble *et al.,* 1971). The Scottish pathologist Ogilvie (1937) noted pancreatic beta cell hyperplasia in non-diabetic obese patients at autopsy, suggesting that obesity demanded excess insulin. When Yalow & Berson (1960) first described the immunoassay for insulin and results in diabetics, the bulk of their diabetic subjects demonstrated hyperinsulinemia. But, in these studies, obesity was not taken into consideration, and since thin, insulin-requiring diabetics developed antibodies to insulin which made the immunoassay difficult to interpret, only maturity-onset type diabetic subjects were studied, and the vast majority were obese. Subsequently Karam (Karam, Grodsky & Forsham, 1963) correlated insulin levels with obesity, and many workers, most recently Genuth (1973), demonstrated that diabetic obese subjects could have insulin levels higher than those in the non-diabetic, non-obese, but their levels for any given glucose concentration were still less than those in a non-diabetic subject with the same degree of obesity, meaning a relative insulin deficiency in the obese. Rabinowitz & Zierler (1962) had clearly demonstrated that forearm tissues in obese man were less responsive to elevations in insulin levels than those of non-obese man, and that the hyperinsulinism of the obese was an adaptive response to this tissue's unresponsiveness.

Beta cells in obesity

As mentioned, Ogilvie (1937) noted beta cell hyperplasia in non-diabetic obese subjects, suggesting that beta cell replication can compensate for the increased insulin need in obesity. Thus why do some subjects develop diabetes and others do not? One explanation is the degree of the obesity; the more obese the greater the prevalence of diabetes. Nothing is known of beta cell kinetics in man, and for that matter, little is known in experimental animal preparations. Induction of diabetes with antibody (Logothetopoulos & Bell, 1966), by steroid (Like & Chick, 1974), or challenging with changes in caloric intake (Chick & Like, 1971), results in beta cell replication, but the reserve is greatly limited. Mitoses in beta cells in man are noted from time to time especially in subjects with liver disease (Warren, LeCompte & Legg, 1966), but there is probably a very limited replicative capacity, similar to the capacity for compensatory renal hypertrophy. Like the hair follicle in balding men, or the melanocyte in older individuals with graying hair, or as the best example, the ovarian cortex in menopausal females, progressive senescence of beta cells occurs with aging, with a decreased number of beta cells, fibrosis, hyaline accumulation and other age-related processes. Numerous pathological studies summarized by Warren & co-workers (1966) show prematurely senescent changes in the islets in the majority of diabetics developing their disease in midlife. In juvenile-onset type diabetics, the lesion appears to be an early and rapid demise of the beta cells associated with lymphocytic infiltration, and after several years, disappearance of all or nearly all beta cells. A viral and/or autoimmune etiology has been suggested (Nerup *et al.,* 1974; Thomsen *et al.,* 1975; Craighead, 1975; Nerup *et al.,* 1971; MacCuish *et al.,* 1974; Lendrum, Walker & Gamble, 1975). In the maturity-onset type diabetic, the beta cell lesion appears to be a combination of decreased cellularity as well as alterations indicative of premature senescence.

Are there other pieces of evidence indicative of premature cellular senescence in diabetics? Other diseases usually associated with aging, such as senile cataract (Marble *et al.*, 1971), osteoporosis (Levin, Boisseau & Avioli, 1976), dental problems and certainly atherosclerosis, are much more prevalent in the diabetic. A direct chemical analysis of collagen from diabetics has revealed characteristics of accelerated aging (Hamlin, Kahn & Luschin, 1975) and fibroblasts from diabetics in tissue culture (Goldstein, Littlefield & Soeldner, 1969; Rowe *et al.*, 1976) behave as if they were derived from a chronologically much older subject.

It is tempting to speculate that all of us have a limited potential for replication of beta cells, and with the increased insulin requirement of obesity, or, for that matter, of pregnancy, or of glucorticoid or growth hormone excess, if the insulin need surpasses this potential, diabetes ensues. This is a gross over-simplification, and fails to answer why the release of insulin from beta cells is defective, not only quantitatively but also qualitatively, in the obese diabetic. In other words, the acute or first phase of insulin release is relatively more impaired in the obese diabetic, or for that matter, any maturity-onset diabetic, obese or non-obese. One can only speculate that there is either a selective loss of the more sensitive, rapidly responding beta cells, and this has been supported by experimental animal work in which small doses of beta cell toxins have been administered and loss of first phase insulin release noted (Pupo *et al.*, 1976). The other possibility is an exhaustion of the remaining beta cells due to overwork, if indeed this does occur in man as in cats (Dohan & Lukens, 1947) and a resulting loss of first phase due to this cellular fatigue.

The high rate of concordance in identical twins for maturity-onset type diabetes (Gottlieb & Root, 1968; Tattersall & Pyke, 1972) strongly enforces a genetic component to this beta cell deficiency. Longevity, baldness, graying hair, time of menarche and menopause, are also all genetically programmed but modified by environment, and it is logical that beta cell kinetics should be likewise influenced.

Insulin responsiveness

Turning to the other half of the problem; why is the capacity for insulin to be metabolically effective in tissues from the obese animal or man decreased? In experimental animals, a number of tissues such as liver, muscle and especially adipose tissue, demonstrate decreased metabolic effectiveness of insulin on a number of parameters. Rabinowitz & Zierler (1962) clearly showed this to be true in human forearm tissues, and Felig, Wahren & Hendler, (1974) characterized the blunted response of the human liver to glucose and insulin in obese man.

In the past few years, a number of workers, led by Roth and his associates (Roth *et al.*, 1975; Bar & Roth, 1977) at the National Institutes of Health, have shown that for insulin to be effective on cells, the first step in a binding of insulin to highly specific receptors on the membrane of the responsive cell. A decrease in the number of receptors have been characterized on the surface of cells from obese animals and man, including liver, muscle, adipocytes and, as an easily available model for study, the circulating monocyte. Thus, should the number of receptors be halved, twice the insulin concentration would be necessary for a given effect on a responsive cell.

The nature of the receptor is highly complex as well as the kinetics of binding and release of insulin and its degradation. There is also evidence, especially as recently reported by Czech, Richardson & Smith (1977), and previously by Cuatrecasas 1974, and by Amatruda, Livingston & Lockwood, 1975), that the insulin resistance of obesity involves more than simply a binding defect. Since insulin's second message, namely, the event or events inside the cell after initiation of insulin binding to the cell surface, are still not characterized, controversy will continue over the precise locus of the insulin resistance in obesity. In fact, even the nature and variability of the binding itself, especially to white cells, remains controversial (Kahn *et al.*, 1977; Helderman & Strom, 1977) and specific binding to primitive unicellular organisms has been described (Legros *et al.*, 1975). In any case, cells responsive to insulin need higher levels of insulin in obese animals and man for any given response. That this decrease in response can be experimentally induced in man by forced-feeding to induce obesity was shown by Sims & co-workers (Salans *et al.*, 1974) in their classic series of experimentally-produced obesity in man.

How does the cell surface, or the inside of the responsive cell, if one believes that the intracellular events are more at fault in obesity, result from increased adopisity? Or more simply, how does the monocyte know that it is circulating in the blood stream of a fat man or animal? The Roth concept of 'down regulation' suggests that in the presence of excess quantities of hormones, receptors diminish, producing a kind of induced tachyphylaxis, endocrinologically speaking. This places the hyperinsulinemia as a primary event. The increased number of receptors after brief starvation of obese individuals supports this concept. But on the other hand, if one overfeeds a normal non-obese, non-diabetic individual, their tissues become more and more sensitive to insulin, similar to the response of the adrenal gland to ACTH after chronic exposure to high levels of ACTH. Why then the 'down regulation' to insulin, if, indeed, it does exist as a true physiologic phenomenon?

Obesity and diabetes – balanced polymorphisms?

The author has spent the major proportion of his scientific efforts in the study of the interrelationships between hormones, particularly insulin, with body fuel homeostasis. Primitive man, and unfortunately modern man in certain areas of the world, is still challenged by the nutritional requirements for survival: calories and protein. Natural selection has done a remarkable feat in making man almost as efficient as any other homotherm in meeting the challenges of surplus and deficit in calories and nitrogen in his environment. The first priority in times of surplus is to optimize the body's protein mass, meaning enzymes, structural proteins, and especially muscle. Protein is so important that all is used as part of the machinery; there are no storage depots. Man probably did never have the luxury of excess protein to be able to afford storage. Equally as important, were it to be stored, it would need to be accumulated with four to five parts of water and would create a gravimetric problem, and mobility would be compromised. Hence what storage of protein there is, is as functioning muscle. Physical exercise, either work or play, augments this effect. It in interesting how important vigorous dancing and games are in primitive societies at times of harvest, perhaps a selective advantage to accumulate excess muscle during times of plenty. Also supporting the concept that protein was probably never available in excess to primitive man is the fact that the maximal rate of urea synthesis is insufficient to handle all the amino groups were man to eat solely protein as a source of energy (Rudman *et al.*, 1973).

Surplus calories as carbohydrate or as lipid are handled by man differently to protein. First, there is a very small reserve supply of carbohydrate, and this is maintained for emergency anaerobic energy, especially in muscle, should the occasion arise (muscle glycogen = circa 200 to 400 grams) or in liver, to maintain glucose in the blood for use by brain or exercising muscle (liver glycogen = circa 100 grams in the fed state). Any excess carbohydrate intake is converted into fatty acids in liver and adipose tissue and eventually will be stored in adipose tissue as triglyceride. The extra-aqueous nature of triglyceride makes it the ultimate fuel for energy storage in any mobile creature, particularly one which has to work against gravity. Storage of carbohydrate as glycogen, like protein storage, necessitates accumulation of several parts of water for each part of glycogen and this is as uneconomical as storage as protein. Thus in man, just enough glycogen is stored for the anaerobic emergencies mentioned above. Primitive man thus optimized his muscle and glycogen stores and stored hydrocarbon in his adipose tissue as his defence against prolonged starvation.

In starvation, the strategy for survival is to withdraw calories solely from fat, and to conserve but a small amount of emergency glycogen, especially in muscle, and, most

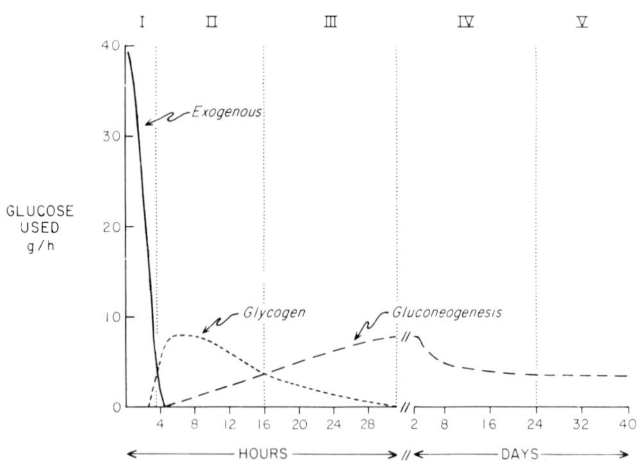

Fig. 2. Phases of glucose utilization by tissues, during transition from the fed state to prolonged starvation

important, to conserve as much muscle protein as possible to be able to defend himself from aggressors as well as to capture his next meal (Cahill, 1970; 1971). Man thus goes through a series of metabolic events during progressive starvation as the strategic plan is brought into play (Fig. 2). The first phase, of course, follows the absorptive phase; glucose begins to be excluded from peripheral tissues, especially muscle and adipose tissue, and hepatic glycogen provides sufficient glucose to provision brain. Liver glycogen is then gradually depleted over 12 to 20 hours, and blood glucose begins to be maintained by gluconeogenesis in liver from amino acids released from muscle. By three or four days of starvation, muscle breakdown amounts to approximately 0.5 kg daily, a phenomenon obviously incompatible with survival if the starvation were to be continued for several weeks. However, there is a gradual reduction in the rate of muscle proteolysis and hepatic gluconeogenesis as the levels of the ketone bodies, β-hydroxybutyrate and acetoacetate, increase in blood. Hepatic ketone production is maximal by day 2 of starvation (Owen & Reichard, 1971), but the subsequent increase (Fig. 3) in blood levels is secondary to progressive diminution in utilization of the ketone bodies by muscle (Reichard, Owen & Itaff, 1974).

Brain readily utilizes the ketone bodies, providing their concentration in blood is sufficient to maintain a good diffusion gradient across the blood brain barrier (Pardridge & Oldensorf,

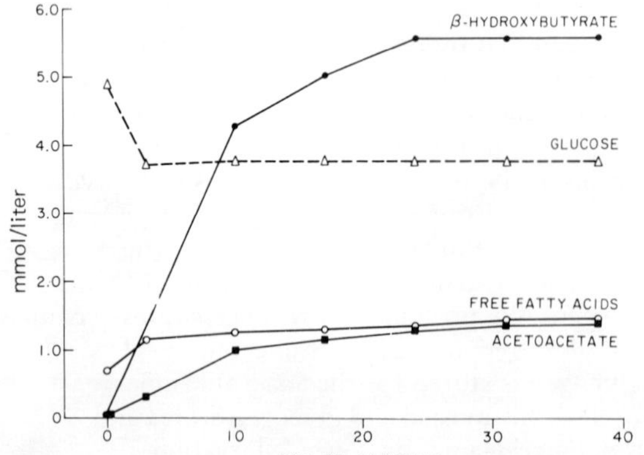

Fig. 3. Circulating substrate levels in prolonged fasted man

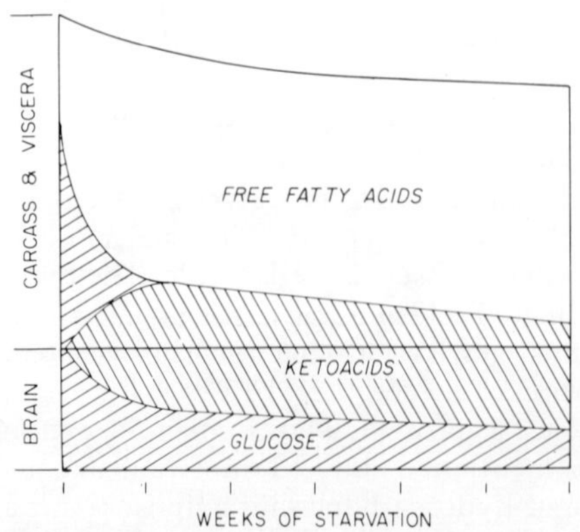

Fig. 4. Substrate utilization by brain and the remaining body during prolonged starvation in man

1977). Thus by 1 to 2 weeks of starvation, brain is mainly using ketoacids as fuel and diminishing its use of glucose accordingly (Fig. 4). The net effect is the sparing of muscle protein as the entire body selectively draws on fat as its source of fuel, either directly as free fatty acids to be used by muscle or liver, or as modified, water-soluble fatty acid products produced by liver, the ketoacids, to be used by brain. There are other tissues, such as red cells, renal medulla, peripheral nerve and to a limited degree brain itself which still use some glucose, but the glycolysis goes no further than pyruvate and its reduced equivalent, lactate, which are then returned to the blood for resynthesis back to glucose by liver and kidney, hence there is no net loss of carbohydrate or potential carbohydrate (Cahill, 1970, 1971; Owen & Reichard, 1971). After several weeks of fasting, muscle loss is but 80 to 100 g daily. Some animals, such as the black bear in winter sleep (Nelson *et al.*, 1973), the nesting Emperor penguin (Pinshow *et al.*, 1976), or certain other carnivores like the elephant seal pup (Ortiz, Costa & LeBoeuf, in press) can do even better than man with no detectable net nitrogen loss, and what glucose is metabolized is derived solely from the glycerol moiety of the lipolyzed triglyceride.

What these animals and fasted man have done is to become operationally diabetic in excluding glucose utilization, but, unlike the diabetic, without hyperglycemia and glucosuria, which would be not only detrimental but fatal. If the transition state, from feeding to fasting, were to be made more quickly, or even, if the individual had a head start by being slightly diabetic, but still without elevated glucose levels, the slight diabetes being only reflected by more efficient glucose exclusion from peripheral tissues, some nitrogen would be spared with each feeding-fasting cycle. Two mildly diabetic subjects, totally fasted, did lose less nitrogen than did six non-diabetic subjects on the same starvation regimen, but the meaning of this single observation can only be speculative (Figs. 5 & 6).

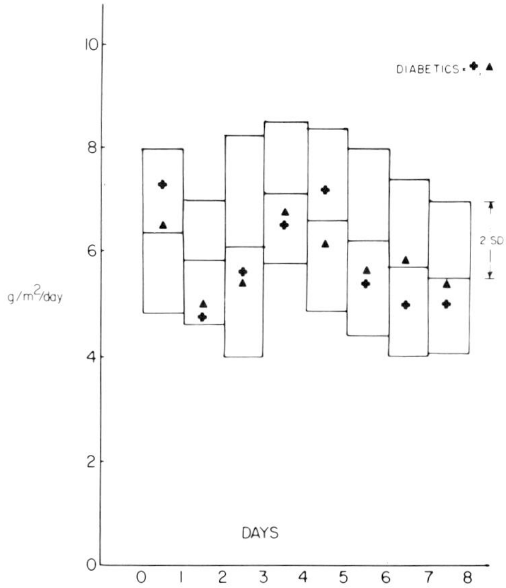

Fig. 5. Urinary nitrogen loss of two mild maturity-onset diabetics fasted for eight days compared to the mean ± 2 s.d. of six normals

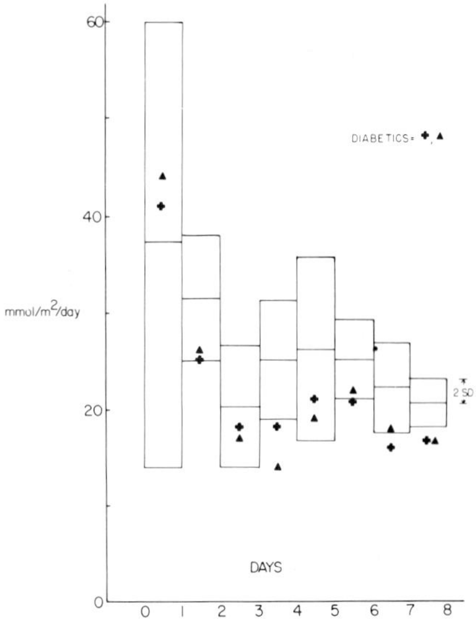

Fig. 6. Urinary potassium loss in the two diabetic subjects in Fig. 5., corroborating the sparing of lean tissue mass

The question, of course, is whether this slight advantage, or some similar process, could explain the preservation of such a prevalent genetic disorder as maturity-onset type diabetes in the population. Neel (1962, 1976) has questioned whether such a balanced polymorphism could exist, analogous to the protective effect of sickling hemoglobin or deficient glucose-6-phosphatase dehydrogenase activity against malaria. Some comfort to the defender of the hypothesis is the variable predisposition to maturity-onset type diabetes amongst different populations, the American Pima Indian so far being not only the best studied, but also the highest prevalence (Karam, Grodsky & Forsham, 1963; Genuth, 1973).

Against the hypothesis is the age of onset of mild maturity-onset type diabetes, which, in primitive populations, was after the reproductive age. However, a grandparent, whom one did not have to give very much food, especially protein, was of survival benefit to a primitive cluster or family group, in which case there would be a selective effect for the group at large, and thereby to the individual. The age-related decrease in metabolic rate would also provide a selective advantage. Certainly obesity and its unmasking of the relative beta cell deficiency was a rare event, and confined probably only to the nobility.

Juvenile type diabetes which more and more appears to come from a separate genetic pool, would certainly be a lethal factor in any primitive society and, prior to the present day scrupulous management of the pregnant diabetic, was still a semi-lethal factor. It is of interest to point out the reciprocal or minimal prevalence of juvenile-onset type diabetes in those populations with remarkedly high rates of maturity-onset diabetes. Could this also have some rational basis? With the recent correlations of juvenile-onset type diabetes with alleles in the major histocompatibility complex and the demonstration of both cell-mediated (Nerup *et al.*, 1971; MacCuish *et al.*, 1974) and circulating (Lendrum *et al.*, 1975) autoimmune phenomena, one must ask whether this might not be an expression of a hyperactive immune process which provided survival advantage (deVries *et al.*, 1977) during plagues or against endemic tuberculosis or measles or syphilis, in the so-called more 'civilized' cultures. These impediments of civilization were never brought to the more centripetally located man (Armelagos, Goodman & Jacobs, in press) until the era of colonization.

These speculations fall more into the 'soft-science' realm of philisophy, but this larger scale type of thinking of medical problems has occasionally provided direct insight into day-to-day clinical care. What still has not been discussed, however, is the major point of why over-nutrition and obesity necessitate a higher concentration of insulin for insulin to exert its metabolic effects. How does the monocyte know it is floating around in the blood of a fat man and not a thin man? The message must be hormonal, or via a hormonal type of signal transmitted by one or more substrate levels, or other factors in the circulation (Leibel, 1977). Others in this volume have addressed themselves to the quantification of adipose tissue triglyceride and its effect on appetite mechanisms, so the problem is not unique to the insulin receptor, if that be the altered process in the decreased sensitivities of tissues in the obese to insulin's metabolic effects. The selective advantage of this phenomenon escapes this philosopher, and again, in primitive man, the problem never arose. It is possible, however, that the decreased insulin receptor process in obesity is either directly or indirectly involved in the feedback system for total body lipid homeostasis (Leibel, 1977). That such a system exists in animals is indubitable, and it is also probably present in man, but markedly suppressed by his intellectual processes. Unlike the instinctual pre-hibernation or pre-migratory hyperphagia, in which environmental cues are interpreted into changes in eating behavior, man is probably the only organism whose thinking processes, if they overrode any fundamental instinctual patterning of caloric homeostasis, could be advantageous. The Polynesians boarding their sailing canoes were far better obese, and the fatter ones survived the journey. In the canoe there was little need for mobility, so the gravimetric disadvantage was minimal. And, certainly, the better he retained his muscle mass, the better the struggle on reaching the shore, especially if the mission was hostile. One could not make a better case for both obesity and a 'touch' of diabetes.

In summary, obesity and diabetes are strange bedfellows, and one might add hyperuricemia, atherosclerosis, hyperlipidemia, gall-bladder disease and many others as closely-related intimates. In primitive societies, a touch of diabetes, as long as hyperglycemia did not occur, might have been slightly advantageous, perhaps, but is this enough to explain its prevalence?

On the other hand, it might just be the fringe of a normal distribution pattern of selective tissue aging: baldness, graying hair, senile cataracts and hyperkeratosis, and perhaps beta cell senescence!

Acknowledgement – The work in this paper has been supported in part by U.S.P.H.S. Grants Nos. AM-15191 and RR-05673.

References

Ajgaonkar, S.S. (1972): Diabetes mellitus as seen in the ancient Ayurvedic medicine. In *Insulin and metabolism*, ed S.S. Bajaj, pp. 1-19. Bombay: Bhatkal.
Amatruda, J.M., Livingston, J.N. & Lockwood, D.H. (1975): *Science* **188**, 264.
Armelagos, G.J., Goodman, A.H. & Jacobs, K.H. (in press): The ecological perspective in disease. In *Health and human conditions: perspectives on medical anthropology*, ed M.H. Logan & E. Hunt. Duxbury Press:

Bar, R.S. & Roth, J. (1977): *Archs Intern. Med.* **137**, 474.
Bennett, P.H., Rushforth, N.B., Miller, M. & LeCompte, P.M. (1976): *Rec. Prog. Horm. Res.* **32**, 333.
Booyens, J., Frank, M. deV., de Waal, V.M., Campbell, G.D. & Goldberg, M.D. (1970): *S. Afr. Med. J.* **44**, 271.
Bouchardat, A. (1883): *De la glycosurie ou diabète sucre.* Paris: Germer-Baillière.
Boyer, J., Clement, M., Vague, Ph., & Vague, J. (1968): Le taux de production du cortisol dans les obesites faminines. Atti del XII Congresso Nazionale della Societa Italiana di Endocrinologia, Cantania, p. 197, Sept. 1968.
Butler, L. & Gerritsen, G.C. (1970): *Diabetologia* **6**, 163.
Cahill, G.F., Jr. (1971): *Diabetes* **20**, 785.
Cahill, G.F., Jr. (1970): *New Engl. J. Med.* **282**, 668.
Cameron, D.P., Stauffacher, W. & Renold, A.E. (1972): Spontaneous hyperglycemia and obesity in laboratory rodents. In *Handbook of physiology,* Section 7, Endocrinology, ed D. Steiner, N. Freinkel, R. Greep & E. Astwood, p. 611. Baltimore: Williams & Wilkins.
Campbell, G.D. (1963): *S. Afr. Med. J.* **37**, 1195.
Chick, W.L. & Like, A.A. (1971): *Am. J. Physiol.* **221**, 202.
Cleave, T.L. (1974): In *The saccharine disease.* Bristol: John Wright.
Cohen, A.M., Teitelbaum, A. & Saliternik, R. (1972): *Metabolism* **21**, 235.
Craighead, J.E. (1975): *Prog. Med. Virol.* **19**, 161.
Cuatrecasas, P. (1974): *Ann. Rev. Biochem.* **43**, 169.
Czech, M.P., Richardson, D.K. & Smith, C.J. (1977): *Metabolism* **26**, 1057.
deVries, R.R.P., Kreeftenberg, H.G., Loggen, H.G. & vanRood, J.J. (1977): *New Engl. J. Med.* **297**, 692.
Doeblin, T.D., Evans, K., Ingall, G., Frohman, L.A. & Bannerman, R.M. (1969): *Diabetologia* **5**, 203.
Dohan, F.C. & Lukens, F.D.W. (1947): *Science* **105**, 183.
Feldman, R., Sender, A.J. & Siegelaub. (1969): *Diabetes* **18**, 478.
Felig, P., Wahren, J. & Hendler, R. (1974): *J. Clin. Invest.* **53**, 582.
First Brook Lodge Workshop on spontaneous 'diabetes' in animals (1967): *Diabetologia* **3**, 63.
Genuth, A.M. (1973): *Ann. Intern. Med.* **79**, 812.
Goldstein, S., Littlefield, J.W. & Soeldner, J.S. (1969): *Proc. Natn. Acad. Sci. U.S.A.* **64**, 155.
Goto, Y., Nakayma, Y. & Yagi, T. (1958): *Diabetes* **7**, 133.
Gottlieb, M.S. & Root, H.F. (1968): *Diabetes* **17**, 693.
Hamlin, C.R., Kahn, R.B. & Luschin, J.H. (1975): *Diabetes* **24**, 902.
Helderman, J.H. & Strom, T.B. (1977): *J. Clin. Invest.* **59**, 338.
Himsworth, H.P. (1935): *Clin. Sci. J.* **2**, 117.
Himsworth, H.P. (1949): *Proc. R. Soc. Med.* **43**, 323.
Issenberg, P. (1976): *Fed. Proc.* **35**, 1322.
Kahn, C.R., Megysi, K., Bar, R.S., Eastman, R.C. & Flier, J.S. (1977): *Ann. Int. Med.* **86**, 205.
Kahn. H.A., Herman, J.B., Medalie, J.H., Neufeld, H.N., Riss, E. & Goldbourt, U. (1971): *J. Chron. Dis.* **23**, 617.
Karam, J.H., Grodsky, G.M. & Fosham, P.H. (1963): *Diabetes* **12**, 197.
Legros, F., Wytdenhoef, P., Dumont, I., Hanson, B., Jeanmart, J., Massant, B., & Conard, V. (1975): *Protoplasma* **86**, 119.
Leibel, R.L. (1977): *J. Theor. Biol.* **66**, 297.
Lendrum, R., Walker, G. & Gamble, D.R. (1975): *Lancet* **1**, 880.
Levin, M.E., Boisseau, V.C. & Avioli, L.V. (1976): *New Engl. J. Med.* **294**, 291.

Like, A.A. & Chick, W.L. (1974): *Am. J. Path.* 75, 329.
Logothetopoulos, J. & Bell, E.G. (1966): *Diabetes* 15, 205.
MacCuish, A.C., Jordan, J., Campbell, C.J., Duncan, L.J.P. & Irvine, W.J. (1974): *Diabetes* 23, 693.
Marble, A., White, P., Bradley, R.F. & Krall, L.P. (1971): *Treatment of diabetes mellitus,* 11th edn. Philadelphia: Lea & Febiger.
Medalie, J.H., Papier, C.M., Goldbourt, U. & Herman, J.B. (1975): *Archs Intern. Med.* 135, 811.
Medley, D.R.K. (1965): *Q. Jl. Med.* 34, 111.
Mering, J. von. & Minowski, O. (1890): *Archs. Exp. Path. Pharmakol.* 26, 371.
Miki, E., Like, A.A., Soeldner, J.S., Steinke, J. & Cahill, G.F., Jr. (1966): *Metabolism* 15, 749.
Mouratoff, C.J. & Scott, E.M. (1973): *J. Am. Med. Ass.* 226, 1345.
Neel, J.V. (1976): Diabetes mellitus, - a geneticist's nightmare. In *The genetics of diabetes mellitus,* ed Creutzfeldt, W., Kobhaling, J. & Neel, J.V., p. 1. Berlin: Springer-Verlag.
Neel, J.V. (1962): *Am. J. Hum. Genet.* 14, 353.
Nelson, R.A., Wahner, H.W., Jones, J.D., Ellefson, R.D., Zollman, P.E. (1973): *Am. J. Physiol.* 224, 491.
Nerup, J., Anderson, O.O., Bendixen, G., Egeberg, J. & Poulsen, J.E. (1971): *Diabetes* 20, 424.
Nerup, J., Platz, P., Anderson, O.O., Christy, M., Lyngse, J., Poulsen, J.E., Ryder, L.P., Nielsen, L.S., Thomsen, M. & Svejgaard, A. (1974): *Lancet* 2, 864.
Ogilvie, R.F. (1937): *Q. Jl. Med.* 30, 287.
Ortiz, C.L., Costa, D. & LeBouef, B.J. (in press): Water and energy flux in elephant seal pups fasting under natural conditions.
O'Sullivan, J.B. & Mahan, C.M. (1965): *J. Am. Med. Ass.* 194, 587.
Owen, O.E. & Reichard, G.A.J. (1971): *J. Clin. Invest.* 50, 1538.
Pardridge, W.M. & Oldensorf, W.H. (1977): *J. Neurochem.* 28, 5.
Pinshow, B., Fedak, M.A., Battles, D.R. & Schmidt-Nielsen, K. (1976): *Am. J. Physiol.* 231, 903.
Prior, I.A.M. & Davidson, F. (1966). *N.Z. Med. J.* 65, 375.
Pupo, A.A., Ursich, M.J.M., Lauraguchi, E. & Vasioncellos, F.G. (1976): *Diabetes* 25, 161.
Pyorala, K., Lehtovirta, E. & Llomaki, L. (1974): *Acta Endocr., Suppl.* 181, 23.
Rabinowitz, D. & Zierler, K.L. (1962): *J. Clin. Invest.* 41, 2173.
Reichard, G.A., Owen, O.E. & Itaff, A.C. (1974): *J. Clin. Invest.* 53, 508.
Renold, A.E., Muller, W.A., Mintz, D. & Cahill, G.F. (1977): Diabetes mellitus. In *Metabolic basis of inherited disease.* 4th edn, ed Stanbury, J.B., Wyngaarden, J,B. & Fredrickson, D.S. New York: McGraw-Hill.
Renold, A.E. & Dulin, W.E. (1967): *Diabetologia* 3, 63.
Rimm, A.A., Werner, L.H., van Iserloo, B. & Bernstein, R. (1975): *Publ. Hlth. Rep.* 90, 44.
Roth, J., Kahn, C.R., Lesniak, M.A., Gorden, P., deMeyts, P., Megyesi, K., Neville, D.M., Jr., Gavin, J.R., III, Soll, A.H., Freychet, P., Goldfine, I.D., Bar, J.S. & Archer, J.A. (1975): *Rec. Prog. Horm. Res.* 31, 95.
Rowe, D.W., Starman, B.J., Fujimoto, W.Y. & Williams, R.H. (1976): *Diabetes 25,* Suppl. 1, abst. No. 62.
Rudman, D., DiFulca, T.J., Galambos, J.T., Smith, R.B. III, Salam, A.A. & Warren, W.D. (1973): *J. Clin. Invest.* 52, 2241.
Rushforth, N.B., Bennett, P.H., Steinberg, A.G., Burch, T.A. & Miller, M. (1971): *Diabetes* 20, 756.
Salans, L.B., Bray, G.A., Cushman, S.W., Danforth, E., Jr., Glennon, J.A., Horton, E.S. & Sims, E.A.H. (1974): *J. Clin. Invest.* 53, 848.
Schliack, V. (1954): *Z. Klin. Med.* 151, 382.
Second Brook Lodge Workshop on spontaneous 'diabetes' in animals (1970): *Diabetologia* 6, 153.
Stauffacher, W., Orci, L., Cameron, D.P., Burr, I.M. & Renold, A.E. (1971): *Rec. Prog. Horm. Res.* 27, 41.
Stein, J.H., West, K.M., Robey, J.M., Tirador, D.F. & MacDonald, G.W. (1965): *Archs Intern. Med.* 166, 842.
Tattersall, R.B, & Pyke, D.A. (1972): *Lancet* 2, 1120.
Third Brook Lodge Workshop on spontaneous diabetes in laboratory animals (1974): *Diabetologia* 10, 493.
Thomsen, M., Platz, P., Anderson, O.O., Christy, M., Lyngse, J., Nerup, J., Rasmussen, K., Ryder, L.P., Nielsen, L.S. & Suejgaard, A. (1975): *Transplant Rev.* 22, 125.
Trowell, H. (1974): *Lancet* 2, 998.
Vague, J. (1956): *Am. J. Nutr.* 4, 20.
Warren. S., LeCompte, P.M. & Legg, M.A. (1966): *The pathology of diabetes mellitus,* p. 231. Philadelphia: Lea & Febiger.
West, K.M., Bailey, C.P., Coniglione, T.C., Smith Jr., W.O., Scroggins, K.R., Ellison, M.G., Maxwell, E.L., Sanders, M.L. & Whayne, T.F. (1974): Diabetes in nineteen Oklahoma Indian tribes. *Diabetes* 23, 285 abstract.
Westlung, K. & Nicolaysen, R. (1972): *Scand. J. Clin. and Lab. Invest.* 30, suppl. 127, 1.
Yalow, R.S. & Berson, S.A. (1960): *J. Clin. Invest.* 39, 1157.

12
An overview of experimental models of obesity

B. JEANRENAUD*
Laboratoires de Recherches Médicales et Département de Médecine, Geneva University, 64 Avenue de la Roseraie, 1205 Geneva, Switzerland.

During this lecture, I should like to summarize the main pathological traits of the syndromes of obesity in animals, as I see them. Figure 1 illustrates the syndromes of obesity that we shall consider, and which can be either inherited (as is the case for various types of mice and rats designated by a double symbol eg, *ob/ob*, indicating that their overall abnormalities are due to a double recessive gene) or experimentally produced by chemicals (eg, administration of goldthioglucose) or by electrolytic lesions of the ventromedial hypothalamus (VMH) (for rev.: Assimacopoulos-Jeannet & Jeanrenaud, 1976; Bray, 1977). It is interesting to realize that whatever the cause of the obesities mentioned in Fig. 1, ie whether the syndromes are inherited or acquired, the main metabolic and hormonal abnormalities observed are very similar (Assimacopolous-Jeannet & Jeanrenaud, 1976). Due to this, and for the sake of clarity, I shall consider all the types of obese animals indicated in Fig. 1 as a single entity. Beside their increased body weight due to excessive fat depots, the principal characteristics of these animals are the existence of an hyperinsulinemic state and, in spite of this, hyperglycemia together with an abnormal glucose tolerance, indicating the prevalence of resistance to the action of insulin (Assimacopoulos-Jeannet & Jeanrenaud, 1976; Jeanrenaud, 1976).

Genetic obesities – *ob/ob* mice
– *db/db* mice
– *mdb/mdb* mice
– *fa/fa* rats

Hypothalamic lesions
– chemical lesions
(goldthioglucose, GTG)
– electrolytic lesions
of mice and rats

OB/OB GTG

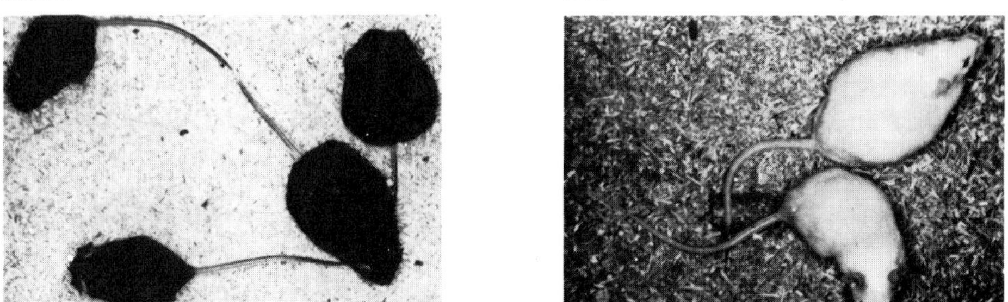

Fig. 1. Summary of some genetic and hypothalamic obese mice and rats. (Assimacopoulos-Jeannet & Jeanrenaud, 1976; Bray, 1977)

**The work summarized in this lecture has been a joint effort that included the collaboration of: F. Assimacopoulos-Jeannet, H.R. Berthoud, D. Bereiter, A.C. Hochstrasser-Dufour, C. Karakash, E.G. Loten, F. Rohner (Geneva); P. Freychet and Y. Le Marchand (Nice); B. Hustvedt and A.Løvø (Oslo), as cited in the literature*

By this summary, I shall attempt to answer three questions: (1) why are these animals obese? (2) why are they hyperglycemic since, being hyperinsulinemic, they should be hypoglycemic? (3) what is the possible cause of their hyperinsulinemia?

Possible etiology of animal obesities

Let us first consider why these animals are obese. It is useful to recall that lipogenesis and lipid accretion are due to the metabolic activity of two organs, the liver and the adipose tissue. Liver synthesizes triglycerides, stores them in part as small lipid droplets, oxidizes or secretes them out as triglycerides contained in very low density lipoproteins (VLDL) (Müller *et al.*, 1976; Assimacopoulos-Jeannet *et al.*, 1977). Adipose tissue synthesizes triglycerides mainly from glucose, and takes up TG-VLDL originating from the liver (Jeanrenaud & Hepp, 1970). Under normal conditions, these pathways of lipid metabolism are under the control of several hormones, particularly insulin (Jeanrenaud & Hepp, 1970; Assimacopoulos-Jeannet *et al.*, 1977; Hems, 1977). If an animal becomes obese, it is thus likely to have abnormalities at the level of these two tissues. We and others (for rev.: Assimacopoulos-Jeannet & Jeanrenaud, 1976) therefore studied liver and adipose tissue metabolism in various types of obese animals.

Let us consider these hepatic abnormalities (Assimacopoulos-Jeannet *et al.*, 1974; Loten, Rabinovitch & Jeanrenaud, 1974; Karakash *et al.*, 1977; Le Marchand *et al.*, 1977*a;* Le Marchand, Freychet & Jeanrenaud, 1977*b*). One should emphasize that whether genetically obese mice *(ob/ob* type) or hypothalamic obese mice or rats were investigated, using either *in vivo* or *in vitro* techniques, very similar hepatic abnormalities were recorded. These abnormalities were the following: (1) increased lipogenesis from various substrates; (2) increased triglyceride secretion; (3) decreased ability to oxidize fatty acids to ketone bodies; (4) accumulation of triglycerides within the hepatocytes. Fatty livers often develop due to the imbalance between lipogenesis and the lipid oxidizing capacity. All of these types of obese animals are hyperinsulinemic, and since insulin normally influences hepatic lipid metabolism (Assimacopoulos *et al.*, 1977; Hems, 1977), we hypothesized that these abnormalities could be due to an overstimulation of the liver by excessive amounts of circulating insulin. To demonstrate this, several indirect approaches were used. Hyperinsulinemia was reduced, prior to studying liver metabolism, either by treating the animals with the B-cytotozic agent, streptozotocin; by submitting them to a fast of varying duration; or by injecting them with anti-insulin serum (AIS). In all instances, as summarized in Table 1, the abnormalities of liver metabolism were restored to or towards normal when hyperinsulinemia of obese animals was corrected.

When adipose tissue metabolism was considered, similar conclusions were reached (Loten *et al.*, 1974; Loten *et al.*, 1976; Le Marchand *et al.*, 1977*b*). Lipogenesis of untreated obese

Table 1. Hyperinsulinemia: a key factor in liver and adipose tissue abnormalities of obese animals

	Liver abnormalities in obese animals	**Corrected by correcting hyperinsulinemia**
1.	Increased lipogenesis	yes
2.	Increased VLDL secretion	yes
3.	Decreased fatty acid oxidation to ketone bodies	yes
4.	Increased triglyceride content	yes
5.	Decreased number of insulin receptors per unit plasma membrane	yes
	Adipose tissue abnormalities in obese animals	
1.	Increased lipogenesis	yes
2.	Increased lipoprotein lipase activity	?
3.	Decreased number of insulin receptors per unit plasma membrane	yes

animals was much higher than that of lean controls. Furthermore, when obese animals were treated with streptozotocin or AIS, lipogenesis in adipose tissue was reduced to values that were similar to those of controls (Table 1). In a similar fashion (Table 1), the activity of adipose tissue lipoprotein lipase (an enzyme needed for the actual uptake of circulating lipids) was found to be high in untreated obese animals, correlating with a marked degree of hyperinsulinemia (Rath, Hems & Beloff-Chain, 1974). To summarize the first question as to why these animals are obese, we can tentatively conclude, as depicted in Fig. 2, that hyper-

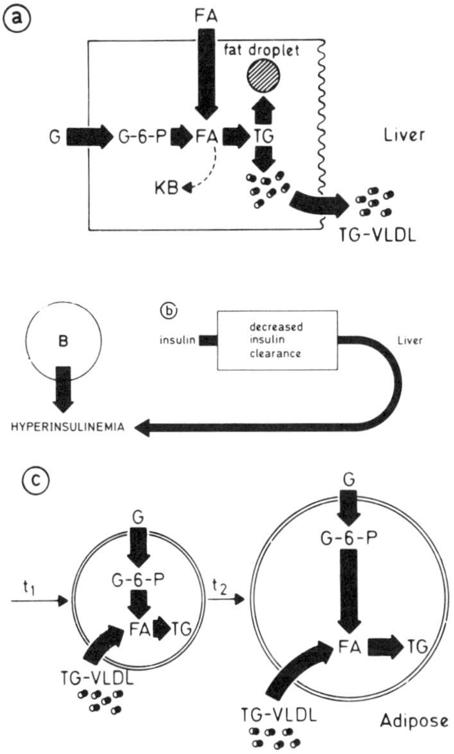

Fig. 2. Schematic representation of the consequences of hyperinsulinemia upon liver and adipose tissue metabolism in obese animals. (Jeanrenaud, 1976). G=glucose, G-6-P=glucose-6-phosphate; FA= fatty acids; KB=ketone bodies; TG=triglycerides; VLDL= very low density lipoproteins

insulinemia: (1) stimulates hepatic oversynthesis of triglycerides, together with oversecretion of TG-VLDL, while less lipids are oxidized, and hence a fatty liver develops; and (2) stimulates adipose tissue oversynthesis of lipids, mainly from glucose, and takes up excessive amounts of VLDL derived from the liver. This contributes to triglyceride secretion in fat cells with a resulting increase in the size of TG-overloaded adipocytes and, eventually, obesity. Figure 2 schematizes another abnormality of livers of obese animals, ie the existence of a lesser clearance of insulin. It is known (Mortimore & Tietze, 1959) that under normal conditions the liver 'clears', ie removes from circulating blood, a sizeable amount of insulin when the hormone passes through the organ. We were interested in determining whether the 'clearance' capacity of the liver would be altered in syndromes with obesity. That this appears to be the case is illustrated by Fig. 3 (Karakash, Assimacopoulos-Jeannet & Jeanrenaud, 1976). In these experiments, insulin was radioimmunologically determined just before entering and upon leaving perfused livers during a single passage through the organ ('flow-through experiments'). We observed that, in normal livers, the percentage of the total insulin infused into the portal vein, and that was removed after one passage, decreased when the concentration of the hormone was raised from 2.5 to 20 ng/g/min. Of more importance was

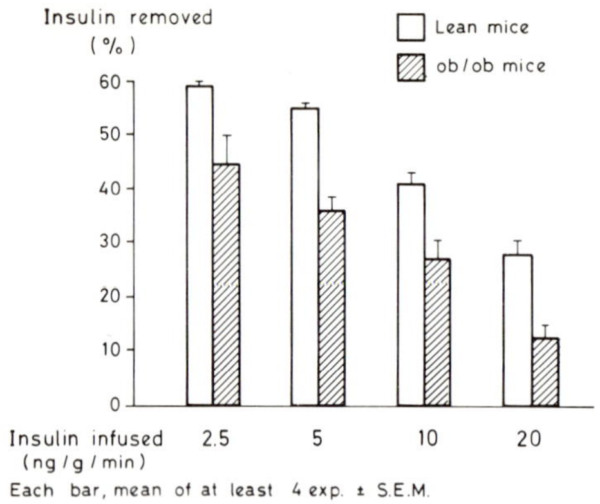

Fig. 3. Effect of increasing concentrations of portal insulin upon its removal by perfused livers of lean and obese *(ob/ob)* mice during one passage of the hormone through the organ ('flow through experiments'). (Karakash *et al.,* 1976)

the observation that, for all insulin concentrations tested, livers of the obese mice always removed significantly less of the hormone than controls. Although the precise nature of this defect in hepatic insulin removal is unknown, one can speculate that such an abnormality could further favor hyperinsulinemia since, whatever the concentration of the hormone that reaches the liver of the obese animal, a greater percentage of it is prone to be recovered peripherally as compared to controls. It is interesting to note that this abnormailty is related to hyperinsulinemia, as it disappears or is attenuated when hyperinsulinemia of obese animals is corrected by prior streptozotocin treatment, AIS administration or fasting.

The importance of hyperinsulinemia in bringing about an increase in liver and adipose tissue lipogenesis was further supported by carrying out experiments in genetic C57BL/ks *mdb/mdb* mice (Le Marchand & Jeanrenaud, 1977). In the *mdb/mdb* mice, the animals that will become obese and hyperglycemic can be recognized (prior to overt obesity) by the fact that the gene responsible for the coat color (*m*) is linked with that responsible for the obesity syndrome (*db*) (Coleman & Hummel, 1974). Thus, the misty (*m*), ie greyish pups, will become fat, while the black ones will remain non-obese. Such mice can thus be investigated as a function of their age until they actually become obese. It was observed that the body weight of controls (*mdb*/++; ++/++ mice) and the potentially obese animals (*mdb/mdb*) was identical both before weaning and, following weaning, up to about 30 to 40 days of age. An overt increase in body weight in *mdb/mdb* mice was evident only from two months onwards. It was, therefore, of interest to find (Fig. 4, 5) that, before weaning, hepatic as well as adipose tissue lipogenesis was small and identical in both control and *mdb/mdb* mice. Lipogenesis became markedly greater in weaned *mdb/mdb* mice than in weaned controls at about 30 days of age. This actually coincided, as shown by Fig. 6, with the occurrence of hyperinsulinemia which, after weaning and at about 30 days of age, reached values that were two to three times higher than normal. Insulin increased further thereafter and, subsequently, always remained much greater than control values. In contrast, only a 25 per cent increase in insulinemia was recorded in the *mdb/mdb* animals prior to weaning (Coleman & Hummel, 1974). Figure 7 schematizes these and other data obtained with *mdb/mdb* mice. We have observed that the *mdb/mdb* mice were apparently not hyperphagic. However, from the 12th day of age onwards they were chemically obese, as their carcass lipid content was increased when compared to controls, even though their body weight was normal.

The early pre-weaning excess in body lipids of the *mdb/mdb* pups,which cannot be explained by an increase in either hepatic or adipose tissue lipogenesis, appears to be due in part to an augmented uptake, by adipose tissue, of circulating lipids derived from mother's milk (Le Marchand & Jeanrenaud,1977). On the basis of these experiments we have hypothesized that there might be two phases in the development of genetic obesity of the *mdb/mdb* type (Fig. 7). In the pre-weaning phase, pups are exposed to the high lipid (16.7 g/100 ml)

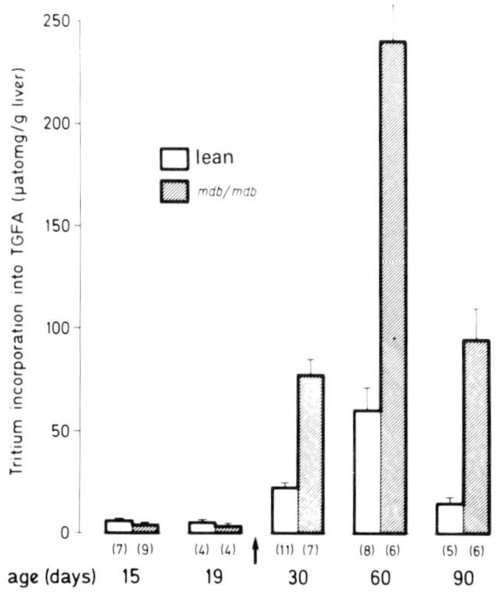

Fig. 4. ***In vivo*** **liver lipogenesis from tritiated water in lean controls and** ***mdb/mdb*** **mice.** ^{3}H incorporation into triglyceride fatty acids (TGFA) was determined. Each column is the mean ± s.e., the number of animals being in parenthesis (Le Marchand & Jeanrenaud, 1977) Arrow=weaning time (21 days of age)

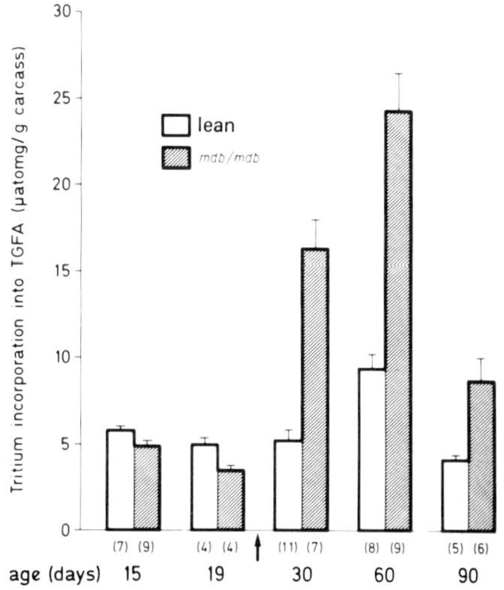

Fig. 5. ***In vivo*** **carcass lipogenesis from tritiated water in lean controls and** ***mdb/mdb*** **mice.** Exptl. design as in Fig. 4. Each column is the mean ± s.e., the number of animals being in parenthesis (Le Marchand & Jeanrenaud, 1977). Arrow=weaning time (21 days of age)

and low carbohydrate (1.3 g/100 ml) diet of the mother's milk. It is conceivable that due to this, the underlying abnormality of the B-cells of the *mdb/mdb* mice is kept to a minimum, allowing only slight hyperinsulinemia that might be sufficient, however, to stimulate lipoproteinlipase that would favor lipid deposition originating from mother's milk. The slight hyperinsulinemia of the pre-weaning phase, together with the low carbohydrate availability, would keep both adipose tissue and liver lipogenesis to a minimum. After weaning, due to the switch from the high fat to the high carbohydrate diet of the laboratory chow (and possibly to other unknown factors), the underlying defect of the B-cells of the *mdb/mdb* mice would become overt. Thenceforth, gross hyperinsulinemia, together with an ample carbohydrate availability, would overstimulate the liver and adipose tissue lipogenesis, thus bringing about the full syndrome of obesity.

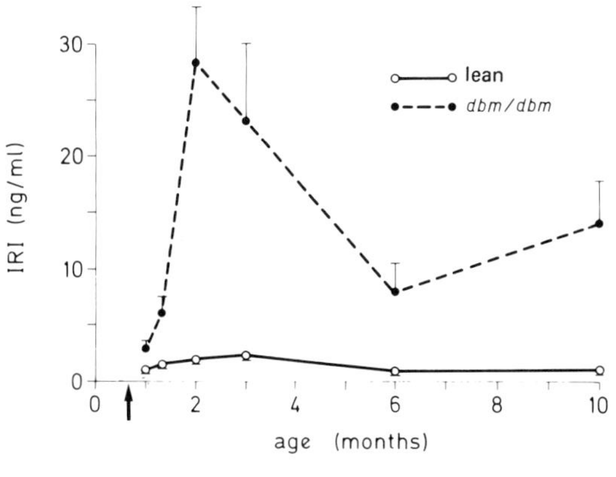

Fig. 6. Insulin levels of lean and ***mdb/mdb*** **mice.** Mean of 6-15 values ± s.e. (Le Marchand & Jeanrenaud, 1977). Arrow=weaning time (21 days of age). IRI: immunoreactive insulin

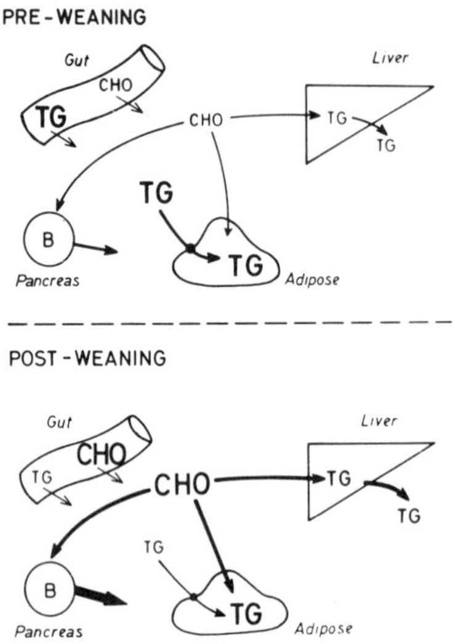

Fig. 7. Schematic representation of the abnormalities of the *mdb/mdb* obese mice in the pre-weaning and post-weaning phases (see text). (Le Marchand & Jeanrenaud, 1977)

Possible etiology of hyperglycemia in animal obesities

This leads us to the second question of why the obese animals are hyperglycemic and usually intolerant to carbohydrate. From several sets of data it seems that the appearance of an insulin resistance state is progressive, and related to the degree of hyperinsulinemia (for rev.: Assimacopoulos-Jeannet & Jeanrenaud, 1976; Le Marchand *et al.*, 1977*b*). Such an evolution is depicted in Fig. 8 for adipose tissue. When glucose metabolism and insulin responsiveness were tested in adipose tissue, two observations were made (Le Marchand *et al.*, 1977*b)*: (1)

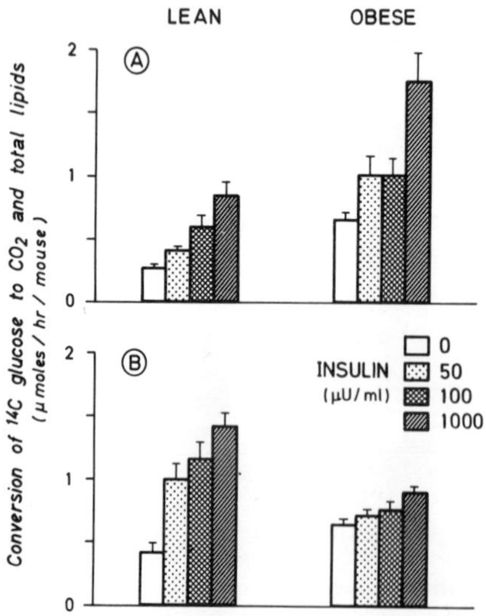

Fig. 8. Total glucose metabolism by fat pads of 9-weeks (A) or 20 weeks old (B) lean and goldthioglucose obese mice. Occurrence of insulin resistance in the 20 week old obese animals (Le Marchand *et al.*, 1977). Krebs-Ringer bicarbonate buffer with 1% bovine albumin and 7.5 mmol glucose. Total glucose metabolism, sum of CO_2 + total lipids. Each column, mean of 8 values ± s.e.

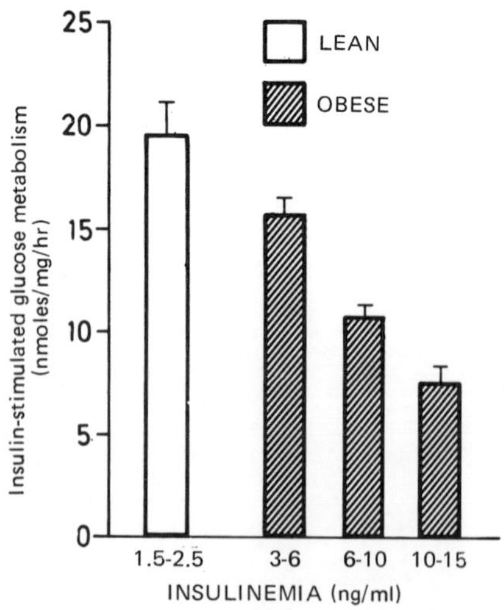

Fig. 9. Apparent correlation between insulinemia, and *in vitro* response of soleus muscles to insulin of 20 week old goldthioglucose obese mice. (Le Marchand *et al.*, 1977*b*). Krebs-Ringer bicarbonate buffer containing 3% albumin, 5 mmol glucose. Glucose metabolism: glycogen synthesis + glycolysis. Insulin 1mU/ml. Each column, mean of 6-10 values ±s.e.

adipose tissue from young or older lean mice responded to insulin added *in vitro* by an increase in glucose metabolism; (2) adipose tissue from young and moderately hyperinsulinemic obese mice also responded and even overresponded, to insulin *in vitro*. However, when obesity persisted and the hyperinsulinemia became grossly abnormal, the adipose tissue failed to be influenced by the hormone. The tissue had become insulin resistant. In a similar way (Fig. 9), insulin was capable of stimulating glucose metabolism in soleus muscles of lean mice but, in muscles of obese mice, the hormone was much less effective in doing so (Le Marchand *et al.*, 1977*b*). Muscles of obese animals thus had also become insulin resistant, a resistance that was related to the degree of hyperinsulinemia prevailing *in vivo* just prior to the experiment (Fig. 9) (Cuendet *et al.*, 1976; Le Marchand *et al.*, 1977*b*). Thus as summarized in Fig. 10, hyperinsulinemia of obese animals initially results in alterations of both hepatic and adipose tissue metabolism. Subsequently, it is accompanied by a state of resistance

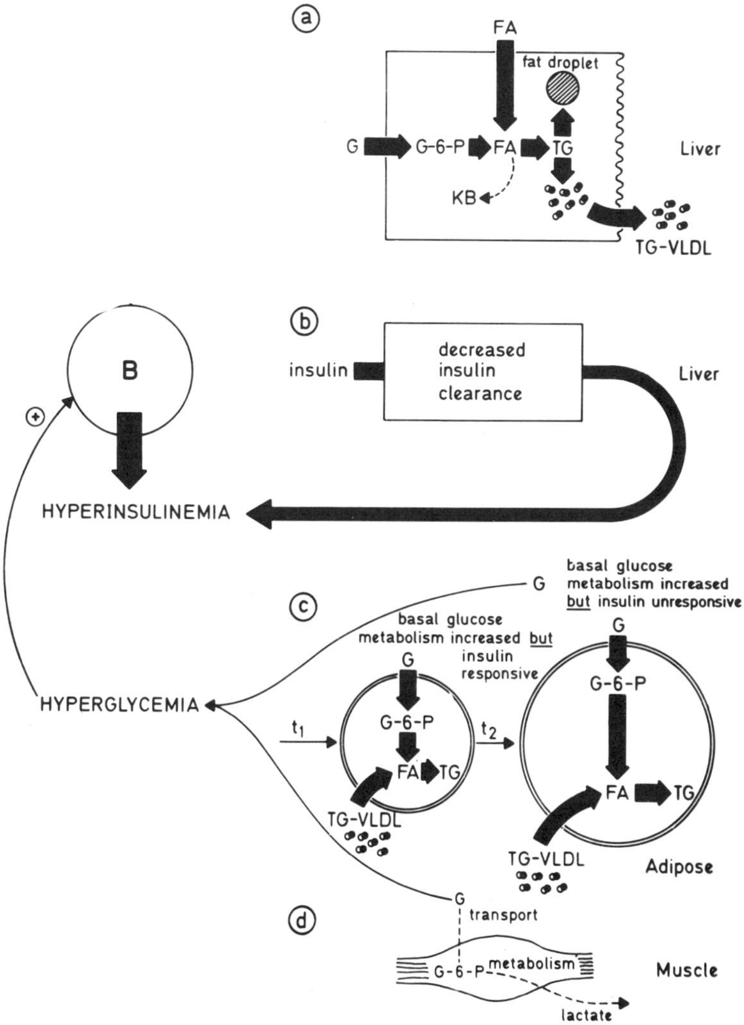

Fig. 10. Schematic representation of the consequences of hyperinsulinemia upon liver, adipose and muscle tissue metabolism in obese animals (Jeanrenaud, 1976). G=glucose; G-6-P=glucose-6-phosphate; FA=fatty acids; KB=ketone bodies; TG=triglycerides; VLDL=very low density lipoproteins. Insulin resistance brings about hyperglycemia that further favors hyperinsulinemia (see text)

to the effect of the hormone, particularly at the level of adipose tissue and muscle, a defect that produces hyperglycemia. As glucose is a powerful stimulus of insulin secretion, hyperinsulinemia is further favored, placing obese animals in obvious metabolic and hormonal vicious circles.

The nature of insulin resistance is complex (Archer *et al.*, 1973; Salans *et al.*, 1974; Olefsky & Reaven, 1975; Amatruda, Livingstone & Lockwood, 1975; Freychet, 1976; Olefsky, 1976), and I shall attempt to illustrate it by using experiments carried out in soleus muscles (Le Marchand, Jeanrenaud & Freychet, 1978). Analogous, although not identical, alterations have been noted in adipose tissue. Muscles of obese animals are characterized by a marked decrease in the specific binding of insulin that can be attributed to an actual decrease in the number of insulin receptors per unit plasma membrane. It can be further demonstrated that the decreased insulin binding, ie the decrease in receptors number, is most marked when hyperinsulinemia of obese animals *in vivo* is greatest. Thus hyperinsulinemia appears to exert a suppressive influence upon receptors of target tissues via mechanisms that are still largely unknown (Freychet, 1976). What are the metabolic consequences of such a decrease in the number of receptors in obese animals? If the number of receptors (R) per unit membrane is decreased, the formation of an adequate hormone (H) receptor (R) complex (HR) to exert biological activity will now require a higher concentration of the hormone. As a consequence, the target tissues for insulin in obese animals will become less sensitive to the hormone. This was indeed shown to be the case (Le Marchand, Jeanrenaud & Freychet, 1978). When glucose uptake was measured in muscles from lean and obese animals, it could be seen that half-maximal stimulation was achieved at a much lower concentration of insulin in muscles of normal than in muscles of obese mice. Another abnormality could be detected in muscles of obese mice (Le Marchand *et al.*, 1978). When overall glucose metabolism was tested *in vitro* in the presence of insulin, the latter was always less in muscles of obese animals than in those of lean controls. This was true even when very high concentrations of insulin were tested. At this point, two comments should be made: (1) it can be demonstrated that in normal muscle, maximal stimulation of overall glucose metabolism can be obtained when only about 20 per cent of total available insulin receptors are filled by the hormone (Le Marchand *et al.*, 1978); (2) on the basis of insulin binding studies one can estimate that the decrease in the number of receptors (R) in muscles of obese mice is such that about 30 per cent of the initial 'stock' appears to remain available (Freychet, 1976; Le Marchand *et al.*, 1977*a*). Thus, in muscles of obese mice there are theoretically enough receptors left to obtain maximal stimulatory effect of insulin at maximal concentrations of the hormone. However, as noted above, this does not appear to be the case. This suggests that in muscles of obese mice, there must be a defect either at the level of the coupling between the HR complex and the insulin sensitive pathways, or at a site more distal than the HR complex, eg an intracellular defect that might interfere with normal glucose utilization (Czech, 1976; Le Marchand *et al.*, 1977*a*; Le Marchand *et al.*, 1978). The overall abnormalities in muscles of obese animals that bring about an insulin resistant state are summarized in Table 2. As shown in this table, insulin resistance appears to be a multifactorial phenomenon and, in addition, is likely to change from one type of obesity to another and from one target tissue to another.

Table 2. Abnormalities of muscles of obese animals responsible for the occurrence of insulin resistance. (Analogous alterations are observed in adipose tissue)

1. Decreased insulin binding (ie decreased number of insulin receptors per unit plasma membrane)
2. Decreased insulin sensitivity
3. Decreased maximal effect of insulin possibly due to:

    Defect in coupling between hormone-receptor complex and insulin-sensitive pathways
    Intracellular factors inhibiting glucose utilization
    Other factors

Possible etiology of hyperinsulinemia in animal obesities

Let us now consider the third and last question, namely, why are obese animals hyperinsulinemic? In hypothalamic obesity, it is evident that the defect originates in the hypothalamus (Hustvedt & Løvø, 1972; York & Bray, 1973; Goldman *et al.*, 1974). As depicted by Fig. 11,

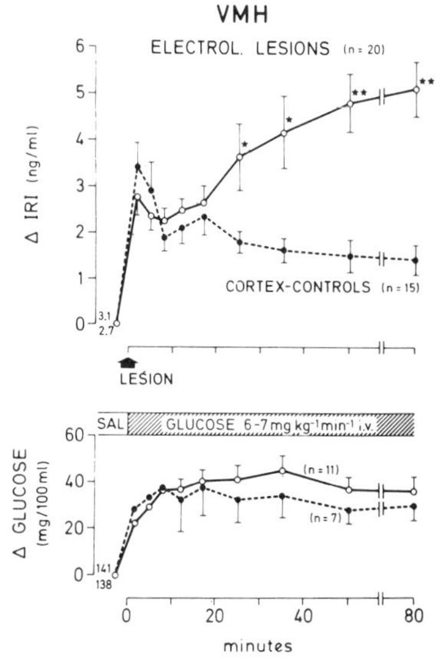

Fig. 11. Role of the hypothalamus in the insulin secretion *in vivo* (Berthoud & Jeanrenaud, unpublished data). Acute electrolytic lesions of the ventromedial hypothalamic (VMH) area were made in anesthetized rats, immediately followed by a glucose infusion. Controls were lesioned in the cortex area. IRI: immunoreactive insulin

when acute lesions were placed in the VMH area and were immediately followed by a glucose infusion or by a glucose bolus, a marked increase in insulin secretion was obtained when compared to that obtained in sham-operated controls similarly treated (Berthoud & Jeanrenaud, in preparation; Rohner *et al.*, 1977). Of note was the observation that hyperinsulinemia obtained by such acute lesions of the VMH area persisted thereafter even when hyperphagia was prevented (Karakash *et al.*, 1977). The functional relationships that may exist between the hypothalamus and the activity of the endocrine pancreas are still poorly understood. It is noteworthy, however, that the oversecretion of insulin that follows acute lesioning of the hypothalamic area can largely be prevented by concomitantly cutting the vagus nerve (Dufour, Berthoud & Jeanrenaud, in preparation).

Since hypothalamic lesions produce hyperinsulinemia, it is conceivable that they would result in alterations not only of B-cell activity but in the relationships possibly existing between the A (glucagon)-cells and the D- (somatostatin) ones. Indeed, when electrolytic lesions were placed in the hypothalamus of normal rats, and when resulting hyperphagia was prevented by feeding VMH-lesioned rats with a diet matching exactly that of controls, the following changes were observed in subsequently isolated and perfused pancreases: (1) an increase in overall insulin secretion following a glucose load (Fig. 12), without qualitative alterations of the pattern of the hormone output; (2) an increase in basal glucagon secretion; (3) an increase in pancreatic content of both insulin and glucagon (Rohner & Jeanrenaud, in preparation; Bierwolf, Blech & Weiss, in preparation).

When one considers genetic obesity, it is fascinating to realize that the changes in the endocrine pancreas observed are rather analogous to those just described in animals with experimental hypothalamic lesions (Table 3). Thus, it has been shown, both *in vivo* and *in vitro*, that pancreases from *ob/ob* mice oversecrete insulin when the organ is challenged by glucose (Stauffacher *et al.*, 1971; Beloff-Chain, Newman & Mansford, 1973). Similarly, pancreatic insulin (Stauffacher *et al.*, 1971; Loten *et al.*, 1974) and pancreatic glucagon contents (Patel *et al.*, 1976) were increased while that of somatostatin was decreased in both *ob/ob* and *db/db* mice (Patel *et al.*, 1976).

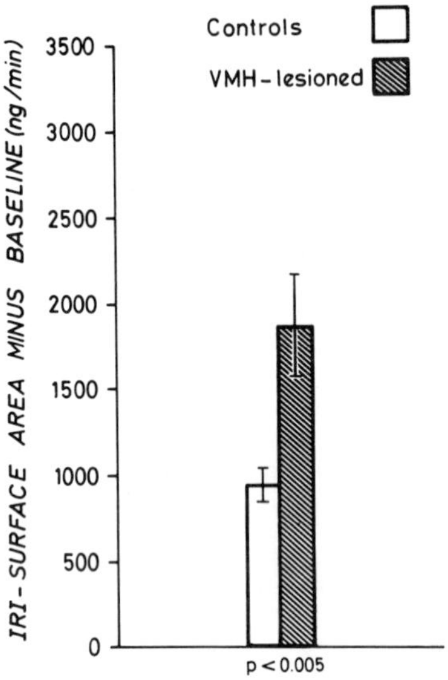

Fig. 12. Glucose-induced (20mmol) **insulin secretion by perfused pancreases of control and immediately food-restricted ventromedial hypothalamic (VMH)-lesioned rats** (Rohner & Jeanrenaud, unpublished data). IRI: immunoreactive insulin. KRB buffer-Glucose 20mmol-Perfusion time: 20 min. Mean of 7-5 experiments±s.e.m.

Table 3. Apparent similarities in the changes of endocrine pancreases from genetically-obese and hypothalamic-obese animals

Type of obesity	**Insulin secretion**	**Pancreatic content of:**		
		Insulin	**Glucagon**	**Somatostatin**
Hypothalamic	increased	increased	increased	?
Genetic	increased	increased	increased	decreased

As schematized in Fig. 13, and on the basis of the available observations that point to the existence of at least some similarities between the function of the endocrine pancreas of genetically obese and of hypothalamic obese animals, one could speculate that genetic obese animals might have a defect in the hypothalamus (Bray & York, 1971). Although this concept is still poorly substantiated, an abnormal hypothalamic regulation of food intake has been proposed (Coleman & Hummel, 1969; Coleman, 1973). Similarly, neurotransmitter contents have been shown to be abnormal in some genetic obese animals (Lorden, Oltmans

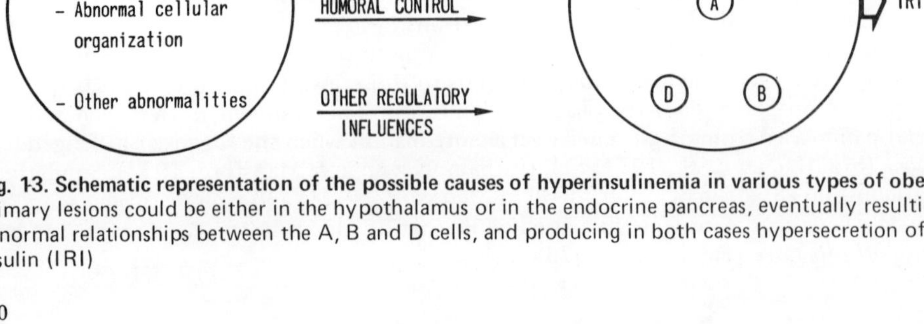

Fig. 13. Schematic representation of the possible causes of hyperinsulinemia in various types of obesities. Primary lesions could be either in the hypothalamus or in the endocrine pancreas, eventually resulting in abnormal relationships between the A, B and D cells, and producing in both cases hypersecretion of insulin (IRI)

& Margules, 1976; Lorden & Oltmans, 1977). Finally, preliminary results from our laboratories (Bereiter & Jeanrenaud, in preparation) suggest that the anatomical organization of the hypothalamus of the *ob/ob* mice might differ from that of controls. Such hypothalamic disorders of obese animals could, via neural, humoral or other distorted control mechanisms, affect the normal regulation of the endocrine pancreas, and alter in particular the functional relationship between the A, the B and the D cells, with resulting portal hyperinsulinemia and hyperglucagonemia. However, a primary etiology of the hypersecretion of insulin, including abnormal A-B-D cell relationships in genetic obese animals, could also reside in the endocrine pancreas *per se*. Indeed, it has been shown that the implantation of normal islets into *ob/ob* mice (Strautz, 1970) or to New Zealand obese mice (Gates *et al.*, 1972) resulted in a partial normalization of the hyperinsulinemia of the obese animals. When normal islets had their B-cell destroyed by streptozotocin, they nevertheless retained their ability to bring about amelioration of the hyperinsulinemia of the New Zealand obese animals (Gates, Hunt & Lazarus, 1974). This suggested the possible existence of some diffusible and relatively stable endocrine pancreatic factor(s) that would eventually regulate and coordinate the function of the pancreas leading to insulin secretion.

It is evident that considerable research efforts must now be placed in defining the normal functional relationships that may exist between the hypothalamus and the endocrine pancreas, and the normal functional relationships between the various cell types within the endocrine pancreas, in order to subsequently decide which of these relationships might be primarily abnormal in spontaneous obesity syndromes. This is all the more crucial if one tends to think, as I do, that most of the abnormalities of the obesity syndromes in general are secondary to a key factor, hyperinsulinemia.

Acknowledgements – Work supported by grants of the Fonds National de la Recherche Scientifique, Berne, Switzerland; and by a grant-in-aid of Nestlé-Alimentana, Vevey, Switzerland.

References

Amatruda, J.M., Livingston, J.N. & Lockwood, D.H. (1975): *Science* **188**, 264.
Archer, J.A., Gorden, P., Gavin, J.R., Lesniak, M.A. & Roth, J. (1973): *J. Clin. Endoc. Metab.* **36**, 627.
Assimacopoulos-Jeannet, F., Singh, A., Le Marchand, Y., Loten, E.G. & Jeanrenaud, B. (1974): *Diabetologia* **10**, 155.
Assimacopoulos-Jeannet, F. & Jeanrenaud, B. (1976): *Clins Endoc. Metab.* **5**, 337.
Assimacopoulos-Jeannet, F., Karakash, C., Le Marchand, Y., & Jeanrenaud, B. (1977): *Biochim. Biophys. Acta* **498**, 91.
Beloff-Chain, A., Newman, M.E. & Mansford, K.R.L. (1973): *Diabetologia* **9**, 447.
Bray, G.A. & York, D.A. (1971): *Physiol. Rev.* **51**, 598.
Bray, G.A. (1977): *Fed. Proc.* **36**, 148.
Coleman, D.L. & Hummel, K.P. (1969): *Am. J. Physiol.* **217**, 1298.
Coleman, D.L. (1973): *Diabetologia* **9**, 294.
Coleman, D.L. & Hummel, K.P. (1974): *Diabetologia* **10**, 607.
Cuendet, G.S., Loten, E.G., Jeanrenaud, B. & Renold, A.E. (1976): *J. Clin. Invest.* **58**, 1078.
Czech, M.P. (1976): *J. Clin. Invest.* **57**, 1523.
Freychet, P. (1976): *Diabetologia* **12**, 83.
Gates, R.J., Hunt, M.I., Smith, R. & Lazarus, N.R. (1972): *Lancet* **2**, 567.
Gates, R.J., Hunt, M.I. & Lazarus, N.R. (1974): *Diabetologia* **10**, 401.
Goldman, J.K., Bernardis, L.L. & Frohman, L.A. (1974): *Am. J. Physiol.* **227**, 88.
Hems, D.A. (1977): FEBS Letters **80**, 237.
Hustvedt, B.E. & Løvø, A. (1972): *Acta Physiol. Scand.* **84**, 29.
Jeanrenaud, B. & Hepp, D. (eds) (1970): Adipose tissue. Regulation and metabolic functions. *Horm. Metab. Res.* Suppl. 2. Stuttgart: G. Thieme Verlag.
Jeanrenaud, B. (1976): Diabetes research today, ed Renold, A.E., Creutzfeldt, W., & Pfeiffer, E.F. *Symposia Medica Hoechst* 12, p. 153. Stuttgart & New York: Schattauer Verlag.
Karakash, C., Assimacopoulos-Jeanner, F. & Jeanrenaud, B. (1976): *J. Clin. Invest.* **57**, 1117.
Karakash, C., Hustvedt, B.E., Lovo, A., Le Marchand, Y., & Jeanrenaud, B. (1977): *Am. J. Physiol.* **232** (3), E286.
Le Marchand, Y. & Jeanrenaud, B. (1977): *Am. J. Physiol.* (in press).

Le Marchand, Y., Loten, E.G., Assimacopoulos-Jeannet, F., Forgue, M.E., Freychet, P. & Jeanrenaud, B. (1977*a*): *Diabetes* 26, 582.
Le Marchand, Y., Freychet, P. & Jeanrenaud, B. (1977*b*): *Endocrinology* (in press).
Le Marchand, Y., Jeanrenaud, B. & Freychet, P. (1978): *Am. J. Physiol* (in press).
Lorden, J.F., Oltmans, G.A. & Margules, D.L. (1976): *Brain Res.* 117, 357.
Lorden, J.F. & Oltmans, G.A. (1977): *Brain Res.* 131, 162.
Loten, E.G., Rabinovitch, A & Jeanrenaud, B. (1974): *Diabetologia* 10, 45.
Loten, E.G., Le Marchand, Y. Assimacopoulos-Jeannet, F., Denton, R.M. & Jeanrenaud, B. (1976): *Am.J. Physiol.* 230, (3), 602.
Mortimore, G.E. & Tietze, F. (1959): *Ann. N.Y. Acad. Sci.* 82, 329.
Müller, P., Singh, A., Orci, L., & Jeanrenaud, B. (1976): *Biochim. Biophys. Acta* 428, 480.
Olefsky, J.M. & Reaven, G.M. (1975): *Endocrinology* 96, 1486.
Olefsky, J.M. (1976): *J. Clin. Invest.* 57, 842.
Patel, Y.C., Orci, L., Bankier, A. & Cameron, D.P. (1976): *Endocrinology* 99, 1415.
Rath, E.A., Hems, D.A. & Beloff-Chain, A. (1974): *Diabetologia* 10, 261.
Rohner, F., Dufour, A.C., Karakash, C., Le Marchand, Y., Ruf, K.B. & Jeanrenaud, B. (1977): *Diabetologia* 13, 239.
Salans, L.B., Bray, G.A., Cushman, S.W., Danforth, E. Jr., Glennon, J.A., Horton, E.S. & Sims, E.A.H. (1974): *J. Clin. Invest.* 53, 848.
Stauffacher, W., Orci, L., Cameron, D.P., Burr, I.M. & Renold, A.E. (1971): *Recent Prog. Horm. Res.* 27, 41.
Strautz, R.L. (1970): *Diabetologia* 6, 306.
York, D.A. & Bray, G.A. (1973): *Metabolism* 22, 443.

13
Dietary obesity

A. SCLAFANI
Department of Psychology, Brooklyn College of the City, University of New York, Brooklyn, New York 11210, USA.

Several different experimental models of obesity have been identified in animals. The most pronounced and also the most extensively investigated include the syndrome produced by medial hypothalamic damage and the various forms of genetically transmitted obesity. Models of dietary obesity have been studied less, although they are perhaps the most relevant to our understanding of human adiposity. The present paper will review those dietary conditions which lead to the excessive accumulation of body fat in laboratory animals, the two primary factors being diet composition and diet availability. Dietary effects on adipose tissue morphology will not be discussed in detail, since this topic has recently been reviewed by Stern & Johnson (in press).

Lab chow diets

In most studies of dietary obesity the control group of animals is given access *ad lib.* to a standard laboratory chow diet, usually in pellet form. The body weight and fat content of animals maintained on this diet are usually taken as the normal baseline and weights in excess of this baseline are considered to represent obesity. However, on lab chow diets adult rats contain 10 to 20 per cent body fat, depending upon their age, and some investigators consider these levels to be excessive (Berg, 1960). Furthermore, compared to rats maintained on restricted amounts of food, rats given lab chow *ad lib.* not only weigh more and contain more body fat, but also have a decreased longevity, reduced fertility, and impaired health (Berg, 1960; Berg & Simms, 1960; Ross, 1959). Therefore, it does not seem unreasonable to consider the so-called normal body weight maintained by chow-fed rats to be a mild form of obesity, especially since the amount of body fat that constitutes obesity is ill-defined (Berg, 1960). Obesity has also been observed in wild species, including the sand rat (Schmidt-Nielsen, Haines & Hackel, 1964), spiny mouse (Gonet *et al.*, 1965), and woodchuck (Young, 1976) when the animals are laboratory reared on *ad lib.* chow diets.

High fat diets

In one of the first laboratory reports of dietary obesity Ingle (1949) noted that adult male rats restricted to small cages and fed a palatable semi-liquid diet reached body weights almost twice as great as that of rats maintained in standard size cages and on a stock diet. Mickelsen, Takahashi & Craig (1955) confirmed these findings, but also observed that male rats would get just as fat when kept in standard size cages and fed either Ingle's medium carbohydrate diet or a high fat diet (60 per cent Crisco). Early studies by Fenton & Carr (1951) also revealed that high fat diets promoted excessive weight gains in mice and most subsequent dietary obesity studies have employed such diets.

The obesity-promoting effect of high fat rations results from both increased caloric intake and increased feed efficiency, defined in terms of body weight gain per calorie of food ingested. Rats prefer greasy diets to lab chow and tend to overeat when offered high fat diets (Hamilton, 1964). That is, although rats typically decrease their food intake when given high fat rations, this decrease is not sufficient to compensate for the increased caloric density of the diet, and thus their daily caloric intake is increased (Corbit & Stellar, 1964; Schemmel, Mickelsen & Gill, 1970). It has also been reported that animals are more efficient in converting dietary energy into body energy (fat) when maintained on high fat diets (Schemmel, Mickelsen & Motawi, 1972). Increased feed efficiency may account for cases in which animals become obese on high fat rations even though their caloric intake is not elevated (Herberg *et al.*, 1974; Lemonnier, 1972). Food intake, feed efficiency, and ultimately body weight gain are influenced by the concentration and type of fat in the diet. Weight gains tend to be proportional to the fat concentration, and are enhanced by diets containing long-chain triglycerides rather than medium chain triglycerides and by diets containing solid fats rather than vegetable oils (Barboriak *et al.*, 1957; Fenton & Carr, 1951; Schemmel, 1976). The strain, age, and sex of the animal are also important factors determining the degree of obesity attained on high fat diets.

There are substantial differences between the various strains of laboratory rodents in their susceptibility to dietary obesity. In a study of seven strains of rats, male Osborne-Mendel rats fed a high fat diet for 20 weeks gained 63 per cent more weight than did their grain-fed littermates, whereas males of the S 5B/P1 strain gained only 16 per cent more than did their littermate controls (Schemmel *et al.*, 1970). The S 5B/P1 rats given the high fat diet showed not only less of an increase in caloric intake compared to the Osborne-Mendel rats, but also less of an increase in feed efficiency (Schemmel & Mickelsen, 1974). The weight gains of the remaining five strains fell between these extremes. Excluding the genetically obese Zucker rat, the Osborne-Mendel rat appears to be the strain most prone to obesity. When fed a high fat diet from weaning, these rats reach a mean body weight near 1200 g (individual rats may exceed 1700 g), while the mean weight of the littermates fed a grain diet remains under 600 g (Schemmel, Mickelsen & Mostosky, 1969*a*; Schemmel & Mickelsen, 1974). It has also been reported (Maller, 1967) that wild rats gain less weight on high fat diets than do laboratory rats, but this finding is not conclusive since the laboratory rats were heavier than the wild rats to begin with (see below). Strain differences in the development of dietary obesity have also been observed in mice (Fenton & Carr, 1951).

In addition to elevating the mean body weight, feeding laboratory animals high fat rations also increases the variability in body weight (DeLaey, 1975; Schemmel *et al.*, 1970). Furthermore, there are strain differences in body weight variability. Of the seven strains studied Schemmel & co-workers (1970) observed that Hoppert rats displayed the greatest variability in weight gain on the high fat diet. In males, for example, the range in body weights was 384 to 700 g after 20 weeks on the high fat ration (mean = 495.9 g vs 402.5 g for grain-fed controls). Why some rats of the same strain and sex gain considerably more weight than others when fed high fat diets is not known and is an important question.

The age at which high fat feeding begins is another determinant of body weight gain. Rats fed a high fat diet since weaning tend to reach higher body weights than do rats fed the diet only during adulthood (Peckham *et al.*, 1962). Feeding the high fat food prior to weaning, however, does not significantly potentiate the effect of post-weaning access to the diet, at least not in the obesity prone Osborne-Mendel rat (Schemmel, Mickelsen & Fisher, 1973). Adult rats often display only modest weight gains when offered high fat diets (Corbit & Stellar, 1964; Kanarek & Hirsch, 1977; Lemonnier & Alexiu, 1974; Mickelsen *et al.*, 1955; Sclafani & Springer, 1976; Gale & Sclafani, 1977), although here again the age at which the diet is introduced is a relevant variable. Older, heavier rats tend to put on weight faster than do younger, lighter adult animals when switched to a high fat diet (Peckham *et al.*, 1962).

Another effect of early exposure to high fat rations is that, while it does not permanently elevate body weight, it appears to predispose the animal to dietary obesity. Peckham & co-workers (1962) reported that rats who were fed a high fat diet from weaning lost weight, when switched to lab chow at age 34 weeks, to levels similar to that of rat fed the lab chow from weaning. However, when subsequently given the high fat diet at age 68 weeks, the rats which had previously been fed this diet ate more food, and gained more weight than did the rats without such previous experience. The enhanced effectiveness in promoting obesity of early exposure to high fat rations has been attributed to changes in adipose cellularity and long-term behavioral effects of early feeding habits (Lemonnier & Alexiu, 1974; Peckham *et al.*, 1962), but further research is needed to resolve this question.

Although the greatest weight gains are produced when high fat feeding begins at weaning, animals fed high fat rations typically do not begin to outweigh chow-fed controls until they are approximately 60 days of age (Lemonnier, 1972; Peckham *et al.*, 1962; Schemmel *et al.*, 1969*a*). The body weight differences between the two diet groups then continues to increase as the animals get older. Thus, two age-related factors influence the degree of obesity attained on high fat diets: the age at which the diet is first introduced, and the absolute age of the animal.

Sex seems to be of limited importance in the development of fat-induced obesity. Male rats normally gain more weight and body fat than do females following weaning, and these differences are exaggerated by a high fat diet (Schemmel *et al.*, 1970). However, when body fat is expressed as a percentage of body weight then females fed a high fat ration accumulate as much or more fat than do males (Schemmel *et al.*, 1969*b*, 1970). Significant sex differences occur in the distribution of fat in the various adipose sites in rats and mice maintained on high fat diets (Lemonnier, 1972. Schemmel *et al.*, 1970). Also, females are reported to be less efficient than males in converting dietary energy into body fat (Schemmel & Mickelsen, 1974).

High carbohydrate diets

Two types of studies have revealed that mild obesity can be produced by increasing the carbohydrate content of the diet. In an experiment by Allen & Leahy (1966) adult male rats were maintained for 26 weeks on a diet containing 80.6 per cent sucrose or a standard chow diet containing 60 per cent carbohydrate, primarily in the form of starch. Despite its high sugar content, the sucrose diet was apparently not very palatable since the rats fed this diet ate significantly less than did the chow-fed rats. Nevertheless, the sucrose group gained slightly more weight than did the chow group (139 vs 127 g) and by the end of the experiment contained significantly more body fat (23.2 vs 18.0 per cent). Thus, the effect of the sucrose diet was to increase feed efficiency rather than caloric intake. Other rats fed a fructose diet also consumed less food, but accumulated more body fat (21.8 per cent) than did the chow-fed controls. However, rats fed a glucose diet gained significantly less weight than did the chow-fed rats, although the body content of the two groups was similar (19.7 vs 18.0 per cent). The glucose-fed group also gained less weight and body fat than did the sucrose-fed group, despite the fact that it consumed more food than did the sucrose-fed group. Increased fat accumulation has also been reported in baboons and humans fed high sucrose diets (Brook & Noel, 1969; Rath, 1977).

A more effective way of producing carbohydrate induced obesity has recently been reported by Kanarek & Hirsch (1977). Adult male rats were given *ad lib.* access to a 32 per cent sucrose solution in addition to lab chow and water. Compared to controls given only chow and water, these rats consumed 20 per cent more calories and gained 43 per cent more weight over a 125 day period. Increased calorie intake and weight gain were also observed in other groups of rats given access to a 16 per cent glucose, 32 per cent glucose, or 62 per cent glucose solution. The amount of sugar consumed from the various solutions was equivalent and all experimental groups reduced their chow intake such that sugar accounted for 55 to 65 per cent of their total caloric consumption. It is interesting to note, in view of the results obtained by Allen & Leahy (1966), that the group given 32 per cent sucrose tended to gain more weight than those given 32 per cent glucose although the caloric intakes of the two groups were similar.

In other studies, sugar solutions have been offered to young rats. Muto & Miyhara (1972) observed that male weanling rats given to a 40 per cent sucrose solution, in addition to a normal diet, consumed consistently more calories and gained slightly more weight (320 *vs* 290 g) over a nine-week period, compared to controls given only the high protein diet. At the end of the experiment the sucrose-fed rats contained slightly, but significantly more body fat than did the control group (4.5 vs 3.1 per cent). Rats given the sucrose solution, and a low protein diet (9 per cent) showed impaired rather than facilitated growth compared to rats given the low protein diet only. Kanarek & Hirsch (1977) have also reported that rats given access to a sucrose solution and lab chow from the time of weaning have elevated caloric intakes, but, like rats fed high fat diets (see above), do not begin to outweigh controls until they are about 70 days of age. The greater weight gain produced by presenting sugar in solution, rather than mixed in the diet, is presumably related to the palatability difference between the two forms of presentation, although other factors may also be involved.

Snack food diets

Sclafani & Springer (1976) have recently reported that feeding adult rats a variety of palatable snack food is a particularly effective way of producing dietary obesity. Female rats given, in addition to lab chow and water, a food assortment including cookies, salami, cheese, bananas, marshmallows, candy, peanut butter, and sweetened milk gained over 2.6 times as much weight in a two-month period as did females fed only lab chow (weight gains = 124 vs 46 g). This diet, sometimes disrespectfully referred to as a 'junk-food' diet, was used because attempts to produce obesity in young adult rats using a high fat diet resulted in only modest weight gains. Food intake was not systematically recorded, but it was obvious that the rats ate considerable quantities of the milk and other snack foods, and ate little of the lab chow. The milk was supplemented with vitamins and minerals and it is unlikely that nutritional deficiencies contributed to the development of obesity. The excessive weight produced by the snack foods was also not dependent upon the barren living conditions typical of laboratory rearing, since group housing the rats in a large multilevel cage did not alter the development of dietary obesity. Allowing rats access to a running wheel, however, resulted in a 27 per cent reduction in the weight gain produced by the snack food diet (see Fig. 1).

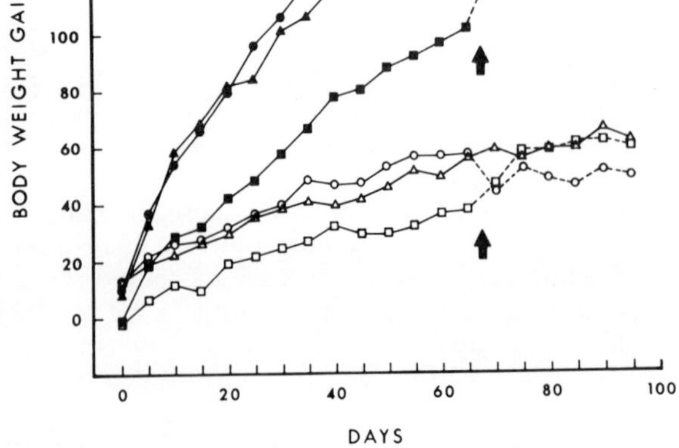

Fig. 1. The effect of housing condition on the development of dietary obesity. Adult female rats were housed either individually in standard size cages (I=isolated/inactive condition), individually in activity wheel cages (E=enriched condition), and were fed either a snack diet (S) or Purina Chow (P). On Day 65, indicated by arrow, the isolated/inactive groups (I-S, I-P) were transferred to the activity wheels thus becoming groups IA-S and IA-P, while the active groups (A-S, A-P) were transferred to the isolated/inactive condition, thus becoming groups AI-S, AI-P). (From Sclafani & Springer, 1976)

A second study by Sclafani & Gorman (1977) found that adult male rats gained as much or more weight as did females on the snack food diet, and estimates of body fat (Lee Index) indicated that males and females attained equivalent levels of obesity (Fig. 2). However, when compared to the controls of the same sex fed lab chow, the female rats gained more weight on the snack foods than did the males. It was also observed that the weight promoting effect of the snack food diet was more pronounced in older (180 days) than in younger (90 days) adult rats. In the case of the females, for example, young rats fed the snack foods gained 2.7 times as much weight in 60 days as did the chow-fed controls, while the older rats gained 9.4 times as much as controls in an equal period of time. Within the same sex and age range, however, the rats were not equally susceptible to the weight promoting effect of the snack foods, although they all outgained the control rats maintained on lab chow (Sclafani & Springer, 1976; Sclafani & Gorman, 1977). Thus, as in the case of high fat rations, the snack food diet increases both mean body weight and body weight variability.

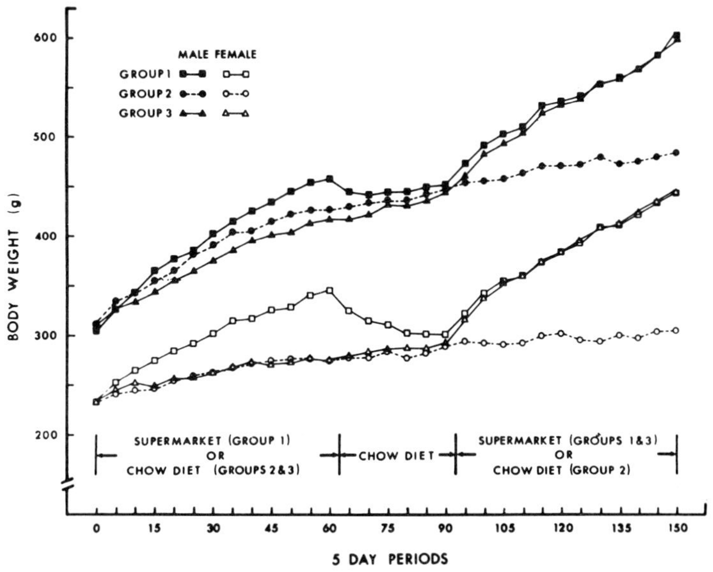

Fig. 2. The effects of sex, age, and previous dietary experience of the development of dietary obesity. Adult male and female rats (approx. 90 days old at Day 0) were individually housed in standard size cages and fed either a supermarket (snack) food diet or Purina Chow during the periods indicated in the figure. (From Sclafani & Gorman, 1977).

The overweight produced by snack foods was not a permanent effect since dietary obese rats readily lost weight when given only lab chow to eat (Sclafani & Springer, 1976; Sclafani & Gorman, 1977). Similar findings have been obtained by Gale & Van Itallie (in preparation) and these results are consistent with previous reports that the obesity induced by high fat diets is reversed when the animals are switched to lab chow (Corbit & Stellar, 1964; Peckham *et al.*, 1962). Rowe & Rolls (1977), however, have recently reported that adult rats fed a snack food diet not only became obese, but also maintained their elevated weights when given only lab chow to eat. Furthermore, when their body weights were reduced by food restriction the rats subsequently regained weight on the lab chow diet. These results are difficult to reconcile with those obtained by other investigators and the irreversibility of dietary obesity requires further documentation.

Sclafani & Springer (1976) also examined motivational changes in eating associated with snack food induced obesity. Compared to control animals, the rats with dietary obesity worked less for food when deprived, ate less of quinine-adulterated diets, and regained their body weight at a slower rate following a fast. The obese rats, unlike the controls, also did not increase their running activity during a short fast (Sclafani & Springer, 1976), although their activity eventually increases when their body weight falls below normal levels (Sclafani & Rendel, in preparation). In several respects, therefore, animals with dietary obesity behave like hypothalamic obese animals: they overeat and gain weight when the feeding conditions are very favorable, but are not motivated to maintain their excess weights when less favorable conditions exist. Sclafani (1976; Sclafani & Springer, 1976) has proposed, therefore, that both types of obesity involve an increase in appetite rather than in hunger drive or regulated body weight level.

The medial hypothalamic feeding system appears to have an important inhibitory function on appetite which normally serves to limit the development of dietary obesity. Thus, damage to the medial hypothalamus greatly potentiates the weight gains produced by high fat diets, sucrose solutions, and snack foods (Berner & Sclafani, in preparation; Gale & Sclafani, 1977; Sclafani, 1973). The lateral hypothalamic feeding system, in contrast, although it may determine the regulated body weight level (set point), does not appear to have a critical function in the development of dietary obesity (Keesey *et al.*, 1976; Powley & Keesey, 1970). This is suggested by the finding that lateral hypothalamic lesions, although they permanently depress body weight on chow diets, do not interfere with the obesity-promoting effect of a palatable liquid diet (Keesey *et al.*, 1976). It has also been found that removal of the olfactory bulbs in rats has relatively little effect either in normal rats or hypothalamic obese rats on the weight gains induced by snack foods (Berner & Sclafani, in preparation). This finding was unexpected, given the presumed importance of olfaction in the rat, and apparently the gustatory and textural stimuli provided by the diet are sufficient to promote overeating and obesity. Little is known about the role of other neural systems in the development of dietary obesity and this remains a fruitful area of research.

As mentioned above, it is well known that the weight gains produced by palatable foods are exaggerated in hypothalamic obese rats. The interaction between dietary obesity and other syndromes of obesity has also recently been studied. Ovariectomy in adult female rats significantly elevates body weight and fat content and Gale & Van Itallie (in preparation) have observed that the weight promoting effects of ovariectomy and a snack food diet are additive. In a 12-week period, ovariectomized and intact rats fed snack foods gained 202 g and 145.3 g, respectively, while chow-fed ovariectomized and intact rats gained only 123 g and 65.4 g, respectively. These results are consistent with an earlier report that ovariectomy, unlike medial hypothalamic damage, does not potentiate the weight promoting effect of a high fat diet (Gale & Sclafani, 1977). Not surprisingly, forced exercise (1 hr/day) reduced the dietary, ovarian, and combined obesities, although body weights rapidly recovered following the termination of exercise. In another study Gale & Van Itallie (in preparation) compared the weight promoting effect of a snack food diet in genetically obese Zucker rats and their lean littermates. Obese female Zucker rats offered the snack foods for 50 days gained 198 g, while the lean littermates exposed to the same diet gained 87.8 g. The chow-fed obese and lean controls gained 48.3 g and 14.5 g, respectively, during the same time period. Thus, the snack food diet produced greater weight gains in the genetically obese rats than in their lean littermates, although both groups displayed similar increments in relation to their baseline body weights (obese = 34.4 per cent, lean = 31.9 per cent). The dietary induced weight gains were reversed when the snack foods were withdrawn, and both the obese and lean Zucker rats gradually lost weight to the level of their respective chow-fed controls.

Thus, snack food diets can induce excessive weight gains not only in normal rats, but also in animals with preexisting obesity due to other causes, The effectiveness of this diet is no doubt due to the palatability of the individual foodstuffs used as well as to the variety of foods available to the animal. Variety is widely recognized to be an important component of human diets (Pilgrim, 1967), but has been largely ignored in studies of laboratory animals (Le Magnen, 1974). However, because of the variety and composition of the foods used it is difficult to obtain accurate measures of caloric consumption, and this represents a major drawback to the snack food diet. One promising approach to this problem, taken by Gale, Yang & Van Itallie (personal communication), is to offer animals, in addition to lab chow and water, snack foods in a pellet form and a palatable liquid diet. Mice offered such a diet overate and gained 17.5 g in 60 days, compared to chow-fed controls who gained only 4.8 g.

Preweaning overfeeding

Under normal rearing conditions laboratory animals are given food *ad lib.* following weaning. Prior to weaning, however, food is not available *ad lib.* since rat and mouse pups must compete with their littermates for the mother's milk. Altering the size of the litter, therefore, can significantly affect the food intake and weight gain of pups (Aubert, Suquet & Lemonnier, 1971). More importantly, the preweaning nutritional experience of the animal will determine its adult body weight and size. Widdowson & Kennedy (1962) have reported, for example, that compared to rats reared in large litters (17 to 21 pups) male rats raised in small litters (three pups) not only weighed more at the time of weaning (44 vs 19 g), but also reached higher maximum weights during adulthood (451 vs 334 g). Since the weight difference between animals reared in small and large litters increased with age, even though both groups had free access to the same diet after weaning, preweaning nutrition must affect postweaning food intake. These differences are not simply the result of stunting of the animals reared in the large litter, since rats and mice raised in small litters will, as adults, outweigh animals raised in normal size litters (eight to ten pups) (Aubert *et al.*, 1971; Johnson *et al.*, 1973; Lemonnier *et al.*, 1973).

Although it is well documented that preweaning overfeeding leads to increased body weights during adulthood, there is some question as to whether or not it produces obesity. Some investigators describe their rats in small litters as being fast growers and do not consider them to be obese, since both lean body mass and body fat are increased (Widdowson & McCance, 1960; Widdowson & Kennedy, 1962). Other workers, however, have observed changes in adipose cell size and number, and in body fat content in small litter reared animals that are indicative of obesity (Aubert *et al.*, 1971; Johnson *et al.*, 1973; Knittle & Hirsch, 1968; Lemonnier *et al.*, 1973). In any event, preweaning overnutrition does not by itself lead to the excessive weight gains that are produced by postweaning exposure to high fat diets or other foods rich in calories. Schemmel & co-workers (1973), in fact, have reported that in the Osborne-Mendel rat the diet fed after weaning can completely overshadow the effects of preweaning nutrition. In other strains less prone to obesity, however, pre and postweaning overnutrition may have additive or synergistic effects on adult body weight.

Meal-feeding

As documented above, giving laboratory animals food *ad lib.* results in varying degrees of obesity depending upon the particular diet used. Under some conditions, however, restricted access to food may lead to greater body fat deposition than does unrestricted access. Laboratory rodents normally eat about 8 to 14 small meals per 24 h when food is continuously available. If they are forced to take fewer, but much larger meals (meal-feeding pattern), rats and mice will gain more body fat than if they are allowed to eat the same amount, or even slightly more food, in numerous small meals (nibbling pattern) (Fabry, 1967).

Cohn and his associates (Cohn & Joseph, 1959; Cohn *et al.*, 1965), for example, have demonstrated that rats force-fed two large meals a day by gavage gained more body fat, although not more body weight, than did controls eating the same amount of food *ad lib.* This increased fat deposition, termed adaptive hyperlipogensis by Tepperman & Tepperman (1965), was obtained using various diets, although the composition of the diet influenced the amount of fat that was deposited (Cohn *et al.*, 1965). In the case of a high fat ration, force-fed rats accumulated 75 per cent more body fat than did rats with free access to the diet (Cohn *et al.*, 1965). Force-feeding mice two meals a day has also been found to increase body fat content, as well as body weight gain, relative to controls fed *ad lib.* (Kekwick & Pawan, 1966). It is not necessary to force-feed by gavage to produce hyperlipogenesis, since rats given access to a fixed amount of food one or two times a day have been reported to gain more weight than do rats given continuous access to the same amount of food (Florence & Quarterman, 1972). In another study (Hollifield & Parson, 1962), rats given unlimited amounts of food for 2 h/day gained considerably more weight over a ten-week period than did rats given food 24 h/day (weight gains = 259 *vs* 163 g, respectively). The weight difference was not due solely to hyperlipogenesis, however, since the 2 h fed rats ate 5 to 15 per cent more than did the *ad lib.* fed group. This finding is unusual since, in most other experiments, animals fed for only 2 h/day tend to undereat, rather than overeat, relative to *ad lib.* fed controls (Fabry, 1967).

Another feeding regime which produces large meals and hyperlipogenesis is intermittent starvation. Rats given food every other day, or three or two days a week, will overeat on the days that food is available and will convert more of the ingested food into body fat compared to rats fed continuously (Fabry, 1967). However, since the total weekly food intake of the intermittently starved rats may be considerably below that of the *ad lib.* fed controls, they do not necessarily accumulate more body fat than do controls (Fabry, 1967).

The physiological changes produced by meal-feeding have been extensively studied, and include gastric and intestinal hypertrophy, enhanced intestinal absorption, increased insulin release, and enzymatic adaptations in adipose tissue and liver (Cohn *et al.*, 1965; Fabry, 1967; Tepperman & Tepperman, 1965). All of these changes favor increase fat deposition and they apparently represent an adaptive mechanism that increases the animal's chances to survive periods of food scarcity in its environment.

Conclusions

As is evident from the studies reviewed above, obesity can be induced in animals by a variety of dietary manipulations. The adiposity may result from increased food intake due to the palatability of the diet or to its increased availability in the case of preweaning animals. Increased efficiency of food utilization due to changes in diet composition or feeding patterns may also lead to the excessive accumulation of body fat. In most instances dietary obesity is associated with increases in body weight, although in some cases it may be accompanied by normal weight gains. Depending upon the age of onset dietary induced obesity may involve increases in adipose cell size only, or increases in both cell size and number (Stern & Johnson, 1977). Thus, several different forms of the dietary obesity model can be produced in the laboratory.

The fact that obesity can be readily induced by dietary means in otherwise normal animals indicates that the excessive accumulation of fat is not always the result of some specific genetic, neural, or hormonal disorder. Moderate obesity, in fact, can be considered to be a natural response to unnatural diet conditions, such as the unlimited availability of very palatable foods. Such diet conditions not only increase body weight in normal animals, but also potentiate the adiposity produced by specific disorders, as in the cases of ovarian, hypothalamic, and genetic obesity in the rat. However, animals are not all equally susceptible to dietary-induced weight gains, and important strain and age differences exist. Even within the same group of identically treated, genetically related, animals there is considerable variability in the degree of obesity produced by high fat or snack food diets. An interesting and potentially useful line of research is to explore the physiological basis for these individual differences.

The same dietary factors that promote adiposity in experimental animals are implicated in the pathogenesis of obesity in humans. The prevalence of human obesity has been attributed to the abundance of highly palatable and high energy processed foods and the sedentary activity levels which are characteristic of affluent societies (Yudkin, 1963). The availability of such foods not only stimulates appetite, but also makes possible feeding habits that promote lipogenesis, and increases the likelihood of infant and childhood overfeeding. Therefore, while recognizing the importance of genetic and physiological factors, it is difficult not to conclude that the dietary conditions of the environment have a pervasive influence in the etiology of human obesity.

Acknowledgements – The preparation of this report was supported by a National Institute of Mental Health Research Fellowship (MH07299) and Grant 11182 from the Faculty Research Award Program of the City University of New York.

References

Allen, R.J.L. & Leahy, J.S. (1966): *Br. J. Nutr.* **20**, 339.
Aubert, R., Suquet, J-P. & Lemonnier, D. (1971): *C.R. Acad. Sci., Paris.* **273**, 2636.
Barboriak, J.J., Krehl, W.A., Cowgill, G.R. & Whedon, A.D. (1957) *J. Nutr.* **64**, 241.
Berg, B.N. (1960): *J. Nutr.* **71**, 242.
Berg, B.N. & Simms, H.S. (1960): *J. Nutr.* **71**, 255.
Brook, M. & Noel, P. (1969): *Nature* **222**, 562.
Cohn, C. & Joseph, D. (1959): *Am. J. Physiol.* **196**, 965.
Cohn, C., Joseph, D., Bell, L. & Allweiss, M.D. (1965): *Ann. N.Y. Acad. Sci.* **131**, 507.
Corbitt, J. & Stellar, E. (1964): *J. Comp. Physiol. Psychol.* **58**, 63.
DeLaey, P. (1975): *Archs Int. Pharmacodyn,* **216**, 288.
Fabry, P. (1967): Metabolic consequences of the pattern of food intake. In *Handbook of physiology,* Sect. 1, Vol. 1, ed C.F. Code, p. 31. Washington: American Physiological Society.
Fenton, P.F. & Carr, C. (1951): *J. Nutr.* **45**, 225.
Florence, E. & Quarterman, J. (1972): *Br. J. Nutr.* **28**, 63.
Gale, S.K. & Sclafani, A. (1977): *J. Comp. Physiol. Psychol.* **91**, 381.
Gonet, A.E., Stauffacher, W., Pictet, R. & Renold, A.E. (1965): *Diabetologia* **1**, 162.
Hamilton, C.L. (1964): *J. Comp. Physiol. Psychol.* **58**, 459.
Herberg, L., Doppen, W., Major, E. & Gries, F.A. (1974): *J. Lipid Res.* **15**, 580.
Hollifield, G. & Parson, W. (1962): *J. Clin. Invest.* **41**, 245.
Ingle, D.J. (1949): *Proc. Soc. Exp. Biol. Med.* **72**, 604.
Johnson, P.R., Stern, J.S., Greenwood, M.R.C., Zucker, L.M. & Hirsch, J. (1973): *J. Nutr.* **103**, 738.
Kanarek, R.B. & Hirsch, E. (1977): *Fed. Proc.* **36**, 154.
Keesey, R.E., Boyle, P.C., Kemnitz, J.W. & Mitchel, J.S. (1976): The role of the lateral hypothalamus in determining the body weight set point. In *Hunger: basic mechanisms and clinical implications,* ed D. Novin, W. Wyrwicka & G. Bray, p. 243. New York: Raven Press.
Kekwick, A. & Pawan, G.L. (1966): *Metabolism* **15**, 173.
Knittle, J.L. & Hirsch, J. (1968): *J. Clin. Invest.* **47**, 2091.
Le Magnen, J. (1974): Advances in studies in the physiological control and regulation of food intake. In *Progress in physiological psychology,* ed E. Stellar & J.M. Sprague, p. 204. New York: Academic Press.
Lemonnier, D. (1972): *J. Clin. Invest.* **51**, 2907.
Lemonnier, D. & Alexiu, A. (1974): Nutritional, genetic and hormonal aspects of adipose tissue cellularity. In *The regulation of the adipose tissue mass,* ed J. Vague & J. Boyer, p. 158. New York: American Elsevier Publishing Co.
Lemonnier, D., Suquet, J-P., Aubert, R. & Rosselin, G. (1973): *Horm. Metab. Res.* **5**, 223.
Maller, O. (1967): Specific appetite. In *The chemical senses and nutrition,* ed M.R. Kare & O. Maller, p. 201. Baltimore: Johns Hopkins Press.
Mickelsen, O., Takahashi, S. & Craig, C. (1955): *J. Nutr.* **57**, 541.
Muto, S. & Miyhara, C. (1972): *Br. J. Nutr.* **28**, 327.
Peckham, S.C., Entenman, C. & Carrol, H.W. (1962): *J. Nutr.* **77**, 187.
Pilgrim, F.J. (1967): Human food attitudes and consumption. In *Handbook of Physiology,* Sect. 1, Vol. 1, ed C.F. Code, p. 139. Washington: American Physiological Society.
Powley, T.L. & Keesey, R.E. (1970): *J. Comp. Physiol. Psychol.* **70**, 25.
Rath, R. (1977): *Prog. Food Nutr. Sci.* **2**, 307.
Ross, M.H. (1959): *Fed. Proc.* **18**, 1190.
Rowe, E.A. & Rolls, B.J. (1977): Dietary obesity: permanent changes in body weight. Paper presented at the Sixth International Conference on the Physiology of Food and Fluid Intake, Jouy en Josas, France.

Schemmel, R. (1976): *Amer. Zool.* 16, 661.
Schemmel, R. & Mickelsen, O. (1974): Influence of diet, strain, age and sex on fat depot mass and body composition of the nutritionally obese rat. In *The regulation of the adipose mass,* ed J. Vague & J. Boyer, p. 238. New York: American Elsevier Publishing Co.
Schemmel, R., Mickelsen, O. & Mostosky, U. (1969*a*): *Clin. Orthop.* 65, 89.
Schemmel, R., Mickelsen, O. & Tolgay, Z. (1969*b*): *Am. J. Physiol.* 216, 373.
Schemmel, R., Mickelsen, O. & Gill, J.L. (1970): *J. Nutr.* 100, 1941.
Schemmel, R., Mickelsen, O. & Motawi, K. (1972): *J. Nutr.* 102, 1187.
Schemmel, R., Mickelsen, O. & Fisher, L. (1973): *J. Nutr.* 103, 477.
Schmidt-Nielsen, K., Haines, H.B., & Hackel, D.B. (1964): *Science* 143, 689.
Sclafani, A. (1973): *Physiol. Behav.* 11, 771.
Sclafani, A. (1976): Appetite and hunger in experimental obesity syndromes. In *Hunger: basic mechanisms and clinical implications,* ed D. Novin, W. Wyrwicka, & G. Bray, p. 281. New York: Raven Press.
Sclafani, A. & Gorman, A.N. (1977): *Physiol. Behav.* 18, 1021.
Sclafani, A. & Springer, D. (1976): *Physiol. Behav.* 17, 461.
Stern, J.S. & Johnson, P.R. (in press): Size and number of adipocytes and their implications. In *Advances in modern nutrition,* ed H. Katzen & R.J. Mahler.
Tepperman, J. & Tepperman, H.M. (1965): *Ann. N.Y. Acad. Sci.* 131, 404.
Widdowson, E.M. & McCance, R.A. (1960): *Proc. R. Soc.* Ser. B. 152, 188.
Widdowson, E.M. & Kennedy, G.C. (1962): *Proc. R. Soc.* Ser. B. 156, 96.
Young, R.A. (1976): *Amer. Zool.* 16, 699.
Yudkin, J. (1963): *Lancet* 1, 1335.

14
The syndrome of hypothalamic obesity

LAWRENCE A. FROHMAN, M.D.
Division of Endocrinology and Metabolism, Department of Medicine, Michael Reese Hospital and the Pritzker School of Medicine, University of Chicago, Chicago, Illinois 60616, USA.

The first report that electrolytic destruction of the ventromedial hypothalamus was followed by the development of obesity appeared nearly 30 years ago (Hetherington & Ranson, 1940). The association between ventromedial hypothalamic (VMH) destruction and hyperphagia was characterized shortly thereafter (Brobeck, Tepperman & Long, 1943) and for a considerable period of time it was believed that the obesity and associated metabolic changes were a consequence of the increased food intake (Tepperman, Brobeck & Long, 1943; Brobeck, 1946; Mayer, 1955). In the first report of hyperinsulinemia after VMH lesions (Hales & Kennedy, 1964) a similar explanation was offered. The question of the role of hyperphagia became a central issue and led for a period to the classification of hypothalamic obesity as a 'regulatory' obesity, related to excessive food intake, as contrasted to the 'metabolic' obesity presumed to exist in genetically obese animals (Mayer, 1955).

Evidence soon appeared, however, to suggest that hypothalamic obesity was not merely the result of hyperphagia. Kennedy (1957) first observed that destruction of the ventromedial hypothalamus of the weanling female rat produced obesity, here defined as an increase in carcass fat rather than in total body weight and growth retardation. However, in contrast to the mature rat, the weanling rat did not develop hyperphagia. These studies were confirmed by Han and co-workers (1965), who observed that although weanling rats with extensive VMH lesions did not develop hyperphagia nor gain excessive weight, their carcass fat content was significantly increased. Bernardis & Skelton (1965, 1967) subsequently demonstrated that the degree to which hyperphagia developed was both age and sex related, being more readily demonstrable in females. The explanation for the lack of hyperphagia in weanling rats is unknown. It was originally postulated that the weanling rat is already eating at a maximal rate, due to its rapid growth, and that it cannot further increase its food intake (Kennedy, 1957). It has also been proposed that the satiety function of the ventromedial nucleus (VMN) is underdeveloped in the weanling rat (Groome-Kurtz, Rozin & Teitelbaum, 1972). However, the recent demonstration that the lack of hyperphagia persists for at least six months (Bernardis *et al.*, 1975) does not support this hypothesis. It was subsequently shown that obesity and the associated hormonal metabolic changes could occur in mature rats with VMH lesions in which food intake was restricted (Han, 1968*a*; Han & Frohman, 1970). Thus, it appears that there is nothing unique about the obesity which develops in the weanling rat. As a result, workers desirous of studying the hormonal and metabolic alterations which followed VMH destruction, and needing to distinguish those changes attributable to the loss of normal hypothalamic function from those secondary to hyperphagia, had two basic models from which to choose. The author's experience, and that of his colleagues, related to the weanling rat with VMN destruction and the results of these studies provide the basis for many of the concepts to be presented. However, it should be emphasized that others, using the diet-restricted adult rat with VMH lesions or the diet-restricted mouse with chemical destruction of the hypothalamus, found similar changes and arrived at identical conclusions in nearly all instances.

Characterization of hypothalamic obesity

Food intake

Food intake following VMH destruction is altered in many ways and for a detailed discussion of the subject the reader is referred to an excellent review which has recently appeared (Novin, Wyrwicka & Bray, 1976). For our present purpose it is important to note that the alterations include not only quantitative changes but qualitative ones as well. In addition to the hyperphagia, the pattern of food intake is dramatically altered. The rat is normally a nocturnal eater and a nibbler. Following hypothalamic destruction there is a reversal of the nocturnal preference for food intake (Brooks, 1946) and a number of moderate to large-sized meals are consumed in place of the frequent nibbling. The nocturnal eating preference also disappears in the weanling rat, although the changes are not as marked as in the adult rat (Bernardis, 1973) and a tendency towards meal eating in contrast to nibbling occurs as well. This latter change by itself has been shown to exhibit a contributory role in the development of obesity in intact, meal-fed rats (Cohn, 1966) though the extent of its contribution following hypothalamic destruction is uncertain.

In both weanlings (Bernardis & Border, 1975*a*) and adult rats (Panksepp, 1973) it has been suggested that the VMN is not involved in short-term regulation of satiety, but rather in the long-term regulation of food intake. Finally, the taste preference alterations favoring sweetened solutions seen in adult rats with VMH lesions (Panksepp, 1973) are also present in weanling rats (Bernardis & Border, 1975*b*)

Activity

A marked reduction in spontaneous locomotor activity is seen in mature rats following VMH lesions. This decreased energy expenditure undoubtedly contributes to the development of obesity (Hetherington & Ransom, 1942; May & Beaton, 1966) though obesity develops in animals subjected to both forced restraint and to tube feeding (Han, 1968*b*).

Weanling rats begin to decrease their activity about 24 hours after VMN lesions, and hypoactivity also appears to be a contributory factor (Bernardis, 1972). It is of interest that survival of animals in activity cages is reduced compared with that in standard housing, possibly related to the development of hypoglycemia.

Somatic changes

The effect of hypothalamic destruction on linear growth, weight gain and body composition varies with age and sex. Electrolytic or chemical lesions which destroy the VMH result in impaired linear growth and are most readily demonstrated in weanling animals (Kennedy, 1957; Bernardis & Skelton, 1965). Changes in body weight, as already indicated, are also affected by the same two factors and reflect the extent of hyperphagia. In normophagic weanling rats body weight may actually be subnormal at times. Measurement of body composition, rather than weight gain, is the most accurate method of assessing the development of obesity. It has been repeatly demonstrated that carcass fat content is increased in normophagic, normal weight weanling rats with VMN lesions (Han *et al.*, 1965; Bernardis & Skelton, 1965). A very accurate and predictive assessment of carcass lipid content in both weanling and mature rats with VMN lesions can be made using the Lee index (body weight$^{1/3}$/naso-anal length) (Bernardis & Patterson, 1968). This index is highly significant in weanling animals within two weeks after lesioning and provides the investigator with a simple method of assessing the presence of the appropriate hypothalamic destruction. The increase in carcass fat is balanced by a corresponding decrease in the percentage of both water and lean body mass. In the weanling rat and also in the mature rat with restricted food intake the accumulation of protein may cease entirely, and is reflected by the cessation of linear growth.

Hormonal changes
Hyperinsulinemia was first reported in mature rats with VMH lesions by Hales & Kennedy (1964). These authors attributed the findings to the transient hyperglycemia presumed to accompany the hyperphagia. The inadequacy of this explanation was evident, however, from our reports of hyperinsulinemia in the absence of hyperglycemia in normophagic weanling rats with VMN lesions (Frohman & Bernardis, 1968) and in the mature hypophysectomized rats with restricted food intake and activity (Han & Frohman, 1970). The hyperinsulinemia has been shown to be responsive to changes in dietary carbohydrate and fat content and to fasting, although its disappearance after 48 hours of food deprivation is associated with a mild hypoglycemia and therefore a relative hyperinsulinemia still persists (Frohman *et al.*, 1971). The insulin secretory response in normophagic weanling rats to intravenous or intraperitoneal glucose administration is comparable to that in controls (Frohman, Goldman & Bernardis, 1972), whereas the response to oral glucose in hyperphagic mature animals is increased (Steffens, 1970).

The development of hyperinsulinemia following VMH lesions is quite rapid and in the weanling rats can be demonstrated within four days (Frohman *et al.*, 1969). Since these animals are markedly hypophagic immediately after operation, presumably due to transient injury of the nearby lateral hypothalamic feeding center, insulin levels normalized to food intake are elevated even by the second postoperative day. Similar findings have been demonstrated in the tube-fed weanling rat (Slaunwhite, Goldman & Bernardis, 1972) and in the food-restricted adult rat with VMH lesions (Hustvedt & Løvø, 1972).

The development of hyperinsulinemia in the absense of hyperphagia or any evidence of peripheral insulin insensitivity (see below) has suggested a primary neurogenic etiology. Since hyperinsulinemia develops also in hypophysectomized rats (Han & Frohman, 1970; Goldman *et al.*, 1970) the most likely alternative pathways involve the autonomic nervous system, as will be discussed.

Destruction of the VMN also results in a decrease in growth hormone secretion (Frohman & Bernardis, 1968), presumably as a consequence of this locus being the site of or required for the production of growth hormone releasing factor (Frohman, Bernardis & Kant, 1968). Large lesions in the VMH frequently destroy portions of the median eminence as well and thus impair the mechanism for the release of the hypophysiotrophic hormones into the hypothalamic-pituitary portal vessels. The lack of growth hormone, with its lipolytic effects, clearly contributes to the development of obesity. Treatment of VMH-lesioned rats with growth hormone has been shown to reduce the extent of obesity and, in weanling rats, to restore partially the impairment in linear growth (Goldman *et al.*, 1970). However, the major features of hypothalamic obesity persist even in growth hormone treated animals, thus indicating that the development of obesity is independent of the effects of growth hormone deficiency.

Lesions confined to the VMN do not in general impair the hypothalamic-pituitary-thyroid axis and serum thyroid hormone levels have been shown to be normal in weanling rats with VMN lesions (Frohman & Bernardis, 1968). With more extensive lesions involving the median eminence, it is possible to produce partial thyroid deficiency and also adreno-cortical insufficiency. The contribution of these hormone deficiencies to the obese state must therefore be considered ancillary. The ventromedial hypothalamus exerts a role in the tonic secretion of gonadotropin and its destruction is associated with decreased gonadol function.

Metabolic changes

Blood glucose regulation
In the mature animal with ventromedial hypothalamic destruction, hyperphagia frequently leads to mild hyperglycemia whereas in the weanling, normophagic rat, hyperglycemia does not occur. With extreme hyperphagia, and in a species such as the mouse, overt diabetes

frequently develops (Katsuki *et al.*, 1962). This has also been reported in the rat (Hausberger, Broadhed & Hausberger, 1964) but it is extremely rare. During periods of hypophagia, which occur spontaneously for the first few days after lesioning or with fasting, hypoglycemia can be demonstrated. The basis for the hypoglycemia appears to be multifactorial. Hepatic glycogen levels are normal in the fed state and glycogen mobilization during fasting is also normal (Frohman *et al.*, 1971). The glucose removal rate from plasma which is increased as a result of hyperinsulinemia (Frohman, Goldman & Bernardis, 1972) appears to be the most important factor. There is evidence for increased gluconeogenesis, even in the fed state (Goldman & Bernardis, 1975), which appears necessary to maintain normoglycemia and a further increase during fasting probably does not occur.

Hyperlipidemia

Hyperlipidemia was originally reported to occur in mature hyperphagic rats (Brobeck *et al.*, 1943). It is, however, also present in normophagic rats (Frohman & Bernardis, 1968), can be detected four days after lesioning at a time when animals are still hypophagic (Frohman *et al.*, 1969) and consists of both endogenous and exogenous components (Schnatz, Frohman & Bernardis, 1971). The basis for the exogenous hypertriglyceridemia is not entirely clear since plasma lipoprotein lipase activity is increased rather than decreased, there are no detectable lipase inhibitors, and the circulating lipoprotein exhibits normal sensitivity to hydrolysis. The possibility of an impaired tissue uptake of circulating triglycerides has been raised but remains to be confirmed. The etiology of endogenous hypertriglyceridemia is more apparent and is related to the enhanced hepatic triglyceride synthesis, which is the source of endogenous plasma triglyceride (Goldman *et al.*, 1972*b*). A mild hypercholesterolemia is also present in rats with VMN lesions (Bernardis & Schnatz, 1971) but has been less extensively studied. Plasma free fatty acids, in contrast, are not elevated (Hales & Kennedy, 1964; Nishizawa & Bray, 1977), reflecting the presence of hyperinsulinemia.

Intermediary carbohydrate and lipid metabolism

The first suggestion that hypothalamic obesity was associated with a primary metabolic disturbance dates to the report by Han (1968*a*) which indicated that hypophysectomized, tube-fed rats with VMH lesions exhibited mild hypothermia, decreased activity and a reduction of the resting oxygen consumption rate. The decreased energy expenditure attributed to the latter was equivalent to the calculated calorie requirement for lipogenesis. An increase in lipogenesis, the metabolic prerequisite for obesity in the absence of hyperphagia, implies an alteration of substrate utilization and such changes have been repeatedly demonstrated. Initial experiments indicated that glucose oxidation and incorporation into triglyceride is enhanced in adipose tissue of lesioned weanling rats (Goldman *et al.*, 1970). This change was originally attributed to the hyperinsulinemia and decreased growth hormone secretion but it has subsequently been shown to be at least partially independent of each of the hormonal changes. The enhanced lipogenesis persists both following hypophysectomy and after growth hormone treatment indicating its independence from growth hormone secretion. Dissociation of the metabolic responses from hyperinsulinemia can be accomplished by dietary alteration, using high fat or high carbohydrate diets, and by starvation where the enhanced lipogenesis persists despite exaggeration or normalization of the hyperinsulinemia (Frohman *et al.*, 1971).

If animals are rendered diabetic by streptozotocin treatment prior to hypothalamic destruction, in order to exclude the persistent effects of preexisting hyperinsulinemia, the characteristic metabolic changes still occur (Goldman *et al.*, 1972*a*). Although the absolute changes in glucose oxidation and lipogenesis are markedly reduced in diabetic animals, an increase relative to that of controls was observed despite the absence of hyperinsulinemia which is similar to that seen in non-diabetic, lesioned animals. Thus, although the enhancement of lipogenesis following hypothalamic destruction is accentuated by hyperinsulinemia, it is at least in part independent of the hormonal change and most likely represents a primary effect of the lesion.

Studies using selectively labelled glucose have indicated greater enhancement of 1-^{14}C-glucose than of 6-^{14}C-glucose oxidation, suggesting a preferential increase in the activity of the hexose monophosphate shunt, leading to increased NADPH generation which would be utilized in lipogenesis (Goldman & Bernardis, 1974). Pyruvate oxidation by the citric acid cycle is reduced as is its incorporation into glyceride glycerol, implying a decrease in glycerol-phosphate formation as well as a decreased activity of the dicarboxylic acid shuttle. Similar findings have also been reported in the genetically obese mouse (Chakrabarty & Leveille, 1968), though their role in the development of obesity is uncertain.

While the majority of the *in vitro* studies have focused on adipose tissue, similar changes in intermediary metabolism have been shown in both liver and muscle, although with a slightly different chronology. This difference supports the hypothesis that hyperinsulinemia and enhanced lipogenesis are primary consequences of hypothalamic destruction, while the hyperphagia and adipose tissue accumulation lead to the development of insulin resistance.

Protein metabolism

A direct role for the VMH in the regulation of protein metabolism has been suggested by several observations. First, the decrease in linear growth in weanling rats with VMN destruction is not entirely corrected by treatment with growth hormone (Goldman *et al.*, 1970), indicating that other factors also contribute to the growth retardation. Calculations have indicated that although weight gain during the first two weeks following VMN destruction in weanling rats is comparable to that in controls, it consists almost entirely of fat (Frohman *et al.*, 1971). In addition, nitrogen balance studies have indicated an alteration in protein metabolism within 24 hours of hypothalamic destruction (Holm, Hustvedt & Løvø, 1973). Second, the enhanced plasma glucose appearance (Frohman *et al.*, 1972), together with normophagia, implies an increased glucose production from endogenous sources. These findings suggest that, in an attempt to compensate for the increased lipogenesis due to both primary tissue metabolic changes and the hyperinsulinemia, enhanced glucose production from amino acids (gluconeogenesis) occurs and the protein lost as a result contributes to the impaired net protein accumulation and linear growth.

Evidence for increased gluconeogenesis has been demonstrated by several techniques. Plasma urea levels are increased in rats with hypothalamic lesions and rise more rapidly after nephrectomy than in intact rats (Goldman & Bernardis, 1975). In addition, there is increased conversion of ^{14}C-alanine and ^{14}C-bicarbonate to plasma glucose and liver glycogen in rats with VMN lesions. Finally, an increase in amino acid incorporation into hepatic protein and in muscle protein breakdown have been demonstrated, which suggest that much of the impairment in skeletal protein accumulation is secondary to the increased utilization of muscle protein for gluconeogenesis (Goldman & Bernardis, 1976).

Anatomic features

Central nervous system localization and techniques of tissue destruction

Initial studies of hypothalamic obesity involved the destruction of much of the ventromedial hypothalamus, including the median eminence. Subsequent work by Bernardis and colleagues (Bernardis & Skelton, 1965; Bernardis & Frohman, 1970, 1971) revealed the critical area to be the VMN. Lesions dorsal and interior to the VMN were ineffective in producing either obesity or hyperinsulinemia in weanling rats (Bernardis & Frohman, 1971). Increasing the extent of VMN destruction by increasing the size of the lesions or increasing their number results in progressive hormonal-metabolic alterations and accumulation of carcass fat (Bernardis & Frohman, 1970; Bernardis & Schnatz, 1971).

Two adjacent hypothalamic loci, the ventrolateral area and the dorsomedial nucleus, also participate in the regulation of food intake and their destruction leads to hypophagic syndromes. In rats with VMN lesions, concomitant destruction of each of these loci failed to alter the hormonal metabolic disturbances with VMN destruction alone (Schnatz, Frohman & Bernardis, 1973; Bernardis *et al.*, 1974). Thus, the efferent pathways from the VMN appear to be independent of these hypothalamic loci.

The syndrome of hypothalamic obesity has classically been produced by passage of a direct anodal current through a stainless steel electrode which results in an electrolytic lesion. Both platinum electrodes and radiofrequency current have been used to produce similar lesions. Parasagittal knife-cuts, which interrupt the connections between the ventromedial and ventrolateral hypothalamus and which transsect the ventral noradrenergic bundle have also been reported to produce hyperphagia and obesity (Gold & Kapatos, 1975). Chemical agents which produce destruction on a functional rather than an anatomic basis include goldthioglucose, monosodium glutamate, and bipiperidyl mustard. Goldthioglucose injections in mice produce extensive destruction of the VMN as well as varying degrees of destruction of the surrounding arcuate nucleus, median eminence, ventrolateral hypothalamus and supraoptic nucleus (Marshall, Barnette & Mayer, 1955) and is followed by a syndrome of hyperphagia-obesity. Similar changes are seen in rats, though the nephrotoxicity in this species precludes the drug's usefulness. The tissue destruction is related to gold deposition, with the glucose moiety serving to enhance accumulation in the ventromedial hypothalamus. Bipiperidyl mustard has been reported to cause similar VMH destruction in mice associated with the development of a hyperphagic obesity, though it has been less extensively investigated (Rutman, Lewis & Bloomer, 1967). Monosodium glutamate in newborn mice produces VMH lesions, growth retardation and obesity, though the most heavily damaged structure is the arcuate nucleus rather than the VMN (Olney, 1969). Recent studies aimed at altering the function of neurotransmitters associated with the regulation of food intake have had variable degrees of success in the production of experimental obesity. Intracerebroventricular injection of 5,7-dihydroxytryptamine, a serotonin analog, administered in conjunction with desmethylimipramine, a monoamine reuptake inhibitor, damages serotonin-containing neurons and causes persistent hyperphagia, though gross obesity has not been observed (Saller & Stricker, 1976). Transient hyperphagia and obesity have also been observed after the injection of *p*-chlorophenylalanine, a serotonin synthesis inhibitor (Breisch, Zemlan & Hoebel, 1976). It is not currently known whether the neurons primarily affected by these agents are in the ventromedial hypothalamus. Selective destruction of the ventral bundle of the ascending noradrenergic fibers which project to the ventral hypothalamus, by injection of 6-hydroxydopamine, also produces hyperphagia and obesity (Ahlskog & Hoebel, 1973) although there are differences in the manifestations of hyperphagia from those observed after electrolytic destruction of the hypothalamus (Ahlskog, Randall & Hoebel, 1975).

Autonomic nervous system

The two major pathways involved in the systemic expression of alterations in hypothalamic function involve (1) the neural and vascular components of the pituitary stalk leading to the secretion of pituitary hormones, and (2) the lower brain centers and the autonomic nervous systems. The role of the pituitary must be considered to be of secondary importance, since hypophysectomy does not prevent nor reverse hypothalamic obesity. The importance of the autonomic nervous system in the neurometabolic disturbances following VMH destruction is well recognized. There is, however, still some uncertainty as to the relative contribution of the sympathetic as compared with the parasympathetic components.

The VMH is considered to be in the sympathetic zone of the hypothalamus (Ban, 1966) and stimulation of this region results in an acute elevation of plasma glucose, free fatty acids and glucagon levels and a suppression of insulin secretion (Frohman & Bernardis,

1971; Barkai & Allweis, 1972). It would therefore be anticipated that destruction of VMN would lead to a diminished sympathetic tone resulting in impaired glucose, fatty acid and glucagon levels - either under basal conditions or in response to neurogenic stimulation, and an increase in insulin levels. Centrally mediated stimulation of free fatty acid release does appear to be impaired (Nishizawa & Bray, 1977) though the sympathetic nervous system mediated hyperglycemic response to central glucopenia remains intact after VMH destruction (Muller *et al.*, 1974). There is also a suggestion of enhanced insulin responses to stress (Frohman *et al.*, 1972).

The parasympathetic nervous system has also been implicated in the mediation of the hormonal-metabolic response to VMH destruction, on the basis of the known effects of vagal stimulation on insulin secretion (Frohman, Ezdinli & Javid, 1967). Attempts to reverse the obesity by vagotomy have yielded conflicting results. Powley & Opsahl (1974) claimed that subdiaphragmatic vagotomy abolished hypothalamic obesity. However, Inoue & Bray (1977) demonstrated impaired gastric emptying in vagotomized rats with hypothalamic lesions and concluded that the absence of hyperinsulinemia and obesity was a consequence of inadequate absorption of nutrients. In preliminary studies, we (Carpenter, R., Grossman, S.E. & Frohman, L.A.) have also shown that if VMH lesions are placed in rats following recovery from vagotomy, hyperphagia and obesity will be produced. Thus, enhancement of the parasympathetic tone by itself is an inadequate explanation for the hormonal-metabolic effects of hypothalamic destruction. The most impressive evidence for the role of the autonomic nervous system and the pathogenesis of both the hyperinsulinemia and obesity has been provided by Inoue, Bray & Mullen (1977) who reported that diabetic rats which received pancreatic islet transplants did not develop hyperinsulinemia or obesity following VMH lesions. If the insulin secretory capacity of these animals to humoral stimuli can be shown to be intact, the results will provide strong evidence for a major role of neurogenic hyperinsulinemia in the pathogenesis of obesity.

Conclusions

The syndrome of hypothalamic obesity which was originally thought to be a primary consequence of hyperphagia has now been shown to be independently associated with alterations in activity, hormonal secretion, and intermediary metabolism of carbohydrate, lipid, and protein. The mediation of the hormonal metabolic changes appears to occur primarily through the autonomic nervous system. Although elimination of any single component can be demonstrated to influence the final manifestation of the obesity syndrome, all appear to interact with one another to enhance the development of obesity. Suppression of the obese state, therefore, requires consideration of each of these factors and an effort to counteract the various perturbations induced by hypothalamic destruction.

The relationship of this model of obesity to human obesity is less clear. There are occasional individuals with disordered hypothalamic function in whom obesity develops and where the analogy with the animal model appears reasonable (Bray & Gallagher, 1975). However, it is not known whether a subtle regulatory defect (ie at an enzymatic level) in hypothalamic function is present in the majority of obese individuals in whom no other evidence of hypothalamic disease can be demonstrated. The recognition of hormonal-metabolic responses unique to hypothalamic obesity, if they exist, in obese humans, may help to answer this question.

Summary

Destruction of the ventromedial hypothalamus of the rat is followed by the development of obesity associated with altered behavioral, feeding, hormonal and metabolic activity. Hyperphagia, finicky eating behavior, changes in taste preference and in the pattern of food intake and hypoactivity were the first features recognized. Subsequently, hyperinsulinemia, growth hormone deficiency, decreased energy expenditure (basal metabolic activity) and increases in lipogenesis, protein turnover, gluconeogenesis, and glucose oxidation have been noted. It has been shown that the hormonal and metabolic changes are independent of the hyperphagia since weanling rats in which hyperphagia does not develop and food-restricted mature rats become obese. The metabolic changes appear to be a combination of primary effects of hypothalamic destruction and effects secondary to hyperinsulinemia. During the dynamic phase of obesity, animals exhibit normal sensitivity to exogenous insulin and only subsequent to the development of marked obesity is there evidence for insulin resistance.

The mechanism for the altered neurometabolic control appears to involve both the sympathetic and parasympathetic components of the autonomic nervous system. Removal of the pancreatic islets from their neural control prevents at least some of the manifestations of obesity following hypothalamic destruction. The specific biochemical reactions within the hypothalamus which are responsible for maintaining normal energy metabolism and body nutrient stores, however, remain to be determined.

Acknowledgement – The work in this paper was supported in part by USPHS Grant AM17046.

References

Ahlskog, J.E. & Hoebel, B.G. (1973): *Science* **193**, 166.
Ahlskog, J.E., Randall, P.K. & Hoebel, B.G. (1975): *Science* **190**, 399.
Ban, T. (1966): In *Progress in brain research,* Vol. 21A, ed T. Tokizane & J.P. Schade, p. 1. Amsterdam: Elsevier Publishing Co.
Barkai, A., & Allweis, C. (1972): *Metabolism* **21**, 921.
Bernardis, L.L. & Patterson, B.D. (1968): *J. Endocrinol.* **40**, 527.
Bernardis, L.L. & Skelton, F.R. (1965): *Neuroendocrinology* **1**, 265.
Bernardis, L.L. & Skelton, F.R. (1967): *J. Endocrinol.* **38**, 351.
Bernardis, L.L. & Frohman, L.A. (1970): *Neuroendocrinology* **6**, 319.
Bernardis, L.L. & Frohman, L.A. (1971): *J. Comp. Neurol.* **141**, 107.
Bernardis, L.L. & Schnatz, J.D. (1971): *Experientia* **27**, 1082.
Bernardis, L.L. (1972): *Can. J. Physiol. Pharmacol.* **50**, 370.
Bernardis, L.L. (1973): *Physiol. Behav.* **10**, 855.
Bernardis, L.L., Chlouverakis, C., Schnatz, J.D. & Frohman, L.A. (1974): *Brain Res.* **69**, 67.
Bernardis, L.L. & Border, J.R. (1975*a*): *J. Neurosci. Res.* **1**, 377.
Bernardis, L.L. & Border, J.R. (1975*b*): *J. Neurosci. Res.* **1**, 485.
Bernardis, L.L., Goldman, J.K., Chlouverakis, C. & Frohman, L.A (1975): *J. Neurosci. Res.* **1**, 95.
Bray, G.A. & Gallagher, P.F., Jr. (1975): *Medicine* **54**, 301.
Breisch, S.T., Zemlan, F.P. & Hoebel, B.G. (1976): *Science* **192**, 382.
Brobeck, J.R., Tepperman, J. & Long, C.N.H. (1943): *Yale J. Biol. Med.* **15**, 831.
Brobeck, J.R. (1946): *Physiol. Rev.* **26**, 541.
Brooks, C.M. (1946): *Am. J. Physiol.* **147**, 708.
Chakrabarty, K. & Leveille, G.A. (1968): *Archs Biochem. Biophys.* **125**, 259.
Cohn, C. (1966): In *Endocrines and the central nervous system,* Vol. 23, ed R. Levine, p. 212. Boston: Williams & Wilkins.
Frohman, L.A., Ezdinli, E.Z. & Javid, R. (1967): *Diabetes* **16**, 433.
Frohman, L.A. & Bernardis, L.L. (1968): *Endocrinology* **82**, 1125.
Frohman, L.A., Bernardis, L.L. & Kant, K.J. (1968): *Science* **162**, 580.
Frohman, L.A., Bernardis, L.L., Schnatz, J.D. & Burek, L. (1969): *Am. J. Physiol.* **216**, 1496.
Frohman, L.A. & Bernardis, L.L. (1971): *Am. J. Physiol.* **221**, 1596.
Frohman, L.A., Goldman, J.K., Schnatz, J.D. & Bernardis, L.L. (1971): *Metabolism* **20**, 501.
Frohman, L.A., Goldman, J.K. & Bernardis, L.L. (1972): *Metabolism* **21**, 799.
Gold, R.M. & Kapatos, G. (1975): *J. Comp. Physiol. Psychol.* **88**, 202.
Goldman, J.K., Schnatz, L.L. & Frohman, L.A. (1970): *Metabolism* **19**, 995.
Goldman, J.K., Schnatz, J.D., Bernardis, L.L. & Frohman, L.A. (1972*a*): *Metabolism* **21**, 132.
Goldman, J.K., Schnatz, J.D., Bernardis, L.L. & Frohman, L.A. (1972*b*): *Diabetologica* **8**, 160.
Goldman, J.K. & Bernardis, L.L. (1974): *Horm. Metab. Res.* **6**, 370.
Goldman, J.K. & Bernardis, L.L. (1975): *Horm. Metab. Res.* **7**, 148.
Goldman, J.K. & Bernardis, L.L. (1976): *Proc. Soc. Exp. Biol. Med.* **151**, 155.
Groome-Kurtz, R.I., Rozin, P. & Teitelbaum, P. (1972): *J. Comp. Physiol. Psychol.* **80**, 19.

Hales, C.M. & Kennedy, G.C. (1964): *Biochem. J.* 90, 620.
Han, P.W., Lin, C.H., Chu, K.C., Mu, J.Y. & Liu, A.C. (1965): *Am. J. Physiol.* 209, 627.
Han, P.W. (1968*a*): *Am. J. Physiol.* 215, 1343.
Han, P.W. (1968*b*): *Proc. Soc. Exp. Biol. Med.* 127, 1057.
Han, P.W. & Frohman, L.A. (1970): *Am. J. Physiol.* 219, 1632.
Hausberger, F.X., Broadhed, C.L. & Hausberger, B.C. (1964): *Acta Endocrinol.* 45, 600.
Hetherington, A. & Ranson, S.W. (1940): *Anat. Rec.* 78, 149.
Hetherington, A. & Ranson, S.W. (1942): *Am. J. Physiol.* 136, 609.
Holm, H., Hustvedt, B.E. & Løvø, A. (1973): *Metabolism* 22, 1377.
Hustvedt, B.E. & Løvø, A. (1972): *Acta Physiol. Scand.* 84, 29.
Inoue, S. & Bray, G.A. (1977): *Endocrinology* 100, 108.
Inoue, S., Bray, G.A. & Mullen, Y. (1977): *Nature* 266, 742.
Inoue, S. & Mullen, Y.S. (1977): Progr. 59th Meeting, Endocrine Society, p. 187.
Katsuki, S., Hirata, Y., Horino, M., Ito, M., Ishimoto, M., Makino, N. & Hososako, A. (1962): *Diabetes* 11, 209.
Kennedy, G.C. (1957): *J. Endocrinol.* 16, 9.
Marshall, M.B., Barnett, R.J. & Mayer, J. (1955): *Proc. Soc. Exp. Biol. Med.* 90, 240.
May, K.K. & Beaton, J.R. (1966): *Can. J. Physiol. Pharmacol.* 44, 641.
Mayer, J. (1955): *Nutr. Abstr. Rev.* 25, 597.
Muller, E.E., Pecile, A., Cocchi, D. & Oligiati, V.R. (1974): *Am. J. Physiol.* 226, 1100.
Nishizawa, Y. & Bray, G.A. (1977): *J. Clin. Invest.* (in press).
Novin, D., Warwicka, W. & Bray, G.A. editors (1976): *Hunger: basic mechanisms and clinical implications.* New York: Raven Press.
Olney, J.W. (1969): *Science* 164, 719.
Panksepp, J. (1973): *Behav. Biol.* 9, 65.
Powley, T.L. & Opsahl, C.A. (1974): *Am. J. Physiol.* 226, 25.
Rutman, R.J., Lewis, F.S. & Bloomer, W. (1967): *Trans. N.Y. Acad. Sci.* 30, 244.
Saller, C.F. & Stricker, E.M. (1976): *Science* 192, 385.
Schnatz, J.D., Bernardis, L.L., Frohman, L.A. & Goldman, J.K. (1971): *Diabetes* 20, 655.
Schnatz, J.D., Frohman, L.A. & Bernardis, L.L. (1973): *Proc. Soc. Exp. Biol. Med.* 142, 256.
Slaunwhite, W.R., Goldman, J.K. & Bernardis, L.L. (1972): *Metabolism* 21, 619.
Steffens, A.B. (1970): *Physiol. Behav.* 5, 147.
Tepperman, J., Brobeck, J.R. & Long, C.N.H. (1943): *Yale J. Biol. Med.* 15, 855.

15
Genetics of obesity in rodents

D.L. COLEMAN
The Jackson Laboratory, Bar Harbor, Maine 04609, USA.

Several different animal models are available for metabolic studies on the development of obesity (Table 1). Although many studies have been conducted by many investigators in attempts to understand the various syndromes, no one has as yet defined the primary lesion involved in any one of these conditions. This review will briefly describe these syndromes, compare one with the other, and attempt to delineate areas in which productive research could be done in the light of our most current knowledge. For comprehensive bibliographies and excellent reviews of the various studies carried out with each of these syndromes see: Renold & Dulin (1967), Renold, Cahill & Gerritsen (1970) and Renold, Chang & Muller (1974) in three Brook Lodge publications; Bray & York, 1971; Assimacopoulos-Jeannet & Jeanrenaud, 1976; and Herberg & Coleman, 1977.

Table 1. Genetic obesity of laboratory rodents

Single gene mutations		
Gene name	**Inheritance**	**Chromosome**
Mice:		
Yellow *(A^y, A^{vy}, A^{iy})*	Autosomal dominant	2
Obese *(ob)*	Autosomal recessive	6
Diabetes *(db, db^{2J}, db^{3J}, db^{ad})*	Autosomal recessive	4
Fat *(fat)*	Autosomal recessive	?
Rats:		
Fatty *(fa, fa^k)*	Autosomal recessive	?
Inbred strains		
Mice:		
NZO	Polygenic	?
KK	Polygenic	
Other species:		
Acomys cahirinus (spiny mouse)	Polygenic, strongly influenced by environmental and nutritional factors	
Psammomys obesus (sand rat)		
Genomys tolarum (tuco-tuco)		

Although the abnormalities associated with each obesity type have many similarities with regard to their overall development, the documentation of several different single genes being involved in each obesity condition makes it unlikely that the various syndromes will be reduced to disturbances in a single metabolic pathway. Of most interest to the biochemical geneticist are those syndromes caused by single gene mutations. Although each causes massive obesity, rather than the social obesities dealt with most often in the human population, we hope that with sufficient models one can elaborate the number and nature of the metabolic insults that can cause obesity and establish the independent action of each of the individual genes. Those mutations on inbred strains are particularly useful in that appropriate matings can be made that will produce predictable numbers of unaffected and obese mice, all of which are of the same strain, differing only by a single gene. These single gene mutations should involve only one pathway or one primary defect and should be easier to unravel than those syndromes inherited in a polygenic fashion.

Not only hereditary but environmental factors, particularly the effects of diet and pharmacotherapeutic agents on the time of manifestation and the severity of the disease can be evaluated. The availability of congenic histocompatible controls permits organ and tissue transplantation, without concern for tissue rejection. Such transplantation experiments have already proved invaluable in examining the role of specific organs (islets of Langerhans, fat pad) on the development of the obesity syndrome (Strautz, 1970; Ashwell *et al.*, 1977).

For most of the obesities listed in Table 1 a genetic component has been clearly established. In the cases of the desert rodents a clear-cut genetic determinant is not obvious; apparently these species have been selected for increased feed efficiency in a desert environment and when introduced into the laboratory and fed diets of high caloric density become obese. It is quite likely that if sufficient breeding studies were made with these rodents, under laboratory conditions, the genetic component(s) could be established.

The obesity syndromes in mice vary in the degree rather than the developmental profile of the disease. In most cases, the syndrome includes hyperphagia, coupled with marked accumulation of fat, some degree of hyperinsulinemia, and hyperglycemia (either transient or sustained). Increased rates of lipogenesis and glycolysis reflect the degree of hyperinsulinemia. The most notable exceptions occur with those enzymes involved in gluconeogenesis that remain elevated in spite of high plasma insulin concentrations. Hyperplasia and hypertrophy of the islets of Langerhans are associated with all of the obesities. Insulin resistance associated with a loss of receptor sites causes excessive insulin demand. The ability to sustain the mutants' abnormal demand for insulin once the initial increase in number and size of the islets has occurred depends upon the inbred background on which the mutation is maintained (Hummel, Coleman & Lane, 1972; Coleman & Hummel, 1973).

The agouti (A) locus (Chromosome 2)

Several alleles (A^y, A^{vy}, A^{iy}) at the agouti (A) locus change the normal agouti (black and yellow banded) pattern to a complete yellow. These alleles also cause mild glucose intolerance and excess accumulation of adipose tissue (Cuénot, 1905; Danforth, 1927). The condition is inherited as an autosomal dominant. Homozygous (A^y/A^y) mice are lethal, developing only until the blastocyst stage (Robertson, 1942). In contrast, viable yellow (A^{vy}) and intermediate yellow (A^{iy}) are viable in the homozygous state (Dickie, 1962). These latter mutants produce progeny with a coat color pattern ranging from a clear yellow, to a yellow splotched with typical agouti patches, or to a complete agouti pattern (Wolff, 1965). The degree of adiposity that develops in genetically yellow mice seems to be proportional to the percentage of yellow in the coat. Phenotypically agouti, but genetically viable yellow mice, attain weights no larger than their normal siblings. Yellow obese mice are maintained on many inbred and non-inbred backgrounds in several laboratories. The degree of obesity and metabolic changes vary depending on the genetic background. In general, yellow obese mice have only moderate hyperphagia and hyperglycemia coupled with mild hyperinsulinemia and some hypertrophy and hyperplasia of the islets of Langerhans (Hellerström & Hellman, 1963). The hyperphagia is coupled with, or caused by, hyperinsulinemia and both are probably closely associated with the primary lesion. However, thermoregulatory disturbances have been documented (Turner, 1948) which, coupled with faulty regulation of food intake, may suggest a hypothalamic defect.

The obese (ob) mouse (Chromosome 6)

The obese mutation occurred in a non-inbred stock (Ingalls, Dickie & Snell, 1950) but was established later, and has been maintained, in the C57BL/6J (BL/6) strain. BL/6 obese mice are characterized by marked obesity, hyperphagia, transient hyperglycemia and markedly elevated plasma insulin concentrations associated with an increase in number and size of the beta cells of the islets of Langerhans (Genuth, Pryzybylski & Rosenberg, 1971; Coleman & Hummel, 1973). The mutation is an autosomal recessive and homozygous mutants of both sexes are infertile. Obese mutants are obtained by mating known heterozygotes. The rate of liver and adipose tissue lipogenesis is more than doubled (Loten, Rabinovitch & Jeanrenaud, 1974), although this increase is not strictly proportional to the circulating insulin concentration (10 to 20 times normal). Marked insulin resistance is associated with a loss of insulin receptors in several tissues (Kahn *et al.,* 1972; Kahn, Neville & Roth, 1973). This loss of receptor sites with obesity seems general in all mutants with obesity and may be an attempt by the animal to protect itself against the hypoglycemic effect of massive levels of circulating insulin (Assimacopoulos-Jeannet & Jeanrenaud, 1976). Those enzymes involved in gluconeogenesis, which normally are decreased in the hyperinsulinemic state, remain elevated in obese mice. This abnormality occurs early in development in most mutants with obesity and may be associated with the loss of insulin receptor sites in target cells, or may represent a primary defect, but in either event would contribute to the hyperglycemia. A primary metabolic disturbance in the adipocyte has been postulated as the primary lesion in obese mice since increased adipocyte size has been observed as early as 14 days of age well before any obesity or hyperinsulinemia are observed (Joosten & van der Kroon, 1974).

The diabetes (db) mouse (Chromosome 4)

Diabetes *(db)*, an autosomal recessive mutation, occurred in the C57BL/KsJ (BL/Ks) inbred strain and on this background is characterized by obesity, hyperphagia, and a severe diabetes with marked hyperglycemia (Hummel, Dickie & Coleman, 1966; Coleman & Hummel, 1967). Increased plasma insulin concentration is observed as early as ten days of age (Coleman & Hummel, 1974). The concentration of insulin peaks at six to ten times normal by two to three months of age, then drops precipitously to near normal levels. Prior to the drop in plasma insulin concentration, the most consistent morphological feature of the islets of Langerhans appears to be hyperplasia and hypertrophy of the beta cells in an attempt to produce sufficient insulin to control blood sugar concentration at physiological levels. The drop in plasma insulin concentration is concomitant with islet atrophy and rapidly rising blood glucose concentrations remaining over 400 mg per 100 ml until death at five to eight months (Coleman & Hummel, 1967). Compared with other mutants with obesity the diabetic condition is more severe and the lifespan is markedy decreased.

A second allele (db^{2J}) arose shortly after the original mutation was discovered at the Jackson Laboratory. This mutation on the strain of origin exhibited mild diabetes with markedly elevated plasma insulin concentrations sustained throughout a nearly normal lifespan. The phenotypic expression was identical to that observed with the BL/6 obese mutant and was distinctly unlike the original diabetes mutation on the BL/Ks background (Hummel *et al.,* 1972). When the db^{2J} allele was introduced to the BL/Ks background, no differences in gene expression were observed between it and the original *db* mutation, suggesting a marked effect of genetic background on the expression of the gene. Another spontaneous mutation (db^{3J}) occurred in the 129/J strain at the Jackson Laboratory and presented as a severe obesity with hypoglycemia rather than hyperglycemia, coupled with marked hyperinsulinemia and massively enlarged islets of Langerhans (Leiter & Coleman, unpublished). This allele has not been placed on the BL/Ks background and the unusual clinical manifestations may be due to the allele itself or the background on which it is maintained. Falconer & Isaacson (1959) described a mutant in a heterogeneous stock that was named adipose *(ad).* This was subsequently found to be an allele of diabetes and the gene symbol was changed from *ad* to db^{ad}. No differences have been observed between *db* and db^{ad} when the alleles are maintained in the same inbred background (Lane, 1965).

Homozygous diabetes mice are sterile and heterozygous carriers must be used to propagate these mutants. In this regard, use has been made of the close linkage of the coat color gene, misty (*m*), to diabetes to develop two new congenic strains, BL/6 *m db* and BL/Ks *m db*, in which the misty gene is maintained in repulsion on the opposite chromosome from the diabetes gene. This facilitates identification of the heterozygotes (+ *m/db* +) required for breeding, which are thin and black as opposed to normals (+ *m/* + *m*) thin and gray, and mutants (*db* +/*db* +), fat and black. Maintenance of misty and diabetes in coupling on the same chromosome permits identification of future diabetes (*db m/db m*) mice by the expression of the misty (gray) coat color as early as four days post-partum well before any hyperinsulinemia, obesity or other clinical symptoms are apparent.

The fat (fat) mouse

This recessive mutation (linkage unknown) occurred in the HRS/J stock at the Jackson Laboratory and produces a slowly developing but severe obesity (Coleman, unpublished). Prenounced hyperglycemia is not typical of any stage of the disease. Hyperinsulinemia is marked and the islets of Langerhans show enlargement coupled with marked degranulation of the beta cells. The obesity extends all over the body rather than being confined more specifically to the axial and inguinal regions. Attempts have been made to place this mutation on the BL/Ks background to see if severe diabetes would develop. With four generations of backcrossing completed, the condition remains a simple obesity syndrome with no diabetes symptoms. In this regard, fat is distinctly different from obese and diabetes which manifest markedly different syndromes when on different inbred backgrounds (see next section).

Effects of inbred background

The syndrome produced in BL/Ks diabetes (*db*) mice, while similar in early development to that of BL/6 obese (*ob*) mice, has a more severe diabetes-like condition and a less pronounced obesity. However, both mutations when maintained on the same inbred background exhibit identical syndromes from three weeks of age (Hummel *et al.*, 1972; Coleman & Hummel, 1973). Both diabetes and obese mice of the BL/Ks strain have the severe diabetes characterized by insulinopenia and islet atrophy, whereas both mutations maintained on the BL/6 strain have mild diabetes characterized by islet hypertrophy and hyperplasia of the beta cells. Islet hypertrophy is either sustained or followed by atrophy depending on modifiers in the genetic background rather than the specific action of the mutant gene. The markedly different obesity-diabetes states exhibited when obese and diabetes mice are on different backgrounds points out the importance of strict genetic control in studies with all types of obese-hyperglycemic mutants. Genetic studies (Coleman & Hummel, 1975) have shown that the modifiers leading to islet hypertrophy and well-compensated diabetes compatible with a near normal lifespan are dominant to those factors causing severe diabetes.

The BL/Ks strain is the only strain to date that consistently shows a near 100 per cent incidence of severe diabetes. Most strains exhibit a milder syndrome with males being most severely afflicted. Studies with cultured postnatal islet cells have revealed increased secretion of glucagon as early as five days of age in cells isolated from pancreases of BL/Ks diabetes mice but not those of BL/6 diabetes mice (Leiter & Coleman, unpublished). This abnormality, if present *in vivo*, could cause excess glucagon secretion early in development and predispose the beta cell to the typical degeneration characteristic of BL/Ks diabetes mice.

The inbred background may be implicated in the control of the number and size of the fat cells in obesity mutants. The obese (*ob*) mutation on the BL/6 background is one of two rodent models characterized by a hypertrophic-hyperplastic type of obesity with both an enlargement and an increase in number of individual fat cells contributing to the obesity. In contrast the phenotypically similar diabetes (*db*) mutation, maintained on the BL/Ks background, is characterized by adipocyte hypertrophy only (Johnson & Hirsch, 1972). This difference may be related to the effects of the obese and diabetes genes themselves, or may be related to the different genetic background on which these mutants are maintained.

Parabiosis experiments

Having obese and diabetes on same histocompatible backgrounds has permitted critical studies of parabiotic unions of normal with mutant mice and provided some insight into the nature of primary lesions in these mutants. Unions of diabetes (*db/db*) with normal mice resulted in the death of the normal mouse, apparently of starvation, within three to four weeks after surgery (Coleman & Hummel, 1969). Our interpretation of this finding is that the diabetes partner produces, but does not respond to, a satiety factor that prevents overeating. In parabiosis this factor crosses into the circulation of the normal partner where it acts on the normal partner's satiety center to inhibit eating, producing subsequent starvation and death. Parabiosis of two diabetes mice is not lethal to either, presumably because both have defective satiety centers. When obese (*ob/ob*) mice were parabiosed with diabetes (*db/db*) mice, the obese partner lost weight and died of starvation, while no abnormal changes were observed in the diabetes partner (Coleman, 1973). This suggests that obese mice are like normal mice with normal satiety centers responsive to satiety factor. Both partners survive in unions of obese with normal mice, suggesting that the obese partner, unlike the diabetes mouse, does not produce sufficient satiety factor to turn off the normal partner's eating drive. However, obese mice in such pairs eat less and gain weight less rapidly than obese with obese pairs (Coleman, 1973). This observation suggests that the normal partner provides a humoral (satiety) factor that regulates food consumption and weight gain in the obese partner. These experiments suggest that the obese mouse is unable to produce sufficient satiety factor to regulate its food consumption, whereas the diabetes mouse produces satiety factor, but cannot respond to it because of a defective satiety center. This would explain the identical obese-hyperglycemic syndromes produced by these two unrelated genes when they are acting in identical genetic backgrounds.

The New Zealand obese (NZO) mouse

This strain of mouse was developed by selection of obese animals from a mixed colony (Bielschowsky & Bielschowsky, 1953). The mode of inheritance is not understood, although it is considered polygenic. For this reason, a normal congenic line is unavailable for the critical comparison. The obesity in NZO mice is slower in development than that for obese or diabetes mutants. Hyperglycemia is not severe (maximum 250 mg/100 ml at four to six months). Plasma insulin increases slightly with age corresponding with increased deposition of adipose tissue. Hypertrophy and hyperplasia of the islets of Langerhans is marked; islet tissue may consist of up to 90 per cent beta cells (Bielschowsky & Bielschowsky, 1956). Although the inheritance of the obesity is controlled by several genes, the primary lesion may involve a pancreatic factor. Gates, Hunt & Lazarus (1974) reported that intraperitoneal implantation of islets from normal mice normalizes the diabetes-like disorder and is followed by an increase in binding capacity of ^{125}I insulin to liver plasma membranes. Islets treated with streptozotin to destroy beta cells before implantation were equally as effective as untreated islets, suggesting that the missing factor was contributed by pancreatic cells other than beta cells. The obesity produced in the NZO mouse is hypertrophic in contrast to the obese mouse and the cellular type of obesity can be modified by diet. A high fat diet produces adipocyte proliferation, increasing both cell number and cell size (Herberg *et al.*, 1972).

The KK mouse

Moderate obesity and polyuria were observed in a Japanese mouse strain (KK) bred for large body size (Nakamura, 1962). This strain has a slowly developing obesity, mild hyperglycemia coupled with hyperinsulinemia, and associated increases in the number and size of the pancreatic islets. The genetics of the syndrome is not understood but it is felt to be polygenic. Characterization of the metabolic disturbance is complicated by the several different lines of KK mice that have been developed and bred by various breeding systems. Again, because of the polygenic nature of the inheritance, there is no congenic control mouse with which to make the most critical comparisons. Hyperphagia, obesity, hyperglycemia and hyperinsulinemia are consistent findings in most strains. These parameters normalize around one year of age (Dulin & Wyse, 1970).

The fatty (fa) rat

The fatty rat (Zucker & Zucker, 1961) is a mutant with obesity caused by an autosomal recessive gene. Obesity is recognizable at four to five weeks of age by excess subcutaneous and intraperitoneal fat deposits. In most respects the fatty rat is very similar to the obese mouse on the BL/6 inbred background. Females are infertile. Obesity, hyperphagia, hyperinsulinemia and insulin resistance are consistent findings (Bray, 1977; York, Steinke & Bray, 1972). Hypertrophy and hyperplasia of the islets of Langerhans coupled with hyperinsulinemia suggest both increases in the rate of synthesis and secretion of insulin (York *et al.*, 1972). Hyperglycemia is not usually found in these mutants whereas hyperinsulinemia and lipemia are pronounced (Bray, 1977).

The fatty rat is characterized by hypertrophic-hyperplastic obesity. Adipocyte proliferation continues after weaning (Johnson *et al.*, 1971) resulting in an obesity that is characterized by increases in both number and size of adipocytes. This may be a reflection of the mutant gene itself, or a manifestation of the interaction of the gene with the host background. Subdiaphragmatic vagotomy of fatty rats was without effect in preventing obesity, whereas obesity in rats caused by lesioning the ventromedial nucleus was prevented by this procedure (Powley & Opsahl, 1974; Opsahl & Powley, 1974; Inoue & Bray, 1977). These data show that the etiology of this obesity is distinct from that observed in lesioned rats, and that the hyperphagia and obesity are not caused by overstimulation of the pancreas by signals coming from the lateral hypothalamus via the vagus nerve. Indeed, a defective beta cell, over responsive to normal stimuli, may reflect the primary lesion.

The obese spontaneously hypertensive rat (fa^k)

This obese rat mutant is similar in most respects to the fatty rat. The inheritance is autosomal recessive, and obesity, endocrine disturbances, and hyperlipidemia are consistent features (Koletsky, 1975). Hypertension and premature atherosclerosis are features not seen in the fatty rat. Albuminuria appears at an early age and is associated with the later development of nephrosclerosis. Allelism tests (Yen, Shaw & Yu, 1977) establish this mutant as an allele of fatty with minor differences in expression, probably due to the inbred background.

Obesity in other species

Three species of rodents (*Psammomys obesus*, the sand rat; *Acomys cahirinus*, the spiny mouse; and *Genomys tolarum*, tuco tuco) are found in hot arid areas of the world and must constantly forage for food to eke out a bare subsistence. When these species are introduced into the laboratory with a readily available supply of chow diet of high caloric density, hyperphagia, obesity, hyperglycemia and hyperinsulinemia develop.

The syndrome in the sand rat (Haines, Hackel & Schmidt-Neilson, 1965; Hackel *et al.*, 1970) begins with an attempt to cope with increased caloric load by compensatory increased insulin production sufficient to maintain blood sugar concentration within the normal range and to prevent ketosis. Thus, in younger animals, there is a normal number of well-granulated beta cells of the islets of Langerhans. Degranulation is observed in the intermediate stages of the disease development. This is followed in some instances by beta cell degeneration and necrosis with resultant insulinopenia and fatal ketosis (Like & Miki, 1967). In contrast, if sand rats are maintained on a low calorie vegetable diet they remain thin and develop normally.

The appearance of diabetes and obesity in the spiny mouse was originally reported by Hefti & Flückiger (1961) and has been described in detail by Gonet *et al.* (1965). Variants of the syndrome have been described which are markedly different in the severity and incidence of obesity. Some animals show obesity, hyperinsulinemia, glucose intolerance and glycosuria. Others have frank hyperglycemia and glucosuria without ketosis that eventually develops into a ketotic form of diabetes with marked life-shortening. All spiny mice have extreme beta cell hyperplasia, regardless of stage of disease or whether they will ultimately become either obese or diabetic. Beta cells are well-granulated and beta cell hyperplasia seems congenital. These findings, coupled with the decreased insulin secretion in response to glucose, suggests a relative unavailability of insulin in the insulin pool (Gonet *et al.*, 1965; Pictet *et al.*, 1967; Trueheart *et al.*, 1976). Obesity was frequent in the early studies, but the incidence seems to have decreased in recent reports. The diabetes-like condition still appears with no clear correlation between the development of obesity and subsequent derangements in carbohydrate metabolism. Although conditions of housing and feeding of these mice have remained constant, there appears to have been some adaptation to laboratory conditions after a few generations, resulting in normalization of metabolism.

Tuco tucos in the laboratory develop cataracts within six months and this development correlates with the incidence of hyperglycemia. Many animals, especially males, become hyperphagic and obese. Pancreatic histology shows degranulation of the beta cells of the islet of Langerhans (Wise *et al.*, 1969).

These three desert rodents represent a group of mammals that, through evolution under extreme conditions, have developed more efficient ways of processing the limited food available. As a consequence, when presented with unlimited amounts of high caloric diets, they cannot cope and become obese, or diabetic, or both.

Discussion

Although studies with models of obesity have been extensive and exhaustive in scope, no primary lesion has been defined for any of the syndromes described. Several possibilities have been suggested and many remain acceptable in the light of present data. One primary defect applicable to several mutants involves a possible hypothalamic abnormality. Most of the models are infertile, have defects in thermoregulation, and are hyperphagic, all of which supports a hypothalamic defect. The best evidence for a hypothalamic defect is found in the diabetes (*db*) mouse which may have a defective satiety center preventing it from responding to satiety factor (Coleman & Hummel, 1969). Although these studies appear very clear-cut, they must be interpreted with caution since the syndrome in the diabetes mouse differs in many respects from the classical syndrome in which the ventromedial nucleus (VMH) is destroyed by electrolytic lesioning. The genetic lesion possibly involves a defect in a much more discrete area of the hypothalamus than is destroyed by chemical or electrolytic lesions and many of the normal functions of the region other than satiety may be preserved.

The obese (*ob*) mouse is phenotypically identical to the diabetes mouse, when maintained on the same genetic background, suggesting that this syndrome might also be caused by a defect in the hypothalamus. However, our results with obese mice in parabiosis with diabetes mice suggest that obese mice can respond to satiety factor and that at least that part of the hypothalamus involving satiety is normal (Coleman, 1973). Studies with obese (*ob/ob*) and normal mice in parabiosis have established that food consumption and rate of weight gain were regulated in the obese partner by something coming from the normal partner. This suggested that the obese mouse cannot produce satiety factor in sufficient amounts to control its appetite. Strautz (1970) has shown that transplantation of normal islets to obese mice stabilized rate of weight gain and reduced both hyperglycemia and hyperinsulinemia. These studies imply that the missing satiety factor may be pancreatic in origin. Similar islet transplant studies undertaken by others with obese mice have not been able to repeat these results, and this hypothesis, until confirmed, must be considered with caution. Studies by Gates

& co-workers (1974) using the genetically dissimilar NZO mice have established the existence of a pancreatic, but non-beta cell factor, that will cure NZO mice. It is hard to see how a single missing factor could alleviate the syndrome entirely in NZO mice since the condition is caused by the interaction of several genes and must represent more than one primary defect. Still to be evaluated as potential curative factors are somatostatin, pancreatic polypeptide, and serotonin, all compounds contained in various cells of the pancreas.

The hypothalamus regulates food consumption via two mechanisms. The ventromedial region (satiety center) exerts an inhibitory influence on the lateral hypothalamus (feeding center) thereby regulating food intake. The lateral hypothalamus (LH) stimulates insulin secretion by the pancreas via impulses through the vagus nerve. A defective satiety center, as postulated in the diabetes mouse, would cause the LH to fire continuously causing excess insulin secretion very early in development, prior to any hyperphagia or signs of obesity. Our studies (Coleman & Hummel, 1974) with preclinical diabetes (*db*) mice showed this to be the case and support the hypothesis of a defective satiety center. Severing the vagus nerve (Opsahl & Powley, 1974) prevents the obesity from developing in VMH lesioned rats, whereas vagotomy in the mutant fatty rat was without effect.These experiments demonstrated that production of obesity in the fatty rat was independent of stimulation of the pancreas by the LH via the vagus. The hyperinsulinemia of this type of obesity may represent a primary defect in the insulin releasing mechanism of the pancreas rather than a hypothalamic defect. Similar studies with the other models of obesity would establish any involvement of either the lateral hypothalamus or the pancreas as being associated with the primary lesion.

Another attractive hypothesis regarding the primary defect in the obese mouse is a defect intrinsic to the adipocyte itself. Joosten & van der Kroon (1974) showed that increases in the size of the individual fat cells in obese mice could be observed as early as 14 days, prior to any evidence of either obesity or hyperinsulinemia (24 to 30 days). These data suggested that the primary defect may be in the metabolism of the individual fat cell. Recent studies (Ashwell *et al.*, 1977) using fat pads from obese or normal mice transplanted beneath the kidney capsule of obese or normal mice showed that the transplanted fat pad took on the morphological characteristics of the host, ie normal fat to an obese host caused marked enlargement of the fat cells, whereas obese fat to normal host cause normalization of fat tissue. The same results were obtained with fat pads from diabetes and yellow mice and as well as those made obese with the goldthioglucose (GTG) (Ashwell, personal communication). These authors conclude that none of the obesities (*ob, db,* A^y *or GTG)* are caused by defects in the fat pad but rather the nature of the fat cell depends on the environment in which it is located. The availability of the congenitically athymic nude mouse, which does not reject either allografts or xenografts and will accept tissue grafts from unrelated strains, and even other species, should make this technique applicable to all obesity models as well as human beings.

The yellow mouse represents the only single gene mutation that has multiple pleiotropic effects that affect viability and pigmentation as well as obesity. This obesity model, caused by an autosomal dominant gene, is less severe than any of the others, being only moderately hyperphagic, and then only for discrete periods in its development. Body weight may be regulated more by controlling energy utilization rather than energy (food) intake. Further studies on feed efficiency and energy utilization will be required in all of these models. The yellow mouse is particularly intriguing because the yellow (A^y) gene is lethal in homozygotes, preventing development past the blastocyst stage. Thus, we can conclude that the gene controls a metabolic pathway essential to normal development, as well as being involved in producing obesity. Also, the phenotype expressed is subject to very subtle environmental influences even *in utero.* Genetically yellow ($A^{vy}/?$) mice may be phenotypically wild type (agouti) on maturing. If the phenotype is agouti, regardless of the genotype, insulin secretion is normal, and the mouse does not become obese. In those mice, phenotypically yellow or mottled, the degree of hyperinsulinemia and obesity correlates nicely with the extent of yellow pigmentation of the pelage. Defining the nature of the environmental insults that can occur *in utero* to change subsequent hair development from yellow to agouti, and also prevent obesity, should shed much light on factors involved in the control of both pigmentation and obesity.

We have found a marked effect of inbred background on the expression of diabetes and obese genes. In contrast, the yellow and fat mutations appear to have identical syndromes on the two usually divergent inbred backgrounds. This may suggest that the primary insult initiating the obesity is not as strong as that for obese and diabetes and that this more gradual initiation of obesity permits the host genome to make a response (islet hypertrophy) compatible with life rather than islet atrophy, insulinopenia, and life-shortening diabetes.

The fatty rat has no glucose intolerance or hyperglycemia, yet has a marked hyperinsulinemia and obesity. The obesity is unusual in that fat cell proliferation occurs beyond the normal developmental period. Thus, the obesity is of the hypertrophic-hyperplastic type, involving an increase in both number and size of the adipocytes. With the exception of the obese mouse, all of the other obesities represent solely an enlargement of fat cells rather than increase in their number. Whether the type of obesity produced, hypertrophic or hypertrophic-hyperplastic, is related to the mutant allele itself or the background genome remains to be elucidated. The NZO mouse fed a normal laboratory diet develops hypertrophic obesity; but, when provided with high fat diets, a hypertrophic-hyperplastic type of obesity is produced. The mechanisms responsible for the shift from hypertrophic to hyperplastic growth in adipose tissue are unknown. The potential of this strain should be to establish those environmental factors that initiate or suppress adipoçyte proliferation.

The uniqueness of desert rodents lies in their having been selected for those factors which allow better utilization of available food in semi-arid environments with limited food supplies. More efficient pathways of lipogenesis presumably were developed to build up fat stores, when food was plentiful, for utilization when food became scarce. These models are of particular interest in understanding diabetes-prone human populations that, in primitive environments, have almost no diabetes, but, on emigrating to regions or countries with higher standards of living, develop a high incidence of diabetes. Thus, the concept of a predisposition to diabetes being caused by a 'thrifty gene' (Neel, 1964) is realized in desert rodents. This 'thrifty gene', while an asset under subsistence conditions, becomes a liability in times of affluence when environmental changes no longer favor thrift. When these rodents are introduced to the laboratory and are exposed to high calorie food *ad lib.* instead of limited amounts of seeds and grasses, the heretofore beneficial thrifty gene becomes detrimental. Fat stores are increased far beyond normal, excess insulin secretion taxes the pancreatic supply and severe diabetes and premature death ensue. If the diet fed is limited to vegetables, the obesity-diabetes syndrome will not develop.

All of the syndromes described are characterized in the earliest stages by varying degrees of hyperphagia and hyperinsulinemia. Which comes first? Hyperphagia could initiate changes in the pancreatic islet cells leading to hyperinsulinemia or, alternatively, a primary defect in an islet cell could lead to excessive insulin secretion, thereby causing the hyperphagia. Either mechanism sets up the cycle of overeating, increased secretion of plasma insulin and further overeating. The question of which comes first is probably academic since neonatal rodents are hyperphagic from birth until weaning. The only satiety signal that is recognizable by the neonate is fullness of gut (Epstein, 1976). Growth rate and fat deposition of the pup is regulated solely by competition for milk among siblings, which varies greatly with the size of the litter. Satiety mechanisms develop in a systematic fashion around the time of weaning and thereafter. In the case of the diabetic mouse, hyperphagia persists because it cannot recognize satiety factor, whereas in the obese mouse hyperphagia persists because satiety factor is never produced. Accordingly, the hyperinsulinemia detectable by 12 days in diabetes mice would be a result of an unregulated lateral hypothalamus providing overstimulation to the pancreas rather than resulting from hyperphagia.

Hyperphagia is not necessarily a prerequisite to obesity. Experiments undertaken with normal and mutant (*ob, db*) mice, and fatty rats pair-fed the same amounts of food on similar time schedules, have established that whereas the rate of weight gain was not necessarily increased in the mutant, the amount of lipid deposited was in the same proportion as that seen in mutants fed *ad lib.* (Cox & Powley, 1977; Goldman, Bernardis & Frohman, 1974; Zucker, 1975; Coleman, unpublished). Even if hyperphagia is prevented, the mutation causes a more efficient utilization of foodstuffs and conversion to fat than that observed in the normal animal. Decreased energy expenditure, although a factor, cannot totally account for this increased feed efficiency.

Hyperphagia or hyperinsulinemia would lead to obesity and beta cell hyperactivity causing either compensatory hypertrophy and hyperplasia of the beta cells, or beta cell exhaustion and atrophy. The events leading to the obesity-diabetes states follow this sequence. A vicious circle is established with hyperinsulinemia encouraging hyperphagia and hyperphagia favoring further secretion of insulin. The target organs for insulin become maximally stimulated. Insulin resistance intervenes, probably to protect the animal against what should be the hypoglycemic effect of the hyperinsulinemia. The pancreatic output of insulin can either be sustained, thus maintaining grossly elevated concentrations of insulin and producing a massive obesity, or islet atrophy occurs causing insulinopenia, severe diabetes and premature death.

Summary

Several different models in rodents are available for metabolic studies on the development of obesity. Although the abnormalities associated with each type of obesity have many features in common, the documentation of several different genes being involved makes it unlikely that the various syndromes will be reduced to a single disturbance in one metabolic pathway. The best studied models and those for which the most complete information is available are those caused by single genes eg, yellow, obese, diabetes, and fat in mice, and fatty in rats. In the other models the inheritance is either polygenic or otherwise unclear, features which interfere with the interpretation of the data. This review briefly summarizes the developing syndrome in each model, points out any obvious differences, and suggests the most appropriate areas where future research should be most productive in the light of contemporary knowledge.

Acknowledgements – Supported in part by Research Grants AM 14461, AM 20725 from the National Institute of Arthritis, Metabolism, and Digestive Diseases; by Research Grant CA 05873 from the National Cancer Institute; and by a grant from the Juvenile Diabetes Foundation. The Jackson Laboratory is fully accredited by the American Association for the accreditation of Laboratory Animal Care.

References

Ashwell, M., Meade, C.J., Medawar, P. & Sowter, C. (1977): *Proc. R. Soc. Ser. B.* 195, 343.
Assimacopoulos-Jeannet, F. & Jeanrenaud, B. (1976): *Clins Endoc. Metab.* 5, 337.
Bielschowsky, M. & Bielschowsky, F. (1953): *Proc. Univ. Otago Med. Sch.* 31, 29.
Bielschowsky, M. & Bielschowsky, F. (1956): *Aust. J. Exp. Biol. Med.* 34, 181.
Bray, G.A. (1977): *Fed. Proc.* 36, 148.
Bray, G.A. & York, D.A. (1971): *Physiol. Rev.* 51, 598.
Coleman, D.L. (1973): *Diabetologia* 9, 294.
Coleman, D.L. & Hummel, K.P. (1967): *Diabetologia* 3, 238.
Coleman, D.L. & Hummel, K.P. (1969): *Am. J. Physiol.* 217, 1298.
Coleman, D.L. & Hummel, K.P. (1973): *Diabetologia* 9, 287.
Coleman, D.L. & Hummel, K.P. (1974): *Diabetologia* 10, 607.
Coleman, D.L. & Hummel, K.P. (1975): *Isr. J. Med.* 11, 708.
Cox, J.E. & Powley, T.L. (1977): *J. Comp. Physiol. Psychol.* 91, 347.
Cuénot, L. (1905): *Archs Zool. T.* 3, 123.
Danforth, C.H. (1927): *J. Hered.* 18, 153.

Dickie, M.M. (1962): *J. Hered.* 63, 84.
Dulin, W.E. & Wyse, B.M. (1970): *Diabetologia* 6, 317.
Epstein, A.N. (1976): In *Hunger: basic mechanisms and clinical implications*, ed D. Novin, W. Wyrwicka, & G. Bray, p. 193. New York: Raven Press.
Falconer, D.S. & Isaacson, J.H. (1959): *J. Hered.* 50, 290.
Gates, R.J., Hunt, M.I. & Lazarus, N.R. (1974): *Diabetologia* 10, 401.
Genuth, S.M., Pryzbylski, R.S. & Rosenberg, D.M. (1971): *Endocrinology* 88, 1230.
Goldman, J.K., Bernardis, L.L. & Frohman, L.A. (1974): *Am. J. Physiol.* 227, 88.
Gonet, A.E., Stauffacher, W., Pictet, R. & Renold, A.E. (1965): *Diabetologia* 1, 162.
Hackel, D.B., Mikat, E., Lebovitz, H.E., Schmidt-Neilson, K., Horton, E.S. & Kinney, T.O. (1967): *Diabetologia* 3, 130.
Haines, E.S., Hackel, D.B. & Schmidt-Neilson, K. (1965): *Am.J. Physiol.* 208, 297.
Hefti, F. & Flückiger, E. (1961): *Rev. Suisse Zool.* 74, 562.
Hellerström, C. & Hellman, B. (1963): *Metabolism* 12, 522.
Herberg, L., Bergmann, M., Hemmings, U., Major, E. & Grier, F. (1972): *Isr. J. Med. Sci.* 8, 822.
Herberg, L. & Coleman, D.L. (1977): *Metabolism* 26, 59.
Hummel, K.P., Coleman, D.L. & Lane, P.W. (1972): *Biochem. Genet.* 7, 1.
Hummel, K.P., Dickie, M.M. & Coleman, D.L. (1966): *Science* 153, 1127.
Ingalls, A.M., Dickie, M.M. & Snell, G.D. (1950): *J. Hered.* 41, 317.
Inoue, S. & Bray, G.A. (1977): *Endocrinology* 100, 108.
Johnson, P.R. & Hirsch, J. (1972): *J. Lipid Res.* 13, 2.
Johnson, P.R., Zucker, L.M., Cruce, J.A.F. & Hirsch, J. (1971): *J. Lipid Res.* 12, 706.
Joosten, H.F.P. & van der Kroon, P.H.W. (1974): *Metabolism* 23, 59.
Kahn, C.R., Neville, D.M. Jr. & Roth, J. (1973): *J. Biol. Chem.* 248, 244.
Kahn, C.R., Neville, D.M. Jr., Gorden, P., Freychet, P. & Roth, J. (1972): *Biochem. Biophys. Res. Commun.* 48, 135.
Koletsky, S. (1975): *Am. J. Path.* 80, 129.
Lane, P.W. (1973): *Mouse News Letter* 48, 34.
Like, A.A. & Miki, E. (1967): *Diabetologia* 3, 143.
Loten, E.G., Rabinovitch, A. & Jeanrenaud, B. (1974): *Diabetologia* 10, 45.
Nakamura, M. (1962): *Diabetologia* 6, 317.
Neel, J.V. (1962): *Am. J. Human Genet.* 14, 353.
Opsahl, C.A. & Powley, T.L. (1974): *Am. J. Physiol.* 226, 34.
Pictet, R., Orci, L., Gonet, A.E., Rouiller, C. & Renold, A.E. (1967): *Diabetologia* 3, 188.
Powley, T.L. & Opsahl, C.A. (1974): *Am. J. Physiol.* 226, 25.
Renold, A.E. & Dulin, W.E. (1967): *Diabetologia* 3, 63.
Renold, A.E., Cahill, G.F. Jr. & Gerritsen, G.C. (1970): *Diabetologia* 6, 153.
Renold, A.E., Chang, A.Y. & Muller, W.A. (1974): *Diabetologia* 10, 491.
Robertson, G.C. (1942): *J. Exp. Zool.* 89, 197.
Strautz, R.L. (1970): *Diabetologia* 6, 306.
Trueheart, P.A., Maldonato, A., Kaelen, D., Renold, A.E. & Sharpe, G.W.G. (1976): *Diabetologia* 12, 463.
Turner, M.L. (1948): *Am. J. Physiol.* 152, 197.
Wise, P.H., Weir, B.J., Hime, J.M. & Forrest, E. (1969): *Diabetologia* 5, 59.
Wolff, G.L. (1965): *Science* 147, 1145.
Yen, T.T., Shaw, W.N. & Yu, P.L. (1977): *Heredity* 38, 373.
York, D.A., Steinke, A.J. & Bray, G.A. (1972): *Metabolism* 21, 277.
Zucker, L.M. (1975): *Proc. Soc. Exp. Biol. Med.* 148, 498.
Zucker, L.M. & Zucker, T.F. (1961): *J. Hered.* 52, 275.

16
THE FAT CELL: A CLINICAL VIEW

P. BJÖRNTORP
Department of Medicine I, Sahlgrenska Hospital, University of Göteborg, Göteborg, Sweden.

The main function of adipose tissue is to store and release triglyceride. This energy store is by far the largest in the body. The functional unit of adipose tissue is the fat cell, the adipocyte, which is efficiently equipped both functionally and morphologically for this purpose. The dominating activities of fat uptake and release are executed by two lipase systems, each with a specific regulation. The unique ability of these cells to cover a thousandfold change in volume of the triglyceride vacuole represents a very marked flexibility of the capacity of the adipose tissue organ to store fat. This capacity is due not only to the variation of the volume of each cell but also to the number of adipocytes.

Research during the recent past 20 years has elucidated the functional characteristics of adipose tissue. Also, during the last decade, methodological developments have made possible studies on the two-dimensional morphological characteristics of adipose tissue, viz. its capacity to store triglyceride by adipocyte multiplication or expansion. It has proved necessary to reinvestigate much of the basic information from the rat adipocyte before this knowledge is used in the clinic because of the marked species variation in adipocyte metabolism. The human adipocyte does not seem to develop or function in a similar way to the rat adipocyte.

It seems pertinent to focus the interest on the functional unit of the tissue which is the site for the expression of obesity, although as yet very little indeed has been revealed which would give a suspicion of a primary regulatory defect of adipocyte metabolism as a cause of obesity. Some information in this field is beginning to show promise for use in the clinic. Clearly there are, however, several remaining problems, some of them methodological.

In the following section some of the methodological pit-falls will be brought to light in order to prevent overinterpretation of the presently available information. In this review some recently performed studies will be summarized which facilitate interpretations from clinical and physiological points of view.

Determination of fat cell size

Principally three types of methods are useful for this purpose. One is the osmium method (Hirsch & Gallian, 1968) which is very accurate, determining automatically a large number of cells. However, the smallest fat cells are either not fixed by the osmium or filtered off in the preparation procedure. The next method is microscopic measuring cells *in situ* (Sjöström, Björntorp & Vrana, 1971). Smaller cells are theoretically included in measurements with this method. Finally, cells can be liberated by collagenase and then measured. These methods, however, need careful standardization with one of the methods mentioned above in order to ascertain that selections in preparation and handling do not occur among different classes of cell size (Smith, Sjöström & Björntorp, 1972).

With ar.y of these three methods fat cells can be measured containing enough triglyceride to allow fixation in osmium, to allow recognition in the microscope, or to allow floating for measurements in the collagenase methods. This means that none of these methods include cells without triglyceride in the measurements and counts.

Calculation of the results obtained requires some comment. Most laboratories seem to utilize the formula presented by Goldrick (1967). This formula does not necessarily require a gaussian distribution but rather a symmetrical distribution of particle sizes. It has then to be ascertained that this is always the case in different materials. Some doubt has been expressed about this (Ashwell & Garrow, 1973; Widdowson & Shaw, 1973). In order to test the validity of the formula in question determination of the average fat cell size with this formula was compared with the correct, but time-consuming, method of calculating side by side the true average (Sjöström, 1972). Figure 1 shows such a comparison with the osmium

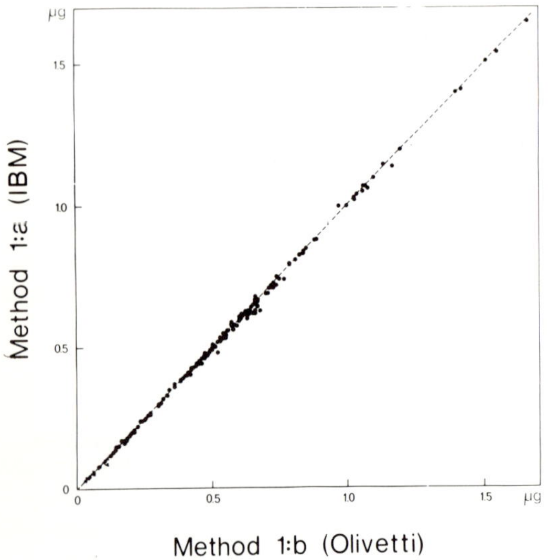

Fig. 1. Relationship between calculations of fat cell weight by the Goldrick (1967) formula (abscissa) and by calculations of a mean of each separate fat cell weight (ordinate). y=0.993 x −0.001. *r:* 0.999. (From Sjöström, 1972)

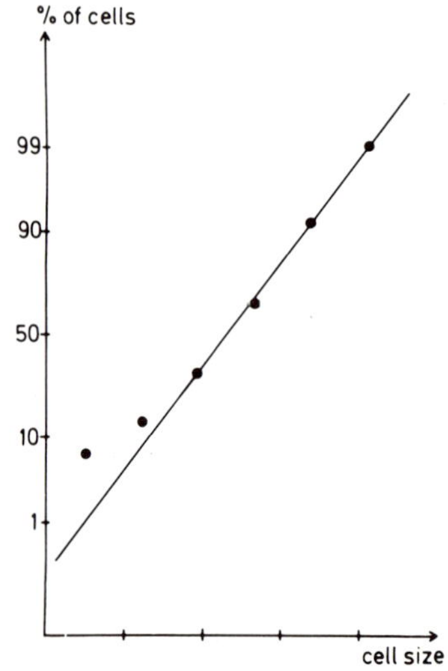

Fig. 2. Deviation from gaussian distribution of fat cell weights in obese women

method, comprising several thousands of measured cells in each point. The result is very close to unity in these samples covering a large range of average fat cell size. Nevertheless, such an analysis should be undertaken in different materials analysed where the fat cell size distribution is not known. In obese subjects for example there is no doubt a skewed distribution of fat cell size with a tailing towards the smaller cells. Figure 2 shows this as a summary of 700 measurements in obese subjects with approximately the same average fat cell size in the abdominal region. Application of the Goldrick formula gives an average fat cell size of 0.660 μg. If the two lowest points are corrected towards the straight line in the plot, and the data recalculated with the assumption of a normal distribution, a new weight of 0.655 μg is obtained. Some skewness can thus be tolerated without a large deviation of the average fat cell size. Nevertheless, the presence of this error should be remembered, particularly in the growing organism, or in conditions with a decreased fat cell size such as after weight decrease treatment in obesity. The correct method of calculating the average from each cell volume is of course to be preferred in these situations.

Determination of fat cell number

The determination of fat cell number is based on the total body fat mass which is divided by an average fat cell size of the whole adipose tissue. This creates several obvious difficulties both as far as body fat determination is concerned and, particularly, in the estimation of the average fat cell size.

Body fat determination has several intrinsic pitfalls because, for obvious reasons, it has to be performed indirectly. The soundest methods theoretically are those using inert fat-soluble gases. These, however, are not yet free from considerable complications (Lesser, Deutsch & Markofsky, 1971). Methods utilizing isotope dilution in different body compartments seem to be useful and comparisons with direct methods in animals, and in a few dead bodies, give acceptable results (Forbes, Gallup & Hursch, 1961; Moore *et al.*, 1963). It seems necessary to take into account shifts in the water spaces in clinical conditions such as dieting otherwise erroneous results may well be obtained. Determinations should also include here the water spaces such as in the four-compartment model described by Berg & Isaksson (1970).

Other uncertainties remain such as the assumption of constant potassium contents in all cells at different ages, a constant relation between extra- and intracellular water and a constant amount of fat-free extracellular solids. These are, however, probably the best methods available for body fat determination.

Determination of body density is simpler than the compartment determinations and seems to give useful measurements if performed carefully (Wilmore & Behnke, 1969).

This methodological dilemma is, however, a fundamental one because the whole field of obesity research is of course based on the diagnosis of the condition, that is the measurements of the amount of fat in the body.

Determination of an average fat cell size, valid for the whole body, is even more difficult. In order to see whether this is at all possible to perform in a meaningful way it is necessary to look into the different sources of error.

The variation of fat cell size within one site of subcutaneous adipose tissue is of the same order as the error of the method (Sjöström *et al.*, 1971). The next problem is the variation between sites and this is analysed in Fig. 3 where determination of fat cell size was performed in several subcutaneous regions in non-obese young and middle-aged men and women, as well as in obese women. The variation around the average is not very pronounced, particularly in the obese women where it would not matter much which site was selected for the calculations of fat cell number if this was to be determined in a group. On an individual basis, however, the problem is much more pronounced (Fig. 4). These fat cell profiles are more or less spread around the average and, clearly, in several of these obese women, determination

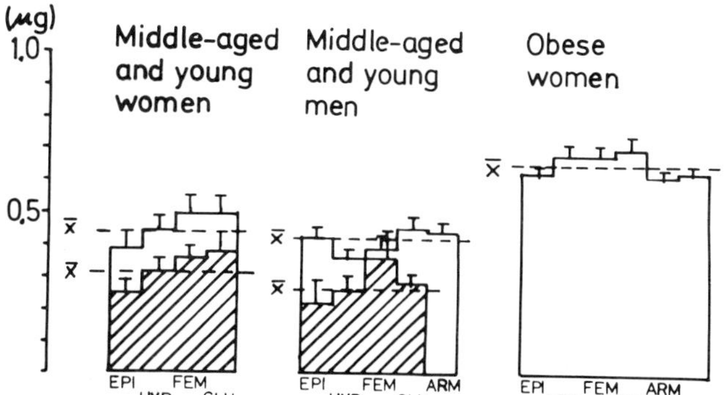

Fig. 3. Regional fat cell size in different populations. Young populations: striped. X: average. Abbreviations of sites: Epi: epigastrial. Hyp: hypogastrial. Fem: femoral. Glu: gluteal. Hip: hip region

in only one site would give a very deviant result from the average of several sites. But with a large variation it is clear that the average also will be somewhat uncertain, due to the fact that each fat cell size here may well represent adipose tissue sites of varying quantity. These

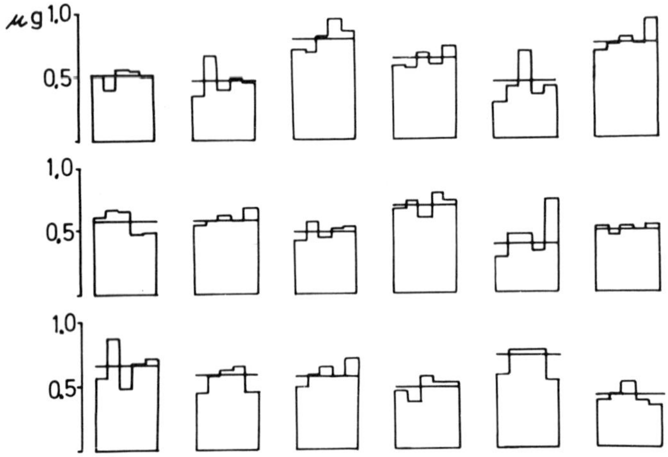

Fig. 4. Individual fat cell size profiles in obese women. Epigastrial, hypogastrial, femoral and gluteal sites

results show, however, as has been pointed out previously by Salans, Cushman & Weismann (1973) that an average of determinations from different sites is necessary if a meaningful average fat cell size is required to be used for determination of fat cell number.

The error obtained by determination in only one site can be analysed by a sort of 'sensitivity test'. The mean of the differences between the largest and smallest observation has been expressed as percentage of the average fat cell volume for all the examined sites in 50 consecutive obese women and found to be 35.6 ± 7.6 per cent. This then means that there is on average about 36 per cent difference between the largest and smallest fat cell size. Assuming a symmetrical distribution of these observations the average would be about 18 per cent distant from the mean. In other words if the determination is performed in only one of these sites the error is of the order of 18 per cent in comparison with the measurement based on all sites. This then again shows the importance of examining several sites.

Another important question is how much adipose tissue is covered by the needle biopsy measurements. After all, 4 to 6 biopsies from different sites weigh 40 to 60 mg which is of the order of one part per million of total adipose tissue weight. A rough estimation of how much adipose tissue is covered by the measurements has been performed in the following way. Using measurements of different distances, ie subcutaneous fat thickness, by ultrasound, and circumference in 100 obese women, subcutaneous adipose tissue can be estimated as a cylinder from the neck to the knees plus two cylinders covering the upper arms. A comparison with the total body fat measured by isotope dilution methods (Berg & Isaksson, 1970) shows that these cylinders comprise 80 to 90 per cent of the total body fat. The remaining fat is mainly the visceral fat.

Figure 3 shows the sites where fat cell determinations were performed. The results are shown in Fig. 3 and also individually in some of the subjects in Fig. 4. The intra-site variation is about 10 per cent (Sjöström *et al.*, 1971) and these sources of error have already been discussed. To sum up, it seems reasonable to state that the variation of fat cell size within the cylinder is small within the group of obese women, and that the measurements are representative for most of the total body fat. Individually, the error is, however, large if several biopsies are not performed.

The remaining error is the contribution of visceral tissue and its fat cell size to the determination of average fat cell size. There is no simple way to include this fat in the measurements. Reports indicate that there is a correlation between the fat cell size of visceral fat and subcutaneous fat (Goldrick & McLoughlin, 1970). The rough estimation of Fig. 5 would indicate that the amount of visceral fat is small in comparison with the subcutaneous fat. Thus the error introduced by an unknown fat cell volume in visceral fat would not change the fat cell number appreciably. To take an example which is unfavourable for the precision of the measurement in question: suppose the subcutaneous fat is 40 kg out of a total of 50 kg, the fat cell weight of the subcutaneous tissue is 0.80 μg and only half (0.40 μg) in the visceral fat. Then the average fat cell weight will be 0.72 μg. The total fat cell number is 6.3×10^{10} and 6.9×10^{10}, respectively, a fairly limited variation in spite of the unfavourable conditions.

This analysis shows that the largest error is introduced in determinations in one individual by the regional variation in fat cell size. The variation here is of the order of 20 per cent. This has to be kept in mind when individuals are classed in groups. In determinations in groups the error is considerably smaller, perhaps of the order of half that in individuals. This does not, however, take into account that small cells might be present which are not measured and counted by presently available methods. This will be discussed below.

Developmental aspects of adipose tissue and errors introduced into fat cell count by 'non-visible' fat cells

The present knowledge of adipose tissue development is based on morphological (Hammar, 1895; Napolitano, 1963; Hirsch & Han, 1969) and DNA-synthesis studies (Hollenberg & Vost, 1968; Greenwood & Hirsch, 1974). The morphological studies suffer from the fact that they are either non-quantitative or only semi-quantitative, because they do not measure the numbers of cells developing into adipocytes. The DNA-synthesis method is not quantitative either but gives information on the periods during life when fat cells or their precursors multiply. This method cannot be used in studies in man because it requires administration of labelled thymidine.

A method is clearly needed to isolate, characterize and quantify not only the mature adipocytes, but also the cells developing into adipocytes, which are called preadipocytes below. Having set out to study the methodological possibilities several years ago, after several unsuccessful attempts, we have now ended up with the following procedures which seem useful for the purpose (Björntorp *et al.*, 1977*a*). First, we needed a method to assay the cells in question in purification procedures. It turned out that morphological and *in vitro* functional tests were not useful. We therefore decided to expose the cells in question to labelled chylomicra *in vivo* before their separation. It seemed reasonable to assume that the labelled chylomicra would be taken up by the mature adipocytes and their precursors, rather than by other cells such as blood cells and fibroblasts. Therefore, small rats (40 to 50 g) were given labelled palmitic acid in corn oil the night before sacrifice followed by sucrose in the drinking water to direct the label as much as possible to adipose tissue. The epididymal fat pads were removed next morning and treated with collagenase under as careful conditions as possible to avoid the formation of ghosts which would disturb the identification of the labelled preadipocytes. Another technical problem was large masses of aggregating cells. These latter cells were removed by filtration after conditions had been worked out for the optimal formation of these aggregates, requiring among other things the presence of calcium. The cells so obtained in the filtrate were further purified by adhesion to the bottom of a tissue culture dish.

These cells were next cultured in medium 199 fortified with serum glucose, insulin, and a triglyceride emulsion. The cells then multiplied and collected coalescing granules ending up in floating 'tissues' from which cells of identical morphology and function could be isolated with collagenase as the adipocytes originally obtained from the rat (Fig. 5). The conversion

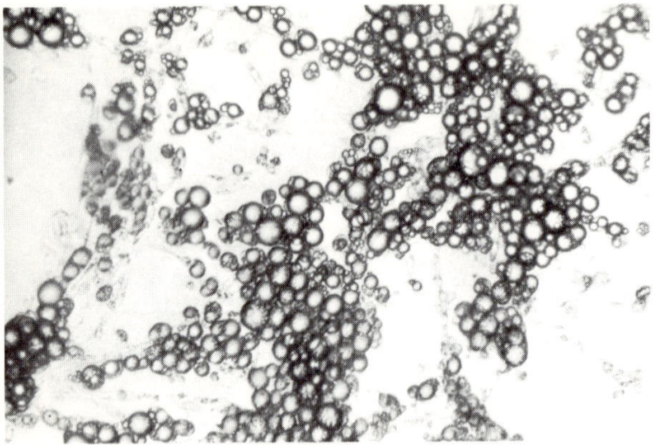

Fig. 5. Adipocyte development in culture (from Björntorp *et al.*, 1977*a*)

of the cells to adipocytes varied from one preparation to another and could be varied both by *in vitro* and *in vivo* conditions. With increasing age the spontaneous development of adipocytes in rats disappeared at about 300 g body weight. Adding isobutylmethylxanthine, cholera toxin or prostaglandin E_1 caused a marked conversion of essentially all cells in the preparation to adipocytes. It is of particular interest that, in preparations from large rats where there was no spontaneous adipocyte formation, isobutylmethylxanthine apparently could induce such formation *in vitro*.

There is another preparation of cells described by Green & Meuth (1974) where adipocytes develop. This is the 3T3-L1 line obtained from mouse embryos. The spontaneous formation of fat cells from this preparation appears less pronounced than in the cells isolated from the fat pad of small rats, probably depending on the source of cells and on the purification procedures.

These studies showed that preadipocytes could be isolated and characterized from the epididymal fat pads of small rats. To allow quantitation of these cells further methodological development was necessary (Björntorp *et al.*, 1977*b*). First, the tissue examined had to be totally disintegrated into its component cells which should be essentially intact. This was accomplished by the development of a method where a mixture of lytic enzymes (collagenase, hyaluronidase and elastase) as well as different mechanical procedures were utilized. In the largest rats an initial brief perfusion with the lytic solution of the epididymal fat pad through the right spermatic artery, followed by the conventional *in vitro* incubation, proved necessary.

The morphological characteristics of the cells so obtained were not so characteristic as to allow counting of preadipocytes. Therefore, the culture technique was again utilized in order to identify the preadipocytes when they had developed into adipocytes. In this culture multiplication had to be prevented to make counting meaningful and this was accomplished by making the culture medium viscous with methyl cellulose. After culture in this medium for several weeks cells developing into adipocytes could be counted and these were assumed to be preadipocytes from the original tissue.

First, preadipocytes in the rat epididymal fat pad were determined. In 40 to 50 g rats the preadipocytes are about twice as numerous as mature adipocytes. At the body weight of about 300 g preadipocytes disappear and adipocytes reach a constant level of about 6×10^6 cells per fat pad.

With these methods available it was now possible to examine to what extent cells were present in human adipose tissue which could multiply and develop into adipocytes. First, adult non-obese tissue from subcutis and omentum was examined in eight subjects operated on for gallbladder disease. These cells multiplied readily and collected granules of lipid but never developed into the characteristic shape of mature adipocytes in cultures for up to eight weeks. In the medium containing methyl cellulose there was no formation of fat cells, indicating the absence of preadipocytes in these tissues.

Next, eight severely obese subjects were examined. The degree of hypercellularity of their adipose tissue varied. In these samples cells were again seen which collected lipid but did not develop into typical adipocytes. In the methyl cellulose system the result was not completely conclusive. In some of the sample there was a formation of multivacuolar cells which possibly were preadipocytes in the process of collecting lipid. They never formed typical adipocytes, however. The number of such cells was very few, amounting to less than one per thousand of the mature adipocytes isolated from the sample during the initial preparation.

Finally, adipose tissue from a few children have been examined. Here also cells with some lipid have been seen. It should be remembered that in these samples the amount of original tissues were so small that there must have been a risk for overgrowth of fibroblasts in the preparation. This risk should have been smaller in the adult tissues where much tissue was available for examination.

In tissues from children typical adipocytes developed in the methyl cellulose cultures. Counting of these cells revealed, however, that their number amounted to less than one per cent of the adipocytes. This included tissues from children of about one month of age. This part of the examination has to be performed on more children before definite conclusions are possible, however.

In human tissues there has thus so far been no conclusive evidence for the presence of cells which can multiply and form adipocytes. The presence of preadipocytes has been established in children, and possibly in some obese subjects. The number of these cells seems, however, insignificant (Fig. 6). It would therefore appear that a bed of preadipocytes which is present

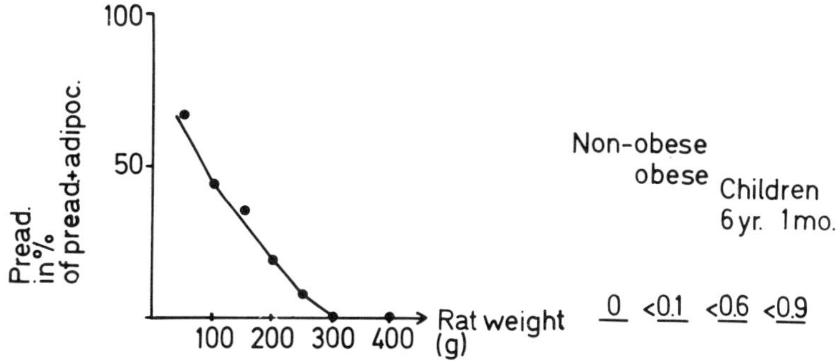

Fig. 6. Relative part of preadipocytes in adipose tissue of rats (left) and different groups of humans (right) (from Björntorp *et al.*, 1977. *a* and *b*)

in young rats is not found in obese or non-obese adults or in non-obese children to any significant extent. This in turn would imply that when the adipose tissue in the new-born child is developing, newly formed cells are immediately filled up with lipid, leaving only a few lipid-free cells. Furthermore, these results imply that, at least in adults, the fat cell measurements and counts so far performed have not been invalidated significantly by errors introduced by non-measurable preadipocytes.

Normal range of adipose tissue cellularity

Definition of normality of body weight and of body fat is arbitrary. Therefore 'normal' limits are often selected from statistical borderlines in more or less well-defined reference populations. The same dilemma exists for adipose tissue cellularity. In our attempts to establish some sort of standard we have mainly utilized randomly selected groups from the city of Gothenburg (Björntorp *et al.*, 1971). An additional difficulty is that age plays a major role here also when only the adult ages are considered. Fat cell size increases over the years (Björntorp, 1974) but probably reaches a steady state, or might even decrease, at higher ages. Fat cell number, in contrast, is dependent on sex, women having more fat cells (Björntorp *et al.*, 1971; Sjöström *et al.*, 1972).

Regional variation of adipose cellularity

Variation in adipose tissue distribution is known to occur with exposure to certain endocrine factors found, for example, in Cushing's syndrome. There is also a typical android-gynoid distribution of fat (Vague,1947). In order to examine these questions more systematically Krotkiewski has administered estrogens, progesterone and dexamethasone to rats and compared the regional effects on adipose cellularity with those of insulin and starvation. Estrogens and progesterone seem to induce a fat cell size increase in the parametrial adipose tissue of female rats (Krotkiewski, 1976; Krotkiewski & Björntörp, 1976). This seems to be independent of the effects of these hormones on energy balance and insulin secretion because these latter effects seem dependent mainly on fat cell size (Krotkiewski & Björntorp, 1975; 1976). Insulin thus primarily promotes fat cell filling in regions with the smallest fat cells, and starvation emptying of fat cells in the regions with largest fat cells. This is in accordance with the known effects of insulin on triglyceride accumulation being more pronounced in smaller cells with remaining intact insulin sensitivity (Salans, Knittle & Hirsch, 1968). Furthermore, large fat cells have a more efficient lipid mobilizing system than small cells (Björntorp & Sjöström, 1972).

With dexamethasone the results are less clear showing no certain characteristics separate from the effects of starvation in rats (Krotkiewski & Björntorp, 1975). This might, however, be dose-dependent because in long-term exposure of humans to adrenal corticosteroids characteristic regional changes have been observed (Krotkiewski *et al.*, 1976).

In man some information is available on this question. The differences between men and women are most clearly seen in young subjects (Sjöström *et al.*, 1972; Krotkiewski *et al.*, 1975) and it seems possible that the fat cell size of the femoral-gluteal region is that characteristic for the sex difference and then possibly directly dependent on estrogen-progesterone effects. This assumption is also supported by the fact that when estrogens are administered to men with cancer of the prostate the fat cells of the gluteal region are those specifically increasing in weight (Krotkiewski & Björntorp, 1977) (Fig. 7).

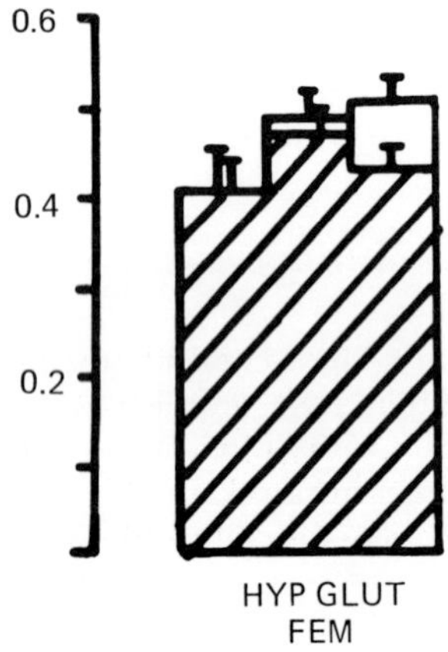

Fig. 7. Fat cell weights before and after estrogen. Effects on regional fat cell size in men treated with estrogens for carcinoma of the prostate. Abbreviations of regions: Hyp: hypogastrial. Fem: femoral. Glu: gluteal. Striped columns: before treatment. Open columns: after treatment. Change in gluteal region: $P<0.05$. (from Krotkiewski & Björntorp, 1977)

By analogy with the results in rats referred to above it seems probable that the fat cells of other regions than those specifically influenced by hormones with specific regional effects should be the primary target for the shifts in energy balance. Some evidence has been obtained along these lines since abdominal fat cell size seems to follow the changes in energy balance (Krotkiewski *et al.*, 1975). Visceral depots are of great interest here but have so far not been examined in man from this point of view.

The metabolic correlates of the described morphologic changes are only partially known. The effects of hormone administration on certain metabolic pathways have been examined in association with the morphologic examinations. These include influences on both the mechanism of lipid accumulation as well as on the lipolytic machinery (Krotkiewski, 1976). It is, however, not known which are the primary effects of the hormones on regulation of fat cell metabolism whether on hormone receptor level, enzyme level or even on the regulation of blood flow.

Obesity

Interest in the cellularity of adipose tissue in obesity is not new. Reh (1953) and Bjurulf (1959) suggested that both ways of storing increased amounts of fat, by an increase in fat cell number or in fat cell size, might be associated with different clinical characteristics of obesity. Studies on these important questions were not possible, however, before methods had been developed for examinations of adipose tissue on a large scale in free-living subjects. A first improvement here was the use of the needle-biopsy technique (Hirsch *et al.*, 1960) allowing non-traumatic examinations on a large scale. The other methodological improvements allowing determination of fat cell size and number in an adequate way have already been reviewed above.

An increase in both adipocyte size and number has now been described from different laboratories (Björntorp, 1974). The presence of subjects with more or less dominating increases of one or the other or both of these variables must now be considered to have been conclusively demonstrated. The remaining question is, however, whether or not the morphologically, descriptive forms of these conditions (hyperplastic and hypertrophic obesity) have associations with biological and clinical findings. This question will be scrutinized below.

Hyperplastic obesity

It has been claimed that hyperplastic obesity is a condition which debuts at a young age (Hirsch & Knittle, 1970; Björnstorp & Sjöström, 1971; Salans *et al.*, 1973; Sjöström & Björntorp, 1974). The first basis for these statements is the finding of hypercellular obesity in childhood, particularly in small children (Brook, Lloyd & Wolf, 1972). These works are, however, not yet conclusive because the development of fat cells has not been possible to follow (preadipocytes). The preliminary work described above seems to suggest that a bed of preadipocytes is not present even in small children. This would increase the validity of the statement of hyperplastic obesity being characteristic of early childhood obesity.

The second basis for these statements is the fact that several laboratories have found an association between juvenile onset of obesity in retrospective weight history and adipose hypercellularity (see above). The association, however, is often not very strong and therefore not very convincing. This might be due to one of several reasons. The first is simply a technical one. It is notoriously difficult to obtain an accurate retrospective weight history. It also seems possible that weights at certain stages of life, such as the first years or immediately before puberty, are the critical ones. The reason for the weakness of the correlation found might of course also be due to the fact that this is truly a very weak or even non-existent association.

The conclusive evidence needed here is a longitudinal study of adipose cellularity from childhood into adult life. Such information is not yet available. Objective weight records instead of weight histories would improve the present situation to some extent. An epidemiological study on the prevalence of obesity in relation to starvation of mothers and probable undernutrition of new-born children during the Second World War (Ravelli, Stein & Susser, 1976) is also in accordance with the concept of the importance of early nutrition for the development of adipose tissue and risk for obesity. The associations found by histories are weak but nevertheless present. These seem to be the arguments which favour the opinion of an early debut of hyperplastic obesity. The child obesity data support this view.

It should be clearly realized that there is a difference between whether or not hyperplastic obesity begins at a young age, or whether obesity beginning at a young age is hyperplastic in adult life. The latter alternative is supported by the evidence given above although as mentioned, longitudinal data are required to settle the question definitely. The possibility still exists that fat cells might disappear during the years, although this is less likely because it has as yet not been possible to demonstrate such a disappearance. The first alternative would require that all hyperplastic obesity began at a young age. This is based on the assumption that adipocyte number would be fixed by a certain age. Work on experimental animals with obesity has shown that fat cell multiplication goes on in certain obesities for an abnormally long period of time (Johnson & Hirsch, 1972) and this may well be similar to some types of human obesity. Furthermore, recent work on the multiplication of fat cell precursors has implied the remaining potential of fat cell multiplication under certain circumstances *in vitro* in rats where the spontaneous formation of new adipocytes has ceased (Björntorp *et al.*, 1977*b*). This might mean that *in vivo* multiplication is still possible.

Suggestions from clinical observations suggest that this might indeed occur. It is a frequent observation that severely obese women have a weight history with stepwise increases in body weight in relation to pregnancies. These women have an obesity which usually is found to be of the hyperplastic type. Two alternatives could explain this hyperplastic obesity; either these women have a number of non-filled adipocytes or an abnormally small average fat cell size, before pregnancy, or their adipocytes multiply during pregnancy. The latter alternative seems at least as probable as the former, particularly since abnormally small fat cells are usually not found in free-living subjects unless some disease or dieting interferes with normal regulation of energy balance (Björntorp *et al.*, 1971). Furthermore, preadipocytes have not been found in adult non-obese subjects.

Another aspect of hyperplastic obesity which is currently debated is whether or not treatment by conventional methods is less successful in this condition. It is a common experience that when obese subjects are placed on an ordinary low-energy diet they initially decrease in weight, then level off, and then often relapse back to their original body weight. In order to study this problem systematically about 100 obese women were treated in an ordinary out-patient program by a 1100 kcal diet and followed through the decrease - steady state - relapse cycle mentioned above (Krotkiewski *et al.*, 1977). It could then be shown that fat cell number was associated with a rapid initial decrease, a steady state level of body fat far from the normal range, and a short period on the steady state level before the relapse which occurred very quickly. This is schematically represented in Fig. 8, which also shows that

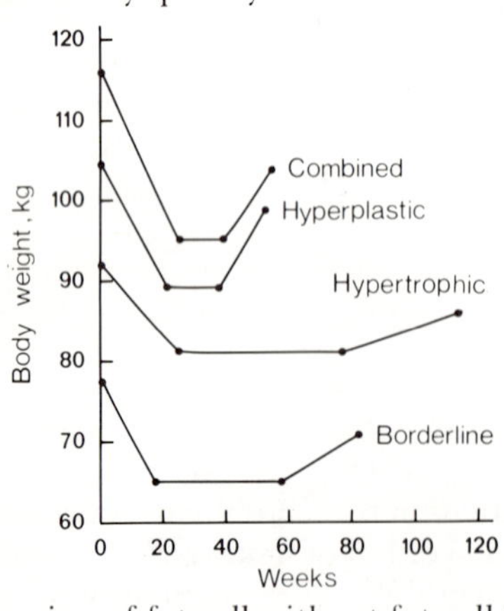

Fig. 8. Schematic summary of results of out-patient dietary treatment of obese women in relation to adipose tissue cellularity (from Krotkiewski *et al.*, 1977)

expansion of fat cell without fat cell hyperplasia was associated with a body fat close to normal on the steady state level, and with a much longer duration on this approximately normal body weight before relapse. These results would imply a poor prognosis for treatment of hyperplastic obesity in terms of ability to decrease to normal weight and to stay reduced for a significant period of time.

This examination describes the actual events in treatment of hyperplastic, hypertrophic and combined obesity. It might be argued that the hyperplastic obese subjects are much more obese than the hypertrophic obese subjects and, therefore, have a poorer treatment prognosis irrespective of adipocytes. When the adipose cellularity variables are examined one by one with multivariate statistical analysis the same findings remain. This is also essentially so when body fat is matched between groups, although by necessity this decreases the size of the groups (Krotkiewski *et al.*, 1977).

These data then strongly indicate that adipose cellularity is of importance for the prognosis of out-patient treatment of obesity by dietary means. How can this be explained? One simple possibility is that appetite regulation is primarily deranged in subjects with hyperplastic obesity, causing fat cell hyperplasia, obesity and difficulties with treatment. An alternative possibility is that fat cell expansion is in some way associated with this phenomenon. This seems to be a more attractive hypothesis because of the rather tight associations between treatment, prognosis and fat cell variables. Dietary treatment seems to be feasible down to a certain defined fat cell size (Björntorp *et al.*, 1975). Other observations support the concept of an association between energy balance and fat cell size. The suggestion by Kennedy (1953) of a lipostat is probably associated with fat cell size in adipose tissue because adipectomy leaving a deficit in body fat with intact fat cell size does not lead to compensatory positive energy balance (Faust, Johnson & Hirsch, 1976; Kral, 1976). This is also the case with a corresponding deficit due to a decrease in fat cell size, leaving number of fat cells intact, such as in starvation or exercise (Kral *et al.*, 1974). This would imply that the decrease in body fat in obese subjects treated with diet becomes more and more difficult the smaller the fat cells. In other words, hyperplastic obesity would have difficulties working against a system which would tend to keep the degree of filling of adipocytes within a certain range.

Analogous difficulties with treatment of hyperplastic obesity have been found with physical exercise where such patients decrease abnormally slowly or not at all (Björntorp *et al.*, 1973) even after prolonged periods of training. Subjects with moderate hypertrophic obesity or non-obese subjects decrease in body fat to a low steady-state level which also seems to be dependent on the fat cell size (Björntorp *et al.*, 1972). This again suggests a role of adipocyte filling in regulation of energy balance particularly since an association between exercise and appetite regulation has been claimed (Mayer *et al.*, 1954). Furthermore, from a practical point of view this again shows the difficulties of treating hyperplastic obesity.

From the therapeutic point of view this shows that severe hyperplastic obesity is a difficult problem. No doubt therapeutic ambitions here have to be restricted. These subjects also have a tendency to a high spontaneous weight increase (Krotkiewski *et al.*, 1977) and a realistic goal would be to prevent this progression.

Hypertrophic obesity

The associations between adipocyte hypertrophy and clinical observations are a more complex question. The descriptive term hypertrophic obesity is characterized by a more moderate increase of body fat mass than hyperplastic obesity. In general terms this form of obesity has been found to be associated with abnormalities in carbohydrate and lipid metabolism (Björntorp, 1974). This problem is, however, complicated and needs some further clarification and comment.

Fat cell size has been found to be positively correlated with plasma insulin in both non-obese and obese groups (Björntorp, Berchtold & Tibblin, 1971; Stern *et al.*, 1972*a, b;* Bjorntorp & Sjostrom, 1972; Brook & Lloyd, 1973). Although less strongly correlated with body fat and fat cell number the association between fat cell size and plasma insulin is not a very firm one with *r*-values about 0.5. Furthermore, it is easily disturbed by diet, physical training and diabetes mellitus (Bjorntorp, 1974). When analysed with fat cell number and body fat kept constant the association is no longer found (Larsson, 1977). Furthermore, in randomly selected moderately obese subjects with the same body fat, enlargement of fat cells is not associated with elevated insulin (B. Larsson, personal communication). The well-known association between obesity and plasma insulin (Karam, Grodsky & Forsham, 1963) thus seems to be best correlated to fat cell size but remains a weak association. It, therefore, seems most likely that other factors are also involved. In an obese population the subjects with the highest insulin levels were those who had gained recently (Sjöström & Björntorp, 1974). The previously mentioned findings that diet, exercise and diabetes disturb the association imply also that other factors than fat cell size are involved. These factors may well be associated with current nutritional status.

Fat cell size has also been found to be associated with plasma triglyceride levels. Endogenous hypertriglyceridemia seems to be associated with enlargement of fat cells (Björntorp, Gustafson & Persson 1971; Stern, Olefsky, Farquhar & Reaven, 1973). This association seems somewhat stronger than that of fat cell size and plasma insulin, and persists when body fat is kept constant both in populations selected at random (B. Larsson, personal communication) and in endogenous hypertriglyceridemia (Stern *et al.*, 1973). Findings of abnormalities in adipocyte metabolism in this condition makes this somewhat stronger association more plausible. Abnormalities in adipocytes metabolism include an increased insensitivity to inhibition of lipolysis by insulin (Larsson *et al.*, 1975) and decreased activity of lipoprotein lipase activity (Persson, Björntorp & Hood, 1966; Larsson *et al.*, 1975), both potentially contributing to hypertriglyceridemia by furnishing the liver with increased free fatty acid substrate for lipoprotein triglyceride formation, and by impairing triglyceride removal by interference with lipoprotein lipase.

It has been claimed that hyperplastic obesity is associated with a juvenile onset, as discussed above. By analogy it has been claimed that hypertrophic obesity is characterized by a late onset. In a way this would follow from the hyperplastic obesity - juvenile onset association leaving the remaining subjects, those with fat cell enlargement, to have begun in later in life. Experimentally this hypothesis finds support in the fact that spontaneous fat cell multiplication has not been found under normal circumstances in adult animals or man, although exceptions could occur.

Direct experimental evidence is presented by Salans, Horton & Sims (1971) who found an increase in fat cell size only in adult young men volunteering to overeat, causing a rather pronounced obesity. These were, however, short-term experiments with an obesity of much shorter duration than that usually seen in the clinic.

A longer term 'experiment' of a similar nature is the known westernization of the food-habits and exercise-habits of certain previously isolated populations, often leading to over-nutrition and obesity, associated with a high prevalence of diabetes mellitus. In the Pacific Islands this occurred after World War II. The time the overnutrition began can be determined with reasonable accuracy (Zimmet *et al.*, 1977). Examinations of such a population exposed to overnutrition at adult age has shown that at approximately the same degree of obesity as in the Vermont study with short-term overfeeding the fat cell size increase was of a similar magnitude (Fig. 9) although in this population the non-obese fat cell size is much smaller than in European or North American populations (Zimmet & Björntorp, 1977). This observation of a population with overnutrition at the adult age for a period of about ten years

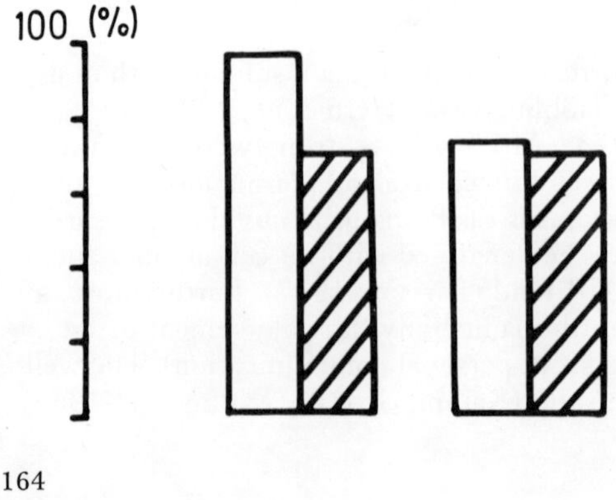

Fig. 9. Body fat (left) and fat cell weight (right) increases in relation to control values in experimental obesity (Vermont) and in an urbanized population from a Pacific island (Zimmet & Björntorp, 1977). Open columns, Pacific; striped, Vermont

implies that fat cell multiplication has not occurred in this population. This then also supports the concept of an adult onset for hypertrophic obesity.

By analogy with hyperplastic obesity it has to be remembered that the observation that hypertrophic obesity is produced by overfeeding at adult ages does not mean that all obesities produced this way become hypertrophic. The observations on the potential for multiplication of fat cell precursors in the adult rat mentioned above, as well as the clinical observations in obesity after pregnancies, are examples of possible hyperplastic obesity beginning in adult life.

Adult onset diabetes mellitus is another condition where the associated obesity seems to be of a hypertrophic type (Björntorp, Jonsson & Berchtold, 1972; Leonhardt *et al.*, 1972). The hyperinsulinemia associated with hypertrophic obesity under certain defined conditions might form the basis for the precipitation of diabetes mellitus by an overload on the insulin producing beta cells. The very high prevalence of diabetes in the urbanized Pacific populations (Zimmet *et al.*, 1977) where hypertrophic obesity is also very prevalent seems to support this possibility, but here other factors probably are of importance as well.

In this connection it might be pertinent to observe that juvenile onset diabetes mellitus is frequently associated with a decrease of fat cell size, probably dependent on the relative insulin deficiency in some of these cases in spite of exogenous adminstration of insulin (Langer *et al.*, 1975). In juvenile as well as poorly controlled adult onset diabetes mellitus metabolic derangements have been found which promote diminution of the adipocyte triglyceride depot. These include increased lipolysis (Östman, 1965; Björntorp, 1967) as well as a decreased fatty acid reesterification (Galton & Wilson, 1970). It has been suggested that fat cell size might be useful as a long-term metabolic variable to follow the metabolic control in diabetes mellitus where blood glucose and urinary glucose output are indicators of short-term control (Langer *et al.*, 1975).

Recent observations have shown that non-selected patients with essential hypertension in an early phase without pronounced secondary complications often have a moderate obesity, a decreased glucose tolerance and high plasma insulin and triglyceride levels (Berglund *et al.*, 1976). Their obesity is characterized by an increased fat cell size (Ljungman *et al.*, 1977; Fig. 10) and is, therefore, by definition a type of hypertrophic obesity. The overlapping metabolic features of endogenous hypertriglyceridemia, adult onset diabetes mellitus and essential hypertension, all characterized by the same type of obesity, give interesting possibilities both for pathogenetic and therapeutic research.

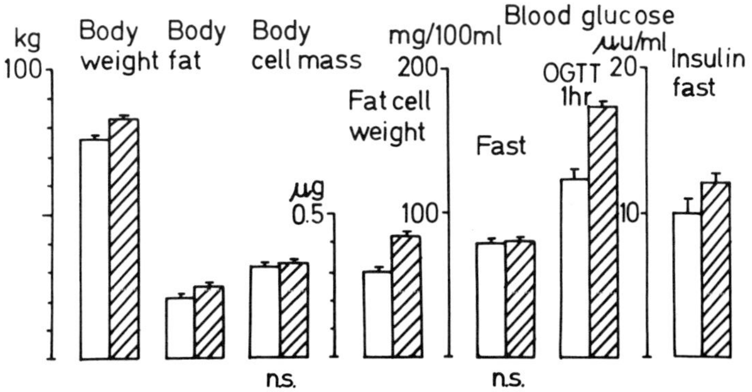

Fig. 10. Body composition and metabolism in non-selected, early essential hypertension in comparison with non-selected controls. OGTT: peroral, 100 g glucose tolerance test. Open columns, controls; striped, hypertensives (from Berglund *et al.*, 1976 and Ljungman *et al.*, 1977)

Summary
The possibility of determining adipose cellularity in human obesity is dependent on fat cell size determinations, where the currently available methodology is adequate for measuring lipid-filled cells. Determination of fat cell number is more difficult methodologically, and requires an adequate determination of body fat and average fat cell size. The former can probably also be determined with reasonable accuracy. An average fat cell size can also be determined in a meaningful way in groups of subjects where the variation between regions of adipose tissue is limited. In individuals, however, the variation is sometimes large and here determinations in several regions are necessary to hold the methodological error within a level of about 20 per cent.

A major problem for this field has been the potential presence of preadipocytes. Methods have now been developed which allow quantification of these cells.

From the epididymal fat pads of small rats, cells other than mature adipocytes which take up labelled chylomicratriglyceride label *in vivo* have been purified and cultured in a substrate rich medium. Here multiplication and formation of cells forming adipocytes is occurring. These cells are formed in young but not spontaneously in old rats, where such formation can only be induced *in vitro*. Quantification of preadipocytes can be performed in culture media where fat cell multiplication is prevented by a high viscosity. A large number of preadipocytes are present in adipose tissue from small rats. Preadipocytes are present at least in adipose tissue from children but only to a minor extent. These results indicate that the presently available results of fat cell counting and measuring in man are not invalidated by the presence of preadipocytes.

Hyperplastic obesity is thought to begin at an early age. The evidence is suggestive and consists of the fact that obesity in children is often hypercellular, and that obesity is usually of early onset. Another feature is the poor prognosis of conventional treatment with diet and exercise. It seems possible that this is associated with a regulatory mechanism of energy balance associated with fat cell expansion, a hypothesis supported by experimental evidence.

Hypertrophic obesity has been claimed to be associated with metabolic disturbances. Hyperinsulinemia is more strongly associated with fat cell size than with number or with total body fat, but the correlation is not very strong and is easily disturbed. Other factors such as the dietary status probably also play a role here. The association with plasma triglycerides seems tighter both in randomly selected subjects and in endogenous hypertriglyceridemia. This might be due to the fact that direct contributory factors in the metabolism of adipose tissue can be found in endogenous hypertriglyceridemia in the form of an increased, non-inhibited outflow of fatty acids with a potential to form liver triglycerides, and a decreased efficiency of lipoprotein lipase.

Hypertrophic obesity is found after acute experiments with overeating. In populations where adult onset obesity has been present for much longer time there is also evidence for fat cell hypertrophy only. This indicates that obesity starting at adult age often is hypertrophic but does not exclude that hyperplastic obesity can also develop in adult life.

Essential hypertension is often associated with hypertrophic obesity, decreased glucose tolerance and elevated plasma insulin and triglycerides. The overlapping features of hypertrophic obesity, endogenous hypertriglyceridemia, adult onset diabetes mellitus and essential hypertension give interesting possibilities for the research of the pathogenesis and therapy of these conditions.

References

Ashwell, M. & Garrow, J.S. (1973): *Lancet* 2, 1036.
Berg, K. & Isaksson, B. (1970): *Acta Paediat. Scand.* Suppl 204.
Berglund, G., Larsson, B., Andersson, O., Svärdsudd, K., Björntorp, P. & Wilhelmsen, L. (1976): *Acta Med. Scand.* 200, 163.
Bjurulf, P. (1959): *Acta Med. Scand.*, Suppl 166.

Björntorp, P. (1967): *Acta Med. Scand.* **181**, 389.
Björntorp, P., Berchtold, P. & Tibblin, G. (1971): *Diabetes* **20**, 65.
Björntorp, P., Bengtsson, C., Blohmé, G., Jonsson, A., Sjöström, L., Tibblin, E., Tibblin, G. & Wilhelmsen, L. (1971): *Metabolism* **20**, 927.
Bjorntorp, P., Gustafson, A. & Persson, B. (1971): *Acta Med. Scand.* **190**, 363.
Bjorntorp, P. & Sjöström, L. (1971): *Metabolism* **20**, 703.
Björntorp, P. & Sjöström, L. (1972): *Europ. J. Clin. Invest.* **2**, 78.
Björntorp, P., Jonsson, A. & Berchtold, P. (1972): *Acta Med. Scand.* **191**, 129.
Björntorp, P., Grimby, G., Sanne, H., Sjöström, L., Tibblin, G. & Wilhelmsen, L. (1972): *Horm. Metab. Res.* **4**, 182.
Björntorp, P., de Jounge, K., Krotkiewski, M., Sullivan, L., Sjöström, L. & Stenberg, J. (1973): *Metabolism* **22**, 1467.
Björntorp, P. (1974): *Metabolism* **23**, 1091.
Björntorp, P., Carlgren, G., Isaksson, B., Krotkiewski, M., Larsson, B. & Sjöström, L. (1975): *Am. J. Clin. Nutr.* **28**, 445.
Björntorp, P., Karlsson, M., Pertoft, H., Pettersson, P., Sjöström, L. & Smith, U. (1977*a*): Submitted for publication.
Björntorp, P., Karlsson, M., Gustafsson, L., Smith, U., Sjöström, L., Cigolini, M., Storck, G. & Pettersson, P. (1977*b*): In prep.
Brook, C.G.D., Lloyd, J.K. & Wolf, O.H. (1972): *Br. Med. J.* **2**, 25.
Brook, C.G.D. & Lloyd, J.K. (1973): *Arch. Dis. Childh.* **48**, 301.
Faust, I.M., Johnsson, P.R. & Hirsch, J. (1976): *Am. J. Physiol.* **231**, 538.
Forbes, G.B., Gallup, J. & Hursch, J.B. (1961): *Science* **133**, 101.
Galton, D.J. & Wilson, J.P.D. (1970): In *Adipose tissue: regulation and metabolic functions*, ed B. Jeanrenaud & D. Hepp. London: Academic Press.
Goldrick, R.B. (1967): *Am. J. Physiol.* **212**, 777.
Goldrick, R.B. & McLoughlin, G.M. (1970): *J. Clin. Invest.* **49**, 1213.
Green, H. & Meuth, M. (1974): *Cell* **3**, 127.
Greenwood, M.R.C. & Hirsch, J. (1974): *J. Lipid Res.* **15**, 474.
Hammar, J.A. (1895): *Arch. Mikrosk. Anat.* **45**, 512.
Hirsch, J., Farquhar, J., Ahrens, E.H. Jr, Peterson, M. & Stoffel, W. (1960): *Am. J. Clin. Nutr.* **8**, 499.
Hirsch, J. & Gallian, E. (1968): *J. Lipid Res.* **9**, 110.
Hirsch, J. & Han, P.W. (1969): *J. Lipid Res.* **10**, 77.
Hirsch, J. & Knittle, J.L. (1970): *Fed. Proc.* **29**, 1516.
Hollenberg, C.H., & Vost, A. (1968): *J. Clin. Invest.* **47**, 2485.
Johnson, P.R. & Hirsch, J. (1972): *J. Lipid Res.* **13**, 2.
Karam, J.H., Grodsky, G.M. & Forsham, P.H. (1963): *Diabetes* **12**, 197.
Kennedy, G.C. (1953): *Proc. Royal Soc.* **140**, 572.
Kral, J.G., Jacobsson, B., Smith, U. & Björntorp, P. (1974): *Acta Physiol. Scand.* **90**, 664.
Kral, J. (1976): *Am. J. Physiol.* **231**, 1090.
Krotkiewski, M. & Björntorp, P. (1975): *Acta Endocrin.* (Kbh) **80**, 667.
Krotkiewski, M., Sjöström, L., Björntorp, P. & Smith, U. (1975): *Metabolism* **24**, 703.
Krotkiewski, M. (1976): Thesis. Gotab, Kungälv, Sweden.
Krotkiewski, M. (1976): *Acta Physiol. Scand.* **96**, 128.
Krotkiewski, M. & Björntorp, P. (1976): *Acta Physiol. Scand.* **96**, 122.
Krotkiewski, M., Blohmé, B., Lindholm, B. & Björntorp, P. (1976): *J. Clin. Endocr. Metab.* **42**, 91.
Krotkiewski, M. & Björntorp, P. (1977): In prep.
Krotkiewski, M., Sjöström, L., Björntorp, P., Carlgren, G., & Smith, U. (1977): *Int. J. Obesity* **1**, 395.
Langer, L., Lindholm, B., Örndahl, G. & Björntorp, P. (1975): *Diabetologia* **11**, 101.
Larsson, B., Björntorp, P., Holm, J., Scherstén, T., Sjöström, L. & Smith, U. (1975): *Metabolism* **24**, 1375.
Larsson, B. (1977): Thesis. To be published.
Leonhardt, W., Hanefeld, M., Schneider, H. & Haller, H. (1972): *Diabetologia* **8**, 287.
Lesser, G.T., Deutsch, S. & Markofsky, J. (1971): *Metabolism* **26**, 792.
Ljungman, S., Hartford, M., Berglund, G. & Björntorp, P. (1977): To be published.
Mayer, J., Marshall, N.B., Vitale, J.J. Christensen, J.H., Mashayekhi, M.B. & Stare, F.J. (1954): *Am. J. Physiol.* **177**, 544.
Moore, F.D., Olesen, K.H., McMurray, J.D., Parker, H.V., Ball, M.R. & Boyden, C.M. (1963): *The body cell mass and its supporting environment*. Philadelphia: Saunders.
Napolitano, L. (1963): *J. Cell Biol.* **18**, 663.
Östman, J. (1965): *Acta Med. Scand.* **177**, 639.
Persson, B., Björntorp, P. & Hood, B. (1966): *Metabolism* **15**, 730.
Ravelli, G-P., Stein, Z.A. & Susser, M.W. (1976): *New Engl. J. Med.* **295**, 349.

Reh, M. (1953): *Virchows Arch. (Pathol. Anat.)* 324, 234.
Salans, L-S., Knittle, J.L. & Hirsch, J. (1968): *J. Clin. Invest.* 47, 153.
Salans, L-S., Horton, E.S. & Sims, E.A.H. (1971): *J. Clin. Invest.* 50, 1005.
Salans, L.B., Cushman, S.W. & Weismann, R.E. (1973): *J. Clin. Invest.* 52, 929.
Sjöström, L., Björntorp, P. & Vrana, J. (1971): *J. Lipid Res.* 12, 521.
Sjöström, L. (1972): *Acta Med. Scand., Suppl.* 544, 17.
Sjöström, L., Smith, U., Krotkiewski, M. & Björntorp, P. (1972): *Metabolism* 21, 1143.
Sjöström, L. & Björntorp, P. (1974): *Acta Med. Scand.* 195, 201.
Smith, U., Sjostrom, L. & Bjorntorp, P. (1972): *J. Lipid Res.* 13, 822.
Stern, J., Batchelor, B.R., Hollander, N., Cohn, C.K. & Hirsch, J. (1972*a*): *Lancet* 2, 948.
Stern, M., Olefsky, J., Farquhar, J. & Reaven, G. (1972*b*): *Clin. Res.* 20, 557.
Stern, M., Olefsky, J., Farquhar, J. & Reaven, G. (1973): *Metabolism* 22, 1311.
Vague, J. (1947): *Presse Med.* 55, 339.
Widdowson, E.M. & Shaw, W.T. (1973): *Lancet* 2, 905.
Wilmore, J.H. & Behnke, A.R. (1969): *J. Appl. Physiol.* 27, 25.
Zimmet, P. & Björntorp, P. (1977): In Prep.
Zimmet, P., Taft, P., Guinea, A., Guthrie, W. & Thoma, K. (1977): *Diabetologia* 13, 111.

17
Adipose tissue growth and the development of fat cells

M.R.C. GREENWOOD, R. GRUEN and M.P. CLEARY
The Institute of Human Nutrition and Department of Human Genetics and Development, Columbia University New York City, NY 10032, USA.

Summary
Adipose tissue, like other mammalian organs, displays a characteristic pattern of cellular growth. In normal lean rodents, the hyperplastic period occurs early in development and ultimate adult cellularity can be influenced by both overnutrition and undernutrition during this period. During this early hyperplastic stage enzymes characteristic of proliferation, thymidine kinase and DNA polymerase, are at highest levels early and reach adult levels by the fourth to fifth postnatal week. The onset of differentiation, ie lipid-filling, begins around the third to fourth postnatal week and is characterized by the onset of reciprocal regulation of lipogenic and lipolytic control. In obese rats, the hyperplastic period apparently extends well into adulthood and is not easily restrained by early undernutrition. Alterations in the rate of differentiation may also be present. In advancing our knowledge of the development of the fat cell the techniques of lipectomy and cell culture seem particularly appropriate and promising.

Introduction
If one looks at the plethora of animal models of obesity, it becomes obvious that obesity is not a unitary disorder, but occurs under many diverse conditions. For example, among the naturally occurring obesities in animals there are those thought to be the result of a single dominant gene, a single recessive gene or due to polygenic inbred, or hybrid combinations (Bray & York, 1971). These vary in the degree of obesity, the time of onset of obesity and the type of symptomology. In humans, at least two types of obesity can be identified on the basis of adipose depot morphology: (1) juvenile-onset, characterized by extreme hyperplasia as well as hypertrophy, and (2) adult-onset, characterized primarily by a hypertrophic enlargement (Hirsch & Knittle, 1970). In rats and mice, which are often utilized as animal models for the study of obesity, the depot morphology can be characterized as hypertrophic, hyperplastic or some mixture of the two (Johnson *et al.*, 1971; Johnson & Hirsch, 1972).

Accompanying these morphological distinctions are numerous metabolic correlates. For example, obese humans, rats and mice may by hyperglycemic, hyperinsulinemic, hypertensive, hypercholesterolemic, hypertriglyceridemic (Bray & York, 1972; Zucker & Zucker, 1961; Björntorp, 1972) or any combination of these. In the case of the obese (*ob/ob*) mouse, one of the major animal models utilized in the study of obesity, it has been proposed that the primary genetic lesion occurs in the pancreas (Strautz, 1970). In the case of the yellow ($A^{y}a$) mouse and the NH mouse the primary lesion is thought to result from hypersecretion of corticoids (Hausberger, 1959). Periodically, hibernating animals use a new set of criteria to monitor food intake and become obese during the pre-hibernation period (Mrosovsky, 1974). Gonadectomized rats, mice and humans become obese, particularly if the gonads are removed or destroyed before puberty (Kakolewski, 1968). Many of the above examples strongly point to hypothalamic-hypophyseal involvement in body weight regulation, but the total impression conveyed is that the mechanisms involved are numerous and mediated by a complexly integrated network.

Whatever the behavioral correlates, the symptomology observed, or the experimental manipulation used, in any pathological disturbance of body weight regulation, it is the degree of caloric storage primarily in the adipose depot which changes. The adipose depot grows, shrinks or is maintained as an organism regulates its body weight. Adipose depot size changes as the size and/or number of adipocytes present in it changes.

There are at least two types of obesity that can be distinguished on the basis of their adipose depot morphology. Essentially, all obese rats, mice and humans have enlarged fat cells (hypertrophy) but some, in addition, have an increased number of fat cells (hyperplasia) (Hirsch & Han, 1969; Hirsch & Knittle, 1970; Johnson *et al.*, 1971; Johnson & Hirsch, 1972; Björntorp & Sjöström, 1971). This suggests that even more categories of obesity can be made on the basis of depot morphology.

In normal mature man, rats and mice, adipose depot cellularity is thought to be stable (Hirsch & Knittle, 1970; Johnson *et al.*, 1971; Johnson & Hirsch, 1972; Björntorp & Sjöström, 1971; Hellman, Taljedal & Westman, 1962). Juvenile-onset obesity, in human beings and some strains of rats and mice, shows hyperplasia of the adipose depot. Studies have shown that in mature obese humans, rats and mice, reduction by weight loss of the depot does not reduce the hypercellularity (Hirsch & Han, 1969). In the adult organism, it seeems established that once the number of cells is fixed, the only regulatory parameter of the caloric storage depot that can vary is the size of the adipocytes.

Adipose tissue development in rodents

The coincidence of early onset obesity and hyperplasia of the adipose tissue mass, in both man and animals, has suggested to many investigators that one possible regulatory error in the control of adipose depot size is a failure to fix the number of fat cells at the appropriate point in organogenesis. In the epididymal fat pad of the rat, a depot commonly used in these studies, we and others have shown that there is a continual rise in the quantity of DNA in this tissue, which persists at least until 12 weeks of age (Enesco & Le Blond, 1962) Fig. 1 & 2. Similar results are reported when the number of adipose cells is counted by the electronic method of Hirsch & Gallian (1968), or by visual estimation (Hellman *et al.*, 1962). In mice a similar phenomenon is noted except that cell number determined by electronic counting of osmium fixed cells stops increasing around 40 to 60 days of age (Johnson & Hirsch, 1972). During the postnatal period of growth, before puberty, normal lean rats and mice attain a maximum number of adipose cells. Further growth is normally the result of fat cell enlargement, and not cell proliferation.

Various manipulations, such as starvation, chronic malnutrition and hypothalamically-induced hyperphagia have no lasting effects on the number of fat cells in the adult (Knittle & Hirsch, 1968; Hirsch & Han, 1969). Malnutrition from 6 to 12 weeks post-partum seems to halt the increase in fat cells but, upon refeeding, the numbers return to normal levels. Only when the manipulations in nutritional status occur during the pre-weaning period is there a change in cell number which is maintained into adulthood. These studies have been interpreted as meaning that fat cell number is genetically determined in the normal epididymal fat depot; when it is attained, no further cell addition occurs and only fluctuations in the size of fat cells are possible. Further evidence for this hypothesis is found in the work of Rakow *et al.* (1970) who showed by histologic methods that adipocyte number did not change when postpubertal mice were made obese by goldthioglucose. Connective tissue cells increased, probably indicating an increased need for support and vascularization of the fat cells as fat content increased. Other reports (Rakow *et al.*, 1971*a*) have indicated that an increase in the tissue content of DNA accompanies the

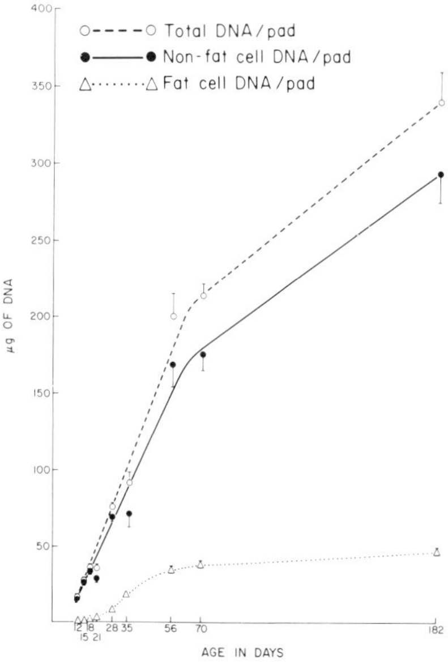

Fig. 1. Total DNA per pad, non-lipid filled tissue DNA per pad, and osmium-fixed fat cell DNA per pad in epididymal pads of Sprague-Dawley rats from 12 to 182 days of age. Data are indicated as $\bar{x} \pm$ s.e.m. (from *J. Nutr.* 1977) (Figs 1 & 2: Cleary *et al.*, 1977)

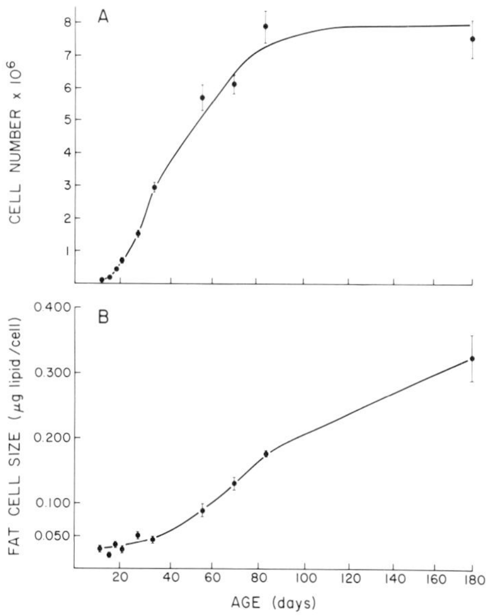

Fig. 2. A. Epididymal fat cell number of Sprague-Dawley rats from 12 to 182 days of age. Data are indicated as $\bar{x}$ + s.e.m.
B. Epididymal fat cell size of Sprague-Dawley rats from 12 to 182 days of age. Data are indicated as $\bar{x}$ + s.e.m. (from *J. Nutr.* 1977)

normal process of adipocyte hypertrophy associated with maturation. Rakow, Benecke & Vogt (1971*b*) also showed that chronic malnutrition and refeeding in the adult resulted in fluctuations in the number of connective tissue cells but not in the number of fat cells.

Although most nutritional manipulations in adult rodents have been demonstrated to affect primarily cell size, there have been some reports that feeding a high fat diet in some strains of rats will result in an increased number of fat cells in some adipose depots. For example, it has been reported (Lemmonier, 1972) that feeding adult lean Zucker rats a high fat diet from five months to one year results in an increase in adipocyte number limited to the retroperitoneal depot. Furthermore, in adult Osborne-Mendel male rats fed a high fat diet (70 per cent of calories), the adipocyte number increased from 14 to 23.5 million in the retroperitoneal depot while the fat cell number of the inguinal depot remained unchanged (Johnson *et al.*, 1976). Such experimental data suggest that some adipose depots either contain a reserve of preadipocytes which remain non lipid-filled unless stimulated or that some adipose depots may respond to dietary stimulation by renewed development of fat cells. In any case, the fact that only some species respond with increasing cellularity points out that a complex interaction of genetic endowment, environmental conditions and developmental stage is at work.

Radiothymidine incorporation into preadipocytes during normal development

One of the primary difficulties in interpreting many of the published reports on changes in adipose tissue cellularity is that there are no satisfactory methods for detecting presumptive fat cells which contain little or no lipid. In an effort to differentiate the early hyperplastic growth period of adipose tissue from lipid-filling of preexistent cells, we conducted a retrospective investigation of ^{3}H-thymidine incorporation into preadipocyte DNA. These experiments utilized the technique first suggested by Hollenberg & Vost (1968). Radiothymidine was injected into rats of various ages ranging from 9 days to 5 months. Appropriate 'chase' injections of unlabelled thymidine followed one hour later. The principle in these experiments is that any preadipocyte being synthesized at the time of thymidine injection will incorporate radiothymidine into DNA. Obviously, many other cells in adipose tissue during early development would also do so. However, only those 'destined' to become fat cells, the preadipocytes, will subsequently fill with lipid; and when they do, they can be separated and the specific activity of the fat cell fraction at later ages can be used as an index of preadipocyte proliferation on the day of radioisotope injection. At the time of sacrifice, isolated fat cells and stromalvascular cells, presumably including any preadipocyte fraction, were isolated. The specific activity of both fractions (dpm/μg DNA) was measured and recorded over time. The results of these experiments indicated that proliferation of adipocytes occurs until between 28 to 35 days postnatally in the epididymal pad of the rat with the majority of the proliferation taking place before the end of the suckling period (Fig. 3). The data further suggested that the proliferative process provided a 'bed of preadipocytes' which could take as long as 30 days to mature into the typical adipocyte.

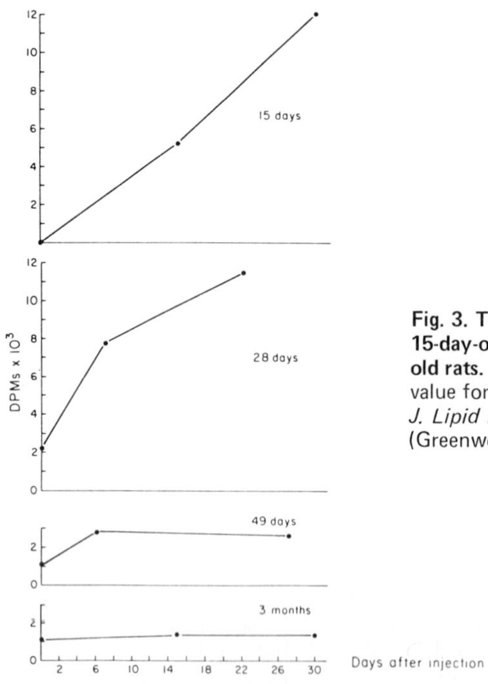

Fig. 3. Total dpms in adipocyte DNA for 15-day-old, 28-day-old, 49-day-old and 3-month-old rats. Each data point represents the mean value for the 2 pools sampled at each time (from *J. Lipid Res.,* 1974)
(Greenwood & Hirsch, 1974)

Adipose tissue cellularity in the development of genetic obesity

Obese rats of the Zucker strain (*fa/fa*) differ from the normal Sprague-Dawley rat in that adipocyte number, measured by electronic counting of osmium-fixed cells, as well as adipocyte size, continues to increase beyond the 14th week of the rat's life (Table 1). This pattern of apparent fat cell hyperplasia beyond the first few postnatal weeks is also evident in the *ob/ob* mouse (Johnson & Hirsch, 1972). We have shown that early undernutrition of Zucker fatty rats does not reduce fat cell number and that early overnutrition stimulates further increases in their already elevated cell numbers (Johnson *et al.*, 1973). This observation suggests that failure to regulate adipose cellular proliferation early in life can augment the predisposition to hyperplastic obesity. In both female and male Zucker fatty rats, fat cell number, determined by electronic counting of osmium-fixed fat cells, has been shown to increase in three depots until at least 26 weeks of age. Cleary *et al.* (1976) have shown that this apparent increase in fat cell number is preceded by increased

Table 1. **Total adipose tissue cellularity in lean and obese female Zucker rats** (from *Nutritional disorders of American women,* ed·M. Winick. New York: Wiley & Co., 1976)

Age (wk)	*n*	Lean Cell Number x 10^6	Lean Cell size μg lipid	*n*	Obese Cell Number x 10^6	Obese Cell size μg lipid
5	6	17.583 ±0.703	0.0461 ±0.0105	6	30.012 ±1.611	0.6013 ±0.0255
8	3	41.480 ±5.421	0.0668 ±0.0000	3	40.486 ±3.744	1.0241 ±0.0954
9	6	37.407 ±3.407	0.0799 ±0.0114	6	48.413 ±2.813	1.1595 ±0.0941
14	6	44.671 ±1.634	0.1141 ±0.0221	4	60.996 ±3.861	1.8888 ±0.1173
24	6	47.585 ±3.406	0.2558 ±0.0868	5	126.849 ±20.220	1.3555 ±0.0974
36	6	51.014 ±3.418	0.2852 ±0.0404	5	141.422 ±16.035	1.3834 ±0.1452
52	6	50.115 ±4.881	0.2110 +0.0230	2	174.457 ±3.456	1.3700 ±0.1416

enzymatic activity of adipose tissue, DNA polymerase and thymidine kinase. Thus, it seems clear that in some strains of rodents there is a genetic predisposition to adipose tissue hyperplasia, above and beyond what may be induced by early nutritional intervention.

The use of lipectomy as an investigative tool

It has occurred to some investigators that, if fat cell number is an important regulated feature of the adipose mass, as the lipostatic theory of Kennedy (1952) would suggest, and if fat cell number is relatively constant in the adult, then the removal of excess adipose cells by surgical means might result in the maintenance of weight loss in the reduced obese individual. In addition, it has occurred to several investigators that the use of lipectomy as an investigative tool might provide a means of teasing apart the respective roles of adipocyte size, adipocyte number and total lipid mass in the regulation of body weight. Thus, the surgical removal of fat has been accomplished in both human beings and other animals, and the effects on adipose tissue cellularity have been reported.

Although a number of investigators have reported on adipectomy in human beings, the rationale for these studies was essentially cosmetic and no data on body composition, fat cell number or size were reported. In one study reported by Kral (1975), however, cellularity data are presented on three female patients who underwent surgical removal of adipose tissue from three areas: the abdominal, lumbar and femoral areas. Prior to surgery, the three patients had sustained a mean weight loss of 42.3 kg resulting from a conventional weight loss regimen of diet and exercise. Prior to surgery, the three subjects were hyperplastic, having a mean cell number of 75 x 10^9 cells. Eight, 15 and 12 x 10^9 fat cells, respectively, were removed from the three patients, representing approximately 16 per cent of their total number of adipose cells. Loss of these fat cells did not prevent regain of the lost weight after the surgery, but there was apparently no recurrence of obesity at the scar sites. These limited findings imply that cell number is not as crucial for the regulation of energy balance as cell size or total adipose mass may be. This interpretation is greatly strengthened by recent data reported by Faust, Johnson & Hirsch (1976) and by Kral (1976) on the results of lipectomy in normal rats and mice. Kral lipectomized normal adult Sprague-Dawley rats, removing approximately 24 per cent of their total body fat from the inguinal and epididymal adipose depots. After 12 weeks there was no evidence of compensatory regrowth at the site of removal, nor of compensatory hypertrophy in the remaining adipose depots.

In another study, Faust, Johnson & Hirsch (1977) observed that if Sprague-Dawley rats are lipectomized at weaning and followed for up to seven months, total regenerative regrowth of the inguinal fat depot occurs. Both cell size and cell number of the dissectable subcutaneous fatty sheath are found to be equivalent in lipectomized animals and their sham-operated controls. The difference between these results and those of Kral (1976) may be explained by the timing of the lipectomy. Kral's animals were lipectomized at 15 weeks of age, which is well beyond the critical period for adipocyte proliferation, while the animals of Faust, Johnson & Hirsch (1976) were lipectomized at three weeks of age, which is still within the critical period for proliferative activity. It may thus be concluded that the surgical removal of fat cells during the critical period provides a sufficient stimulus for the production of precursor cells which are capable of proliferating in numbers sufficient to restore normal cell numbers in the inguinal site. It is obvious that the factors which regulate adipose tissue growth are complex; they are at least age, site and species specific.

Adipose tissue development in humans

Very little data exist on the development of adipose tissue in humans. However, Knittle has reported that in normally growing, non-obese children fat cell number seems to increase from birth to 2 years of age, to be stable until the prepubertal growth spurt, and to increase again between 10 and 16 years of age. Apparently, no further increase in fat cell numbers normally occurs after this pubertal growth period. Fat cell size increases between 2 and 12 years of age and in the postadolescent, changes in fat cell size are the major morphologic change occurring with weight loss or gain. In obese children, fat cell number is increased at all ages studied and some obese children at 2 to 3 years of age have a fat cell number in the range of normal weight adults (Knittle, 1972). These changes in number of fat cells have been confirmed independently by Brook, Lloyd & Wolf (1972). It is not uncommon for obese teenagers, who have a history of obesity from infancy, to have several times the number of fat cells detected in normal weight adults. In nearly all cases of childhood obesity fat cell size is also enlarged (Brook, 1972; Knittle, 1972). The concept that onset of obesity in early childhood is characterized by an inability to control adipocyte proliferation has been further strengthened by the work of Adebonojo, who has reported that cells cultured from adipose tissue of young obese children grow in culture and divide, while those from normal weight children and adults show much less proliferative activity (Adebonojo, 1975*a*.

Identification of the preadipocyte

All of the current methods employed to measure adipose tissue morphology depend upon the cell containing an amount of lipid sufficient to give the cell its characteristic unilocular lipid inclusion. Therefore, the interpretation of most studies has been clouded by the possibility that large numbers of preadipocytes (non-lipid-filled, but predetermined, adipocytes) could exist and remain undetected. In fact, one of the most cogent considerations in attempting to interpret the experimental data on adipose tissue cellularity has been that there are currently no methods available for identifying the preadipocyte and differentiating it from other cells in the non-fat cell compartment. This compartment is composed of the capillary bed, connective supportive cells, leukocytes, etc., as well as preadipocytes. The amount of non-fat cell DNA varies with age and presumably so do the number of preadipocytes. In the adult, greater than 75 per cent of the adipose tissue DNA is contained in the non-fat cell fraction of the tissue (Cleary, Brasel & Greenwood, 1977).

Functional correlates

Investigations of adipose tissue development have been hindered by the lack of functional markers for the preadipocytes. Unlike hematopoietic, muscle or pancreatic beta cells, for which functional correlates can be measured before the cells assume their characteristic morphology, there is, to date, no enzymatic marker for preadipocytes. To date, the clearest demonstrations of a functional marker for the preadipocyte have come from the work of Mohr & Beneke (1969) and Pilgrim (1971). Mohr & Beneke demonstrated the presence of an alpha-napthylacetate esterase in fibrocytic cells which do not yet have lipid accumulations. Since similar appearing cells were also glycogen positive, they suggested that these cells were precursor cells that later became osmophilic and still later assumed the appearance of mature adipocytes. The accumulation of glycogen has been shown by Wertheimer & Shapiro (1948) to precede fat deposition in starved and refed rats and may occur during the normal development and lipid-filling of adipose tissue as well. Pilgrim used these reactions to study the prenatal development of subcutaneous adipose tissue and the early postnatal development of the epididymal fat pad of the rat and found that the proliferative index, measured by radiothymidine autoradiography, was highest in esterase and glycogen positive cells, lacking lipid vacoules. He suggested that such cells were preadipocytes. Therefore, although extraordinarily difficult to visualise, it seems likely that the preadipocyte is indeed present in early postnatal development and is difficult to demonstrate in the adult.

The use of cell culture in defining the preadipocyte

The technique of cell culture has proved to be useful in beginning to establish both biochemical and morphological criteria for the preadipocyte. Dixon-Shanies & Knittle (1976) and Adebonojo (1975*b*) have isolated fat cells from adults, infants and rodents and cultured these mature lipid-filled cells. They have been able to show that the cells accumulate lipid in culture, and display enzyme activities consistent with adipose tissue cellular metabolism. More recently, two other types of cell culture systems have been used. Green & Meuth (1974) have shown that clones of 3T3 cells, derived from mouse embryo fibroblasts, can differentiate into fat-filled cells and display morphology characteristic of mature fat cells. Furthermore, this differentiation is enhanced by various substrates (Green & Kehinde, 1975), and hormones (Russel & Ho, 1976). Poznanski, Waheed & Van (1973) reported that cells derived from the human adipose tissue stromalvascular compartments grew in culture and apparently showed multilocular lipid droplets. Van, Bayliss & Roncari (1976) using a similar approach have demonstrated that stromalvascular cells grown in culture, both from humans (Van *et al.*, 1976) and rodents (Van & Roncari, 1977) accumulate lipid and display elevated levels of lipogenic enzymes compared to skin fibroblasts. Our understanding of the cellular differentiation of preadipocytes should be markedly advanced by continued investigation of cells in culture.

Enzymatic correlates of early growth in adipose tissue: studies of fat cell proliferation: proliferative enzymes

Figure 4 illustrates the data obtained for DNA polymerase activity in normally developing epididymal adipose tissue (panel *a*), and compares it to the pattern of thymidine kinase activity (panel *b*) and to the initial specific activity (radiothymidine incorporation in DNA – panel *c*) of the isolated stromalvascular cellular compartment (Greenwood & Hirsch, 1974). It is clear that both DNA polymerase and thymidine kinase display a similar pattern of activity during early tissue development. Enzyme activity in both cases is greatest during early postnatal development, and reaches adult or near adult levels shortly after weaning. Therefore, both of these enzyme activities correlate well with the radiothymidine incorporation data and with each other. In addition, both thymidine kinase and DNA polymerase seem to reflect changes in the rate of preadipocyte proliferation during early postnatal growth. However, since thymidine kinase activity can be measured in very small amounts of adipose tissue (10 to 20 mg), it may be a more useful measurement of proliferative activity, especially when dealing with young animals or needle biopsy samples from humans.

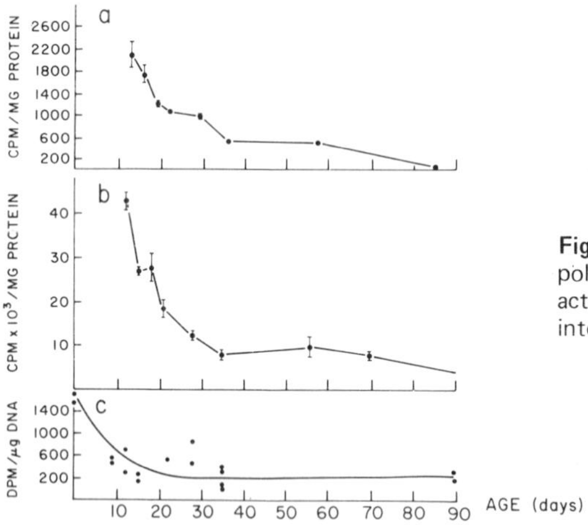

Fig. 4. Normal development. Panel a. DNA polymerase activity; Panel b. Thymidine kinase activity; Panel c. ^{3}H-thymidine incorporation into adipose tissue stromalvascular cells

Proliferative enzymes in the adipose tissue of genetically obese Zucker rats

The Zucker fatty rat was first shown to be hyperplastic by Johnson *et al.* (1971). Johnson *et al.* suggested that hyperplastic obesity in the Zucker fatty rat might derive from a distinctly different pattern of cellular development in adipose tissue. We have shown that the lean Zucker rat, like the normal Sprague-Dawley rat, displays adult levels of thymidine kinase activity around 35 to 38 days of age. In contrast, the enzyme activity in fatty rats is elevated significantly compared to lean littermates at all ages, studied until at least 273 days of age (39 weeks) when enzyme activity in the fatty rat finally reaches the normal lean control adult values (Cleary *et al.*, 1976). The data also show that a 25 to 27-day-old Zucker fatty rat has a thymidine kinase activity similar to that seen in the normal 21-day-old rat. This suggests that the Zucker fatty rat is displaying, not only an extended period of cellular proliferation as originally hypothesized by Johnson *et al.* (1971), but also is showing an increased rate of cell division during the period of hyperplastic adipose tissue growth. In addition to elevated enzymatic activity until at least 182 days of age, an increase over previous levels was noted at 98 days (14 weeks).

Since the DNA polymerase assay requires so much more tissue for determination and provides no better 'monitor' for cellular proliferation than does thymidine kinase, it was not considered feasible to pursue a complete developmental curve in the fatty rat. However, one set of experiments, using 5-week-old and 15-week-old lean and fatty rats, indicated as expected that DNA polymerase in the tissue of the obese rat was elevated compared to the lean rat at 15 weeks of age.

Studies of enzymes associated with adipocyte differentiation: lipoprotein lipase

Although early postnatal regulation of the enzymes associated with cellular proliferation is likely to play a decisive role in determining the size of the ultimate adult adipose tissue mass (Cleary *et al.*, 1976), it seems equally credible that regulation of the rate of lipid-filling during development may also contribute to the pattern of expansion of adipose depots. If a preadipocyte does exist, it may differ from the mature adipocyte with respect to its complement of active lipogenic enzymes, and the process of differentiation of preadipocyte into adipocyte could be marked by the induction and/or activation of those enzymes which are necessary for lipid-filling to occur at appreciable rates. Since little is known about the development of lipogenic enzymes in adipose tissue during normal development, we have conducted a series of experiments to characterize the developmental pattern of lipoprotein lipase (LPL). LPL is the major enzyme catalyzing the breakdown of plasma triglycerides to provide free fatty acids (FFA) for fat cell triglyceride synthesis and storage.

A slight modification of the radioisotopic method described by Schotz *et al.* (1970) was used. The possible correlation between changes in tissue LPL activity and lipid-filling of adipocytes during normal growth is of interest in that it might form a biochemical basis for further evaluation of regulatory disturbances in lipid turnover during development and might suggest a mechanism whereby obesity could occur, particularly that form accompanied by large increases in adipocyte size. When one analyzes adipose tissue growth by examining changes in fat cell size, measured either as the amount of lipid per adipocyte or as the number of adipocytes per gram of tissue, an interesting pattern evolves (Figure 5).

During the early postnatal period from 10 to 35 days of age, cell size (μg lipid/cell) does not change significantly ($P>0.05$); similarly the number of adipocytes per gram of tissue does not change. However, total pad weight and total lipid per pad rise significantly during this same period. Therefore, significant numbers of new cells of the same average size must be added to the pad during this interval. Beginning at approximately 35 days and continuing at least until 100 days of age, marked increases in fat cell size occur. This is reflected both as a decrease in the number of fat cells per gram of tissue and as a sharp increase in the lipid per adipocyte. One might wonder then, whether changes in an enzyme involved with lipid-filling, such as lipoprotein lipase, might precede or be coincident with the marked changes in fat cell size.

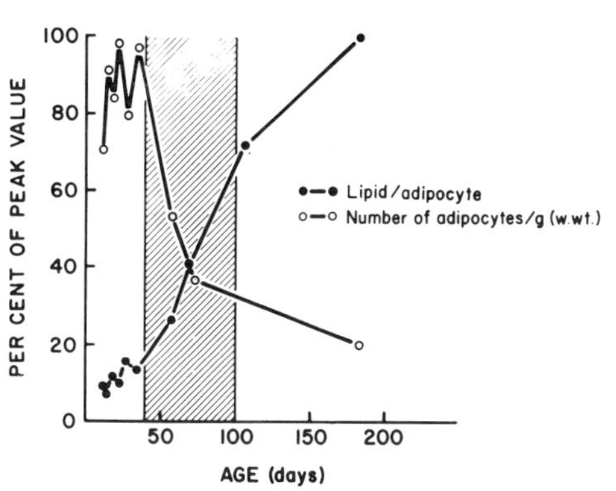

Fig. 5. Changes in adipose tissue cellularity during normal growth. Shaded area represents postweaning - early adult period. (from *J. Lipid Res.* 1974) (Greenwood & Hirsch, 1974)

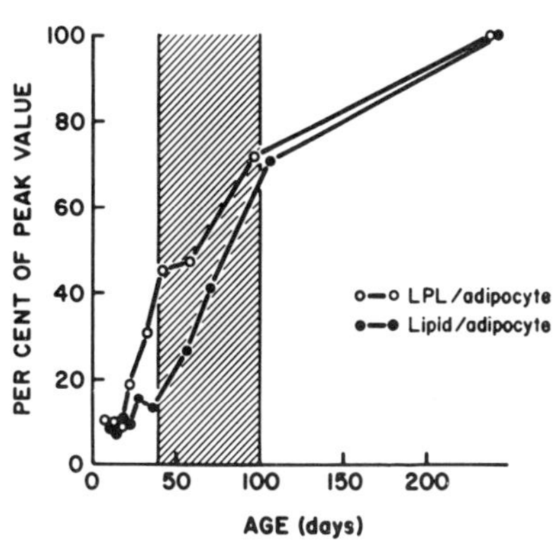

Fig. 6. Changes in LPL/cell and lipid/cell during development of normal adipose tissue. (from *J. Lipid Res.* 1977) (Greenwood & Hirsch, 1974)

The data from our developmental study support the concept that the changes in enzyme activity per fat cell precede the changes seen in fat cell size. The early and marked postnatal increase in the lipoprotein lipase activity per cell occurs between 17 and 35 days of age, which is before the increase in the amount of lipid per cell is noted. Lipoprotein lipase activity per adipocyte shows a significant fourfold increase ($P<0.01$) from the value at 17 days to that at 35 days of age while the fat cell size changes only 40 per cent, which is not a statistically significant increased (Fig. 6). From 10 to 42 days of age the specific activity of the enzyme, expressed per gram wet weight or per mg, supernatant protein also increases markedly. These data suggest that the changes in activity, which precede and are probably causally related to, the active lipid-filling of preadipocytes may have occurred as a result of enzyme activation and/or induction. Further support for the concept that the elevation of LPL activity during early development occurs in the preadipocytes was found in tissue compartmentalization experiments. However, since there are no adequate markers for preadipocytes, it is not possible to separate this pool from the rest of the stromal cells. Nonetheless, there were differences with respect to the distribution of recovered LPL activity between the two fractions. In 10 to 12-day-old rats, all of the activity is present in the stromal fraction. In fact, at this age, there are almost no fat-filled cells large enough to be isolated as an adipocyte fraction. As adipocyte lipid-filling proceeds, increasing amounts of lipoprotein lipase activity are found in the adipocyte fraction (Fig. 7). At 22 days 16 per cent is found in adipocytes; 30 per cent of the LPL activity is in the

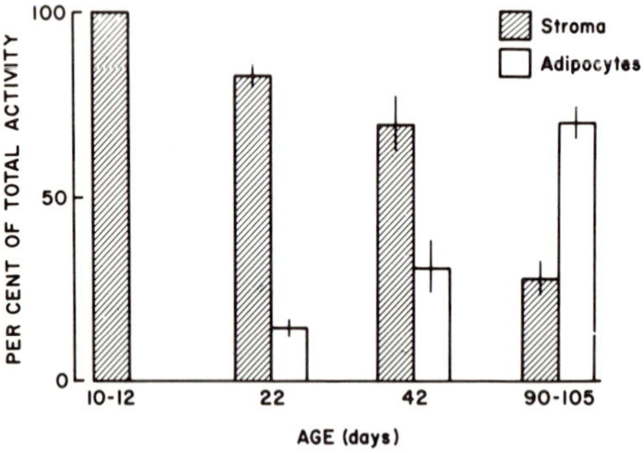

Fig. 7. Distribution of LPL activity between adipocyte and stromal fractions

adopocytes at 42 days, and in the mature rat of 90 to 105 days of age, 72 per cent of the lipoprotein lipase activity is detected in isolated adipocytes. This change in the compartmentalization of LPL activity supports the hypothesis that a 'bed of preadipocytes' is formed during the postnatal hyperplastic growth phase of the tissue which then become lipid-filled as a result of LPL mediated provision of FFA for triglyceride synthesis. Furthermore, the early developmental changes in adipose tissue LPL activity may be among the factors which regulate the rate of triglyceride storage and, therefore, the size of adipose tissue mass in the long term.

In the epididymal fat depot of the Zucker fatty rat excessive adipocyte hyperplasia becomes evident around the time of puberty and, as suggested earlier, is characterized by an extended period of proliferation. Another early morphological change in this type of obesity is the increase in fat cell size, which is detectable as early as the obesity is detectable, usually around 25 days. Therefore, these early increases in fat cell size might be accompanied or preceded by changes in LPL activity in adipose tissue from obese rats.

When LPL activity is determined and expressed per gram of tissue, both lean and obese rats have higher activity at 5 weeks of age than at 11 or 20 weeks of age. However, there were no differences between groups. If the enzyme activity is expressed on a fat cell basis, the 5-week-old Zucker fatty rat shows a fourfold increase in LPL per cell compared to lean controls. Although absolute levels are decreased at both 11 and 20 weeks of age the fatty rats continue to show significantly elevated levels of LPL per fat cell when compared to the lean. Our interpretation of these data is that the development of the early onset obesity in the Zucker fatty rat is characterized by pronounced alterations in the levels of lipoprotein lipase activity in the tissue. In the adult we have confirmed that a persistent increase in LPL activity per fat cell is seen.

General comments on the regulation of adipose tissue size

Several schemes have been presented to explain the normal cellular growth and development of a mammalian tissue but they all have in common the following characteristics (Fig. 8): (1) There are three compartments; proliferative, differentiating and mature, (2) Cells in the proliferative compartment are made at different rates at different times and the rate depends upon a variety of influence such as hormones, temperature, age, and dietary intake, (3) Cells leave the proliferative compartment and enter the differentiating

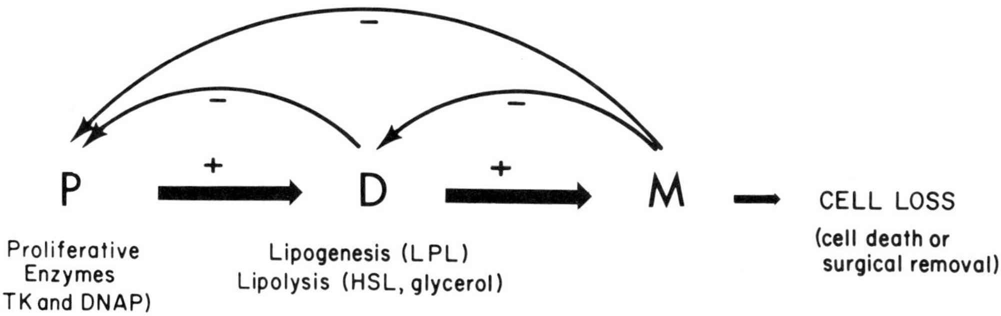

Fig. 8. A general scheme for adipose tissue mass regulation during development: '—' = inhibiting principle; TK = thymidine kinase; DNAP = DNA polymerase; P = Proliferative compartment; D = Differentiating compartment; M = Maturation compartment

compartment where they may stay for varying lengths of time, depending again on the presence of stimuli, such as hormones, substrate availability or temperature changes, (4) Cells that enter the mature compartment may continue to accumulate differentiation products, enlarge or die and be lost from the population, (5) There are several feedback loops that can act to control proliferation or differentiation that are derived from within the system itself. For example, Weiss & Kavanau (1957) postulate that as the maturation compartment enlarges it produces an inhibiting principle that can act to inhibit either proliferation or differentiation, effectively arresting the whole system and maintaining mass. Such a factor has been isolated from skin epidermis.

The currently available data strongly support the concept that during normal postnatal development in rats, particularly in the first two postnatal weeks the proliferation to differentiation to maturation processes are uninhibited and proceed rapidly. From the second to fourth or fifth postnatal week, proliferation to differentiation is very high but differentiation to maturation is relatively slow. After the fourth to fifth postnatal week the rate of differentiation to maturation is the primary regulated variable. The elevated thymidine kinase and DNA polymerase activity and the resistance to early undernutrition seen in the obese Zucker fatty rat may reflect a primary defect in enzymatic control of cellular proliferation. While this is an acceptable interpretation it is at least equally likely that the increased thymidine kinase and DNA polymerase activity and extended proliferation period could result secondarily from an increased rate of movement from the differentiation compartment (D) to the maturation compartment (M). The effect would be an incorrect assessment of the size of the differentiation compartment and lead to excessive proliferation. If one primary defect in the genesis of obesity is either increased substrate availability (LPL) or a decreased lipolytic response (reflected in decreased glycerol release), presumptive (non-lipid-filled cells) might fill with lipid at inappropriately high rates. The enhancement of LPL activity that occurs during early normal development, prior to changes in fat cell size, and the demonstration that LPL is elevated in pre-obese rats suggest that disruption of the normal developmental sequence of adipose tissue mass regulation may well occur at the level of control of differentiation. Much work remains to be done to elucidate whether lipid-filling, lipid-releasing or both are affected.

Even the demonstration that LPL seems to be enhanced at a specific early postnatal stage and is increased in obesity cannot answer the basic question of how this occurs. For example, at least four possible factors could stimulate LPL activity in adipose tissue of young obese rats: (a) diet, (b) increased insulin levels, (c) altered plasma lipoprotein profiles, including abnormal levels of apoVLDL, (d) altered substrate affinity (Fig. 9).

Although one cannot completely rule out the possibility that suckling rats have a primary hyperphagic lesion and are ingesting more calories than needed, this seems unlikely since they do not weigh more and are as active as lean sibs at least until 16 to 18 days of age (Stern & Johnson, 1974). During the first 15 days of suckling, one can also be sure that the diet of lean and pre-obese pups is the same. Therefore, a dietary stimulus as the initiator of increased LPL activity seems unlikely.

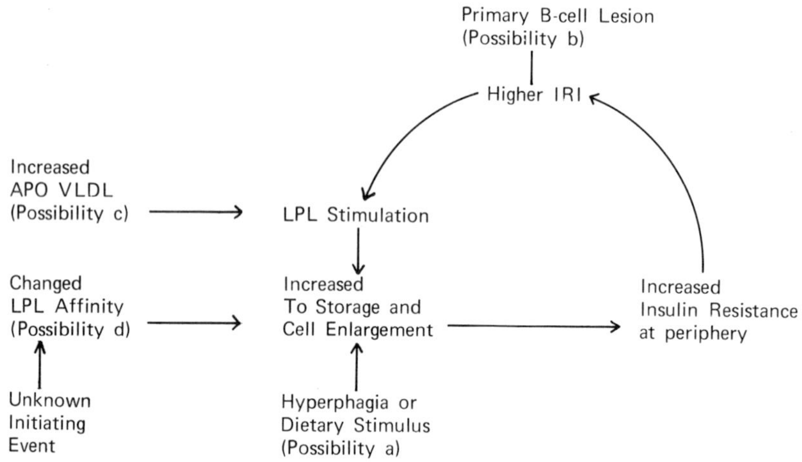

Fig. 9. Four possible factors which could stimulate LPL activity in adipose tissue of young obese rats

Many investigators have suggested that the primary initiating event in the development of obesity is a lesion in the beta cell resulting in hypersecretion of insulin and elevated plasma insulin (Stern & Johnson, 1977). Although early elevated insulin has been looked for in the Zucker fatty rat, it has not been possible to demonstrate that elevated insulin precedes the obesity. Bell & Stern (1976) recently reported that at 13 days of age, they were unable to find differences in plasma insulin among rat pups from breedings of *Fa/fa* males and *Fa/fa* females where 25 per cent of the pups should have been pre-obese. The amount of plasma obtained was at the lower limits of sensitivities of their assay.

The third possibility for early elevation of adipose tissue LPL, which is perhaps the most likely is that there are early changes in the plasma lipoproteins of the obese rat. In adult Zucker fatty rats Schoenfeld *et al.* (1974) have demonstrated that the VLDL fraction of plasma is altered both in quantity (several times greater in obese) and quality (78 per cent TG in obese compared to 60 per cent TG in normal). Furthermore, they found that the apoVLDL levels were five times greater in fatties.

Although other lipoproteins were also elevated in the fatties, the major alterations in plasma lipoprotein profile were related to large changes in VLDL dynamics. Schoenfeld & Pfelger (1974) found that one of the rapidly moving subunit peptides from the apoproteins was disproportionately greater in the fatties and estimated that if this were the rat LPL activator comparable to that found in human apoproteins, the adult Zucker fatty could have up to ten times more LPL activator than the lean rat. To our knowledge, this effect on plasma lipoprotein profile has not been examined intensively during development of obesity. The possibility that the VLDL fraction and its accompanying apoproteins may be elevated early in the development of obesity seems likely since Sullivan, Triscari & Spiegel (1977) have shown that both serum lipid (TG and cholesterol) and rates of liver lipogenesis are elevated as early as 4 to 5 weeks of age in the obese rat. Finally, alterations in substrate affinity may provide another explanation for the developmental changes in LPL activity as well as a possible mechanism, for increased TG storage in obesity.

Although LPL may be only one enzyme (LaRosa *et al.*, 1972; Anfinsen, Boyle & Brown, 1952; Hamosh *et al.*, 1970) with a precursor and active form (Garfinkel & Schotz, 1972; Garfinkel & Schotz, 1973), it reacts differently in different tissues. For example, during fasting, LPL in heart tissue is maximally active, while that of adipose tissue is decreased to minimum levels. In the light of the high tissue LPL activity in early postnatal development of normal rats and its possible enhancement in obesity, it seems most appropriate to consider whether, in addition to being present in a higher concentration, the LPL enzyme may be showing a different affinity for its substrate.

Although there is considerable data to support the notions presented above, considerably more data on enzyme profiles and interactions will be necessary before an understanding of the regulatory mechanisms will be forthcoming. Nonetheless, an approach to the developmental biology of this time which embodies a description of the enzyme patterns seen during normal and abnormal development seems worthwhile.

References

Adebonojo, F.O. (1975*a*): *Yale J. Biol. Med.* **48**, 9.
Adebonojo, F.O. (1975*b*): *In Vitro* **II**, 50.
Anfinsen, C.B., E. Boyle, & Brown, R.K. (1952): *Science* **115**, 583.
Bell, G.E. & Stern, J.S. (1976): *Fed. Proc.* **34**, 657.
Björntorp, P. (1972): *Adv. Psychosom. Med.* **7**, 116.
Björntorp, P. & Sjöström, L. (1971): *Metabolism* **20**, 703.
Bray, G.A. & York, D.A. (1971): *Physiol. Rev.* **51**, 598.
Brook, C.G.D., Lloyd, J.K. & Wolf, O.H. (1972): *Br. Med. J.* **2**, 25.
Brook, C.G.D. (1972): *Lancet* **2**, 624.
Cleary, M.P., Brasel, J.A. & Greenwood, M.R.C. (1977): *J. Nutr.* **107**, 1969.
Cleary, M.P., Klein, B.E., Greenwood, M.R.C. & Brasel, J.A. (1976): *Fed. Proc.* **35**, 502.
Dixon-Shanies, D. & Knittle, L. (1976): *Biochem. Biophys. Res. Comm.* **68**, 982.
Enesco, M. & LeBlond, C.P. (1962): *J. Embroyl. Exper. Morph.* **10**, 530.
Faust, I.M., P.R. Johnson & J. Hirsch (1976): *Am. J. Physiol.* **231**.,538.
Faust, I.M., Johnson, P.R. & Hirsch, J. (1977): *Science* **197**, 391.
Garfinkel, A.S. & Schotz, M.C. (1972): *J. Lipid. Res.* **13**, 63.
Garfinkel, A.S. & Schotz, M.C. (1973): *Biochim. Biophys. Acta* **306**, 128.
Green, H. & Kehinde, O. (1975): *Cell* **1**, 113.
Green, H. & Meuth, M. (1974): *Cell* **3**, 127.
Greenwood, M.R.C. & Hirsch, J. (1974): *J. Lipid Res.* **15**, 474.
Hamosh, M., Clary, T.R. Chernick, S.S. & Scow, R.D. (1970): *Biochim. Biophys. Acta* **210**, 473.
Hausberger, F.X. (1959): *Anat. Rec.* **135**, 109.
Hellman, B., Taljedal, I.B. & Westman, S. (1962): *Acta Anat.* **55**, *286.*
Hirsch, J. & Gallian, E. (1968): *J. Lipid Res.* **9**, 110.
Hirsch, J. & Han, P.W. (1969): *J. Lipid Res.* **10**, 77.
Hirsch, J. & Knittle, J. (1970): *Fed. Proc.* **29**, 1516.
Hollenberg, C.H. & Vost, A. (1968): *J. Clin. Invest.* **47**, 2485.
Johnson, P.R., Zucker, L.M., Cruce, J.A.F. & Hirsch, J. (1971): *J. Lipid Res.* **12**, 706.
Johnson, P.R. & Hirsch, J. (1972): *J. Lipid Res.* **13**, 2.
Johnson, P.R., Stern, J., Greenwood, M.R.C., Zucker, L.M. & Hirsch, J. (1973): *J. Nutr.* **103**, 738.
Johnson, P.R., Faust, I.M., Monahan, J. & Hirsch, J. (1976): *J. Nutr.* **106**, XXIV.
Kakolewski, J.W., Cox, V.C. & Uclenstein, E.S. (1968): *Psychol. Rep.* **22**, 547.
Kennedy, G.C. (1952): *Proc. Roy. Soc. Lond.* Series B. **140**, 578.
Knittle, J.L. (1972): *J. Pediatrics* **81**, 1048.
Knittle, J. & Hirsch, J. (1968): *J. Clin. Invest.* **47**, 2091.
Kral, J.G. (1975): *Scand. J. Plast. Reconstr. Surg.* **9**, 140.
Kral, J.G. (1976): *Am. J. Physiol.* **231**, 1090.
LaRosa, J.C., R.I. Levy, H.G. Windmueller & D.S. Frederickson. (1972): *J. Lipid Res.* **13**, 356.
Lemonnier, D. (1972): *J. Clin. Invest*, **51**, 2907.
Mohr, W. & Beneke, G. (1969): *Virchows. Arch.* B. **3**, 13.
Mrosovsky, N. (1974): *Physiol. Behav.* **12**, 259.

Pilgrim, C. (1971): *Dev. Biol.* **26**, 69.
Poznanski, W.J., Waheed, I. & Van, R. (1973): *Lab Invest.* **29**, 570.
Rakow, L., Beneke, G., Mohr, W. & Brauchle, I. (1970): *Beitr. Pat. Bd.* **141**, 349.
Rakow, L., Beneke, G., Mohr, W. & Brauchle, I. (1971*a*): *Path. Microbiol.* **37**, 261.
Rakow, L., Beneke, G. & Vogt, C. (1971*b*): *Beitr. Path. Bd.* **144**, 377.
Russel, T.R. & Ho, R. (1976): *Proc. Nat. Acad. Sci.* **73**, 4516.
Schotz, M.A., Garfinkel, R.J., Huebotter, & Stewart, J.E. (1970): *J. Lipid Res.* **11**, 68.
Schoenfeld, G. & Pfleger, B. (1971): *Am. J. Physiol.* **220**, 1178.
Stern, J.S. & Johnson, P.R. (1974): *Fed. Proc.* **33**, 67.
Stern, J.S. & Johnson, P.R. (1977): *Metabolism* **26**, 371.
Strautz, R.L. (1970): *Diabetologia* **6**, 980.
Sullivan, A.C., Triscari, J. & Spiegel, H.E. (1977): *Am. J. Clin. Nutr.* **30**, 777.
Van, R.L.R., Bayliss, E. & Roncari, A.K. (1976): *J. Clin. Invest.* **58**, 699.
Van, R.L.R. & Roncari, A.K. (1977): *Cell Tiss. Res.* **181**, 197.
Weiss, P. & Kavanau, J. (1957): *J. Gen. Physiol.* **41**, 1.
Wertheimer, H.E. & Shapiro, B. (1948): *Physiol. Rev.* **28**, 451.
Zucker, L.M. & Zucker, T. (1961): *J. Hered.* **52**, 275.

18
The adipose cell and insulin resistance

L.B. SALANS, L.E. FOLEY and S.W. CUSHMAN
National Institute of Arthritis, Metabolism and Digestive Diseases, National Institutes of Health, Bethesda, Maryland 20014, USA, and Dartmouth Medical School, Hanover, New Hampshire 03755, USA.

An impairment in insulin's ability to influence glucose metabolism in obese humans is well recognized. Hyperglycemia and glucose intolerance in the face of hyperinsulinemia, and a diminished hypoglycemic response of exogenous insulin are characteristic of obesity. Weight loss is associated with an improvement in, and often a restoration to normal of, these metabolic abnormalities. Similar relationships exist in a variety of obese experimental animals.

The hyperinsulinemia of obesity has generally been regarded as a compensatory adaptation to peripheral insulin resistance. It is postulated that a decreased ability of insulin to influence glucose uptake and metabolism in the insulin sensitive tissues of the body leads to hyperglycemia and secondarily to hyperinsulinemia. Research in our laboratories during the past several years has been directed towards defining the nature of this insulin resistance at the cellular level.

Our studies have focused on the adipose cell as a model for examining these relationships. Anatomically the adipose tissue is clearly the most abnormal tissue in obesity. The principal cell of this tissue, the adipocyte, is intimately involved in carbohydrate and lipid metabolism and these functions of the adipose cell are regulated by insulin. Moreover, changes in the size of the adipose mass parallel the systemic metabolic state of obesity as reflected in plasma glucose and insulin concentrations: hyperglycemia, glucose intolerance, and hyperinsulinemia are present when the adipose tissue is expanded, and return to, or towards, normal with reduction in the adipose tissue mass. Finally, the adipose tissue is the most readily accessible insulin sensitive tissue in man and the only one which permits detailed and repeated studies under a variety of different experimental conditions. The use of this tissue as a model for examining insulin-cell interaction, has, nevertheless, been undertaken with full recognition of the complex interdependence among a variety of tissues in regulating the flow of metabolic fuels, and probably more important quantitatively, the role of the liver and skeletal muscle in the systemic metabolic abnormalities of glucose and insulin in obesity. That the adipose tissue does, however, provide a good model for the study of insulin-cell interaction in these quantitatively more important, but less accessible, insulin sensitive tissues is supported by the observation that alterations in the ability of insulin to influence adipocyte glucose metabolism is paralleled by similar changes in the liver (Felig *et al.*, 1974; Le Marchand *et al.*, 1976) and skeletal muscle (Rabinowitz & Zierler, 1962; Horton *et al.*, 1973). Furthermore, there appears to be a close relationship between insulin sensitivity of adipose tissue *in vitro* and the sensitivity of the whole organism to insulin, as reflected in the hypoglycemic effect of exogenously administered insulin (Franckson *et al.*, 1966); thus, the influence of insulin on glucose metabolism in isolated adipose cells *in vitro* may reflect very closely the state of insulin sensitivity in other tissues and the body as a whole.

Studies in experimental animals

There is abundant evidence demonstrating that the influence of insulin on glucose metabolism by adipose cells from various obese experimental animals is impaired. The aging obese rat has been studied in most detail. In that animal, the stimulation *in vitro* of glucose oxidation and glucose carbon incorporation into triglyceride glycerol and fatty acid by insulin, and the antilipolytic effects of insulin are diminished in adipocytes obtained from obese older rats compared to that observed in cells from non-obese younger animals, when the nutritional and growth states of these animals are similar (Salans & Dougherty, 1971; Olefsky, 1976). Weight loss and reduction in adiposity are accompanied by an improvement in the ability of insulin to influence these metabolic functions of the adipose cell. Similar observations have been made in the adipose cells from various genetically obese rats and mice (Assimacopoulos-Jeannet & Jeanrenaud, 1976).

The observations that increased adipose cell size is common to all forms of obesity and that weight loss and reduction in adiposity is always accompanied by reduction in adipose cell size (Hirsch & Batchelor, 1976; Salans, Cushman & Weismann, 1973) have led to the concept that the impairment in the effect of insulin on the metabolism of glucose by the adipocyte is somehow related to enlargement of the adipose cell. This concept receives additional support from the observation that virtually identical relationships between adipose cell size and insulin-stimulated metabolism of glucose are observed when cells of different size are obtained from rates of different body weight and age, or from different fat depots within animals of the same age and weight (Salans & Dougherty, 1971); increasing adipose cell size is associated with a decreasing metabolic effect of insulin.

Detailed studies of the aging rat have been undertaken in this laboratory in an effort to identify the factors responsible for the impairment of glucose metabolism in the presence of insulin in the enlarged adipose cell (Salans & Cushman, 1977). These studies have included an examination of (1) the relationship between insulin dose and glucose metabolism, (2) equilibrium insulin binding, (3) glucose transport, and (4) the distribution of glucose carbon atoms among various glucose metabolites, in adipose cells of widely different sizes obtained from rats of varying body weight, adiposity and age. Glucose metabolism in response to different doses of insulin indicate that the enlarged adipocyte has a normal sensitivity to insulin, as determined by the pattern of the metabolic response and from the dose of insulin required to produce half-maximal stimulation of glucose metabolism, but a diminished capacity to metabolize glucose. Equilibrium insulin binding per cell is greater, not less, in large compared to small adipocytes; per unit surface area, insulin binding is similar irrespective of adipose cell size. Glucose transport has been assessed by measuring the transport of L-arabinose (Foley, Cushman & Salans, 1976); these studies indicate that both basal and insulin-stimulated glucose transport increase with increasing adipose cell size. Thus, when expressed in terms of absolute glucose transport, it is apparent that the decreased rate of glucose metabolism in response to insulin associated with increasing adipose cell size cannot be explained on the basis of an impairment in glucose transport. Basal transport activity, however, increases to a greater degree than does insulin-stimulated transport; therefore, when expressed as the per cent increase above basal, the ability of insulin to stimulate glucose transport is impaired as adipose cell size increases. Nevertheless, the magnitude of the alteration is small compared to the impairment in the ability of insulin to enhance glucose metabolism and it becomes readily apparent that the former cannot explain the latter. The sensitivity of glucose transport to insulin in small and large cells is similar, irrespective of whether absolute rates of transport or per cent increase in transport data are used; this observation parallels, and could perhaps be predicted by, the findings of unaltered insulin binding and normal sensitivity of glucose metabolism to insulin, but a diminished capacity to metabolize glucose by large as compared to small adipose cells. These observations have been interpreted as suggesting that the factor(s) responsible for the impairment in insulin stimulation of glucose metabolism in the enlarged adipose cell from the aging rat lie beyond the site of insulin-receptor interaction and glucose transport, and that they may be located intracellularly in some metabolic process that may or may not be under the direct control of insulin. This concept receives some support from the observation that increasing adipose cell size is associated with alterations in the pattern of glucose metabolism as reflected in the distribution of labelled glucose carbon atoms among the various metabolic end products of glucose. Thus, in the presence of insulin, increasing adipose cell size is associated with increasing rates of glucose carbon incorporated into triglyceride glycerol, but decreasing rates of glucose oxidation and *de novo* fatty acid synthesis. Moreover, examination of the relationships between glucose uptake, utilization and metabolism, using a variety of experimental conditions to enhance glucose uptake, indicate that while the metabolic capacity of small adipose cells is well above that for glucose transport, the capacity for glucose metabolism in large cells is markedly diminished and appears to be well below that which would saturate the transport system (Cushman & Salans, 1977). The factors responsible for these alterations in intracellular metabolism in the enlarged adipose cell remain to be defined. It is, however, quite clear that an impairment of glucose metabolism in response to insulin in the adipose cell can occur with no alteration in the interaction of insulin with its specific cell membrane-located receptor (insulin binding), and that the defect responsible for the impaired effect of insulin on glucose metabolism in the aging rat lies at some intracellular metabolic site within the enlarged adipocyte.

At the same time, it has become evident that adipose cell size is neither the only, nor perhaps the most important factor regulating the metabolic function of this cell; other factors have been shown to alter markedly the ability of insulin to influence glucose metabolism in adipocytes from non-obese and obese animals. Physical activity influences the character of glucose metabolism in the adipose tissue and its regulation by insulin (Björntorp, 1974); physical training improves the stimulation of glucose metabolism by insulin. Both the quantity and quality of calories ingested in the diet influence the metabolism of adipocytes and its regulation by insulin (Salans & Dougherty, 1971; Salans & Cushman, 1977). Thus, basal glucose metabolism and its regulation by insulin are greatly diminished during periods of caloric restriction and weight loss, and markedly enhanced during periods of excessive caloric intake and weight gain, irrespective of adiposity and adipose cell size. Similarly, ingestion of equicaloric diets of different composition is associated in the absence of changes in cell size with changes in metabolism; ingestion of a high carbohydrate, low fat diet stimulates, and ingestion of a high fat, low carbohydrate diet diminishes, both the basal and insulin-stimulated rates of glucose metabolism in the adipose tissue of non-obese, as well as obese, animals. Impairment of glucose metabolism of adipocyte in response to insulin during high fat, low carbohydrate intake, and improvement during high carbohydrate, low fat ingestion, occur in the absence of alterations in insulin binding, a situation similar to that observed when an alteration in the effect of insulin accompanies adipose cellular enlargement. Glucose transport, however, is much more affected by changes in dietary composition than by adipose cell size (Foley, Cushman & Salans, 1977); during high fat, low carbohydrate intake, insulin-stimulated transport decreases in a roughly parallel fashion to metabolism, while the reverse occurs during high carbohydrate, low fat ingestion. The change in transport is one of capacity for glucose transport rather than one of a change in the sensitivity of the transport system to insulin. Thus, ability of insulin to stimulate adipocyte glucose metabolism can be influenced by factors other than adipose cell size, in this case by dietary composition. Once again, an impairment occurs in the absence of alterations in insulin binding; in contrast to that observed with cellular enlargement, however, dietary factors appear to operate at the site of glucose transport.

Studies in man

Studies of human adipose tissue are not as extensive and are considerably less clear-cut than are those in rats. Resistance to the action of insulin on adipose tissue has been demonstrated *in vivo* in obese humans (Rabinowitz & Zierler, 1962; Sims *et al.*, 1973). Infusion of insulin into the brachial artery and measurements of differences in arterial-venous blood glucose concentration in the superficial tissues of the forearm indicates an impairment in the action of insulin on adipose tissue metabolism of glucose in the obese. Weight loss by obese patients improves, and weight gain in non-obese individuals diminishes, the ability of insulin to influence forearm metabolism of adipose tissue. These changes are paralleled by simultaneous alterations in systemic glucose metabolism as reflected in the concentrations of plasma glucose and insulin, and by the blood glucose response to exogenously administered insulin.

It has, however, been most difficult to confirm this indirect *in vivo* evidence for an impaired ability of insulin to stimulate glucose metabolism in adipose tissue of obese patients through direct study of human adipose tissue *in vitro*. The results of studies comparing the metabolism of adipose tissue *in vitro* from non-obese and obese humans have been more disparate than similar. Thus, the ability of insulin to influence glucose metabolism by adipose tissue from obese, compared to non-obese, individuals has been reported to be similar (Davidson, 1975), increased (Björntorp, 1966), or diminished (Salans, Knittle & Hirsch, 1968; Smith, 1971). The explanation for these discrepancies may lie in the extremely small and highly variable *in vitro* effect of insulin on human adipose tissue and the failure to adequately control such variables as antecedent diet, changing body weight, physical activity, and age, factors which are known to influence the function of adipocytes. Studies in this laboratory indicate that when adipose tissue is obtained from subjects during periods of weight maintenance and ingestion of diets of similar composition, increasing adipose cell size is associated with unchanging basal rates of glucose oxidation, increasing basal rates of glucose carbon incorporation into triglyceride glycerol, and decreasing stimulation of glucose oxidation by insulin (Salans *et al.*, 1974); an effect of insulin on triglyceride glycerol or triglyceride fatty acid production from glucose has yet to be demonstrated under these conditions in this laboratory. Weight gain in non-obese individuals, achieved through prolonged overeating, is accompanied by enlargement of adipose cells and is associated with an impairment in the ability of insulin to influence adipocyte glucose oxidation *in vitro* similar to that observed in the spontaneously obese subjects. Weight loss by both spontaneously and experimentally obese individuals and reduction in adipose cell size are accompanied by an improvement in the effects of insulin *in vitro*. Thus, these alterations are neither primary nor permanent changes associated with obesity, but appear to be adaptations to the obese state.

The relationships are observed only when such individuals are maintaining body weight and are ingesting diets of similar composition. The effect of insulin on glucose metabolism by human adipose tissue is influenced by the same environmental factors as described for the rat. Thus, both basal glucose metabolism and the effects of insulin upon it are diminished during periods of caloric deprivation and weight loss, and enhanced during caloric surfeit and active weight gain (Salans & Cushman, 1977). Ingestion of equicaloric diets of different caloric consumption is also associated with marked alterations in adipocyte function (Salans *et al.*, 1974): high fat, low carbohydrate diets diminish, while high carbohydrate, low fat diets enhance, both basal and insulin-stimulated metabolism of glucose in adipose cells from non-obese and obese individuals.

Preliminary studies aimed at defining the factors responsible for these metabolic alterations in the human adipocyte associated with obesity and changes in nutritional state have been undertaken, and like the metabolic studies, disparity in results between laboratories has been reported. Insulin binding in adipose cells from obese patients has been reported to be diminished (Olefsky, 1976*a*), or the same (Salans & Cushman, 1977), compared to that observed in cells from non-obese individuals. The alterations in adipocyte metabolism induced by changes in dietary composition appear to occur without alterations in insulin binding (Salans & Cushman, 1977). Glucose transport has not yet been examined in sufficient detail. Studies of the pattern of glucose metabolism are equally confusing due to the disparity of results between laboratories. Measurement of the rate of insulin-stimulated incorporation of glucose carbon into CO_2, triglyceride glycerol, and triglyceride fatty acids in adipose cells has led to reports of similar, increased, or diminished rates in non-obese compared to obese (Salans *et al.*, 1974; Davidson, 1975; Björntorp, 1966; Nestel & Goldrick, 1976; Bray *et al.*,

1977). Some of these metabolic functions have even been reported to be non-existent; significant rates of *de novo* fatty acid synthesis from glucose have not been demonstrated in the absence or presence of insulin in human adipose cells of any size, when tissue is obtained from adult subjects during periods of weight maintenance (Salans *et al.*, 1974). Incorporation of radioactivity from pyruvate into fatty acids has been used as an alternative means of assessing lipogenic activity by human adipose tissue *in vitro* (Bray *et al.*, 1977); large cells obtained from obese patients during periods of weight maintenance and controlled dietary intake possess lower rates of lipogenesis from pyruvate than small cells from non-obese individuals studies under similar conditions.

Given the current state of the art of assessing the character of human adipose tissue *in vitro*, and of comparing it between non-obese and obese individuals, it appears premature to attempt to draw any conclusions regarding the possible role of the enlarged tissue mass in the development and perpetuation of the abnormalities of glucose metabolism associated with human obesity, let alone the cellular and biochemical mechanisms responsible for these metabolic alterations. An impaired action of insulin on glucose metabolism in isolated adipose tissue from obese human subjects has not been observed with any consistency. Where such an impairment has been demonstrated it has been limited only to the effect of insulin on glucose oxidation; there has been no consistent demonstration of a diminished effect of insulin on the other parameters of glucose metabolism including lipogenesis, glycogen synthesis or lipolysis. The selective impairment of insulin action on only one pathway of glucose metabolism, and the inconsistencies from one laboratory to another, dictate caution in the interpretation of these results and in ascribing a primary role to the adipose tissue.

Furthermore, even if the ability of insulin to influence cellular metabolism in adipose tissue is impaired in obese humans, it is clear that this defect in an increased adipose tissue mass cannot be the sole, or perhaps even the primary, contributor to the development of the altered systemic glucose metabolism of the obese individual. Impaired glucose tolerance and hyperinsulinemia improve substantially with decreased caloric and carbohydrate intake before significant loss of body weight is achieved. Estimates of the distribution of oral glucose to the various tissue of the body suggest that only a small portion of ingested glucose is disposed of in the adipose tissue (Rabinowitz, 1970); even if an alteration in regulation of glucose metabolism by insulin exists in this tissue in the obese, it is unlikely that it would quantitatively contribute more than minimally to the marked alterations in the systemic metabolism observed. It should, however, be noted that these estimations of glucose distribution have been observed in fasting individuals. It remains to determine what proportion of glucose and its precursors escape the liver in the fed state and are delivered to the peripheral tissues. This may be of quantitative importance when one considers that the obese individual is ingesting both excessive amounts of calories and of carbohydrate, and that ten to fifteen per cent of a large amount of glucose escaping the liver represents a significant amount of glucose presented to these tissues.

The liver and skeletal muscle play a major role in the regulation of the flow of metabolic fuels and the control of systemic glucose metabolism; quantitatively these tissues rather than the adipose tissue are likely to be more directly responsible for the alterations of systemic glucose metabolism associated with obesity. An impairment in the ability of insulin to diminish hepatic glucose output in obese patients compared to non-obese individuals has been demonstrated *in vivo* in man (Felig *et al.*, 1974). Studies on the effect of diet and changes in body weight have not yet been reported. However, in view of the fact that this tissue is the most important regulator of glucose economy in the body, and in light of the discussions of dietary effects, such studies seem critical to the understanding of the factors responsible for the impairment of the action of insulin on the liver. Infusion of insulin into the brachial artery of non-obese and obese patients results in a greater difference in the concentration of glucose in the arterial-deep venous blood in non-obese than in obese subjects, indicating an impairment in the effect of insulin on glucose metabolism by the skeletal muscle of the forearm of the obese subjects (Rabinowitz & Zierler, 1962; Horton *et al.*, 1973). This alteration is both reversible through weight loss by obese subjects and inducible through weight gain by non-obese individuals. Furthermore, high carbohydrate, low fat ingestion enhances insulin's effect on forearm muscle *in vivo* (Horton *et al.*, 1973). The similarities between forearm muscle *in vivo* and adipose tissue *in vivo* and *in vitro* are obvious. Taken together, they suggest that what is being observed in these tissues is not a primary event, but rather a reflection of these tissues adapting to their nutrient environment.

Although it is unlikely that the expanded adipose tissue mass plays a primary or direct role in the development of the systemic metabolic abnormalities of obesity, the observations discussed above do not preclude the possibility that the adipose tissue may play some important indirect role in these abnormalities. It remains possible, for example, that the enlarged adipose tissue mass somehow signals other tissues which are quantitatively more important to glucose homeostasis, particularly the liver, such that these tissues are less responsive to insulin; these signals from the adipose tissue may be related to altered adipocyte function. Moreover, the current state of the art of the study of human adipose tissue notwithstanding, the adipose tissue appears to provide a practical and good model for investigating the nature and biochemical character of the impaired action of insulin on tissues in obesity. In this respect it should be borne in mind that in the rat, where the many factors known to influence adipocyte function and its regulation by insulin can be carefully controlled, the finding of an impairment in the ability of insulin to stimulate glucose metabolism in the enlarged adipocyte from the obese animal is consistent and observed for multiple metabolic factors.

Acknowledgement – The authors wish to thank Ms Mary Jane Zarnowski and Ms Ruth Segal for their excellent technical assistance in these studies. The investigators from this laboratory discussed in this report were supported by NIH research grants, AM 13321 and AM 10254, and grants from the Hitchcock Foundation, Weight Watchers, Inc. and the American Diabetes Association.

References

Assimocopoulos-Jeannet, F. & Jeanrenaud, B. (1976): *Clins Endoc. Metab.* 5, 337.

Björntorp, P. (1966): *Acta Med. Scand.* 179, 229.

Björntorp, P. (1974): In *Obesity symposium,* ed W.L. Burland, P.D. Samuel & J. Yudkin, p. 171. Edinburgh: Churchill Livingstone.

Bray, G.A., Glennon, J.A., Salans, L.B., Horton. E.S., Danforth. E. Jr. & Sims, E.A.H. (1977): *Metabolism* 26, 739.

Cushman, S.W. & Salans, L.B. (1977): Presented at annual meeting of the European Society for the Study of Diabetes, Geneva.

Davidson, M.D. (1975): *Diabetes* 24, 1086.

Felig, P., Wahren, J., Hendler, R. & Brundin, T. (1974): *J. Clin. Invest.* 53, 582.

Foley, J., Cushman, S.W. & Salans, L.B. (1976): *Clin. Res.* 24, 360A.

Foley, J., Cushman, S.W. & Salans, L.B. (1977): *Clin. Res.* 25.

Franckson, J.R.M., Malaise, W., Arnould, Y., Rasio, E., Ooms, H.A., Balasse, E., Conrad, V. & Bastenie, P.A. (1966): *Diabetologia* 2, 96.

Hirsch, J. & Batchelor, B. (1976): *Clins Endoc. Metab.* 5, 299.

Horton, E.S., Danforth, E., Jr., Sims, E.A.H. & Salans, L.B. (1975): In *Obesity in perspective,* ed G.A. Bray, p. 323. Washington DC: US Govt. Ptg. Office.

Le Marchand, Y., Loten, E.G., Assimocopoulos-Jeannet, F., Forgue, M.E., Freychet, P. & Jeanrenaud, B. (1977): *Diabetes* 26, 582.

Nestel, P. & Goldrick, B. (1976): *Clins Endoc. Metab.* 5, 313.

Olefsky, J.M. (1976): *J. Clin. Invest.* 57, 842.

Olefsky, J.M. (1976*a*): *J. Clin. Invest.* 57, 1165.

Rabinowitz, D. & Zierler, K.L. (1962): *J. Clin. Invest.* 41, 2173.

Rabinowitz, D. (1970): *Ann. Review Med.* 21, 241.

Salans, L.B., Knittle, J.L. & Hirsch, J. (1968): *J. Clin. Invest.* 47, 153.

Salans, L.B. & Dougherty, J.W. (1971): *J. Clin. Invest.* 50, 1399.

Salans, L.B., Cushman, S.W. & Weismann, R.E. (1973): *J. Clin. Invest.* 52., 929.

Salans, L.B., Bray, G.A., Cushman, S.W., Danforth, E., Jr., Glennon, J.A., Horton, E.S. & Sims, E.A.H. (1974): *J. Clin. Invest.* 53, 848.

Salans, L.B. & Cushman, S.W. (1977): In *Advances in modern nutrition,* Vol. II, ed H.M. Katzen & R.J. Mahler (in press). Washington DC: Hemisphere Publishing Co.
Sims, E.A.H., Danforth, E., Jr., Horton, E.S., Glennon, J.A., Bray, G.A. & Salans, L.B. (1973): *Recent Prog. Horm. Res.* 29, 457.
Smith, U. (1971): *J. Lipid Res.* 12, 65.

19
Human fat cell metabolism

U.SMITH
Department of Medicine II, Sahlgren's Hospital, Göteborg, Sweden.

The most important metabolic function of the adipose cell is to assimilate and store energy in the form of triglycerides and to release energy in the form of fatty acids to be used by the peripheral tissues. The fat cell is well adapted for this function and has the unique ability to vary its degree of filling with triglycerides by at least tenfold. Concomitantly, the cell surface area may change a hundredfold and the cell volume a thousandfold.

The triglyceride fatty acids in the adipocytes may be preformed and directly taken up and esterified from the blood stream (Wilson, Gutman & Galton, 1973; Walldius & Rubba, 1976) or, more importantly, formed by the degradation of the blood triglycerides in the capillary endothelium by the action of the lipoprotein lipase (Korn, 1955; Robinson, 1963) (Fig. 1). However, fatty acids (FA) may also be endogenously formed in the fat cells from different precursors such as glucose and pyruvate (cf Bray, 1972; Sjöström, 1972; Goldrick & Galton, 1974). In experimental animals, such as the rat, a large portion of the triglyceride fatty acids may be endogenously formed in the adipose tissue (Di Girolamo *et al.*, 1974). However, in human fat cells it appears that only a very small part of the fatty acids is directly formed by the fat cells (Sjöström, 1972; Goldrick & Galton, 1974). In fact it has been estimated that, even under optimal conditions, only 1 to 2 g/day can be formed in the total adipose tissue mass (Sjöström, 1972). Consequently, the quantitatively important way for human fat cells to form triglyceride is by esterifying exogenous, preformed FA. The activity of lipoprotein lipase has also been shown to increase postprandially presumably due to increased glucose and insulin levels (Pykälistö, Smith & Brunzell, 1975). Conversely, under conditions

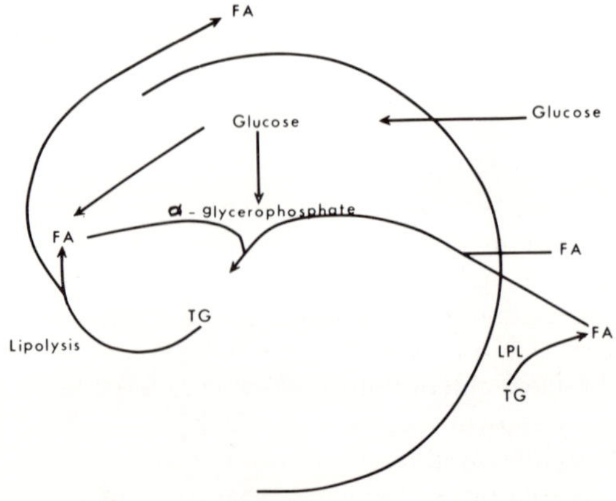

Fig. 1. Metabolism of triglycerides in the adipose cell

when FA are mobilized from the adipose tissue, such as starvation, the lipoprotein lipase activity is reduced. In fact, under almost all conditions so far studied there appears to be a negative correlation between the rate of lipid mobilization from the fat cells and the lipoprotein lipase activity (Table 1).

Table 1. Regulation of adipose tissue lipoprotein lipase activity

Enhanced activity by glucose, insulin, insulin + cortisol, thyroid hormones.
Reduced activity by lipolytic agents such as catecholamines, dibutyryl cAMP, high cortisol levels.

The amount of glucose taken up from the blood stream by the total adipose tissue mass seems very small (a few per cent) and of quantitatively little importance for total body glucose homeostasis (Björntorp *et al.*, 1971). Thus, the association between obesity and reduced glucose tolerance can not directly be explained by reduced effects of insulin on glucose uptake by the fat cells (Salans, Knittle & Hirsch, 1968; Smith, 1971; Davidson, 1975). However, even though it may be a small amount the formation of sufficient α-glycerophosphate from glucose is necessary for adequate reesterification of the FA. Thus, if the α-glycerophosphate formation is reduced this may lead to less FA taken up from the blood stream and, in addition, less reesterification of FA mobilized from the fat cells (Fig. 1). Thus, increased fatty acid levels in the blood will be the result. Since it seems that increased levels of FA are frequently associated with a reduced glucose tolerance via the glucose-fatty acid cycle (Randle *et al.*, 1963) this mechanism may be one way in which adipose tissue glucose metabolism may directly influence total body glucose homeostasis.

Reduced glucose uptake and reduced formation of α-glycerophosphate in the fat cells may be caused by different conditions and hormones. Administration of cortisol leads to increased plasma FA levels and this effect is probably caused to a large extent by the effect of cortisol to reduce glucose uptake (cf Fain & Czech, 1974). Similar effect may be the cause of raised plasma FA levels after administration of growth hormone. We have found that growth hormone added *in vitro* in long-term incubations reduces glucose metabolism, in particular the formation of the glycerol moiety of the triglycerides, without any direct effect of the hormone on the rate of triglyceride breakdown (Nyberg & Smith, 1977). Similarly, the raised FA levels in diabetes may partly be due to an insufficient formation of α-glycerophosphate since increased FA release from the fat cells can be found even in the absence of increased rate of triglyceride breakdown (Gilber, Kaye & Galton, 1974). A decreased glucose uptake in adipose tissue of diabetics has been shown previously (Galton & Wilson, 1970). Finally, evidence for a direct correlation between glucose metabolism and uptake of exogenous FA *in vitro* has recently been presented (Walldius & Rubba, 1976).

In obesity, raised fatty acid levels are frequently found (Balasse, 1968). However, there is no evidence that glucose metabolism is reduced in uncomplicated obesity. In fact, positive correlations between glucose incorporation into triglycerides and fat cell size have repeatedly been reported (Björntorp & Karlsson, 1971; Smith, 1971). The reason for this correlation is not clear at present but may be associated with the larger cell surface area of the enlarged cells. However, since such correlations can disappear after different experimental manipulations (see below) it does not appear to be a fundamental characteristic of large fat cells to have increased rates of glucose metabolism. Consequently, such correlations may reflect some alteration(s) of the hormonal and/or substrate levels associated with obesity. The increased plasma insulin levels found in obesity may be one important cause for this correlation and, in fact, even within an obese group of patients a high degree of correlation between plasma insulin levels and rate of glucose metabolism measured *in vitro* has been found (Fig. 2). We have previously shown that prolonged exposure of human fat cells to insulin *in vitro* (one week) leads to increased basal rates of glucose metabolism. This increase is probably due to both increased rates of glucose transport and increased activities of several glycolytic enzymes (Smith, 1974; Smith *et al.*, 1976*a*). Furthermore, the larger the fat cells

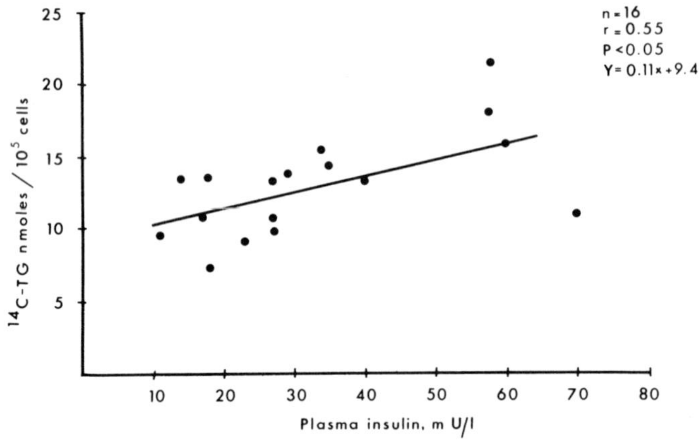

Fig. 2. Correlation between plasma insulin levels and glucose levels

the greater this long-term stimulating effect of insulin *in vitro* on glucose metabolism (Smith, 1974).

In the following, attention will be focused on factors controlling lipid mobilization via direct triglyceride breakdown (lipolysis) in human adipose tissue. Most of our knowledge about fat cell metabolism has come from studies on adipocytes from experimental animals usually the rat. However, very great caution should be exercised in extrapolating data from rat adipose tissue to human fat cells. Several important differences in the responsiveness, metabolic rates and regulatory factors have become evident (Table 2). It is, therefore, important that direct studies with human adipose tissue are carried out before results with rat adipose tissue can be accepted as valid for man.

As exemplified in Table 2 the only hormones which are directly lipolytic in human fat cells are the catecholamines and, as recently described (Gozariu *et al.*, 1974), parathyroid hormone. The physiological role of the catecholamines is clear but not that of parathyroid

Table 2. Some metabolic differences between rat and human fat cells

(1) Human fat cells have lower metabolic rates than fat cells and respond more sluggishly to hormones.
(2) In contrast to human fat cells quantitatively important endogenous fatty acid production in rat cells.
(3) Human cells only respond to acute lipolytic effect of catecholamines (and parathyroid hormones) while rat fat cells respond to glucagon and ACTH as well.
(4) In conventional short-term incubations responsiveness to cortisol and growth hormone shown for rat cells but not for human adipocytes.
(5) Inhibitory α-receptors present in human fat cells but not evident in rat fat cells.
(6) Adenosine possible feed-back regulator and inhibits lipolysis in rat fat cells but not in human fat cells.

hormone. Several hormones, such as glucagon and ACTH, which are lipolytic in rat fat cells do not give an acute lipolytic effect in human cells (cf Galton & Bray, 1967; Nyberg, Häger & Smith, 1977). In addition, responsiveness to other hormones, such as growth hormone and cortisol, has been reported with rat fat cells (Fain, Kovacev & Scow, 1965; Fain & Czech, 1974) but not with human fat cells using conventional incubation techniques (cf Galton & Bray, 1967). However, it has recently been reported that human fat cells also possess glucocorticoid receptors and, consequently, responsiveness to these agents may be anticipated (Feldman & Loose, 1977). However, it seems that human fat cells respond more sluggishly and that longer incubation periods are required to show effects of these hormones. Using the tissue culture technique we have been able to show effects of both growth hormone (Nyberg & Smith, 1977) and cortisol (Cigolini & Smith, 1977). Cortisol in physiologic concentrations antagonizes the effect of insulin (Cigolini & Smith, 1977) and growth hormone reduces glucose metabolism (Nyberg & Smith, 1977) as pointed out above.

Other differences between human and rat fat cell metabolism are the presence of α-receptors with inhibitory effects on lipolysis (Östman & Efendic, 1970; Burns & Langley, 1970) in human fat cells but these do not appear to be present in rat fat cells (Burns & Langley, 1970). Furthermore, adenosine exerts a feedback regulation on rat fat cell lipolysis (Fain, Pointer & Ward, 1972) but this does not appear to be the case with human fat cells (Smith *et al.*, 1976*b*).

Since the only hormones of a clear physiologic importance which exert a direct lopolytic action are the catecholamines, it is of importance to investigate the regulation of catecholamine-stimulated lipolysis. First of all, there does not appear to be catecholamine-resistance in adipocytes from obese individuals. In fact, the sensitivity to these agents, defined as the concentration producing half-maximal effects, is the same in both small fat cells and in large fat cells (Gries *et al.*, 1972; Jacobsson *et al.*, 1976). However, the lipolytic capacity of large fat cells, defined as absolute lipolytic response to a given concentration, is increased in large fat cells (Jacobsson *et al.*, 1976).

Although there have been reports in the literature that catecholamine-responsiveness is reduced in large fat cells from old, fat rats (De Santis *et al.*, 1974), such data can not be directly extrapolated to apply to man due to species differences and to the fact that large adipocytes from rats are usually obtained from fatter and older animals. The age of the rat influences the metabolic rates tremendously (Holm *et al.*, 1975) and also the ability to respond to certain hormones (Holm *et al.*, 1975). Cooper, Weinblatt & Gregerman (1977) have indeed shown that the adenylate cyclase activity decreased with age whether the rats had large fat cells or not.

Since also the effect of dibutyryl cAMP is enhanced in large human fat cells (Gries *et al.*, 1972; Östman, Backman & Hallberg, 1973) the correlation between lipolytic capacity and cell size may well be due to an increased activity or effect of the triglyceride lipase. Again, however, it appears that the correlation between lipolytic capacity and fat cell size is not an obligatory phenomenon since it can be influenced by experimental manipulations. For instance, physical exercise (Holm *et al.*, 1977) and starvation (Reardon, Goldrick & Fidge, 1973) can lead to the loss of such correlations. It, thus, seems that other factors associated with obesity can lead to increased activity or effect of the triglyceride lipase. One such factor may be the increased insulin levels in obesity. Although the acute effect of insulin undoubtedly is to inhibit lipolysis, the effect of chronic exposure to a raised basal insulin level may well be different. Using the tissue culture technique we have maintained human fat cells for several days *in vitro* with different concentrations of insulin. The basal lipolysis as well as the responsiveness to a maximal concentration of catecholamine were studied in conventional 2-hr incubations following the culture period (Smith, 1974; Smith *et al.*, 1976*a*). Results of such studies do indeed demonstrate an increased basal lipolysis in the explants which had been cultured with insulin. Furthermore, the lipolytic effect of catecholamine was enhanced in the cells which had been cultured with insulin, as well (Smith, 1974; Smith *et al.*, 1976*a*). Thus, the chronic exposure to a high insulin level leads to an increased lipolytic capacity, possibly due to an increased activity of the triglyceride lipase since also the effect of dibutyryl cAMP is increased in these cells (Table 3). The sensitivity to insulin, however, was reduced in the cells cultured with insulin, as could be anticipated by the presence of high surrounding

Table 3. Lipolytic effect of dibutyryl cAMP on explants cultured with or without insulin. Explants from two patients were cultured for one week with or without insulin and then incubated for 2 hr as shown

Addition to short-term incubation	Additions during culture —	$+10^3$ μU/ml insulin
	glycerol release, nmoles/10^5 cells	
Basal	59	83
+ 5 x 10^{-5} mol noradrenaline	218	334
+ 1.0 mmol dibutyryl cAMP	291	394

insulin concentrations which, in turn, may modulate the cellular sensitivity to this hormone (cf Olefsky & Reaven, 1977). Thus, based on these and other data, it seems that the high insulin levels in obesity can produce some metabolic alterations found in large fat cells such as increased glucose metabolism and increased lipolysis. In addition to insulin, other hormonal and/or substrate levels may influence catecholamine-responsiveness in human fat cells. For instance, the presence of cortisol seems obligatory to maintain a normal lipolytic capacity (Sjöström, 1977). Furthermore, prolonged exposure to high catecholamine levels leads to a diminished responsiveness to these agents (Smith *et al.*, 1976*b;* Smith *et al.*, 1977), presumably due to several different changes.

Summarizing these data it seems that the release of fatty acids from human fat cells is regulated by different factors: (1) lipolysis stimulated by catecholamines (and parathyroid hormone?), (2) the cellular capacity and sensitivity to respond to catecholamines are influenced by the antecedent hormonal (and/or substrate) levels of insulin in particular. Also antecedent levels of other hormones such as cortisol and catecholamine are of importance for this response, and (3) availability of α-glycerophosphate influences the rate of reesterification.

These three regulatory mechanisms appear to be the most important ones for human adipocyte fatty acid release as judged from presently available data. A change in any of these factors or in the tissue lipoprotein lipase activity is of importance not only in different physiologic conditions but can also be of importance in different pathological conditions. In endogenous hypertriglyceridemia, for instance, we have found increased catecholamine-responsiveness in the fat cells coupled with low lipoprotein lipase activity (Larsson *et al.*, 1975). Both of these changes favor raised blood triglyceride levels. Furthermore, following physical exercise catecholamine-responsiveness of the fat cells is increased and this is also reflected in raised plasma fatty acid levels (Holm *et al.*, 1977). The effect of diabetes on fatty acid release has already been referred to.

References

Balasse, E. (1968): *Diabetologia* 4, 20.
Björntorp, P. & Karlsson, M. (1971): *Europ. J. Clin. Invest.* 1, 112.
Björntorp, P., Berchtold, P., Holm, J. & Larsson, B. (1971): *Europ. J. Clin. Invest.* 1, 480.
Bray, G.A. (1972): *J. Clin. Invest.* 51, 537.
Burns, T.W. & Langley, P.E. (1970): *J. Lab. Clin. Med.* 75, 983.
Cigolini, M. & Smith, U. (1978): Abstr. Second Int. Congress on Obesity 1977. *Int. J. Obesity* 2, (in press).
Cooper, B., Weinblatt, F. & Gregerman, R.I. (1977): *J. Clin. Invest.* 59, 467.
Davidson, M.B. (1975): *Diabetes* 2, 1086.
De Santis, R.A., Gorenstein, T., Livingston, J.N. & Lockwood, D.H. (1974): *J. Lipid Res.* 15, 33.
DiGirolamo, M., Howe, M.D., Esposito, J., Thurman, L. & Owens J.L. (1974): *J.Lipid Res.* 15, 332.
Fain, J.N., Kovacev, V.P. & Scow, R.O. (1965): *J. Biol. Chem.* 240, 3522.
Fain, J.N., Pointer, R.H. & Ward, W.F. (1972): *J. Biol. Chem.* 247, 6866.
Fain, J.N. & Czech, M.P. (1974): In *Handbook of physiology,* 6. Endocrinology. Andrenal gland, p. 169, ed H. Blaschko, G. Sayers & A.D. Smith. Baltimore: Williams and Williams Co.
Feldman, D. & Loose, D. (1977): *Endocrinology* 100, 398.
Galton, D.J. & Bray, G.A. (1967): *J. Clin. Invest.* 46, 421.
Galton, D.J. & Wilson, J.P.D. (1970): In *Adipose tissue. Regulation and metabolic functions,* ed B. Jeanrenaud & D. Hepp. New York: Academic Press.
Gilbert, C.H., Kaye, J. & Galton, D.J. (1974): *Diabetologia* 10, 135.
Goldrick, R.B. & Galton, D.J. (1974): *Clin. Sci. Molecul. Med.* 46, 469.
Gozariu, L., Forster, K. Faulhaber, J.D., Minne, H. & Ziegler, R. (1974): *Horm. Metab. Res.* 6, 243.
Gries, F.A., Berger, M., Neumann, M., Preiss, H., Liebermeister, H., Hesse-Wortmann, C. & Jahnke, K. (1972): *Diabetologia* 8, 75.
Holm, G., Jacobsson, B., Björntorp, P. & Smith, U. (1975): *J. Lipid Res.* 16, 461.
Holm, G., Jacobsson, B., Holm, J., Björntorp, P. & Smith, U. (1977): *Int. J. Obesity.* 1, 249.
Jacobsson, B., Holm, G., Björntorp, P. & Smith, U. (1976): *Diabetologia* 12, 69.
Korn, E.D. (1955): *J. Biol. Chem.* 215, 1.
Larsson, B., Björntorp, P., Holm, J., Schersten, T., Sjöström, L. & Smith, U. (1975): *Metabolism* 24, 1375.

Nyberg, G. & Smith, U. (1977): *Horm. Metab. Res.* 9, 1.
Nyberg, G., Häger, A. & Smith, U. (1977): *Acta Paediatr. Scand.* **66**, 495.
Olefsky, J.M. & Reaven, G.M. (1977): *Diabetes* **26**, 680.
Östman, J. & Efendic, S. (1970): *Acta Med. Scand.* **187**, 471.
Östman, J., Backman, L. & Hellberg, D. (1973): *Acta Med. Scand.* **193**, 469.
Pykälistö, O.J., Smith, P.H. & Brunzell, J.D. (1975): *J. Clin. Invest.* **56**, 1108.
Randle, P.J., Garland, P.B., Hales, C.N. & Newsholme, E.A. (1963): *Lancet* **1**, 785.
Reardon, M.F., Goldrick, R.B. & Fidge, N.H. (1973): *J. Lipid. Res.* **14**, 319.
Robinson, D.S. (1963): *Adv. Lipid Res.* **1**, 133.
Salans, L.B., Knittle, J.L. & Hirsch, J. (1968): *J. Clin. Invest.* **47**, 153.
Sjöström, L. (1972): *Acta Med. Scand.* suppl. 544.
Sjöström, L. (1978): Abst. Second Int. Congress on Obesity 1977. *Int. J. Obesity* 2, (in press).
Smith, U. (1971): *J. Lipid Res.* 12, 65.
Smith, U. (1974): *J. Clin. Invest.* 53, 91.
Smith, U., Boström, S., Johansson, R. & Nyberg, G. (1976*a*): *Diabetologia* **12**, 137.
Smith, U., Isaksson, O., Nyberg, G. & Sjöström, L. (1976*b*): *Europ. J. Clin. Invest.* **6**, 35.
Smith, U., Sjöström, L., Sjöström, G., Isaksson, O. & Jacobson, B. (1977): *Europ. J. Clin. Invest.* (in press).
Walldius, G. & Rubba, P. (1976): *Scand. J. Clin. Lab. Invest.* **36**, 357.
Wilson, J.P.D., Gutman, R. & Galton, D.J. (1973): *Metabolism* 22, 913.

20
Fat cells and infant feeding

C.G.D. BROOK
The Middlesex Hospital, London, W1N 8AA, England.

A major gap in our knowledge of obesity in general and of fat cells in particular results from two facts; first that the majority of studies have been cross-sectional in design and secondly that they are usually retrospective in nature. Taking an obese subject and looking back to antecedent events may give altogether different answers from starting with the infant and following such an infant prospectively. For these reasons, whilst we believe still that the size and number of adipose cells an individual possesses must be important for the genesis of his body fatness and its response to environmental stimuli, there is no proof that this is so. Accordingly, in this paper I shall review what is known of normal adipose cell growth, what is known of adipose cell growth in obese subjects and, quite separately, the effects of genetics and infant feeding on these subjects.

Fat cell growth in the normal subject

White adipose tissue begins to appear in the fetus at the beginning of the third trimester and macroscopically there is a rapid increase in the size of the adipose organ through the first year of life. In infancy and in early childhood it is generally agreed that most of the increase in size of the adipose organ appears to take place through the filling of existing adipocytes with fat (Hager, 1977) so the laying down of adipocytes in normal subjects seems to take place early in adipose organogenesis (Greenwood & Hirsch, 1974). Adipocytes differ both in size and in the chemical composition of the triglyceride they contain according to where they are found in the body (Brook, 1971; Duckerts & Bonnet, 1973); the reason for these site differences are unknown.

During childhood the size of the adipose cells changes much less so that increase in size of the adipose organ has to be accommodated in an increased number of cells. Exactly where in terms of chronological age the changeover from increasing cell size to increasing cell number takes place is a matter of discussion. Bonnet *et al.* (1970) found no change in cell size from age five to 15 years but their youngest subjects were five years old. Hager (1977) found that gluteal fat cell size was the same in 18-month-old infants, eight-year-old girls and 22-year-old women; adipose cell size increased only in the first year of life. These data tallied with those of Knittle (1972) who found adipose cell size stationary between two and ten years and to increase slightly after this age. Recent data from him, however, indicate a progressive increase in cell size during childhood (Knittle, 1977) so the matter is plainly not yet resolved.

Figure 1 shows how body fatness measured by triceps and subscapular skinfold thicknesses changes with age. There are two ages at which growth of subcutaneous fat changes direction. The first is at the end of the skinfold spurt of infancy and the second is around six to eight years when the increases of subcutaneous fat seen in puberty begin. It seems not improbable that the relative contributions which increases in fat cell size and fat cell number make to the changes in body fatness alter at these points of inflexion but such a suggestion is entirely

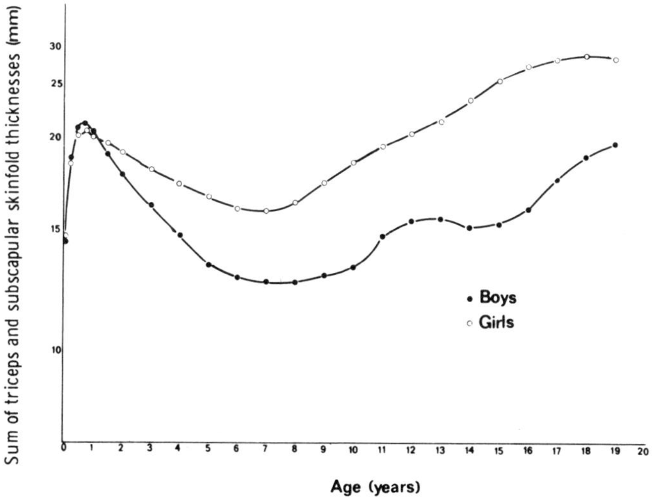

Fig. 1. Growth of body fat

speculative at present. None of the studies reported to date are of sufficient size alone to discern such trends and methodological differences make comparisons between studies very difficult. The resolution of the point awaits reports of longitudinal studies.

Fat cell growth in obese subjects

There is general agreement that obese individuals have larger fat cells than non-obese subjects and that some obese subjects have more fat cells than non-obese subjects. This has led to the concept of hyperplastic obesity, which is thought to originate in childhood, and hypertrophic obesity, which is thought to originate in adult life.

Overnutrition in early life in animals leads to an increase in the number of fat cells and malnutrition causes permanent reduction in the number of fat cells (Knittle & Hirsch, 1968). The same appears to be true of man (Brook, 1972). Whether the number of adipose cells in man can be altered later in life is not clear but the data of Salans, Cushman & Weismann (1973) do suggest that hypercellularity may arise not only in infancy but also in puberty. The finding of pockets of small preadipocytes in animals (Kirkland *et al.*, 1975; Ashwell, Priest & Sowter, 1975) raises the possibility of recruitment of adipose cells later. The point has been well made, however, that how many fat cells there are does not affect how fat an individual may become (Widdowson & Shaw, 1973).

Whatever the mechanisms by which fat cells are laid down it seems unlikely that they can later be lost. There are some data to suggest that the number of fat cells an obese individual has may affect the response of obesity to diet (Hager, 1977) but more studies are required in this area.

If for the moment it is accepted that the adipose organ enlarges by differing combinations of increases in cell size and cell number at different ages, something very different happens in obese subjects. These individuals are on their own from the outset with an increased number of adipose cells, which, according to Knittle (1977), go on increasing. To explain these data it is necessary to consider either a genetic predisposition to increased adipose cellularity or a trigger action of environmental origin.

Genetic and environmental influences

The balance of evidence now suggests that obesity in infancy carries a much better prognosis than obesity in childhood. Thus the likelihood of an environmental stimulus begins to seem less attractive than a genetic predisposition to adipose tissue hypercellularity. Here Knittle (1977) has some interesting new data: examining the number and size of adipose cells of the infants of obese and non-obese parents, he found that the infants of obese parents were identical to their controls up to one year of age but that after that, the number and the size of adipose cells of the infants of obese parents went on increasing at a steady rate whereas adipose cell size and number of infants of non-obese parents ceased increasing rapidly at this age.

Thus far, there are no studies of adipose tissue cellularity which allow any statement of the quantitative genetic contribution to size and number. Body fatness, however, is as strongly genetically determined as most other anthropometric quantities so that it would not be surprising if fat cell number was subject to similar influences. In no way, however, is this to say that environmental influences should be dismissed. All that it means is that the more strongly a characteristic is genetically determined, the more vigorous has an environmental influence to be to change it.

Consequently, it is possible to consider the following hypothesis. Some infants are raised with a genetic predisposition both to obesity and to an increased number of adipose cells. Others, by dint of an extreme environmental stimulus of overfeeding in infancy, can be induced to recruit or replicate adipose cells at a time when most of the enlargement of the adipose organ should be taking place by adipose cell enlargement. Other infants might well become obese with a less strong stimulus and such infants would not have been exposed to an influence strong enough to alter their genetically determined pattern of adipose cellularity. Thus hypertrophic and hyperplastic types of obesity could arise at the same time of life. Such a hypothesis could easily account for variations amongst obese populations and would explain why Ashwell, Priest & Bondoux (1975), for example, failed to differentiate adipose cellularity of obese women on grounds of age at onset of obesity.

In all the studies mentioned the problem is always that of looking at the obese individual and looking backwards to see what went before. What is needed is to follow a large cohort of infants prospectively and if this is done it might be possible to formulate answers to the three basic questions in this field. First, is it possible to have adipose hypercellularity and not to be obese: does the number of fat cells an individual has matter? Secondly, can obesity associated with hyperplasia of adipose cells in infancy be prevented? Thirdly, what is the relation between adipose cellularity of parents and their children?

Summary

Growth of the adipose organ probably takes place through differing combinations of increases in adipose cell size and number at different ages. There is evidence to suggest that infants becoming extremely obese and having many fat cells may be different from other infants. This difference may be partly genetically and partly environmentally determined. Prospective studies of the size and number of adipose cells are required to determine the genetic contribution to adipose cellularity and to determine whether the number of adipose cells an individual has matters to him.

References

Ashwell, M., Priest, P. & Bondoux, M. (1975): In *Recent advances in obesity research:* I, ed. A.N. Howard, p. 74. London: Newman.

Ashwell, M., Priest, P. & Sowter, C. (1975): *Nature* **256**, 724.

Bonnet, F., Gosselin, L., Chantraine, J. & Senterre, J. (1970): *Rev. Europ.Etudes Clin. Biol.* **15**, 1101.

Brook, C.G.D. (1971): *Br. J. Nutr.* **25**, 377.

Brook, C.G.D. (1972): *Lancet* **2**, 624.

Duckerts, M. & Bonnet, F. (1973): *Biomedicine* **19**, 214.

Greenwood, M.R.C. & Hirsch, J. (1974): *J. Lipid Res.* **15**, 474.

Hager, A. (1977): *Pediatric implications for some adult disorders,* ed D. Barltrop, p. 101. London: Fellowship of Postgraduate Medicine.

Kirtland, J., Gurr, M.I., Saville, G. & Widdowson, E.M. (1975): *Nature* **256**, 723.

Knittle, J.L. (1972): *J. Pediat.* **81**, 1048.

Knittle, J.L. (1977): In Proceedings of Serono Symposium No. 17 on Obesity in Childhood, Bologna, Italy (in press).
Knittle, J.L. & Hirsch, J. (1968): *J. Clin. Invest.* 47, 2091.
Salans, L.B., Cushman, S.W. & Weismann, R.E. (1973): *J.Clin. Invest.* 52, 929.
Widdowson, E.M. & Shaw, W.T. (1973): *Lancet* 2, 905.

21
THE REGULATION OF ENERGY EXPENDITURE IN MAN

J.S. GARROW
Medical Research Council, Clinical Research Centre, Watford Road, Harrow, England.

In a recent paper Konishi & Harrison (1977) listed the 'weight gain equivalents of selected foods'. They stated the energy content of, say, an apple, calculated how many apple-equivalents there were in a kilogram of weight gain, and by simple division stated for how many days one would have to eat an extra apple to gain a kilogram of weight.

I wrote to the editors of the journal to say that although the arithmetic was correct, the logic was poor, but I have had no reply, so probably they thought I was another charlatan who denied the laws of thermodynamics. I do not: I have repeatedly stated my faith in the validity of the energy balance equation (Garrow, 1974), namely:

Change in energy stores = energy input minus energy output.

No one can lay down extra fat (energy stored) unless they take in more energy (food) than they expand, nor can they lose stored energy unless the balance is tipped in the other direction. However, the calculations quoted above are false because they incorrectly assume that if you alter two components of the equation the third is unaffected. I hope to convince you that energy expenditure is regulated in many subtle ways, and that changes in energy input or in energy stores, will themselves bring about changes in energy output so that, in fact, an extra apple a day for 267 weeks cannot be expected to convert to 25 kg of adipose tissue. Farmers have known for generations that even the most efficient breeds of livestock have a food conversion efficiency less than 100 per cent, so it should not surprise human nutritionists that our food efficiency is also less than 100 per cent.

For the purpose of this review I shall assume that energy expenditure can be changed only in metabolic rate. This is not quite true, but nearly so, if one excepts abnormal conditions like glycosuria and steatorrhoea. Severely ketotic patients may lose 2 g per day of ketones in the urine (Kekwick, Pawan & Chalmers, 1959) but in terms of energy loss this is trivial. Enthusiasts for high fibre diet (Reuben, 1976) say it will 'impair the ability of the small intestine to absorb calories', but in fact faecal losses remain close to 5 per cent of intake over a wide range of diets (Masterton, Lewis & Widdowson, 1959) and adding 20 g of fibre to the diet increases faecal energy loss by only 4 per cent (Southgate & Durnin, 1970).

The factors which are known to affect human energy expenditure are set out in Table 1. Some, like age, sex and genetic disposition, we cannot do much about. But the others are potentially components of a control system which tends to alter energy expenditure so as to stabilise the energy stores of the body.

Recent advances in the technique of calorimetry (Blaxter, Brockway & Boyne, 1972; Webb, Annis & Troutman, 1972; Spinnler *et al.*, 1973; Garrow *et al.*, 1977) have made it possible to measure energy expenditure in man far more accurately than by intermittent indirect calorimetry (Garrow, 1974), and without the immense labour involved in the

Table 1. Factors known to influence energy expenditure in man

	Inevitable	Va
Resting metabolism	Age Sex (Genes)	Diet Lean Tempe Hormon (Stress)
Muscular work		Level of act Body weight Training (Diet)

pioneering efforts of Atwater & Benedict (1899). It is now possible to show that differences in metabolic rate between people matched for age, sex and surface area are not due to measurement error, but represent a real individual variation of at least 15 per cent above and below the mean value (Warwick, Toft & Garrow, 1978).

Regulation of resting metabolic rate

Individual variation in resting metabolic rate does not constitute regulation, but it makes regulation more difficult to study. The literature on obesity is full of statements which are apparently sound, but which are mutually contradictory. Thus, Newburgh (1944) after an exhaustive review of the available literature concluded that obese people 'produce more heat in the basal state, that they expend more energy to perform a measured amount of work and that their total heat production is greater than that of normal persons of similar age, height and sex under the same circumstances. Since they are unable to absorb more energy from their food, they must eat more than normal people simply to avoid loss of weight.' However, Thomson, Billewicz & Passmore (1961) analysed many dietary surverys, found no evidence that obese people ate more than thin ones, and concluded that 'heaviness is associated with diminished physical activity'. Finally, to complete the cycle, Gwinup (1975) persuaded 11 obese women to walk 70 to 200 minutes per day for a year and observed that they lost less weight than theory might predict, so he concluded that they must have increased their food intake! These examples are given to illustrate the point that the cause of obesity is astonishingly difficult to pin down, and when an investigator fails to find it in the variables he *has* measured he tends to infer that it can safely be ascribed to some factor he has *not* measured.

Lest I fall into the same trap, I will concentrate for the remainder of this review on observations which have been made under well controlled conditions in which serial measurements are made on the same subject, or in which obese subjects and well matched lean controls are subjected to the same test procedure.

Underfeeding

There is ample evidence that when either lean or obese people are put into negative energy balance their resting metabolic rate falls. This was clearly shown by Benedict *et al.* (1919) in their classical study of caloric restriction in normal young men, and confirmed in the Minnesota experiment 30 years later (Keys *et al.*, 1950). The same effect has repeatedly been shown whenever reasonably accurate measurements have been made on obese patients on a reducing diet (Bray, 1970; Apfelbaum, Bostsarron & Lacatis, 1971; Garrow *et al.*, 1978). Here then, is at least a rudimentary control system: when the energy supply is reduced the resting energy expenditure falls, and hence tends to protect the energy stores from excessive depletion. To increase the chance of survival in famine this is a useful adaptation, but for the obese patient trying to lose weight it is a source of frustration. Most of the 1500 kcal or so used by an average person at rest must be used for some housekeeping chore within the cell. The best candidates are either the work involved in maintaining the large concentration gradient between potassium inside the cell and sodium outside (the 'sodium pump'), or the process of turning over tissue protein.

Thyroid hormones increase metabolic rate, but this does not resolve the difficulty, since if [illegible]roid on protein turnover is blocked, the expected increase in metabolic rate [illegible]ur (Tata, 1964), but equally thyroid hormone increases the activity of the [illegible]pump in at least liver, kidney and muscle (Edelman & Ismail-Beigi, 1974). My own [illegible]urite candidate is the effect on protein turnover (Garrow, 1974), since obese patients can be shown to decrease protein turnover during weight loss (Sender, James & Garlick, 1975) and the effect is very marked in malnourished children (Garrow, 1957). However, a definitive answer to this controversy will not be forthcoming until we have better techniques for measuring the rate of sodium pumping and of protein turnover in human subjects in different nutritional states.

Statements in the older literature that obese people have 'no abnormality in thyroid status' mean that the crude test of plasma thyroxin is within normal limits. Recently developed assays for the more potent hormone 3,5,3′-triiodothyronine (T_3) and the inactive analogue reverse 3,3′,5-triiodothyronine (rT_3) provide a much more interesting picture. During a period of total starvation for 10 days, the 12 normal subjects studied by Palmblad *et al.* (1977) showed a marked decrease in T_3, and increase in rT_3, but only a modest decrease in thyroxin or thyroid stimulating hormone. Drs R.L. Himsworth and P. Byfield have been making similar studies on our obese patients on reducing diets, and finding similar effects. It seems, therefore, that we are on the threshold of a better understanding of the endocrine response which mediates the fall in metabolic rate with reduced energy intake.

Thermogenesis and overfeeding

The terms 'specific dynamic action', 'thermic effect of food', 'thermogenesis' and 'luxus-consumption' are used variously by different authors, and it is hard to find a terminology which will suit everyone.

With sufficiently accurate calorimetry it may be shown that the increase in heat production is rather greater with protein than carbohydrate, and with carbohydrate than fat (Blaxter, 1975) but the difference is small and in human subjects we were unable to detect it (Garrow & Hawes, 1972). The term 'specific dynamic action' is inappropriate in human nutrition, since it has come to be associated with a specific action of protein which is not specific at all. I will, therefore, use the term 'thermogenesis' to mean increase in heat production in the resting subject and 'dietary-induced thermogenesis' when it is caused by increased food intake (Miller & Mumford, 1973). Whatever nomenclature is used it is clear that a person who is fed uses more energy at rest than a similar person who is fasted, so this again provides a small measure of regulation. It must be noted that the total extra energy expended as a result of a meal is only about 10 per cent of the energy value of the meal, so in itself this effect would have only a trivial influence on stabilising the energy stores of the body. The point on which there has been heated controversy concerns the cumulative effect of a series of large meals. Does each meal have its thermic effect which dies away, or merges into the thermic effect of the next meal, or is there really a resetting of the level of metabolic rate in the overfed subject so that more energy than usual is expended both at rest and also during exercise?

The conservative view was expressed in an unsigned editorial (1970) which states flatly 'There are no satisfactory experiments on dogs or man indicating that a luxusconsumption mechanism exists. When a subject has been overfed, his metabolism at 8.00 a.m. (some 10 hr after the last evening meal) is at the same level as on normal intake days.' This is hardly a fair summary of the situation in 1970, and more recent work has made this stance still less tenable. In Table 2 the publications relevant to dietary-induced thermogenesis or luxus-consumption are summarised for the past 75 years. All the studies involve experimental overfeeding of human volunteers, of which 57 were initially lean and 23 were already obese before the overfeeding began. In some studies the amount overfed differed between subjects within the group, or can only be indirectly estimated, so the column 'Excess Mcal' is an estimated average which is probably not in error by as much as 10 per cent in any except Neumann (1902), where the estimate of overfeeding depends on how his 'requirements' are assessed. In every paper in which resting metabolic rate was made, it is reported to be raised

Table 2. Is energy expenditure increased by overfeeding in man?

Authors	Date	Subjects Fat	Subjects Lean	Days overfed	Excess (Mcal)	Increased R.M.R?	Unexplained energy loss	Conclusion
Neuman	1902	–	1	365	?100	?	yes	yes
Gulick	1922	–	1	73	51	?	yes	yes
Passmore *et al.*	1955	–	3	14	22	yes	NO	NO
Mann *et al.*	1955	–	3	20	60	?	(no) yes	yes
Ashworth *et al.*	1962	–	3	36	72	?	yes	yes
Passmore *et al.*	1963	2	–	9	10	yes	NO	NO
Miller *et al.*	1967	–	4	50	70	yes	(yes)	yes
Strong *et al.*	1967	9	7	4	6	yes	NO	NO
Sims *et al.*	1968	–	9	160	400	?	yes	yes
Durnin & Norgan	1969	–	4	42	70	yes	no(?)	no
Apfelbaum *et al.*	1971	8	–	15	23	yes	–	yes
Whipp *et al.*	1973	–	4	35	120	yes	–	yes
Garrow & Stalley	1975	–	1	60	80	?	yes	yes
Goldman *et al.*	1975	–	4	83(fat)	72	yes	no	yes
		–	9	18(CHO)	33	yes	no	yes
Glick *et al.*	1977	4	4	5	12	no	NO	NO

during the overfeeding period, with a single exception of Glick *et al.* (1977). The column 'unexplained losses' shows considerable divergence of interpretation. In the 15 publications in which it is possible to draw up a balance sheet of observed increase in metabolic rate plus estimated energy stores as weight gain, and to compare this with the excess intake, seven report that there are no significant discrepancies in the account. Of these, two (Goldman *et al.*, 1975) achieve a satisfactory balance sheet and conclude that there *is* thermogenesis during overfeeding (but less if the overfeeding is with fat than with carbohydrate), while the remaining five papers conclude that their balance sheets show there is no significant thermogenesis. In one of these (Durnin & Norgan, 1969), the arithmetic on the results reported does not support the conclusion that 'only a small part of the excess was burned off'. The relevant data then are, six men overate by 70 Mcal in 42 days and gained 6 kg. There is no known body component which can accomodate 70 Mcal in 6 kg, since 6 kg of anhydrous fat would only store 54 Mcal and at the more probable energy density of tissue stored in such circumstances of 6 Mcal/kg (Garrow, 1974) the weight gain accounts for about half the excess intake, so on conservative assumptions the proportion burned off is about the other half. For this reason the entry 'no' in the unexplained losses column for this paper is marked with a query.

This selection process leaves four studies which provide evidence against any energy wasting mechanism during overfeeding: Passmore *et al.* (1955); Passmore *et al.* (1963); Strong, Shirling & Passmore, (1967); Glick *et al.* (1977). The remaining publications either directly support the idea of some form of luxusconsumption or provide data which are difficult to understand unless some such mechanism exists. It may be possible to resolve the difficulty by examining the size of the energy overload in relation to the conclusion. The largest load which failed to produce demonstrable thermogenesis was that of the three thin men studied by Passmore *et al.* (1955) who ate an extra 22 Mcal, while the smallest load with which this effect was seen was the 23 Mcal fed to the eight women studied by Apfelbaum *et al.* (1971). It might be, therefore, that a certain critical size of overload, around 20 Mcal, is necessary before the thermogenesis effect becomes detectable. This idea is supported by a close inspection of the results of Mann *et al.* (1955). Their experiment was mainly concerned with the effect of exercise on blood lipids during overfeeding, and the part of the experiment abstracted in Table 2 concerns a period, during which their three volunteers were overeating by about 3000 kcal per day but had ceased to undertake the very vigorous exercise programme which had previously prevented weight gain. For the first 10 days of this phase they gained 4.7 kg, so if this represents the excess of 30 Mcal, the energy value of storage tissue is 6.38 Mcal/kg, which is exactly what might be expected if there had been no luxusconsumption.

However, the experiment continued with the same regimen for another 10 days, during which weight increased by only 1.3 kg. An energy value for storage tissue of 23 Mcal/kg is obviously absurb, so it seems that, having stored the first 30 Mcal of excess energy fairly efficiently in the first 10 days, the subjects altered their metabolism in some way so that the next 30 Mcal were largely unaccounted for by weight gain.

It has been argued by Glick *et al.* (1977) that since their own very careful studies, as well as others listed in Table 2, had failed to show thermogenesis during short periods of overeating, 'it appears that it does not play a role in regulating energy balance of those individuals who indulge in overeating periodically', although it may do for those who have long bouts of overeating, or are chronically overfed. This is an important point on which there is no direct experimental evidence: we do not know how the magnitude of the energy overload is integrated by whatever detects it, nor do we know how the thermogenic action is mediated when it does come into action. These are subjects on which there has been much speculation to which I will not add.

Exercise and thermogenesis

Miller, Mumford & Stock (1967) in their study which initiated the new wave of interest in dietary-induced thermogenesis as a factor in regulating energy balance, found little change in the resting metabolic rate of their overfed subjects, and commented: 'The small increase in oxygen consumption in the resting state did not account for the increased heat production of the overeating subjects. However, the consumption of oxygen over the 24 hours was considerably raised while overeating, and the apparent paradox may be resolved by the observation that the thermic effect was greatly increased while exercising.' The effect of exercise on enhancing thermogenesis after a meal has been either confirmed or refuted in the studies listed in Table 3. The question to be answered is: Does the increase in metabolic rate due to food and exercise taken together exceed the sum of the increases of each separately? Miller, Bradfield and Bray, and their associates, conclude it is greater, while Swindells (1972) and Hanson (1973), who looked for this effect, failed to find it. Apfelbaum *et al.* and Glick *et al.* were not specifically testing the theory, but their results do not support it, so apparently the voting is roughly equal, for and against.

Table 3. Is the thermic effect of (food + exercise) greater than that of (food) plus (exercise)?

Author	Date	Subjects		Conclusion
		Fat	Lean	
Miller *et al.*	1967	–	7	yes
Bradfield *et al.*	1968	6	–	yes
Swindells	1972	–	10	no
Hansen	1973	–	4	no
Apfelbaum *et al.*	1971	8	–	(no)
Bray *et al.*	1974	–	6	yes(?)
Glick *et al.*	1977	4	4	no

The problem is that the thermic response to food is variable (Garrow & Hawes, 1972; Bradfield & Jourdan, 1973) and if serial measurements of oxygen uptake are made after a meal in the morning the thermic effect of that meal is superimposed on the diurnal increase in metabolic rate which occurs during the morning and early afternoon (Aschoff & Pohl, 1970). Thus, some publications concerning the thermic effect of food involve a meal at about 10 a.m., show a peak in oxygen consumption about noon, and by 3 p.m. the subject is still far above the 'baseline' which had been carefully established in the early morning (eg, Kaplan & Leveille, 1976). Those investigators who are prudent enough to do a control study without food over the same period show a 'thermic effect' of *no* food of about 64 per cent of basal metabolic rate (Bradfield & Jourdan, 1973). Similarly, it is very difficult to get a subject to do the same amount of exercise on two successive tests. The demonstration that exercise enhances thermogenesis requires at least four experiments, each lasting several hours, for each subject: one to record the thermic effect of the meal, one to record the thermic effect of the exercise, one to record both and the last to record neither. My own unpublished efforts in this field have been unfruitful, since the tendency has been for exercise and food together to produce a smaller thermic effect than the sum of each separately, but in view of the errors discussed above I could not attribute much significance to this observation, except to conclude that the effect, if it exists, must be small.

Two studies which claim to show the enhancement of thermogenesis by exercise deserve to be studied in some detail. Elsewhere (Garrow, 1974) I have gone over the arithmetic of Miller *et al.* (1967) and, having had the opportunity to discuss the problem with those authors, it is probably fair to say that the apparent lack of effect of overfeeding on resting metabolic rate depends on the method of calculation. It is not necessary to postulate exercise-enhanced thermogenesis to explain all their results. However, a direct demonstration of this effect in three subjects is given by Bray, Whipp & Koyal (1974) who, in my opinion, are hoist with their own petard. Fig. 4 of that paper, which is repeated as Fig. 6 of Whipp *et al.* (1975), shows that oxygen consumption is about 0.2 kcal/minute greater, after a breakfast of 1000 or 3000 kcal, in subjects pedalling on a bicycle ergometer, than would be expected from the thermic effect of the meal and the exercise alone. This was consistent for all subjects, and seems to show that these very large breakfasts enhance the thermogenesis of the meal by some 15 per cent of basal heat production. The paper of Bray *et al.* (1974) follows one of Whipp, Bray & Koyal (1973), which is highly critical of a suggestion of Apfelbaum *et al.* (1971) that overeating decreased the efficiency of muscular work, and which contains a homily on the importance of correcting for the weight of the subjects' legs when assessing the effect of weight gain on work efficiency. The paper of Whipp *et al.* (1975) begins the discussion with the statement 'An increase in the O_2 utilization during muscular work does not necessarily mean that work efficiency is reduced.' Elsewhere in the same volume Goldman (1975) explains that heat production for a given task might alter weight gain, either as an effect of the extra weight which must be moved in performing the task, or as a result of the 'hobbling' effect of extra tissue which must be moved around the joints. For example, a man in a seven-layer clothing system uses 16 per cent more energy to perform the same task even when the weight of clothing is allowed for.

If we now apply all this physiological expertise to the subjects before and after a breakfast supplying 1000 or 3000 kcal, it is pertinent to enquire if an increase of 0.2 kcal per minute (according to the figure) or 0.05 kcal/min (according to the text) in the energy cost of pedalling a bicycle, might not represent the 'hobbling' effect of so large a breakfast? This explanation does not seem to have been considered by Whipp *et al.* (1975). I am not an expert in exercise physiology, but conclude that exercise potentiates thermogenesis either very little or not at all.

Does the thermic effect of food differ in lean and obese subjects?

Bradfield & Jourdan (1973) studied four obese subjects, and concluded that the thermic effect of a meal was not different from that which would be expected in lean subjects, and that the importance of the effect in regulating energy balance had been exaggerated. At least the latter part of the conclusion is probably correct, but it is of interest to see if lean and obese people react differently to meals in an effort to understand the physiology of obesity, even though the energy loss involved is trivial. Kaplan & Leveille (1976) claimed to show a greater thermic response in lean than fat subjects, but the results are rather unconvincing, since the metabolic rates do not return to baseline 5 hours after a meal of 823 kcal, and the difference between their four lean and four obese subjects only achieves significance at the 5 per cent level when the results are divided by body weight or fat-free weight.

More compelling evidence that obese people have a smaller thermic response to food comes from the report of Pittet *et al.* (1976) who studied the response to a 50 g load of glucose by ten lean and 11 obese women. They used both direct and indirect calorimetry, since they were interested in thermal balance, but the indirect measurements show that the lean subjects had an increase of 13.0 per cent during the 150 minutes after the load, whereas the obese subjects only increased their metabolic rate by 5.2 per cent: the difference is significant at $P<0.001$ by unpaired *t*-test. There is also a difference in heat storage which may be physiologically important. However, another study which also found a difference between lean and obese tendencies is that of Stordy *et al.* (1977). They studied anorectic women who were being refed to normal weight, and showed that these thin women had a greater thermic response to glucose than normal controls, but also that within the 15 anorectic patients the eight who had been previously obese had a smaller thermic response than the seven who had not been previously obese. Since these differences were found in women who were thin at the time of testing, it may indicate that the women who were previously obese have an inherently smaller propensity to thermogenesis even when the complicating factor of excess body fat is removed.

Response to cold

The layer of subcutaneous fat provides thermal insulation as well as being a chemical store of energy. Many workers have shown that if fat subjects are exposed to low temperatures in near-naked conditions they respond less than thin people at least over a certain temperature range. In the fat and thin subjects, clad only in shorts, which were studied by Wyndham, Williams & Loots (1968), their metabolic rate was similar between 20 to 25° C. When the temperature was decreased to 15° C the fat subject hardly altered his metabolic rate, while the lean subject increased his by 170 ml O_2 per min. While the temperature was progressively lowered this difference decreased, until at 5° C both had an uptake of about 580 ml O_2 per min. Quaade (1963) showed that if fat, average or lean subjects were placed for 30 minutes between blankets containing water cooled to 4° C the lean increased their metabolic rate by 33 per cent, the average subjects by 11 per cent and the obese by 2.5 per cent. There is an interesting analogy with genetically obese (*ob/ob*) mice, which, even before they are obviously obese at the age of 17 days, fail to maintain their temperature by thermogenesis when exposed to an ambient temperature of 4° C (Trayhurn, Thurlby & James, 1977). All this invites the hypothesis that thermal insulation in obese people protects them from the need for thermogenesis, so they do not use energy to keep warm, so they become more obese.

The flaw in this argument is that people in their right mind only rarely expose themselves naked to low temperatures whether they are fat or thin, so, unless these differences can be seen in the temperature range which occurs in real life, it seems unlikely that they are important regulating factors in real life. Jéquier *et al.* (1974) used 20° C as a cold stimulus, and showed interesting differences in thermal insulation between normal controls and people who were 110 to 130 per cent of ideal weight and over 150 per cent of ideal weight: the latter two groups have much greater insulation, which does not depend solely on the thickness of the fat layer. However, when the results of this study are examined with a view to the increased metabolism produced by the cold exposure there is not much difference in the three groups. It is possible that the thermal insulation associated with obesity might diminish the thermic effects of food eaten in the cold, but the work of Buskirk *et al.* (1960) and of Rochelle & Horvath (1969) does not support speculation along these lines. Finally, fat people might habitually chose a different temperature for comfort, and thereby reduce their energy requirements compared with lean people, but Fanger (1972) was unable to find any connection between body build and thermal comfort zone.

Stress and energy expenditure

Stress is difficult to define, and still more difficult to study. Conditions which are acknowledged to be stressful are tiring, and may be associated with increased muscle tone, but I have been unable to find evidence that psychological stress increases metabolic rate more than can be explained by muscular activity. Attempts in my own laboratory to measure oxygen uptake, heart rate and electromyogram in a resting subject, and then to induce stress to study the effect, have been more farcical than informative. If the subject is sufficiently anxious it is easy to demonstrate an increase in heart rate, as Moss & Wynar (1970) reported, but the effect on oxygen uptake is very small.

Patients often ascribe large weight changes, in either upward or downward direction, to stress, but it seems unlikely that this is due to change in energy expenditure, even when it is associated with marked fatigue. The release of adrenalin associated with stress affects lipolysis and the plasma concentration of free tryptophan (Gentil *et al.*, 1977) which may in turn affect food intake and hence body weight, but there is little evidence for this speculation.

Physical activity

Exercise is, I feel sure, good for us. I am prepared to extol its medical, social and metabolic benefits as long as I am not asked to say that it is the major factor determining energy expenditure, or energy intake, or energy balance, because I do not believe this is so. I am often taken to task for this view, and instructed to consult the paper of Mayer, Roy & Mitra (1956) who showed that in man, as in rats (Mayer *et al.*, 1954), there is a range of 'normal activity' in which calorie intake increases with activity, but that below that range there is a 'sedentary zone' in which decreasing activity is associated with increased food intake and increased obesity.

I find it easy to believe that jute workers in West Bengal who are engaged in 'light work' eat about 2800 kcal per day, and that those engaged in heavy work, heaving bales weighing 400 lb each, eat on average about 3500 kcal per day. I suggest that the difference of 700 kcal per day is about the maximum attributable to physical activity on a habitual basis. I am aware that champion cross-country skiers may use 7000 kcal in a day, which is about 5 kcal per minute throughout the 24 hours, but I doubt if they could do it again the following day, and for most non-athletes who have a living to earn, 2 hours a day at 4 kcal per minute is about as much as they can manage within the physical and social constraints which apply in our society. If this 120 minutes is spent walking briskly instead of sitting, and hence using 4 kcal per minute instead of 1 kcal per minute (to use rather generous estimates in both cases) the excess energy spent is 360 kcal, which hardly qualifies as a major factor in energy expenditure when other stimuli, which have been discussed above, may produce greater changes.

Proponents of exercise often use a curious form of accounting when considering the cost of long periods of exercise at low intensity. For example, 12 hours at 2.5 kcal per minute uses 1800 kcal. The arithmetic is correct, but the logic is not. In order to calculate the energy cost of exercise it is necessary to subtract the energy cost of whatever it is you would have been doing if you had not been taking the exercise. Let us take typical figures for a sedentary person, who uses 2400 kcal per day, who sleeps for 8 hours, and has a basal metabolic rate of 1 kcal per minute. If his metabolic rate was basal throughout the day he would use 1440 kcal per day, so that somehow, during his waking hours, he expends about 1000 kcal more than basal. This means that his average energy expenditure while awake is about 2 kcal/minute, the extra 1 kcal above basal being used by the thermic effect of his 2400 kcal intake, minor activity, and other metabolic activity. If this is taken into account the cost of 12 hours at 2.5 kcal per minute is 12 x 60 x (2.5 - 2.0), which is not 1800 kcal but 360 kcal, which is the same figure obtained for a shorter period of activity at a higher intensity.

The conclusion of Mayer *et al.* (1956) that there is a 'sedentary zone', in which with very low levels of activity food intake actually increases, relies on observations on 13 stall-holders, eight supervisors and 22 clerks who lived on the premises of the jute mill in West Bengal. These 43 individuals constituted the 'sedentary' group, and on average ate more, weighed more, and did less than the 'light work' group, which consisted of clerks who had to commute several miles to work on foot or by bicycle, or mechanics who had few power aids. The stall-holders and supervisors differed in income and diet from the clerks, so it is perhaps fairer to compare the 22 clerks who did not have to commute to work (and hence were classed as sedentary) with the clerks who did have to commute. If this comparison is made it appears that the sedentary clerks ate (on average) 500 kcal per day more than the commuting ones, but maintained a body weight of 109 lb (49 kg), while the commuting clerks weighed on average 120 lb (55 kg). Thus the alleged obesity of the sedentary group depends on including the very much heavier supervisors and stall-holders, but if only clerks are considered, inactivity seems to *protect* them from obesity! A more likely explanation is that the errors in data such as these are likely to be large enough to explain this apparent paradox.

So far as I know there has been no serious attempt to repeat this investigation, although there have been several publications relating to the level of activity of obese subjects which I have reviewed elsewhere (Garrow, 1974). Two recent studies are relevant to the effect of extremely low levels of activity on body weight. Greenleaf *et al.* (1977) report weight loss in men kept strictly at bed rest and fed 3073 kcal per day for 14 days, but this is due to loss of lean tissue and not fat. Warnold & Lenner (1977) were investigating the accuracy of heart rate as a measure of energy expenditure, and report an interesting experiment in which six young diabetics were studied for a period of 7 days during which they were 'extremely inactive', and another period of 7 to 11 days when they went to the hospital occupational therapy department and did a few hours of fast walking daily, which the authors rate as 'normal light activity'. Energy expenditure was increased by 25 per cent during the normal light activity period compared with the extremely inactive period, and food intake increased by 35 per cent. This is not what Mayer *et al.* (1956) would predict.

Exercise then, has medical, social and metabolic benefits which will no doubt be clearly stated by Björntorp, Farquhar, Durnin, Nelson and Horton during this Congress, and some of these speakers may even suggest that it is a major factor in regulating energy balance. I remain sceptical on this last point for the reasons stated above, but am open to instruction if there is evidence I have missed. However, if it is accepted that the level of physical activity cannot explain the large differences in energy expenditure which undoubtedly occur between individuals, I hope this may stimulate more work on the factors which affect resting metabolic rate. I believe it is in this sphere that progress is most likely to be made towards a better understanding of the control of energy balance in man. If that is achieved there is hope that by the time we have the next International Congress on Obesity we may have better ways to treat, or prevent, this condition.

Summary

Normal adults differ in energy expenditure, and hence in requirements over a threefold range. Even when matched for age, sex and weight (especially weight of lean tissue) individuals may still differ by 30 per cent.

An energy deficit or excess of about 120 MJ (30 Mcal) causes a decrease or increase in resting metabolic rate of about 15 per cent. The mechanism of dietary-induced thermogenesis is not understood.

Physical exercise in not the main factor in determining energy expenditure or energy intake in affluent societies. Exercise probably does not enhance dietary-induced thermogenesis. It is unrealistic to expect people to increase their energy expenditure by more than about 1.5 MJ (360 kcal) daily, although this may bring considerable benefits.

The economics of the human body, like that of households or nations, is such that a 10 per cent increase (or decrease) in energy intake will always cause less than a 10 per cent increase (or decrease) in the energy available for storage.

References

Apfelbaum, M., Bostsarron, J. & Lacatis, D. (1971): *Amer. J. Clin. Nutr.* 24, 1405.

Aschoff, J. & Pohl, H. (1970): *Fed. Proc.* 29, 1541.

Ashworth, N., Creedy, S., Hunt, J.N., Mahon, S. & Newland, P. (1962): *Lancet* 2, 685.

Atwater, W.O. & Benedict, F.G. (1899): *Bull. U.S. Dep. Agric.* No. 69.

Benedict, F.C., Miles, W.R., Roth, P. & Smith, M. (1919): Carnegie Institution of Washington, publication 280, p. 701.

Blaxter, K.L. (1975): Energy utilization and obesity. In *Obesity in perspective,* ed G. Bray, p. 127. Washington DC: US Gov. Ptg. Office.
Blaxter, K.L., Brockway, J.M. & Boyne, A.W. (1972): *Quart. J. Exp. Physiol.* 57, 60.
Bradfield, R.B. & Jourdan, M.H. (1973): *Lancet* 2, 640.
Bray, G.A. (1970): *Amer. J. Clin. Nutr.* 23, 1141.
Bray, G.A., Whipp, B.J. & Koyal, S.N. (1974): *Amer. J. Clin. Nutr.* 27, 254.
Buskirk, E.R., Thompson, R.H., Moore, R. & Whedon, G.D. (1960): *Amer. J. Clin. Nutr.* 8, 602.
Durnin, J.V.G.A. & Norgan, N. (1969): *J. Physiol. Lond.* 202, 106.
Edelman, I.S. & Ismail-Beigi, F. (1974): *Recent Prog. Horm. Res.* 30, 235.
Fanger, P.O. (1972): *Thermal Comfort,* p. 244. New York: McGraw-Hill.
Garrow, J.S. (1957): ^{35}S methionine uptake in protein-depleted Jamaican children. In *Aminoacid Malnutrition,* ed J.B. Allison, p. 14. New Brunswick: Rutgers University Press.
Garrow, J.S. (1974): *Energy balance and obesity in man.* Amsterdam: North-Holland Publishing Co.
Garrow, J.S., Durrant, M.L., Mann, S., Stalley, S.F. & Warwick, P. (1978): *Int. J. Obesity* 2, (in press).
Garrow, J.S. & Hawes, S.F. (1972): *Br. J. Nutr.* 27, 211.
Garrow, J.S., Murgatroyd, P., Toft, R. & Warwick, P. (1977): *J. Physiol. Lond.* 267, 16.
Garrow, J.S. & Stalley, S. (1975): *Proc. Nutr. Soc.* 34, 84A.
Gentil, V., Lader, M.H., Kantamaneni, B.D. & Curzon, G. (1977): *Clin. Sci. Mol. Med.* 53, 227.
Glick, Z., Shvartz, E., Magazanik, A. & Modan, M. (1977): *Amer. J. Clin. Nutr.* 30, 1026.
Goldman, R.F. (1975): Introduction to bioenergetics. In *Obesity in perspective,* ed G. Bray, p. 119. Washington DC: US Govt. Ptg. Office.
Goldman, R.F., Haisman, M.F., Bynum, G., Horton, E.S. & Sims E.A,H. (1975): Experimental obesity in man. Metabolic rate in relation to dietary intake. In *Obesity in perspective,* ed G. Bray, p. 165. Washington DC: US Govt. Ptg. Office.
Greenleaf, J.E., Bernauer, E.M., Juhos, L.T., Young, H.L., Morse, J.T. & Staley, R.W. (1977): *J. Appl. Physiol.* 43, 126.
Gulick, A. (1922): *Am. J. Physiol.* 60, 371.
Gwinup, G. (1975): *Archs Intern. Med.* 135, 676.
Hansen, J.S. (1973): *J.Appl. Physiol.* 35, 587.
Jéquier, E., Gygax, P-H, Pittet, P. & Vanotti, A. (1974): *J. Appl. Physiol.* 36, 674.
Kaplan, M.L. & Levielle, G.A. (1976): *Amer. J. Clin. Nutr.* 29, 1108.
Kekwick, A., Pawan, G.L.S., Chalmers, T.M. (1959): *Lancet* 2, 1157.
Keys, A., Brozek, J., Hanschel, A., Mickelson, O. & Taylor, H.L. (1950): *The biology of human starvation.* Minneapolis: University of Minnesota Press.
Konishi, F. & Harrison, S.L. (1977): *J. Amer. Diet. Assn.* 70, 365.
Mann, G.V., Teel, K., Hayes, O., McNally, A. & Bruno, D. (1955): *New Engl. J. Med.* 353, 349.
Masterton, J.P., Lewis, H.E. & Widdowson, E.M. (1957): *Br. J. Nutr.* 2, 346.
Mayer, J., Marshall, N.B., Vitale, J.J., Cristensen, J.H., Mashayekhi, M.B. & Stare, F.J. (1954): *Amer. J. Physiol.* 177, 544.
Mayer, J., Roy, P. & Mitra, K.P. (1956): *Amer. J. Clin. Nutr.* 4, 169.
Miller, D.S. & Mumford, P.M. (1973): Luxusconsumption. In *Energy balance in man,* ed M. Apfelbaum, p. 195. Paris: Masson.
Miller, D.S., Mumford, P. & Stock, M.J. (1967): *Amer. J. Clin. Nutr.* 20, 1223.
Moss, A.J. & Wynar, B. (1970): *Ann. Intern. Med.* 72, 255.
Neumann, R.O. (1902): *Arch. Hyg.* 45, 1.
Newburgh, L.H. (1944): *Physiol. Rev.* 24, 18.
Palmblad, J., Levi, L., Burger, A., Melander, A., Westgren, U, von Schenk, H. & Skude, G. (1977): *Acta Med. Scand.* 201, 15.
Passmore, R., Meiklejohn, A.P., Dewar, A.D. & Thow, R.K. (1955): *Br. J. Nutr.* 9, 20.
Passmore, R., Strong, J.A., Swindells, Y.E. & el Din, N. (1963): *Br. J. Nutr.* 17, 373.
Pittet, Ph., Chappuis, Ph., Acheson, K., de Techtermann, F. & Jéquier, E. (1976): *Br. J. Nutr.* 35, 281.
Quaade, F. (1963): *Lancet* 2, 429.
Reuben, D. (1976): *The save your life diet,* p. 160. London: Ebury Press.
Rochelle, R.H. & Horvath, S.M. (1969): *J. Appl. Physiol.* 27, 710.
Sender, P.M., James, W.P.T. & Garlick, P.H. (1975): Protein metabolism in obesity. In *Regulation of energy balance in man,* ed E. Jéquier. Geneva: Editions Medecine et Hygiene.
Sims, E.A.H., Goldman, R.F., Gluck, C.M., Horton, E.S., Kelleher, P.C. & Rowe, D.W. (1968): *Trans. Assn. Amer. Phys.* 81, 153.
Southgate, D.A.T. & Durnin, J.V.G.A. (1970): *Br. J. Nutr.* 24, 517.
Spinnler, G., Jéquier, E., Favre, R., Dolivo, M. & Vanotti, A. (1973): *J. Appl. Physiol.* 35, 158.
Stordy, B.J., Marks, V., Kalucy, R.S. & Crisp, A.H. (1977): *Amer. J. Clin. Nutr.* 30, 138.
Strong, J.A., Shirling, D. & Passmore, R. (1969): *Br. J. Nutr.* 21, 909.
Swindells, Y.E. (1972): *Br. J. Nutr.* 27, 65.

Tata, J.R. (1964): Advances in metabolic disorders. In *Basal metabolic rate and thyroid hormones,* ed R. Levine & R. Luft. New York: Academic Press.
Thomson, A.M., Billewicz, W.Z. & Passmore, R. (1961): *Lancet* 1, 1027.
Trayhurn, P., Thurlby, P.L. & James, W.P.T. (1977): *Nature* 266, 60.
Unsigned editorial (1970): *Amer. J. Clin. Nutr.* 23, 1009.
Warnold, I. & Lenner, R.A. (1977): *Amer. J. Clin. Nutr.* 30, 304.
Warwick, P.M., Toft, R. & Garrow, J.S. (1978): Abstr. Second Int. Congress on Obesity 1977. *Int. J. Obesity* 2, (in press).
Webb, P., Annis, J.F. & Troutman, S.J. (1972): *J. Appl. Physiol.* 32, 412.
Whipp, B.J., Bray, G. & Koyal, S.N. (1973): *Amer. J. Clin. Nutr.* 26, 1284.
Whipp, B.J., Bray, G., Koyal, S.N. & Wasserman, K. (1975): Exercise energetics and respiratory control in man following acute and chronic elevation of caloric intake. In *Obesity in perspective,* ed G. Bray, p. 157. Washington DC: US Govt. Ptg. Office.
Wyndham, C.H., Williams, C.G. & Loots, H. (1968): *J. Appl. Physiol.* 24, 282.

22
The biochemistry of energy expenditure

J.P. FLATT
University of Massachusetts Medical Centre, Worcester, Massachusetts 01605, USA.

The maintenance of adequate ATP levels is of key importance in guaranteeing the viability of cells. Since the pool of adenyl nucleotides is relatively small in comparison to the substrate flux of intermediary metabolism, the rate of ATP generation must be rapidly adjusted to the rate of ATP utilization. Indeed, a complex network of intracellular regulatory phenomena exists which is geared primarily to ensure the maintenance of a high 'adenylate charge' (Atkinson, 1968). The elucidation of the major metabolic pathways of intermediary metabolism has provided means to calculate with stoichiometric precision the amounts of ATP generated in the course of substrate oxidation. On the other hand, the utilization of ATP can only be approximately accounted for (cf. Baldwin & Smith, 1974). In the discussion presented here, various assumptions are made in an attempt to attribute the changes in the rates of resting energy expenditure to some known phenomena, and to the rates of ATP consumption which they imply. This evaluation is subject to future refinements as more precise estimates will become possible. In spite of their approximate nature, however, the evaluations presented here will lead to an overall picture giving a more relevant description of energy metabolism than one not including these considerations.

Figure 1 provides a schematic representation of the types of changes in energy expenditure which are elicited by daily events. The energy expenditure is roughly proportional to the

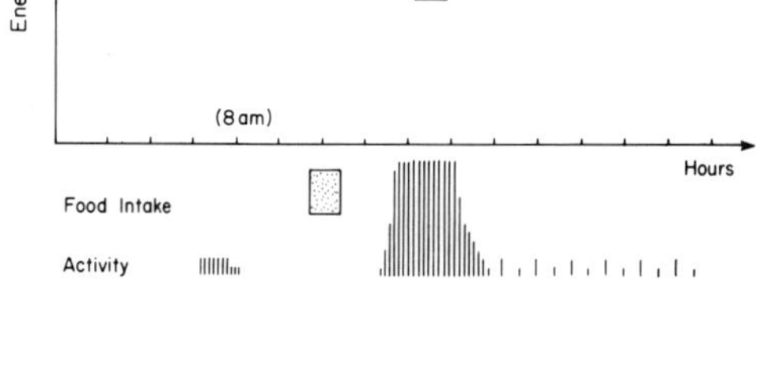

Fig. 1. Type of changes in Energy Expenditure during the day. The Basic Metabolic Rate is measured in the post-absorptive state in the morning, but is typically preceded by a period of increased energy expenditure when the subject is awakened and proceeds towards the laboratory where his oxygen consumption is to be measured. To obtain data truly representative of the Basal Metabolic Rate (BMR), it is important to allow enough time for the energy expenditure to decay after this period of stimulation. Increases in energy expenditure are brought about by consumption of food, ie the 'Specific Dynamic Action' (SDA) and by physical exercise. The figure also indicates that the Minimum Energy Expenditure (MEE) would be observed while the subject is asleep, and that the Resting Energy Expenditure (REE), as determined at rest later during the day, is usually considered to be approximately 20 per cent above Basal Energy Expenditure (BEE = BMR x Body Surface x 24 hours)

consumption of oxygen, since there is a relatively constant relationship between heat release per liter of oxygen consumed (cf. Table 1), as verified by the classical calorimetric studies (cf. Kleiber, 1975). Thus, the energy expenditure of a subject can be calculated quite accurately from data on his respiratory exchanges and urinary, ie nitrogen excretion and, indeed this form of 'indirect calorimetry' is the most commonly employed method for studying overall energy metabolism. Since substrate oxidation is tightly coupled to ATP generation, the determination of a subject's energy expenditure also gives a measure of his ATP production. For this reason, the words energy expenditure and energy production are often interchanged; although illogical in essence (Kleiber, 1975), no confusion usually results from such practice.

Table 1. High-energy bonds produced by substrate oxidation

(1) 1 Glucose + $6\,O_2 \xrightarrow[(5.03\ \text{kcal/l}\ O_2)]{RQ = 1.0} 6\,CO_2 + 6\,H_2O + 673\ \text{kcal}$ [(a)]
(+ 38 – 2 = + 36~)

(2) 1 Palmitate + $23\,O_2 \xrightarrow[(4.68\ \text{kcal/l}\ O_2)]{RQ = 0.70} 16\,CO_2 + 16\,H_2O + 2398\ \text{kcal}$ [(a)]
(+ 131 – 2 = + 129~)

(3) 1 AA + $5.1\,O_2 \xrightarrow[(4.18\ \text{kcal/l}\ O_2)]{RQ = 0.80} 4.1\,CO_2 + 0.7\ \text{Urea} + 2.8\,H_2O + 475\ \text{kcal}$ [(b)]
(+ 28.8 – 5.5 = + 23.3~)

(4) 4.5 Glucose + $4\,O_2 \xrightarrow[(7.06\ \text{kcal/l}\ O_2)]{RQ = 2.75} 1\ \text{Palmityl-} + 11\,CO_2 + 11\,H_2O + 630\ \text{kcal}$ [(c)]
(+ 40 – 34 = + 6~)

(a) Handbook of Chemistry and Physics, 51st edn, 1970, p. D 217.
(b) The stoichiometric coefficients for protein oxidation vary slightly depending on the amino acid composition. The example given here is for the oxidation of 110 g of beefsteak (cf. McGilvery, 1970). The heat of combustion was calculated using a value of 4.32 kcal/g protein (Geigy, Scientific Tables, 1970, page 539).
(c) (4.5 moles Gluc x 673 kcal/mole) – 2398 kcal/mole Palmitate = 630 kcal.
The stoichiometry of the reaction, including the production and utilization of high-energy bonds (~), is based on that reported for the conversion of glucose to fat in rat adipose tissue (Flatt, 1970).

Basal energy expenditure

The energy expended by different subjects is usually compared on the basis of their oxygen consumption measured after an overnight fast in the 'post-absorptive state', when it reflects primarily the subject's endogenous, or 'basal' rate of energy utilization. If a typical mixed diet is eaten, the Respiratory Quotient (RQ) is in the range of 0.80 to 0.84, and the caloric expenditure can be calculated using a value of 4.83 kcal per liter of oxygen consumed. It has long been recognized that resting energy expenditure is related more directly to the body surface (calculated from body weight and height) than to the body weight. Individual energy expenditures are, therefore, most commonly expressed in terms of kcal per square meter of body surface per hour (or in terms of watts per square meter), and referred to as the 'Basal Metabolic Rate' (BMR). The BMR is judged in relation to various tabulations giving values as a function of age and sex (eg, Geigy, Scientific Tables). It may be noted that the minimal energy expenditure would be observed by measuring during a subject's overnight sleep, when it is some 10 per cent less than under basal conditions. When a subject is physically inactive during the day, but after his metabolism has been stimulated intermittently by food consumption, physical activity and in response to diurnal rhythms, his energy expenditure is generally considered to be some 20 per cent higher than under basal conditions. This rate, extrapolated over 24 hours, describes his 'Resting Energy Expenditure' (REE), a value often used to evaluate his energy intake requirements with additional allowances for physical activity (Fig.1).

While the average Basal Energy Expenditure (BEE) of a group of men or women of similar age and body composition can be predicted rather accurately from their body weights and heights, individual variations in BEE can be appreciable (Garrow, 1974). The degree of variability of BEE is still a topic of some dispute. It is an important issue, especially in dealing with the problem of obesity, because differences in resting energy expenditure could have considerable effects on cumulative energy balance, particularly in affluent societies where the physiological regulation of food intake tends to be dominated by social factors (Garrow, 1974).

The variability in BEE suggests that differences in metabolic efficiencies may exist, but such a conclusion must be tempered by the realization that normalizing energy expenditure in relation to body surface is not necessarily an accurate procedure. It does not, for instance, account for differences in body composition. Table 2 illustrates the extent to which changes in body composition may be expected to alter the Basal Metabolic Rate (BMR): the body composition of a hypothetical '70 kg-standard' adult man was modified to cover a range of deviation of ± 40 per cent from Ideal Body Weight (IBW). Calculation A uses the body surface to predict the BMR, whereas calculation B assumes that energy expenditure is proportional to the Body Cell Mass (BCM). The differences between the latter value and the conventional one based on body surface (last column of the table) amount to ± 15 per cent. This suggests that many observations on the variability of BMR, and a trend toward reduced rates in obese individuals, may be attributed to changes in Body Cell Mass in relation to body weight. If one considers further, the possible effects of changes in muscle tone, or residual effects of the preceding day's food consumption, as well as the limitations on the accuracy of respiratory measurements, there are considerable reasons for measured BMRs to be variable, but still within a range 'covered' by present knowledge. Thus, it remains to be established whether the observed variability of the BMR warrants the need to assume the existence of other phenomena capable of modifying metabolic efficiency, particularly if the cost of different rates of 'substrate traffic' or renewal of body components is also considered.

Specific dynamic action of foods

After ingestion of food, an increase in energy expenditure occurs, a phenomenon known as the 'Specific Dynamic Action' (SDA) (or 'Thermic effect of food') (cf. Kleiber, 1975). The increase in energy expenditure is related to the caloric content of the food ingested. SDA values commonly assigned to different nutrients are: 5 to 10 per cent for carbohydrates, 0 to 3 per cent for fat, 20 to 30 per cent for proteins; for mixed diets, an SDA of 10 per cent is usually assumed. The increase in energy expenditure is due primarily to the metabolic cost of transporting and converting the absorbed nutrients into their respective storage forms. The metabolic pathways into which absorbed nutrients may be channelled are shown schematically in Figures 2, 3 and 4, where numbers describe how many moles of ATP are expended and gained per mole of substrate. The amounts of ATP which need to be expended for the processing of the absorbed nutrients can be used to evaluate the SDA. It is necessary at this point to decide how much energy is expended per mole of ATP required for processes such as the synthesis of glycogen, fat, protein and urea (Table 3). The classical value of -7 kcal for the hydrolysis of one mole of ATP under standard conditions has no physiological significance, since the concentration of the reactants is not taken into account. In red blood cells, for example, the concentrations of ATP, ADP and inorganic phosphate are such that the ΔG for the hydrolysis of ATP is -12.9 kcal per mole (Lehninger, 1975). Studies of oxidative phosphorylation indicate that this process occurs at near equilibrium conditions, so that essentially all the energy liberated when reducing equivalents pass a phosphorylating site will be recovered in the high-energy bond of ATP (Wilson *et al.*, 1974). Based on the difference in the redox state between the mitochondrial NAD and cytochrome C couples in isolated liver cells, this corresponds to a ΔG of 12.4 kcal/mole of ATP formed (Wilson *et al.*, 1974). However, chemical energy is lost at most of the many other steps in the degradation of sub-

Table 2. Energy expenditure and changes in body composition

Body weight	Ideal body weight	Skeleton	Interstitial Compartment	Adipose tissue fat	Body cell mass	Body surface	BMR	Energy expenditure 'A'	Body cell mass	Energy expenditure 'B' (f)	B-A/A
(kg)	(%)	(kg)	(kg)	(kg)	(kg)	(m^2)	($kcal/m^2/h$)	(kcal/day)	(kcal/kg)	(kcal/day)	(%)
53[c]	76	7	20	5	21	1.66	36.5	1450	69 !	1230	−15
60[b]	86	7	17.5	5	30	1.75	36.5	1530	51 !	1760	+15
70[a]	100	7	17.5	17.5	28	1.87[a]	36.5[a]	1640	59	1640	(0)
84[d]	120	7	17.5	29.5	30	2.02	36.5	1770	59	1760	−1
98[e]	140	7	17.5	43.5	28	2.16	36.5	1890	68 !	1640	−13

(a) Assuming a 40-year-old male with a height of 178 cm – Geigy, Scientific Tables, 7th edition, Ciba-Geigy, Basel, 1970, p.537 and 540.
(b) 'Active-type', ie decrease in adipose tissue and some increase in Body Cell Mass.
(c) Undernourished individual, with losses of adipose tissue and of Body Cell Mass, and trend towards nutritional edema.
(d) Overweight individual, with appreciable increase in adipose tissue and small increase in Body Cell Mass.
(e) Obese individual, with considerable increase in adipose tissue, but without increased Body Cell Mass.
(f) Assuming energy expenditure to be proportional to the weight of the Body Cell Mass, and amounting to 58.6 kcal/kg Body Cell Mass as in the normal individual.

Table 3. Energy exchange and ATP turnover

		kcal/mole	(kJ/mole)
(1)	$\Delta G = \Delta G^{o\prime}$	$-7.3^{(a)}$	(31)
(2)	$\Delta G = \Delta G^{o\prime} + RT \ln \frac{[ADP]\ [P_i]}{[ATP]}$	$-12.9^{(a)}$	(54)
	$\Delta G = n \cdot z \cdot \Delta E$	$-12.4^{(b)}$	(52)
(3)	Energy released per ATP made [c]		
	Glucose $\longrightarrow 6\ CO_2$: $\frac{673\ \text{kcal}}{38\ \text{ATP}}$	17.7	(74)
	Palmitate $\longrightarrow 16\ CO_2$: $\frac{2398\ \text{kcal}}{131\ \text{ATP}}$	18.3	(77)
	Protein $\longrightarrow CO_2 + (NH_3)$: $\frac{475\ \text{kcal}}{28.8}$	16.5	(69)
(4)	Energy released per ATP gained [d]		
	Glucose $\longrightarrow 6\ CO_2$: $\frac{673\ \text{kcal}\cdot}{(36 \div 34.5)\ \text{ATP}}$	18.7-19.5	(78-82)
	FFA $\longrightarrow CO_2$: $\frac{2398\ \text{kcal}}{(129 \div 122)\ \text{ATP}}$	18.6-19.7	(78-82)
	Protein $\longrightarrow CO_2$ (via Gluc.) + Urea : $\frac{475\ \text{kcal}}{(23.5 \div 23)\ \text{ATP}}$	20.3-20.7	(85-87)

(a) [ATP] = 1.85; [ADP] = 0.14 mmol; [P_i] = 1 mmol, as during steady state conditions in erythrocytes (Lehninger, 1975, p. 432).
(b) One half of ΔG for transfer of two electrons from the mitochondrial NAD to the cytochrome C couples in isolated liver cells (Wilson *et al.*, 1974).
(c) Cf. equations for substrate oxidation given in Table 1.
(d) Based on ATP production and utilization during oxidation of circulating substrates or of endogenous stores, as described in Figures 2, 3 and 4.

strates. The caloric expenditure per mole of ATP formed should, therefore, be based on the heat of combustion of one mole of substrate, divided by the total number of moles of ATP generated in its oxidation. Such values are in the range of 18 kcal/mole (~75 kJ/mole) (Table 3). This means that a daily energy expenditure of 2400 kcal implies that 2400/18 = 133 moles, or 65 kg of ATP are hydrolyzed and regenerated in one day! If one assumes that there are 3 millimoles of ATP/kg of Body Cell Mass, one can calculate that the ATP pool is turned over about once every minute, a value which illustrates that ATP generation must be closely adjusted to ATP utilization.

Since ATP must be expended for the transport and activation of substrates, the metabolic cost incurred for making one mole of ATP available may be evaluated at some 20 kcal (84 kJ). Using this value, the SDA for carbohydrates can be expected to be in the range of 2 to 7 per cent, depending on whether the absorbed glucose is directly oxidized or converted to glycogen (Figure 2). If the ingested carbohydrate were transformed into fat, the predicted SDA would amount to some 25 per cent, since glucose conversion to fatty acids requires an ATP expenditure equivalent to some 20 per cent of the energy of the glucose entering the lipogenic pathway (Table 1). A situation where a very high proportion of ingested carbohydrate is converted to fat is unlikely; but if, for example, 20 per cent of the ingested carbohydrate were converted to fat instead of glycogen, the SDA would be 10 per cent, a value which corresponds to the data in the literature under conditions favoring lipogenesis (cf. Ball, 1965).

As can be seen in Figure 2, the same amounts of ATP are generated, whether glucose is oxidized directly or converted to fatty acids which are oxidized subsequently. This seems at first surprising, since glucose and fatty acid oxidation occur with P:O ratios of 3.17 and 2.85

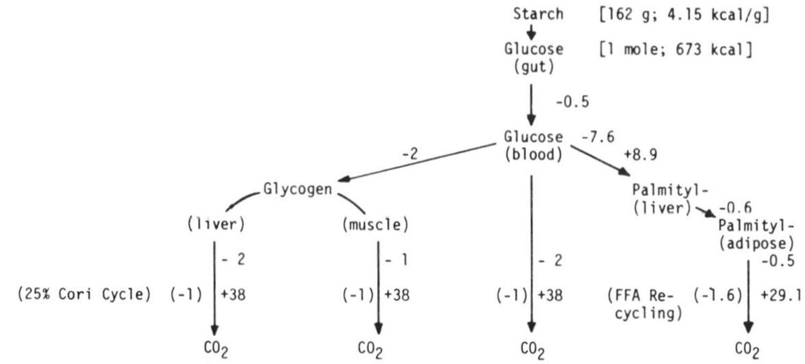

ATP used	-5.5	-4.5	-3.5		-10.8
ATP made	+38	+38	+38		+38
ATP gained	+32.5	+33.5	+34.5		27.2
ATP gained / ATP made from starch	0.86	0.88	0.91		0.72
ATP gained / ATP made from Glycogen	0.92	0.95	-	(from TG stores:)	0.93
ATP used for Absorption, Transport and Storage	2.5	2.5	0.5	8.1	8.7
SDA	7%	7%	2%	24%	26%
Energy dissipated through storage	5%	3%	(0)	-	19%

Fig. 2. Pathways for the metabolism of ingested starch. The numbers indicate moles of ATP formed (+) and utilized (-) per glucose residue. The stoichiometry for glucose conversion to fat is summarized in equation (4) of Table 1. For the oxidation of fat, refer to the details given in Figure 3. 25 per cent of glucose is assumed to be metabolized to lactate and recycled with a net cost of 4 ATP per glucose metabolized via the Cori Cycle. Active transport of glucose in the gut is presumably linked to sodium extrusion, with 3 sodium pumped out of the epithelial cell per ATP consumed (Crane, 1962). The value was rounded to 0.5 to allow for the cost of intestinal enzyme synthesis and gut motility. The ATP utilization and production is summarized below the metabolic scheme, and the balance used to calculate the number of 'ATP gained' per 'ATP made', either from dietary carbohydrate (starch) or from endogenous glycogen or triglyceride stores. The SDA was calculated by assuming an energy expenditure of 20 kcal per ATP required for the absorption, transport and storage of the glucose. This value, divided by the caloric content of the ingested starch, gives the SDA (expressed on a per cent basis). Finally, the energy dissipated through storage is the difference between the SDA observed when absorbed glucose is directly oxidized, or when it is converted to glycogen or fat prior to oxidation

respectively. The high P:O ratio for glucose is in fact due to substrate level phosphorylation in the glycolytic pathway; if only the 34 ATPs produced during glucose oxidation are considered, the P:O ratio is 2.83. Thus, it is substrate level phosphorylation which occurs during carbohydrate, but not during fatty acid oxidation, which explains why the caloric equivalent is 5 kcal/liter of oxygen when the RQ is 1.0, but only 4.7 when the RQ is 0.7. The contribution of energy released by non-oxidative reactions is most strikingly demonstrated during the conversion of glucose to fat (Table 1, equation (4)), when energy release in the glycolytic pathway occurs, but not oxidation of acetyl-CoA, so that 7.1 kcal are released per liter of oxygen consumed in the process of lipogenesis.

In the case of fat, the SDA can be estimated at 2 to 4 per cent, depending on whether the absorbed fatty acids are oxidized or stored (Figure 3). Dietary fat is usually considered to be primarily converted to adipose tissue triglyceride, but some ingested dietary fat probably contributes to the FFA pool and escapes storage.

It is the ingestion of protein which elicits by far the greatest metabolic response. The large SDA of protein has been attributed to the relatively high cost of peptide-bond synthesis.

The scheme of Figure 4 shows that a comparable ATP expenditure is required when ingested amino acids are degraded, because of the metabolic costs of gluconeogenesis and ureogenesis. Thus, the SDA for protein, evaluated at 25 per cent on the basis of the stoichiometry described in Figure 4, is independent of the fate of the ingested amino acids.

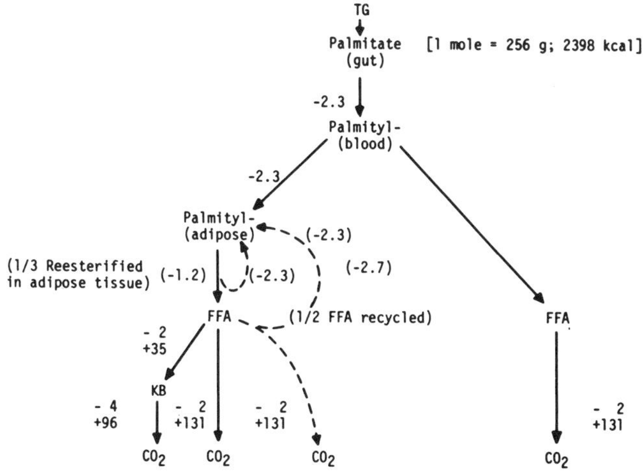

ATP used	-11.8	-7.8	-13.9	-4.3
ATP made	+131	+131	+131	+131
ATP gained	+119.2	+123.2	+117.1	126.7
ATP gained / ATP made from diet. Fat	0.91	0.94	0.89	0.97
ATP gained / ATP made from TG Stores	0.94	0.98	0.93	-
ATP used for Absorption, Transport and Storage	4.6			2.3
SDA	4%			2%
Energy Dissipated through Storage	6%	3%	8%	(0)

Fig. 3. Pathways for the metabolism of ingested fat. The numbers refer to moles of ATP generated (+) and utilized (-) in the course of the oxidation of one mole of palmitate. Palmitate absorption from the gut requires 2.3 ATP for fatty acid activation and esterification; the same cost is incurred for the deposition of fatty-acyl residues in adipose tissue (Ball, 1965). When FFA are converted to ketone bodies, one high-energy bond (GTP) per mole of ketone body is required for activation in the periphery. The dotted line shows the likely recycling and reesterification of free fatty acids, with the related ATP expenditure: it was assumed that one-third of the FFA produced in adipose tissue is reesterified in this tissue, and that half of the FFA reaching the plasma is removed by the liver, esterified and reexported in the form of lipoprotein triglycerides, at a cost of 2.7 ATP per fatty acid (increased from 2.3 to make an allowance for the synthesis of the apolipoprotein). The summary shown at the bottom of the scheme on ATP Production and Utilization was used to calculate 'ATP gained' per 'ATP made' from dietary or endogenous fat. The SDA and the energy dissipated through storage were calculated as in Figure 1

Cost of nutrient storage

Using the information summarized in Figures 2, 3 and 4, it is possible to compare the amounts of 'ATP gained' (ie 'ATP made' – 'ATP used') when ingested nutrients are directly oxidized, or first stored and degraded later. For instance, the ratio of ATP gained to ATP made is 0.91 when glucose from ingested starch is directly oxidized (Figure 2). This 'yield' decreases to 88 per cent or 86 per cent when the glucose is first converted to glycogen in muscle or in the liver, respectively. If ingested carbohydrate is converted to fatty acid, which in turn is oxidized,

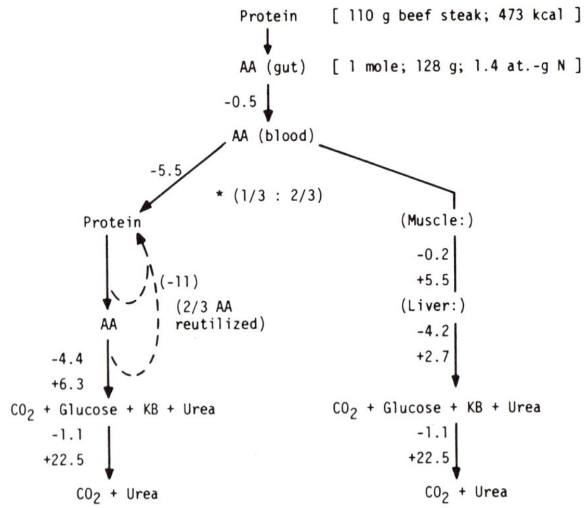

ATP used	-11.5	-22.5	*-11.5	- 6
ATP made	+29	+29	+29	+29
ATP gained	+17.5	+ 6.5	+17.5	+23
ATP gained / ATP made from diet. Prot.	0.60	0.22	0.60	0.79
ATP gained / ATP made from endog. Prot.	0.81	0.43	0.81	-
ATP used for Absorption, Transport and Storage	6		(or for Glucose plus Urea Synthesis)	(6)
SDA	25%		25%	25%
Energy Dissipated through Storage	19%	57%	19%	(0)

Fig. 4. Pathways for the metabolism of ingested amino acids. The numbers show the moles of ATP utilized (-) and generated (+) for 110 grams (1 mole) of an amino acid mixture as found in beef steak (McGilvery, 1970). The cost for the active transport of amino acids in the gut cannot be estimated precisely (Matthews, 1975), and was set at half of a mole of ATP per amino acid (ie same as for monosaccharide uptake, being also linked to sodium extrusion). The stoichiometry for amino acid oxidation, involving the conversion of all the glucogenic residues to glucose and the excretion of nitrogen in the form of urea, is as summarized in Table 1. The cost of protein synthesis is evaluated at 4 ATP for the synthesis of 1 peptide bond, 1 ATP for the synthesis of RNA and 0.5 ATP for amino acid uptake. Amino acids liberated by protein breakdown are in part reutilized for amino acid synthesis as shown by the dotted arrows. The case identified by an asterisk was constructed assuming that one-third of the absorbed amino acids is incorporated into protein and that two-thirds of these will be reutilized for protein synthesis. The ATP production and utilization is summarized at the bottom of the scheme and was used to calculate the number of 'ATP gained' per 'ATP made' from dietary or endogenous protein. The SDA and energy dissipated through storage were calculated as described in Figure 1. It should be noted that the SDA is the same whether amino acids are converted into protein or are directly oxidized, because the cost of gluconeogenesis and ureogenesis is similar to that involved in protein synthesis. The case identified by the asterisk is possible the most likely; it implies that only 60 per cent of the ATP made in the course of amino acid oxidation represents a net gain for the organism

only 72 per cent of the ATP generated represents a net gain. The dissipation of energy due to storing ingested carbohydrate is thus 3 to 5 per cent if the storage form is glycogen, or 19 per cent if it is fat. The dissipation of energy through storage amounts to 8 per cent in the case of fat (Figure 3), and to 19 per cent in the case of protein (Figure 4). Under different nutritional conditions, the amounts of energy dissipated due to the metabolic costs of storage will vary, within ranges summarized in Table 4. Quantitatively, the most important increase in energy dissipation would be brought about if large portions of ingested carbohydrates were converted to fat, because several reactions in the synthesis of fatty acid require ATP, and because carbohydrate represents a major component in the diet. However, *de novo* lipogenesis can be presumed to be a negligible process when a mixed diet is consumed (Masoro, 1962; Sjöström, 1973).

Table 4. Calculated cost of nutrient storage

Nutrient	Storage form	Cost of synthesis	Cost caused by recycling	Energy dissipated through storage
Carbohydrate	Glycogen (liver)	5%	(None)	5%
	Glycogen (muscle)	5%	(None)	3%
	Fat (adipose)	24%	4% (a)	28%
Fat	Fat (adipose)	2%	5% (a)	7%
Protein	Protein	24%	(None)	24%
		8%(b)	16%(b)	24%

(a) Assuming one-third of FFA formed in adipose tissue to be reesterified and one-half of FFA released from adipose tissue to be recycled.

(b) Assuming only one-third of ingested AA converted to protein, but two-thirds of AA liberated by protein breakdown to be reutilized for protein synthesis.

The type of nutrient which yields the least amount of ATP/calorie ingested is protein. Indeed, when amino acids are converted to protein, ATP is utilized in an amount equal to 20 per cent of the ATP generated by oxidation of a like amount of amino acids (Figure 4). Considering, in addition, that 20 per cent of the ATP generated during amino acid degradation is necessary to cover the ATP required for gluconeogenesis and ureogenesis, the energy made available to the organism corresponds to only 60 per cent of that contained in the ingested protein. While it is unlikely that all ingested amino acids are converted to protein, those amino acids which are incorporated into protein are likely to be reutilized for protein synthesis when they reappear in the body's amino acid pool. It seems reasonable to assume that perhaps one-third of the ingested amino acids is converted to protein (two-thirds being oxidized in the hours following the meal), and that two-thirds of the amino acids are liberated by protein breakdown are reutilized for protein synthesis. The ATP consumption would then be comparable to that incurred if all ingested amino acids were converted to protein, but not reutilized for protein synthesis, so that 40 per cent of the energy contained in dietary protein would be necessary to cover the 'handling' costs incurred.

The cost of transporting fat from the intestine to adipose tissue, 3 per cent (Figure 3), is relatively small. Fatty acids, once stored in adipose tissue, will also be reesterified and/or recycled prior to oxidation. These 'handling' costs are estimated at 5 per cent in Table 4, thus exceeding those incurred for their initial storage.

The analysis of the cost of nutrient storage leads to the realization that nutrients once stored have a certain probability of being reutilized in biosynthetic processes. Nutrient intake will therefore increase energy expenditure far beyond the post-prandial phase.

Effect of starvation on energy expenditure

Many investigators have observed during partial or total starvation that the body's energy expenditure declines more rapidly than the decrease in body weight or in body surface (cf. Bray, 1976). That the reduction in Body Cell Mass is not the major factor in explaining the decreasing energy expenditure during short-term, acute caloric deprivation is demonstrated particularly well by studies conducted by Apfelbaum, Bostsarron & Brigant (1969), who reported that the reduction in BEE, of about 1 per cent per day, was similar in totally starved individuals and in subjects receiving 55 grams of casein per day, an amount of protein sufficient to maintain a nearly even nitrogen balance. It appears, therefore, that Basal Energy Expenditure includes a component related to food intake, which manifests itself in a more delayed manner than the Specific Dynamic Action. The quantitative importance of this

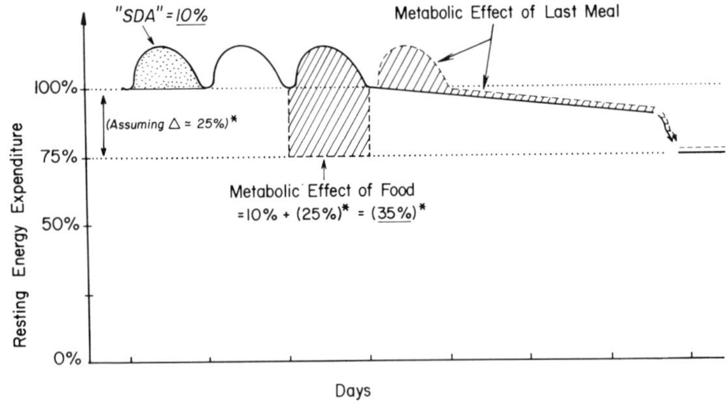

Fig. 5. The 'Metabolic Effect of the Last Meal'. The resting energy expenditure during successive days is shown, with the increases due to food intake (SDA). A decline in energy expenditure occurs upon initiation of total starvation in amounts of approximately 1 per cent per day (Apfelbaum *et al.,* 1969); this decline is assumed to level off, as a value of 75 per cent of the initial post-absorptive energy expenditure is approached. The dotted line shows the energy expenditure if food had been consumed for one more day. The difference between the dotted line and the full line describes the 'Metabolic effect of the last meal'. It includes the SDA (about 10 per cent of the energy consumed) and a more delayed effect, shown graphically by the narrow band between the two lines. The surface of this band is equivalent to a rectangle, whose base has the length of one day, and the height of which is 25 per cent on the vertical energy expenditure during starvation was assumed to level off at 75 per cent). The scheme illustrates that one-third rather than 10 per cent of the daily energy expenditure is due to the food consumed

effect can be appreciated with the help of Figure 5. Energy expenditure in this Figure is shown to decrease at the rate of approximately 1 per cent per day during starvation, the decline being assumed to level off at a value of 75 per cent of that measured initially after an overnight fast. A second line (dotted) shows the decline in energy expenditure had food been consumed for one more day. The narrow band between the two lines thus shows the metabolic effect of the 'last meal', beyond the period during which the SDA is manifested. The surface of this narrow band is equivalent to that of a rectangle, the base of which has the length of one day, and whose height corresponds to 25 per cent of BEE (ie the difference between 100 per cent and 75 per cent). Figure 5 seems useful in providing a frame for a quantitative appreciation of the energy expenditure related to food intake other than the Specific Dynamic Action. The effect of food intake in maintaining Basal Energy Expenditure at a particular level can be attributed, in part, to a certain intensity of 'substrate traffic', with a related consumption of ATP, as well as to the presence in the fed state of larger pools of rapidly turning over substances, particularly proteins.

An attempt to evaluate how much of the decrease in energy expenditure during starvation may be related to changes in protein and amino acid metabolism can be made by comparing daily amino acid fluxes in the fed state, and during prolonged starvation (Figure 6). Rates of protein synthesis were assumed to decrease by 25 per cent in starvation (Winterer *et al.*, 1976) on the basis of protein turnover studies using ^{15}N-glycine. Taking into account the decrease in ATP utilization for gluconeogenesis and ureogenesis (the latter magnified by the shift from urea to ammonia excretion), one can expect a decrease of some 120 kcal/day in the cost of protein metabolism, which corresponds to a fall of some 8 per cent in the Basal Energy Expenditure.

Nutritional surveys in areas where food intake is marginal have revealed that individuals are able to maintain a steady body composition with food intakes appreciably below those believed to be required to cover the Resting Energy Expenditure (Garrow, 1974). These findings suggest that the true nutrient requirements for man are still not known or understood (Durnin *et al.*, 1973). The apparent discrepancy between predicted energy requirement and observed food intake may be easier to accomodate if the metabolic effect of food is

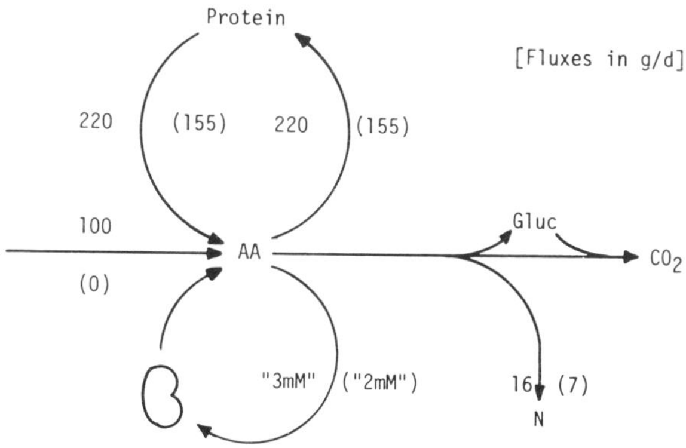

		"Fed"		("Starved")	
	-ATP/mole	moles/d	-ATP/d	moles/d	-ATP/d
AA Absorption	0.5	0.9	0.5	0	0
Protein Synth.	5.5	2	11	1.5	8.3
Gluconeogenesis	4	0.3	1.2	0.13	0.5
Ureogenesis	4	0.6	2.4	0.2	0.8
Renal AA Reabs	3	0.5	1.5	0.3	0.9
- ATP (moles/d)			16.6		10.5
kcal/d (= ATP · 20)			330		210
Δ En. Exp. (kcal/d)					120 (=8% of 1500)

Fig. 6. Major pathways of amino acid and protein metabolism. The numbers describe the fluxes in grams per day, in the fed state, or in the prolonged starved state (in parentheses). The table under the figure describes the ATP required per mole of amino acid entering a particular metabolic process. Renal reabsorption was assumed to occur via the γ-gluamyl cycle (Meister, 1973), at a cost of 3 ATP per amino acid reabsorbed from 120 ml of glomerular filtrate per minute. Protein synthesis in prolonged starvation was considered to be reduced by 25 per cent (Winterer *et al.*, 1976). The decrease in energy expenditure for protein and amino acid metabolism due to starvation was calculated from the change in the daily ATP consumption, considering that 20 kcal are expended by the organism per ATP consumed. This corresponds to a decrease of 8 per cent, if the Basic Metabolic Rate in the fed state is 1600 kcal per day

perceived to include not only the Specific Dynamic Action, some 10 per cent of the calories ingested, but also the more significant component illustrated in Figure 5. If the combined effect of these two phenomena accounts for, say, one-third of the caloric intake, it would imply that only two-thirds of the caloric expenditure is predictable from body size. This may help to understand that individuals are able to maintain a constant body weight while consuming fewer calories than predicted on the basis of the Basal Energy Expenditure of well-fed populations.

Metabolic efficiency

Since even small changes in Resting Energy Expenditure could potentially account for large cumulative effects in energy balance, there has been great interest in studying possible differences in metabolic efficiency, the existence of which is suggested by the variability observed in measuring Basal Energy Expenditure. The very concept of 'Metabolic Efficiency' is difficult to define. In animal husbandry, it is often used to describe the yield in animal tissue in relation to feed consumed (Blaxter, 1971), a notion which seems not applicable to a situation where the difference between energy intake and expenditure is comparatively small, as in adult man. In this case, the notion of metabolic efficiency pertains to the fact that energy balance can be maintained on food intakes which are below or above predicted requirements. In particular, energy expenditure appears to be increased by excessive food consumption, a phenomenon described in terms of 'Luxusconsumption' (Bray, 1976; Sims, 1976; Garrow, this volume).

There is no evidence to suggest that uncoupling of oxidative phosphorylation occurs under physiological conditions, but several metabolic processes are known in which ATP can be dissipated. Examples of such processes are the interconversion of fructose-diphosphate and fructose-6-phosphate, or the hydrolysis of adipose tissue triglycerides followed by reesterification. Because ATP is consumed without apparent change in the system, such interconversions have become known as 'futile cycles'. According to Newsholme & Start (1972), the existence of such ATP-consuming cycles has the advantage of allowing a faster response than would be possible if one reaction were totally inhibited (much as an idling car is more ready to accelerate than a car whose engine is stopped). It seems reasonable to follow Newsholme's suggestion to use the words 'substrate cycle' instead of 'futile cycle', which has the advantage of avoiding to qualify such processes adversely. For instance, free fatty acids are released from adipose tissue in excess of their rate of oxidation, forcing considerable recycling via lipoproteins, but there is the advantage of ensuring an adequate supply of FFA. Some of these processes, which are involved in the general 'substrate traffic', may well be increased when food intake is high.

In studies on overfeeding to induce obesity Sims, Danforth, Horton & collaborators (eg, Sims, 1976)noted that unusually large amounts of food needed to be consumed at the conclusion of a period of overfeeding to maintain the weight attained. The fact that energy intakes far in excess of predictable energy requirements were accommodated without weight gain under these circumstances suggested a significant alteration in metabolic efficiency (ie 'Luxusconsumption'). But constancy in body weight does not imply constancy in caloric content, because replacement of Body Cell Mass by an equal weight of adipose tissue fat increases the body's caloric content to the tune of 8 kcal/gram exchanged. The nitrogen balance would have to be negative, in spite of the high caloric intake. The size of the Body Cell Mass is influenced by the amount of protein consumed, since changing from a low-protein to a high-protein diet, each of which is sufficient to maintain nitrogen balance, leads to a phase of nitrogen retention. Conversely, changing from a high-protein to a lower-protein intake will cause some loss of nitrogen (Fig. 7), until nitrogen balance is again maintained on the lower-protein intake. Thus, a decrease in Body Cell Mass, due to the readjustment of the body's protein (and glycogen) content should in effect be expected upon discontinuation of an overfeeding regimen. If this is to be masked by a compensatory increase in adipose tissue fat, a caloric intake considerably above caloric expenditure will be required. An experimental test of this potential explanation could provide valuable arguments in favor of or against the 'Luxusconsumption' concept.

An area where, by contrast, the metabolic efficiency appears to be very precisely determined is that of physical exercise. For instance, in the case of standing or walking, without or with a load, Pandolf, Givoni & Goldman (1977) have developed the following equation:

$$M = 1.5\ W + 2.0\ (W + L) \cdot \left(\frac{L}{W}\right)^2 + \eta \cdot (W + L)\ (1.5\ v^2 + 0.35\ VG)$$

where M is energy expenditure in Watts; W = Body Weight (kg); L= Load (kg); V= Speed (m/sec); G= Grade (%); and η= Terrain Factor.

According to Goldman (personal communication), the accuracy with which the energy expenditure can be predicted increases with the intensity of the effort, because the driving effect of physical work on energy expenditure will cover up underlying variations in BEE. The equation also shows that energy expenditure when standing (instead of lying as usual during measurement of energy expenditure) is determined by body weight rather than by body surface. When significant parts of the day are spent standing, predictions of daily

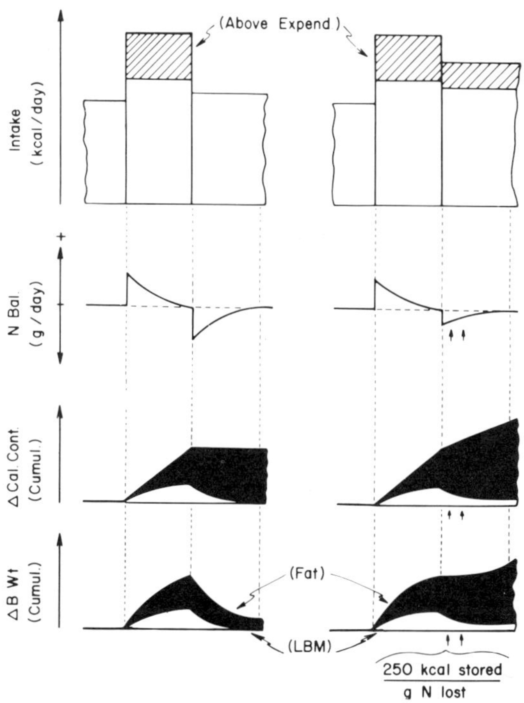

Fig. 7. Changes in protein and fat content during and after periods of acute overfeeding. An increase in energy expenditure occurs during overfeeding. The amount of calories consumed above the increased expenditure is shown by a hatched area, and causes an increase in body weight, partly in the form of lean body mass (LBM) and partly as adipose tissue fat. When a normal food intake is resumed (case on the left side of the figure), the nitrogen retained during the overfeeding is lost, until an even nitrogen balance is again attained. The case illustrated on the right side of the figure is one in which food intake following the period of overfeeding is adjusted so as to avoid a loss in body weight. Since protein intake is reduced, some loss of nitrogen occurs, until a new steady state is achieved with regard to the N balance. The loss in lean body mass (22 per cent protein ≃ 1 kcal/g and 32 mg protein-N/g), however, is compensated by a gain of adipose tissue fat (9 kcal/g). Therefore, while maintaining a constant body weight, the caloric content of the body can increase by 250 kcal per gram of nitrogen lost

energy expenditure based on body surface will be inaccurate (Goldman, personal communication).

During periods of great exertion, the metabolic efficiency is thus very constant. Under resting conditions, a certain variation in ATP dissipation can be expected, of which an important part is related to the prevailing nutritional situation. The existence of changes in metabolic efficiency, which would be due to mechanisms of a nature other than those considered above, remains difficult to establish.

The composition of energy expenditure and its influence on energy balance

The proportions of carbohydrate, fat and protein oxidized by the body under resting conditions are determined primarily by the amount and composition of the food consumed (eg Figure 8). However, these proportions are modified in response to physical activity. Strenuous exercise, for instance, which draws heavily on the muscles' glycogen reserves, is associated with a high respiratory quotient. During sustained physical activity the mobilization of the body's fat reserves is activated, and the relative contribution of glucose, if it is initially important, gradually decreases (Figure 8). In spite of this, the body's glycogen reserves are markedly depleted during prolonged exertion. In the studies shown in Figure 8, carbohydrate oxidation amounted to 400, 167 and 35 grams, depending on whether a high-carbohydrate, a mixed, or a high-fat diet was being consumed.

Among the three components of food (carbohydrate, fat and protein), carbohydrate is clearly the nutrient whose intake must be most closely adjusted to its utilization (and vice versa), because carbohydrate stores are rather limited. Changes in the body's fat reserves, on the other hand, are well tolerated and the body's protein content is maintained relatively constant, because degradation of amino acid can be adjusted to intake over a wide range. Thus, it is in the carbohydrate sector of metabolism that the most powerful regulatory signals on food intake should be expected; the origin of these signals can probably not be based on circulating substrate levels alone (Friedman & Sticker, 1976), since their fluctua-

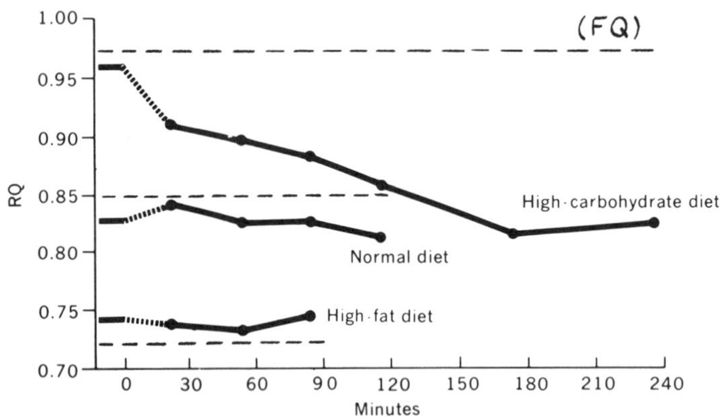

Food Intake to regain CHO oxidized (as % of Cal. Expend.)

Same Diet	High CHO
58	58
92	48
198	7

Fig. 8. The figure was taken from a publication by Christensen & Hansen (1939) on the Respiratory Quotient of a subject working at 1080 kpm per minute on a bicycle ergometer, after one week of adaptation to each of three different diets. The subject was exhausted after 90 minutes when on the high-fat diet, but was able to sustain this work load for 240 minutes when on the high-carbohydrate diet; the experiment was stopped after 120 minutes when the subject was on a normal mixed diet. Horizontal dashed lines have been added to the figure to show the Food-Q for the three diets, as well as a table which shows the caloric intake needed to replenish the carbohydrate oxidized during the exercise (as a percentage of caloric expenditure during exercise), assuming that the subject consumed either the diet to which he had been adapted ('same diet') or the high-carbohydrate (High CHO) diet

tions are dominated by the need to maintain fuel homeostasis (eg, Flatt & Blackburn, 1974) rather than body composition.

We calculated the amount of food which would need to be consumed in order to recover the carbohydrate expended for each of the three dietary situations (Figure 8): intakes equivalent to 58, 92 or 198 per cent of the caloric expenditure would be required. This would correspond to an exercise-induced overall loss of 1200 kcal in one case, but to a gain of 1100 kcal in the other. If the high-carbohydrate regime only were to be consumed following the exercise sessions, the glycogen content could be restored in each case by intakes about 1000 kcal short of the expenditure. These calculations illustrate that the 'composition of expended energy', in relation to that of the diet, should be expected to have a major impact on the energy balance, if one makes the simple assumption that the regulation of food intake is influenced by the need to maintain the body's glycogen content in a given range (which may be high or low, under different nutritional conditions).

Fat content of the diet and energy balance. The 'Food-Q' concept

The incidence of obesity is particularly high in populations consuming a diet in which a large proportion of calories is supplied in the form of fat, and whose level of physical activity is low. The difficulty is maintaining an even balance between energy intake and energy expenditure under these conditions is related to the fact that the caloric density of foods is most markedly increased by their fat content. If, in addition, the energy expenditure is only rarely driven above the resting rate through exercise, the energy balance will all too often become positive. These are well-known considerations. Yet, by dealing only with the balance between energy intake and energy expenditure, they fail to recognize another important aspect of the problem: namely, that the fuel mix oxidized over 24 hours must be the same as that of the food ingested, if body composition, as well as energy content, is to remain in a steady state. Failure to satisfy this condition is likely to generate food intake signals that seek to restore components oxidized in excess, if their depletion can be perceived by the organism (ie carbohydrate).

To address this aspect of the problem, it is convenient to rely on the respiratory quotient to describe the composition of the fuel mix oxidized. The ratio of CO_2 formed to O_2 utilized during the combustion of a representative sample of the dietary nutrient mixture may be called the 'Food Quotient' ('Food-Q' or 'FQ'), by analogy with the Respiratory Quotient (RQ). By comparing RQ to FQ, it becomes possible to assess to which extent the fuel mixture oxidized by the body differs from the fuel mixture in the diet. Since protein contributes only a minor fraction of the metabolic energy, and since the RQ for protein oxidation is 0.80, the RQ and FQ are determined primarily by the carbohydrate-to-fat ratio. The typical 'mixed diet' consumed in affluent countries supplies 45 per cent of calories in the form of carbohydrate, 40 per cent of calories in the form of fat, 15 per cent of calories in the form of protein. The Food-Q for this mixture is 0.85. When this type of diet is consumed, the RQ after an overnight fast is approximately 0.82. When a constant body composition is maintained, the RQ averaged over 24 hours must be equal to the FQ, so that the pattern of RQ changes during the day (Figure 9) is defined quite precisely, simply because periods with RQs below the FQ (Surface B in Figure 9) must offset periods where the RQ is above the FQ (Surface A in Figure 9). The figure suggests the following argument: since the RQ is barely below the FQ even after the overnight fast, it may be difficult to achieve an average RQ as low as the FQ when the fat content of the diet is high, and when physical activity capable of lowering the RQ is not part of the daily routine. If, for instance, the fuel mixture

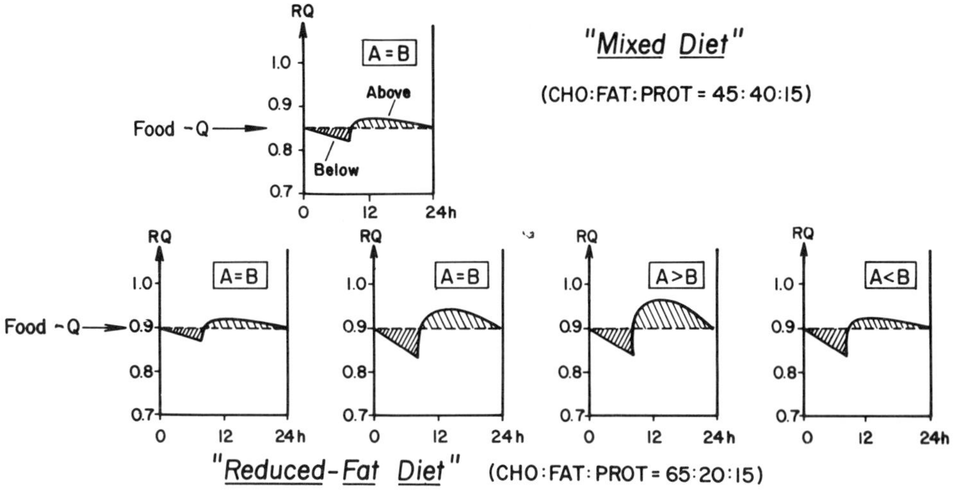

Fig. 9. Daily pattern of RQ changes when a mixed diet is consumed. The pattern at the top was constructed knowing that the Food-Q for a mixed diet (40 per cent of calories in the form of fat) is 0.85, and that the post-absorptive RQ is approximately 0.82 (and assuming no perturbation due to physical activity). During periods of weight maintenance, the surfaces below (B) and above (A) the horizontal dashed line showing the FQ must be equal, if the body composition is to remain constant. The fact that the post-absorptive RQ is only slightly below the Food-Q implies that the increases in RQ elicited during the day by food intake must be rather limited. The lower part of the figure illustrates the possible RQ patterns when the mixed diet is replaced by a diet containing only 20 per cent of calories in the form of fat (Food-Q = 0.85)

oxidized during the day has an average RQ higher than 0.85, the fuel mixture oxidized contains a higher proportion of carbohydrate than the typical 'mixed diet'. In order to recover the oxidized carbohydrate, food would have to be consumed in amounts exceeding the energy expenditure, which is possible by storing a portion of the ingested fat. Accumulation of fat in adipose tissue is in effect particularly likely in obesity (cf. Ashwell, Meade & Medawar, 1977), because high insulin levels must be maintained to achieve fuel homeostasis in the presence of an excessive adipose tissue mass (Flatt, 1972). Failure to replenish the glycogen stores can be expected to elicit hunger, and to cause a shift in the body's metabolism to reduce carbohydrate oxidation during subsequent hours or days so as to recover the initial glycogen levels, or to reach a new steady state with regard to the body's glycogen content.

The perception of the benefit of exercise for weight control has been mitigated, among others, because exercise increases food consumption without it being predictable to what extent this will offset the increase in energy expenditure. But by judging the nature of the exercise, using as a criterion its effect on the RQ, it becomes possible to understand how different forms of exercise could be more or less helpful in facilitating weight control. For instance, prolonged exercise of moderate intensity (eg, walking or running), which is often referred to as 'aerobic exercise' and leads to low RQs, is empirically perceived to be more helpful for weight control than short periods of strenuous exertion at a high RQ. Indeed, in the case of the weight-lifting athlete, exercise seems to be associated with weight gain, whereas the opposite effect is exemplified by the leanness of the long-distance runner.

Search for a strategy for weight maintenance

It follows from the preceding that if a 'general strategy' for facilitating weight maintenance is to be derived, its goal should be to favor the occurrence of periods where metabolism operates at a relatively low RQ by comparison to the FQ. One of the two types of leverages available is to increase physical activity of the type which will depress the RQ; the other is to reduce the fat content of the diet in order to elevate the Food-Q. The possible effects of reducing the fat content of the diet are illustrated in the lower section of Figure 9. The RQ pattern may merely be shifted up from an average of 0.85 to one of 0.90, or it may show a somewhat greater variability above and below the FQ. The third and fourth diagrams from the left illustrate other possible changes, which could either be unfavourable (A > B) or favorable (B > A) for maintaining energy balance. The effects of physical activity are not shown, but reference to Figure 8 will show that the leverage of physical activity in reducing the RQ below the FQ will be far greater when the diet containing less fat (ie the diet with the higher FQ) is consumed.

Experimental data on the variations of RQ brought about by changes in food composition and by various physical activities, be they part of an exercise program or part of a daily routine, could conceivably lead to useful recommendations about dietary and activity habits to ensure that the average fuel mix oxidized during the day is at least as high in fat content as is the diet (cf. Figure 10).

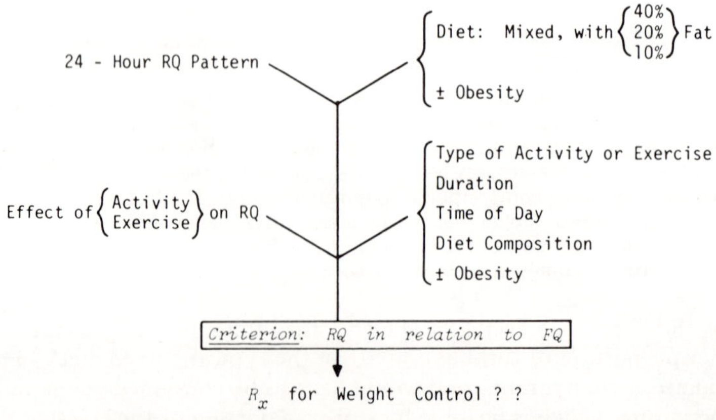

Fig. 10. The figure illustrates the type of experimental data needed to evaluate both whether a reduction in the fat content of the diet, and which types of exercise habits, are likely to help the organism to operate at an average RQ as low as the FQ of the food consumed

Current recommendations for weight maintenance aim at achieving energy balance by limiting energy intake, and increasing energy expenditure. The recommendations envisaged here focus only on the balance between fat intake and fat oxidation, with the hope that by setting a more specific objective, it may become easier to select the components of a winning strategy for weight maintenance. Its rationale provides yet another incentive to reduce the fat content of the diet, and possibly one with considerable appeal.

Summary

Quantitative evaluations of the metabolic cost for the transport, storage, activation and recycling of carbohydrate, fat and amino acids are presented. It is explained that an energy expenditure of 20 kcal should be expected per mole of ATP consumed by these processes. The SDA of different nutrients, calculated on this basis, are in good agreement with observed values. The dissipation of energy through storage, including an allowance for recycling, is estimated at 4 per cent when carbohydrate is stored as glycogen, and 28 per cent when it is stored as fat; comparable figures for fat and protein are 7 per cent and 24 per cent. Considering the additional cost of gluconeogenesis and ureogenesis, it is estimated that only some 60 per cent of the ATP generated from protein represents a net energy gain for the organism. From considerations of the decrease in energy expenditure during starvation, it is tentatively estimated that perhaps 25 per cent of the Basal Metabolic Rate (BMR) is related to the food consumed, so that only a fraction of the BMR can be predicted from body composition. This may serve to reconcile some of the differences between observed and predicted rates of energy expenditure. Attention is drawn to the importance of the 'composition of expended energy' in relation to the composition of the diet. To facilitate this comparison, the concept of a 'Food Quotient' (FQ) is proposed, which describes the ratio of CO_2 produced to O_2 consumed during the combustion of the dietary nutrient mixture. Because the RQ after an overnight fast ($\simeq$0.82) is barely below FQ ($\simeq$0.85) when a typical mixed diet supplying 40 per cent of calories as fat is consumed, it may be difficult for the organism to operate at an average daily RQ as low as the FQ in the absence of physical activities favoring a decrease in RQ. It is suggested that weight maintenance may be facilitated by including physical activities in the daily routine, selected for their effect in lowering the RQ, and to reduce the fat content of the diet in order to elevate the FQ. A strategy for weight maintenance is envisaged, whose goal is to ensure that fat oxidation is at least as great as fat intake. This provides a more specific objective than recommendations aiming at achieving an energy balance by limiting intake and increasing expenditure.

Acknowledgement – This work was supported by Grant #AM 17352 of the National Institute of Health.

References

Apfelbaum, M., Bostsarron, J. & Brigant, L. (1969): *Rev. Franc. Études Clin. et Biol.* **14**, 361.
Ashwell, M., Meade, C.J. & Medawar, P. (1977): *Proc. R. Soc. Lond.* **B 195**, 343.
Atkinson, D.E. (1968): *Biochemistry* **7**, 4030.
Baldwin, R.L. & Smith, N.E. (1974): In *The control of metabolism*, ed J.D. Sink. University Park and London: Pennsylvania State University Press.
Ball, E.G. (1965): *Ann. N.Y. Acad. Sci.* **131**, 225.
Blaxter, K.L. (1971): *Fed. Proc.* **30**, 1436.
Bray, G.A. (1976): *The obese patient*, p. 141. Philadelphia: W.B. Saunders Co.
Christensen, E.H. & Hansen, O. (1939): *Scand. Arch. Physiol.* **81**, 160.
Crane, R.K. (1962): *Fed. Proc.* **21**, 891.
Durnin, J.V.G.A., Edholm, O.G., Miller, D.S. & Waterlow, J.C. (1973): *Nature* **242**, 418.
Flatt, J.P. (1970): *J. Lip. Res.* **11**, 131.
Flatt, J.P. (1972): *Am. J. Clin. Nutr.* **25**, 1189.
Flatt, J.P. & Blackburn, G.L. (1974): *Am. J. Clin. Nutr.* **27**, 175.
Friedman, M.I. & Stricker, E.M. (1976): *Psychol. Review* **83**, 409.

Garrow, J.S. (1974): *Energy balance and obesity in man,* p. 101. Amsterdam and London: North Holland Publishing co.
Geigy, *Scientific Tables* 7th Edition (1970), p. 540. Basle, Switzerland.
Kleiber, M. (1975): *The fire of life.* p. 272. Huntington, New York: R.E. Krieger Publishing Co.
Lehninger, A.L. (1975): *Biochemistry,* 2nd Edition, p. 398. New York: Worth Publishers Inc.
Masoro, E. (1962): *J. Lip. Res.* 3, 149.
Matthews, D.(1975): *Physiol. Rev.* 55, 537.
McGilvery, R.W. (1970): *Biochemistry. A functional approach,* p. 396. Philadelphia: W.B. Saunders Co.
Meister, A. (1973): *Science* **180**, 33.
Newsholme, E.A. & Start, C. (1972): In *Handbook of physiology,* 7. Endocrinology. General aspects of the regulation of enzyme activity and the effects of hormones. Baltimore: Williams and Wilkins Co.
Pandolf, A.N. Givoni, A.N. & Goldman, R.F. (1977): *J. Appl. Physiol.* 43, 577.
Sims, E.A.H. (1976): *Clins Endoc. Metab.* 5, 377.
Sjöström, L. (1973): *Scand.J. Clin. Lab. Invest.* 32, 339.
Wilson, D.F., Stubbs, M., Veech, R.L., Erecinska, M. & Krebs, H.A. (1974): *Biochem. J.* **140**, 57..
Winterer, J.C., Bistrian, B.R., Blackburn, G.L. & Young, V.R. (1976): *Clin. Res.* 3, 373A.

23
Thermogenesis during weight gain

E. DANFORTH, Jr.*, A.G. BURGER**, R.F. GOLDMAN*** and E.A.H. SIMS*
*Metabolic Unit, Department of Medicine, University of Vermont, Burlington, Vermont 05401. ** Unité de Thyroide, Department of Medicine, University of Geneva, Geneva, Switzerland. ***Military Ergonomics Division, U.S. Army Research Institute of Environmental Medicine, Natick, Massachusetts 01760, USA.

The question has again been asked whether individuals utilize energy with the same efficiency at all times and under all dietary conditions. As one of us has noted (Sims, 1976), ever since Lavoisier demonstrated animal respiration, there has been the tendency to assume that animals constantly burn their substrates with the same even flame and with the same efficiency. Clinical situations exist in which there are large discrepancies between the amount of energy predicted to maintain energy balance and that found necessary to achieve such a balance. These are illustrated by post-surgical patients and patients suffering from malignancies who are found to require more calories than predicted to enter positive states of energy retention. While these clinical situations are complicated, they apparently represent altered states of metabolism which are wasteful of administered energy. There is now renewed interest in the possibility in man of an adaptive change in thermogenesis, during both overnutrition and undernutrition, which is responsible for changes in the efficiency with which fuels are utilized for the essential functions of the body.

Demonstration of a change in the net efficiency with which energy is utilized by the body requires accurate estimates of energy balance. Garrow (this volume) discusses energy expenditure and problems involved with its measurement. Flatt (this volume) also considers the biochemistry of energy expenditure, and Durnin (this volume) has discussed the importance of changes in body composition in estimating energy balance. In this paper, we review the evidence for an adaptive increase in thermogenesis during overnutrition and discuss some of the mechanisms which might be responsible for such an adaptation.

Undernutrition

The adaptive changes in thermogenesis which occur during starvation have been more extensively studied than the changes in thermogenesis which follow overnutrition. It is possible to conclude from the classic studies of starvation by Benedict *et al.* (1919) and Keys *et al.* (1950) that adaptive mechanisms not only spare the lean body mass, but also modify the efficiency with which calories are utilized. Cahill *et al.* (1966) have extended these studies to clarify the metabolic changes which take place during starvation. These have the net effect of reducing dependence on gluconeogenesis for energy, thus sparing breakdown of body protein. This, in addition to the reduction in metabolic rate which the earlier workers described, allows the essential functions of life to continue for longer periods than would be predicted if such an economy were not part of the adaptation. Early during starvation, the decline in the metabolic rate is out of proportion to the loss of weight or to the loss of lean body mass. During more prolonged starvation, subsequent adaptations occur and the metabolic rate again becomes appropriate to the remaining respiring mass of the individual. Keys *et al.* (1950) estimated that approximately 65 per cent of the initial decline in metabolic rate during starvation results from the loss of the respiring mass, while 35 per cent results from a decline in the rate of metabolism of the remaining tissues. In other words, a change in the net efficiency of metabolism has occurred. As Garrow indicates (Garrow, 1974), one of the most interesting observations made by Benedict during his long-term studies of undernutrition was the rapid return of the lowered metabolic rates toward normal when his starving subjects interrupted their restricted diets for short periods of 'holiday overeating' followed by a rapid decline to the initial low values when they resumed their fast. No single mechanism or concert of mechanisms has unequivocally been shown to explain this change in efficiency; however, the fact that it occurs seems clear. There is a similar increase in metabolic rate during refeeding of undernourished children (Ashworth, 1969), which is out of proportion to either the gain in weight or the size of the infant's lean body mass. This increased oxygen utilization following refeeding was attributed to the requirements of a burst of synthesis of new tissue. These examples of 'catch-up metabolism' are different from normal growth. A normally growing organism as well may be expected to have a higher thermic response to food than a mature organism, which is simply renewing tissue and maintaining energy stores without net gain. Thus, as Rubner (1902) pointed out many years ago, one must consider the relative state of nutrition of an animal when evaluating the response to feeding. Certainly, variations in the rates of synthesis and renewal of the cellular components can explain some of the differences in thermogenesis measured during these situations.

Overnutrition

Our studies of experimental obesity in man (Sims *et al.*, 1973) stimulated renewed interest in the possibility that overnutrition was associated with an adaptive increase in thermogenesis. An unexpected finding in these studies of weight gain during overfeeding of normal lean volunteers was the relatively increased number of calories needed for the subjects to maintain their added weight. It was also clear that there was great individual variation in the ability of the subjects to gain weight. These observations restricted older and generally discredited theories to the effect that man can adapt to excess intake by expending calories inefficiently. This phenomenon was originally described by Rubner (1902) in dogs. Neumann (1902) later found that he could maintain his weight, albeit at a new level, in spite of sustained increases in his caloric intake, and termed the phenomenon 'Luxuskonsumption'. This is the term, therefore, used by him for the increased expenditure of energy found in response to chronic overnutrition. In this discussion, luxuskonsumption and the 'thermic effect of a meal' are considered separate phenomena. The 'thermic effect of a meal' is used here and by most modern writers to replace the older phrase 'specific dynamic action' (SDA). Both represent the increase in oxygen consumption and heat production over a period of a few hours following a meal. Rubner had originally believed that the thermic response was specific for protein. The more general term was adopted when it was realized that carbohydrate and fat likewise produced this thermic response.

As Garrow has observed (this volume), most investigators have found increased energy expenditure following overnutrition and gain in weight. However, it is not always agreed that this increased expenditure is out of proportion to the accompanying gain in active tissue and increased energy required for moving this increased weight. In other words, is there a change in net efficiency of energy utilization? A major difficulty arises in the ability to measure accurately changes in body composition. Not all the weight gained during periods of overnutrition is of equal caloric content. Fat has more calories per unit weight than lean mass, which has less than a third the caloric content of fat. The proportions gained as fat and lean tissue may vary with the length and type of overfeeding, and change in calories stored may, therefore, not be reflected accurately by the change in body weight.

Strong, Stirling & Passmore (1967) and Glick *et al.* (1977) respectively overfed both lean and obese subjects for 4 or 5 days and were unable to measure an increase in thermogenesis. Passmore *et al.* (1955*a*; 1955*b*; 1963) overfed lean subjects for 2 weeks and obese subjects for 9 days and found an increased energy expenditure. However, they did not consider this respresented a change in net efficiency of weight gain after the results had been corrected for the energy stored. Apfelbaum, Bostsarron & Lacatis (1971) studied normal volunteers following dietary periods of 15 days and estimated energy expenditure by measurement of oxygen consumption throughout the entire day. They found decreased expenditure during undernutrition and increased during overnutrition.

In our initial studies of long-term overfeeding, there was a marked difference between individuals in ability to gain weight (Sims *et al.*, 1973). In our fourth group, who had gained weight by taking a mixed diet, we were able to confirm our previous observation that more calories are required to maintain the added weight than are required by the spontaneously obese by the use of rigidly controlled diets. In this study, which was designed to include a phase of weight maintenance after weight was gained, there was an increase of 50 per cent in the number of calories per square meter required for maintenance at the new weight.

We have subsequently studied the effects of short-term overfeeding, with increase in intake of carbohydrate, fat or protein (Goldman *et al.*, 1973; Burse *et al.*, 1977*a*; 1977*b*). Basal and resting metabolic rates, corrected for either gain in weight or surface area, were increased 6 to 18 per cent after overfeeding. The responses to overfeeding carbohydrate, fat or protein were similar. In these studies, lasting 14 to 20 days, we found no augmentation of the thermic effect of a meal and no increase in the cost of exercise in the lean subjects. However, in four spontaneously overweight subjects (Burse *et al.*, 1976) who had lifelong obesity with measured hyperplasia of their adipocytes, the increment in oxygen consumption following treadmill exercise could not entirely be accounted for by the increment in weight or the cost of moving this increased weight. Whether this observation is reproducible or specific for all forms of obesity is unknown, and further studies will be necessary to confirm this point. Apfelbaum, Bostsarron & Lacatis (1973) have reported a similar increase in cost of bicycle riding in normal subjects following 2 weeks of overfeeding, but this remains to be confirmed. Miller, Mumford & Stock (1967) were unable to find an increased cost of exercise during overfeeding. However, when exercise was associated with a meal they reported an enhanced thermic effect of the meal. Bray, Whipp & Koyal (1973) were unable to find an increased cost of exercise or an enhancement of the thermic effect of a meal by exercise in normal weight subjects overfed for 4 weeks. Glick *et al.* (1977) were also unable to confirm either of these observations in lean or obese subjects, but in this study the overfeeding was maintained for only 5 days and, therefore, may not have been long enough to produce such an effect.

In our studies in both lean and obese subjects the increased thermic effect of overnutrition appeared as an increment in the basal or resting oxygen consumption. Since the subjects had continued to overeat during these studies of thermogenesis, one may question whether the increased thermogenesis might represent a prolongation of the thermic effect of the meals and supplements. Therefore, in the last studies in 16 subjects, we repeated our measurements after overfeeding had been discontinued for 24 hours. By this time, some but not all of the excess thermic effect had disappeared. After 26 days, in one group of subjects overfed protein, all of the excess thermogenesis had disappeared. From these observations it seems unlikely that the thermic effect of overnutrition is identical to the thermic effect of a meal.

Several conclusions can be drawn from the above. First, if an adaptive increase in thermogenesis occurs during overfeeding in man, it develops only after approximately 2 weeks of substantial overfeeding. Second, the magnitude of change is small, probably representing no more than 15 per cent of the resting metabolic rate. Third, the expected changes in thermogenesis in these studies test the limits of sensitivity of the methods used to assess these changes and may account for some of the disagreement in the literature on this subject.

It is tempting to speculate that, if normal people react to overfeeding by using some of the calories inefficiently, spontaneously obese people may lack such a protective mechanism against obesity. Even if the difference in ability to waste calories were small, over a long period of time the result could be considerable. However, there is no convincing evidence to date in the literature that there is a lack of this sort in any of the syndromes of obesity.

Clearly, however, this is an area which requires further investigation. It may well be that the initial state of nutrition of the subject is an important factor in determining the thermic response.

Mechanisms

The site of heat production in the body is intimately related to mitochondrial respiration. It is currently debated whether the efficiency of this process (coupled versus uncoupled or loosely coupled oxidative phosphorylation) is the same at all times and under all conditions. An important point, which does not depend on whether metabolism is 'coupled' or 'uncoupled', is that the heat produced depends on the rate of mitochondrial respiration. Therefore, adaptive thermogenesis, whether decreased as in starvation or increased as in overnutrition, depends on an alteration in the rate of these processes. In the coupled state, the rate of mitochondrial combustions depends on the availability of ADP for phosphorylation, and subsequently, on the rate of utilization of ATP formed by this process for the production of more ADP, thus linking production of the ATP with its utilization. It follows from this that the utilization of ATP must be increased for an adaptive increase in thermogenesis to occur during overnutrition in the coupled state.

In the uncoupled or loosely coupled state the relationship between ATP utilized and, therefore, the ADP available for phosphorylation does not hold. In this case, substrate availability or other factors apparently regulate the rate of respiration. Substrates available for oxidation are increased following overfeeding. It is unknown whether this increased substrate availability by itself or through a direct effect on coupling could increase thermogenesis. There is evidence that high concentrations of fatty acids may produce loose coupling. It should be stated, however, that in man, except for the well-known effect drugs such as dinitrophenol have on oxidative phosphorylation, there are few syndromes in which uncoupled metabolism has been demonstrated. The two reported cases of Luft's syndrome (Luft *et al.*, 1962), in which there is functional and anatomical abnormality of mitochondria and the syndrome of malignant hyperthermia (Gordon, Britt & Kalow, 1973), which occasionally follows inhalation anesthesia, are examples.

If uncoupled respiration rarely occurs in man, then those cellular processes which utilize ATP inefficiently in the coupled state are the most likely mechanisms to explain adaptive thermogenesis during overnutrition. Hegsted (1974) has suggested a few examples, including the loss of restraint of cellular phosphatases which could release the chemical energy from ATP without yielding useful work. This is an interesting possibility, and like other examples discussed below, is not excluded by presently available evidence. As Milligan (1971) has noted and Baldwin (1968) recorded years ago, man is a periodic eater and a constant metabolizer. Hence, it is necessary not only in meal eaters, but also during periods of overfeeding, that considerable dietary metabolites be stored prior to their utilization as sources of energy. The cost of glucose storage as triglyceride prior to utilization is estimated as 20 per cent of the energy which would be available were it oxidized directly. Flatt (this volume) examines the cost of storage of excess nutrients. Although inefficient, the cost of storage during overnutrition should be proportional to the amount overeaten. However, the shuttling of fuels in and out of storage may be increased during overnutrition. It has been suggested that during overnutrition, the rate of cycling of glucose, fatty acids and amino acids may be accelerated because of conflicting signals for both storage and utilization (Himms-Hagen, 1976). If this were so, it would add an additional cost over and above that of storage alone. Examples are the local cycling of fatty acids and triglyceride or the longer more costly cycling of fatty acids from the adipose tissue to the liver for reesterification, followed by transport out of the liver and back into the fat depot. Besides the cost of lipolysis and reesterification, this cycle would also require the added cost of lipoprotein synthesis. In this manner, ATP is utilized without the production of useful work and with the generation of heat.

In a similar fashion, there are several reversible steps in metabolism which, like the above 'loops' of metabolism, could waste energy as heat through cycling. These so-called 'futile cycles' include, for example, cycling between glucose and glucose-6-phosphate, fructose-6-phosphate and fructose 1,6-disphosphate and phosphenol pyruvate and pyruvate. Another inefficient mechanism which is often cited is the hydrogen 'shuttle'. An example is the glycerol phosphate shuttle, where the hydrogen from α-glycero-phosphate, like succinate, is transferred to FAD in the mitochondria as its hydrogen-acceptor. When oxidized, FAD then yields two rather than three moles of ATP as would have happened had cytoplasmic NAD served as a co-factor. The extent to which this pathway functions during overnutrition is unknown. It is known to be decreased in obesity (Galton & Bray, 1967) and accelerated by thyroid hormones (Bray, 1969), by diets low in protein (Sterling & Stock, 1968), and during cold-induced increase in thermogenesis (Smith & Hoijer, 1962).

Protein synthesis is expensive in terms of the energy requirements. The question should be asked whether the rates of protein synthesis and degradation (turnover) might be altered by overnutrition, as it most certainly is during starvation. An increase in the rate of synthesis and renewal of membranes, enzymes and other cellular components, if coupled with an equally increased rate of degradation, could be responsible for increased rates of ATP utilization without a change in the steady state of the organism. This would result in an increased cost to the organism as a result of a decrease in the net efficiency of energy utilization. Several investigators (Miller & Payne, 1962; Sterling & Stock, 1968; Tulp *et al.*, 1976) have found either inefficient food utilization, increased thermogenesis or both, when growing animals are fed low protein, high carbohydrate diets. These studies were performed in growing organisms. It is obvious that the equilibrium reached between synthesis and degradation of cellular components in the growing animals must be different from the fully mature organism, or growth would not occur. However, in the above studies the metabolic cost of this growth was increased. Ashworth (1969) found an increased thermic response to meals during the refeeding of undernourished children and attributed this to a burst of synthesis of new tissue stimulated by the meals. Whether the cost of this synthetic activity was out of proportion to the increase in the new cell mass associated with this refeeding is not known. Blaxter (1971) has noted that growth of lean mass continues even in calorically restricted growing animals, while this growth does not take place in the mature organism. Clearly, the growth response of tissues of the growing animal is different than that of the mature organism. An interesting hypothesis is that intake above maintenance in the mature organism is accompanied as in starvation with a tendency to maintain the lean mass. In contrast to the situation in starvation, maintenance during periods of overnutrition might be at the expense of an increased protein turnover and, therefore, at a decreased metabolic efficiency to the organism. In other words, since hormones and changes in the level of nutrition are known to affect the rates of synthesis and degradation of numerous cellular proteins, one may ask whether the equilibrium reached by these two processes might be at the expense of an increased rate of turnover which would then result in decreased net efficiency of caloric utilization. In the case of a growing animal, this point of equilibrium is not reached, since there is continued growth.

Another process, costly in energy and productive of heat, is the osmotic work of the cell and its membranes. Whittam (1961) suggested that the requirement for sodium-potassium transport might serve as a pacemaker of cellular respiration. Homeothermy, or regulation of body temperature at a constant level above environmental, requires a source of heat for dissipation down the thermal gradient. Edelman (1976) has suggested that modulations of the rate of utilization of ATP by the membrane Na-K-ATPase might serve to maintain this homeostatic function of the body and that this is controlled by thyroid hormones. The mechanism by which thyroid hormones might regulate heat production through an effect on the Na-K-ATPase is not entirely clear. Giving hypothyroid animals thyroid hormone increases the number of Na-K-ATPase transport sites of several thyroid sensitive tissues (Edelman, 1976; Lo & Lo, 1977; Liberman *et al.*, 1977). However, simply increasing the number of sites would not affect the utilization of ATP. Only if this increased capacity were stimulated would increased ATP utilization and thermogenesis occur. We know that the intracellular sodium concentration influences the rate of function of these transport sites, and that the intracellular concentration is itself affected by a number of hormones, substrates and products. There is the possibility, for instance, that the increased fluxes of substrates or change in hormonal profile during overfeeding may affect intracellular sodium concentrations or may even stimulate the Na-K-ATPase directly.

Recent findings have shown a possible further link between adaptive changes in thermogenesis of dietary origin and the calorigenic action of thyroid hormones. Overfeeding and underfeeding alters the peripheral metabolism of thyroxin. Thyroxin (T_4) is the major secretory product of the thyroid gland and its peripheral metabolism occurs largely through monodeiodinative degradation in either ring. If the phenolic ring is monodeiodinated, 3,5,3′-triiodothyronine (T_3) is produced with a three to fivefold increase in activity, while deiodination of the tyrosine ring yields the biologically inactive reverse T_3 (3,3′,5′-T_3). In healthy, normally-fed subjects approximately 60 to 80 per cent of T_4 is metabolized in the periphery in this manner and approximately 40 per cent is then converted to T_3 and 60 per cent to rT_3.

We have found that both overnutrition and undernutrition alter this peripheral metabolism of thyroid hormone (Vagenakis *et al.*, 1975; Danforth *et al.*, 1975). Serum concentrations of T_3 are decreased and rT_3 increased when obese volunteers are fasted, and the opposite changes occur in the serum concentrations of T_3 and rT_3 when lean or obese volunteers are overfed. We have also discovered that the carbohydrate content of the diet may play an important role in these dietary-induced changes in thyroid hormone metabolism. In man the changes produced in T_3 and rT_3 during fasting are mimicked when isocaloric carbohydrate-free diets are provided (Danforth *et al.*, 1976). Also in man, the increased T_3 and decreased rT_3 produced by overfeeding is mimicked by increasing the relative amount of carbohydrate in the diet. Refeeding carbohydrate but not fat to fasted rats returns the lowered T_3 concentrations toward normal (Burger *et al.*, 1977). It is clear from these observations that both the level and composition of ingested calories have an effect on thyroid hormone metabolism.

We have used kinetic techniques to investigate the quantitative significance of these changes in the peripheral metabolism of thyroid hormones. In 16 volunteers overfed for 3 weeks with either carbohydrate, protein, or fat, we have found an increase of approximately 80 per cent in the production rate of T_3 (Danforth *et al.*, 1977). No change in the production rate of T_4 occurred in these same subjects, suggesting that a shift in metabolism of T_4 had occurred with increased production of T_3. Similar studies have been performed by Vagenakis (1977) in subjects during starvation. In these studies T_3 production was decreased and rT_3 production increased.

One small group of four subjects later gave results which were apparently at variance with those from the short-term overfeeding experiments. One would expect that if overfeeding were predominantly with fat, weight gain would be more efficient, since the synthetic requirements for fat storage would be less than for carbohydrate. Such was the case when these volunteers gained weight with comparative ease when adding 1100 calories as fat to their diet (Goldman *et al.*, 1975). They differed from the preceding groups in that they failed to show the increased caloric requirement to maintain weight. There was no evidence of an increased expenditure of calories after weight gain over that predicted for maintenance of the increased body mass in contrast to the findings in short-term overfeeding with fat. No comparable measurements of energy expenditure following long-term overfeeding with mixed diets are yet available. Consistent with the unchanged energy expenditure in those who had undergone long-term overfeeding with fat, there was no change in the concentration of T_3 in the serum. Since there were important differences in the circumstances of the respective long-term studies, such as time, location, and habits of the subjects with respect to coffee drinking, a valid comparison of the effects of long-term overfeeding with varying dietary composition must await further studies.

Clinical implication

It is a frustrating experience for both patient and physician when the rate of loss of weight gradually declines after some weeks of conscientious following of a hypocaloric diet. The survival mechanism, in which the resting metabolic rate declines and thus reduces the caloric demands during starvation, as Bray (1976) has pointed out, explains the smaller net deficit of calories and slower rate of loss. Björntorp (this volume) has shown that this tendency of the rate of weight loss to reach a plateau tends to occur when a normal lipid content of the adipocytes is reached. It is sometimes suggested that it is logical to give thyroid hormone in amounts sufficient to restore the original rate of metabolism, so that weight loss may be speeded. However, as discussed above, the decline in serum T_3 which occurs in undernutrition probably provides an important survival mechanism, namely, the slowing of the rate of protein turnover and hence preservation of the lean body mass. Thus, it seems unwise to consider restoring the original rate of thyroid hormone at the cost of disturbing protein balance.

Summary

Whether the net efficiency of substrate utilization is constant during changes in the level of nutrition is a recurrent question and one which is important in connection with gain and loss of weight in man. There is a new body of evidence that changes in thermogenesis do occur in response to overfeeding. This adaptation develops only after approximately 2 weeks of overfeeding and is associated with overfeeding of either carbohydrate, fat or protein. The increased thermogenesis during overfeeding of either lean or moderately obese volunteers is explained by an increase in the resting metabolic rate and appears to be a phenomenon independent of the thermic effect of meals. There is disagreement in the literature as to whether prior overfeeding increases the cost of exercise.

No single mechanism has been found to explain the increased thermogenesis following overnutrition. Uncoupled or loosely coupled oxidative phosphorylation rarely occur in man and are unlikely explanations. Metabolic pathways which are wasteful of energy during coupled respiration are more likely to account for this phenomenon. The turnover of cellular proteins and pumping of ions across membranes are two of the most costly homeostatic processes of the body, and, if accelerated by overfeeding, could, either singly or together, account for the increased thermogenic response to overnutrition. Other examples, including efficient generation of ATP by 'hydrogen shuttles' or inefficient utilization of ATP by 'futile cycles', may also contribute to the increased thermogenesis.

The production rate of triiodothyronine is increased in overfeeding. This may well be responsible for the increased thermogenesis following overnutrition through a direct or permissive effect on one or more of the above processes. Since thyroid hormones have well-known effects on protein synthesis, their modulation by the state of nutrition could represent an important physiologic adaptation to feast or famine through regulation of the rate of protein turnover and the expenditure of calories.

Acknowledgement – Supported by NIH (NIAMDD) grants AM 18535 (Danforth), AM 10254 (Sims), and the General Clinical Research Center RR109, University of Vermont, Burlington, Vermont 05401.

References

Apfelbaum, M., Bostsarron, J. & Lacatis, D. (1971): *Am. J. Clin. Nutr.* 24, 1405.

Apfelbaum, M., Bostsarron, J. & Lacatis, D. (1973): Adaptation of energy expenditure to the level of intake in man. In *Energy balance in man*, ed M. Apfelbaum. Masson: Paris.

Ashworth, A. (1969): *Nature* 223, 407.

Baldwin, R.L. (1968): *J. Dairy Sci.* **51**, 104.
Benedict, F.G., Miles, W.R., Roth, P. & Smith, M. (1919): Human vitality and efficiency under prolonged restricted diet. Carnegie Institution of Washington, Publication 280.
Blaxter, K.L. (1971): *Fed. Proc.* **30**, 1436.
Bray, G.A. (1969): *J. Clin. Invest.* **48**, 1413.
Bray, G.A., Whipp, B.J. & Koyal, S.N. (1973): *Am. J. Clin. Nutr.* **27**, 254.
Bray, G.A. (1976): *The obese patient.* W.B. Saunders Co: Philadelphia.
Burger, A.G., Wimpfheimer, C., Alliod, C. & Danforth, E., Jr. (1977): Abstr. Second International Congress on Obesity 1977. *Int. J. Obesity* **2**, (in press).
Burse, R.L., Goldman, R.F., Crowley, W., Danforth, E., Jr. & Sims, E.A.H. (1976): *Fed Proc.* **35**, 402.
Burse, R.L., Goldman, R.F., Danforth, E., Jr., Horton, E.S. & Sims, E.A.H. (1977*a*): *Fed. Proc.* **36**, 546.
Burse, R.L., Goldman, R.F., Danforth, E., Jr., Robbins, D.C., Horton, E.S. & Sims, E.A.H. (1977*b*): *American Physiologist* **20**, 13.
Cahill, G.F., Jr., Herrera, M.G., Morgan, A.P., Soeldner, J.S., Steinke, J., Levy, P.L., Reichard, G.A., Jr. & Kipnis, D.M. (1966): *J. Clin. Invest.* **45**, 1751.
Danforth, E., Jr., Sims, E.A.H., Horton, E.S. & Goldman, R.F. (1975): *Diabetes* **24**, 406.
Danforth, E., Jr., Tyzbir, E.D., Horton, E.S., Sims, E.A.H., Burger, A.G., Braverman, L.E., Vagenakis, A.G. & Ingbar, S.H. (1976): *Clin. Res.* **26**, 271A.
Danforth, E., Jr., Horton, E.S., Sims, E.A.H., Burger, A.G., Vagenakis, A.G., Braverman, L.E. & Ingbar, S.H. (1977): *Acta Endocr.* **85** (Suppl. 212), 84.
Edelman, I.S. (1976): *Fed. Proc.* **35**, 2180.
Galton, D.J. & Bray, G.A. (1967): *J. Clin. Endocr.* **27**, 1573.
Garrow, J.S. (1974): *Energy balance and obesity in man.* New York: American Elsevier Publishing Co. Inc.
Glick, Z., Shvartz, E., Magazanik & Modan, M. (1977): *J. Clin. Nutr.* **30**, 1026.
Goldman, R.F., Haisman, M.F., Bynum, G., Danforth, E., Jr ., Horton, E.S. & Sims, E.A.H. (1975): Experimental obesity in man. VII. Metabolic rate in relation to dietary intake. In *Obesity in perspective,* ed G.A. Bray, p. 165. Washington, DC: US Govt. Ptg. Office.
Gordon, R.A., Britt, B.A. & Kalow, W. (1973): *Malignant hyperthermia,* Springfield, Il: Thomas.
Hegsted, D.M. (1974): *Nutr. Rev.* **32**, 33.
Himms-Hagen, J. (1976): *Ann. Rev. Physiol.* **38**, 315.
Keys, A., Brozek, J., Hanschel, A., Mickelson, O. & Taylor, H.L. (1950): *The biology of human starvation.* Minneapolis, Minnesota: University of Minnesota Press.
Liberman, U.A., Asano, Y., Lo, C. & Edelman, I. (1977): *Experientia* (in press).
Lo, C. & Lo, T. (1977): *Experientia* (in press).
Luft, R., Ikkos, D., Palamieri, G., Ernster, L. & Apzelius, B. (1962): *J. Clin. Invest.* **41**, 1776.
Miller, D.S. & Payne, P.R. (1962): *J. Nutr.* **78**, 255.
Miller, D.A., Mumford, P. & Stock, M.J. (1967): *Am. J. Clin. Nutr.* **20**, 1223.
Milligan, L.P. (1971): *Fed. Proc.* **30**, 1454.
Neumann, R.O. (1902): *Arch. Hyg.* **45**, 1.
Passmore, R., Meikeljohn, A.P., Dewar, A.D. & Throw, R.K. (1955*a*): *Brit. J. Nutr.* **9**, 20.
Passmore, R., Meikeljohn, A.P., Dewar, A.D. & Throw, R.K. (1955*b*): *Brit. J. Nutr.* **9**, 27.
Passmore, R., Strong, J.A., Swindells, Y.E. & El Din, N. (1963): *Brit. J. Nutr.* **17**, 373.
Rubner, M. (1902): Die Gesetze des Energie Verbrauchs bei die Ernahrung. Leipzig: Franz Deuticke. U.S. Army Research Institute of Environmental Medicine. Translation (Natick, Massachusetts). R.J.T. (1968).
Sims, E.A.H., Danforth, E., Jr., Horton, E.S., Bray, G.A., Glennon, J.A. & Salans, L.B. (1973): *Recent Prog. Horm. Res.* **29**, 457.
Sims, E.A.H. (1976): *Clins Endoc. Metab.* **5**, 377.
Smith, R.E. & Hoijer, D.J. (1962): *Physiol. Rev.* **42**, 60.
Sterling, J.L. & Stock, M.J. (1968): *Nature* **200**, 801.
Sterling, K. & Milch, P.O. (1975): *Proc. Nat. Acad. Sci.* **72**, 3225.
Strong, J.A., Stirling, D. & Passmore, R. (1967): *Brit. J. Nutr.* **21**, 909.
Tulp, O., Horton, E.S., Tyzbir, E.D., Danforth, E., Jr., & Bollinger, J. (1976): *Clin. Res.* **24**, 371A.
Vagenakis, A.G., Burger, A.G., Portnay, G., Rudolph, M., O'Brien, J.I., Azizi, F., Arky, R., Nicod, P., Ingbar, S.H. & Braverman, L.E. (1975): *J. Clin. Endoc.* **41**, 191.
Vagenakis, A.G. (1977): Thyroid hormone metabolism in prolonged experimental starvation in man. In *Anorexia nervosa,* ed R.A. Vigersky, p. 243. New York: Raven Press.
Whittam, R. (1961): *Nature* **191**, 603.

24
Possible interaction between physical activity, body composition and obesity in man

J.V.G.A. DURNIN
Institute of Physiology, The University, Glasgow, G12 8QQ, Scotland.

Our understanding of the biological and medical significance of the changes which occur in body composition as a result of 'obesity' seems to be still inadequate, and indeed perhaps becoming even more unclear. Certain areas of importance are frequently neglected.

One such area concerns the role of physical activity in the prevention or treatment of obesity. Often this role is either ignored or relegated very much to the background. It seems to me that there are some clear-cut considerations to bear in mind in this subject area.

If an individual has excess adipose tissue and if weight loss in the body is produced entirely by reducing the energy intake, the weight loss is *not* of fat alone but is adipose tissue together with some muscle tissue and possibly skeleton (Keys *et al.*, 1950; Entenman *et al.*, 1958; Buskirk *et al.*, 1963), that is, not only is fat lost, but the fat-free mass (FFM) of the body is also reduced. The loss of FFM can often be considerable so that in complete starvation it may constitute as much as 30 to 50 per cent of the weight lost (Barnard *et al.*, 1969; Durnin & Womersley, 1973); in average weight loss by dietary restriction the FFM accounts for between 15 and 35 per cent of the total tissue discarded by the body (Brozek *et al.*, 1963; Entenman *et al.*, 1958).

In relation to this loss of fat and fat-free mass from the body, there are some simple facts in the energy equation which justify re-emphasizing. In an average obese individual, energy expenditure is low. If this obese individual has read John Garrow's book (Garrow, 1974), he or she might even be reinforced in the attitude that a low level of physical activity was an unimportant factor in his or her obesity. Thus, if energy expenditure is low the extent of the energy deficit is the difference between that low level and the energy intake - say 2000 kcal (8.4 MJ) or less per day of energy expenditure minus 1000 kcal (4.2 MJ) per day of intake, ie about 1000 kcal (4.2 MJ) or less. In other words, for an effective treatment of the condition, energy intake must be kept, often for very long periods of time, at very low levels - with all the problems arising from this long-continued unsatisfying meagre diet. As weight is discarded, a further act of God deals another blow at the unfortunate obese person - a reduction in basal or resting metabolic rate occurs, making the extent of the energy deficit less than it was in the early stages and, therefore, the rate of weight loss slows down.

What role can exercise play in all this? Firstly, from animal studies and from some of the studies on man, (Buskirk *et al.*, 1963; Parizkova, 1969; Lamb *et al.*, 1969) it is clear that physical activity will either prevent, or at least minimize the loss of FFM when weight loss occurs. This resultant higher FFM in turn will tend to reduce the effects of the lowered BMR which usually accompanies weight loss. And lastly, the extra energy expenditure of the physical activity - which, in spite of Garrow's assertions, can often be of the order of 500 to 1000 kcal (2.1 to 4.2 MJ)/day - will either allow a considerable increase in the negative energy balance or will permit a larger energy intake with the same deficit.

In practice, we have frequently found that our moderately obese subjects can maintain their diet (their reduced dietary intake) *better* if they are also involved in an exercise programme.

Of course, in making these statements I am deliberately avoiding the trap so blindly fallen into by many people in discussing obesity. I have not been considering a *grossly obese* individual when referring to the role of physical activity. I do not think that exercise has much relevance to grossly obese people, who may have great difficulty in even walking. But if by referring to 'obesity' this were meant to be synonymous with the condition found only in grossly obese people, then this position ought to be carefully defined beforehand. 'Obesity' should, in general, refer to a condition which usually means the presence of moderate to large amounts of fat in the body, say from 20 to 40 per cent of the body weight as fat, and only at the extreme end of the range would 'obesity' include the very obese person with 50 per cent or more of fat in the body weight.

A strong plea might well be made for at least a rational approach to the measurement of obesity. To assess obesity as 'overweight' seems to me to epitomize a most unsatisfactory state which would not be tolerated in most other areas of medical investigation. Surely, with a little more knowledge, we should be able to find some relatively easy and reasonably accurate way to use skinfold thickness, perhaps along with some girth measurements, to estimate body fat. We ought not to need much persuasion to adopt this approach. Skinfold thicknesses undoubtedly measure subcutaneous fat. The fat in the body is deposited, in variable but relatively predictable proportions, between the subcutaneous and the internal depots. What needs emphasizing now is not that skinfolds are usually very difficult to measure (which they are not, except in the extremely obese person) or that their measurement varies to a large and important degree between different observers - which several publications demonstrate is clearly not the case (Edwards *et al.*, 1955; Imbimbo *et al.*, 1968; Burkinshaw, Jones & Kaupowicz, 1973; Womersley & Durnin, 1973) - or that they are insufficiently accurate in assessing fat, which is true at present but no other technique, applicable on a large scale, is even as satisfactory. What is required now is: the much more thorough investigation of the variation in the proportions of fat which may be found between the subcutaneous and the internal depots; how much of this variation is a reflection of changes due to age, sex, weight gain or weight loss; and how variable is the distribution within the subcutaneous tissues. We might thus eventually be able to predict not only total fat in the body, but also fat distribution, from some simple skinfold measurements.

For very obese people, with their excessive and often unsightly distribution of fat, what is the probability that this is the consequence of a metabolic disorder? And such a peculiar disorder at that, with the disability that the body is more efficient than normal.

I am largely unconvinced up to the present about the relevance to man of the animal studies on feed utilization. I do not find it very helpful to remind myself that farmers are well aware of differences in feed efficiency of animals. These animals are not comparable to any humans I can think of: they are, and have been for many generations, highly inbred for the specific purpose of producing meat or milk at maximum efficiencies. They are rarely allowed a life span beyond the equivalent of a fairly young adult human. In any case, even if we knew that variability was present in man related to the efficiency of food utilization, this is still a far cry from being sure that it would be a phenomenon of importance in obesity.

Some indication of the possible significance of individual variability in the energy derived from food may be obtained from some studies carried out by Southgate and myself some years ago (Southgate & Durnin, 1970). We studied 12 young men, 12 young women, 13 elderly men and 14 elderly women. Different types of diet, with differing amounts of 'roughage' (or unavailable carbohydrate) were investigated. We showed that not only was the net energy available from diets inversely proportional to the amount of 'roughage', but there was also a 3 per cent difference between individuals in the 'availability' of energy from the same diet. On intakes of between 8.4 and 12.5 MJ (2000 to 3000 kcal/day) this is equivalent to 250 to 375 kJ (60 to 90 kcal) per day, or 90 to 135 MJ (22 000 to 33 000 kcal) per year or at least 2 to 3 kg of adipose tissue per year or 20 to 30 kg of adipose tissue in 10 years. For apparently comparable individuals eating the same quantities of the same diet, this is a formidable difference in the amount of fat which might be acquired in a relatively short part of a normal life span. Since much subjective evidence indicates that many adults retain energy balance only by consciously altering their life-style, either by eating less or exercising more, when they are aware of an uncomfortable change in their body weight, one of these two individuals, eating the same quantities of the same foods and having the same amount of physical activity, could sail through life on a dietetically well-balanced ship, whereas the other would require recurrent spells of self-discipline and self-denial to regain the same body weight. Unhappily, there is no way of proving this at the present stage of our methodology.

Another possible important variable, sometimes rather cavalierly dismissed, concerns the influence of environmental temperature on thermogenesis and the smaller amount of energy expended by the obese individual compared to the lean person when exposed to cold. There is a sizable body of information by Buskirk, Iampietro & Welch (1957) and by others showing quite large differences between the obese and the lean in the metabolic rates on exposure to cold.

However, perhaps the most significant factors which cause large variations in body composition between individuals may well be related to apparently small differences in net energy intake or energy expenditure. If we markedly reduce our food intake or markedly increase our energy expenditure, we have sensors which can adequately inform us of our altered state of energy balance and presumably will enable compensation if this is possible. In both situations of a lowered intake or a higher energy expenditure, we will feel hungry and tend to eat more. On the other hand, if we have small quantitative differences in our energy balance - 200 to 400 kJ (50 to 100 kcal) per day - there is no mechanism that I know of which is sensitive enough to detect this. Thus, in the example quoted earlier of the 3 per cent variation in the net energy availability from a diet, our control mechanisms would be unable to monitor this other than as a long-term effect. The long-term effect of small differences can be illustrated by an example of Garrow's. A fellow-countryman of mine, a William Campbell, died in Glasgow in 1878 at the age of 22 having established a British record for obesity. At death he weighed 341 kg: so by making reasonable assumptions about his body composition when he died, we can estimate that in his 22 years he acquired fat representing an excess of intake over expenditure of about 7000 MJ (1.75 million kcal) and if we calculate the daily average excess required to achieve his record-breaking status in 22 years, the answer comes out to about 900 kJ or about 200 kcal per day. Perhaps more apposite to the short-duration measurements which we usually employ for estimating metabolic rate, this represents 0.6 kJ or 0.15 kcal/min. It would require more care in controlling the experimental conditions than most of us employ, to be sure that our measurements of metabolic rate on our obese patients were accurate to this degree of precision. I think we can obtain such accuracy only by long-term calorimetric studies, by incarcerating individuals in a sufficiently spacious direct calorimeter so that a reasonably normal existence may be permitted during several days. The practical difficulties of doing this are daunting at present. If we accept that measurements of the required accuracy virtually do not exist, we are indeed in a quandry. We are admitting that energy differences large enough to result in record-breaking obesity are beyond our ability to detect.

A problem of great interest, both in the causation and the treatment of obesity, concerns whether or not the human body can adapt its level of energy expenditure as a result of varying energy intakes. Much interesting and useful information on adaptation to low energy intakes is contained in the excellently documented volumes, 'The biology of human starvation' by Keys, Brozek and their colleagues (Keys *et al.*, 1950). However, I am bound to reiterate that, again because of methodological problems, we are not at all certain of the frequency or of the degree of adaptation to low energy intakes which occurs in obese patients.

Much evidence, from several studies on very different types of population, demonstrates that there are groups of healthy active muscular men who exist in energy balance on about 8.4 MJ (2000 kcal) per day. There are relatively few studies on whether or not comparable low metabolic rates may occur in obese people. We have recently investigated body composition, and the metabolic rate at rest and in exercise, on a group of refractory obese patients.

The measurements were made on 86 women, mean weight 93 kg with a mean body composition (by densitometry and skinfold thicknesses) of fat equal to 43 per cent of body weight, and 13 men of equivalent weight 75 kg and 38 per cent fat. The mean metabolic rates were equivalent to 7.7 MJ (1840 kcal) per day for the women and 9.2 MJ (2200 kcal) per day for the men. Clearly, most of these supposedly refractory obese people did not have unusually low metabolic rates at rest, but there was some variation between these and *some* metabolic rates were low. On the other hand, they were a highly selected group and were not at all representative of the average obese person.

In conclusion, it is possible to generate a reasonably acceptable philosophy about the maintenance of a normal body composition having more or less general applicability. This philosophy might be contrasted to that proposed by Hirsch in his stimulating introductory talk to this conference.

In that highly biassed way in which one gathers information and becomes emotionally attached to it, reinforced in my case by the two years we spent in our nutritional studies in two New Guinean villages, I think it is possible to argue plausibly that throughout almost the whole of man's long development he has rarely been exposed to severe food shortage. His population of any area was limited - restricted by disease and high infant and child mortality - and his way of life, as a nomad or as a relatively settled hunter-gatherer, of necessity required a constant supply of food. The food was there for the hunting and the gathering.

The contrasting philosophy which this generates is that there was no particular advantage in eating to obesity and living for weeks or months on the stored fat. Man does nor hibernate and in any case mostly populated the warmer parts of the earth's surface. He might have, from time to time, gorged himself on a killed animal and lain back for a day or two, before taking up the hunt again, but that is not quite the same thing as accumulating large depots of fat.

The mode of existence for man (I use the word in a restricted but more important sense as referring to the male) involved much physical activity, occasionally of a very strenuous nature, and the ability to perform physical activity was an important stimulus to his evolutionary development. Mild degrees of fatness had little influence on this ability, and within these limitations the regulation of his food intake was organized on a rather flexible basis. On the other hand, for woman, physical activity was necessary, but less necessary than for the male (hence her lower Hb, blood volume, 0_2 consumption, muscle mass etc.) but *she* had a use for a fat store - to provide for pregnancy and lactation. A normal body composition for a woman, I submit, would include a sizable fat store. The question might then be asked, is obesity really likely to be a health problem for more than a very small percentage of women?

For both sexes, but especially for men, physical activity is the essential component for a properly adjusted equation. Energy balance is difficult in its absence and its absence implies an unphysiological state. When energy balance is disturbed, which may often happen because of the cumulative action of small factors, the imbalance may be detectable only by a conscious self-disapproval in relation to appearance or to bodily comfort. The therapy may also be self-applied, with physical activity opening up the options: the exercise itself burns up more energy, it increases or maintains FFM which also raises metabolic rate, and combined with restricted food intake it enhances the loss of the body's stored energy.

Physical activity has the further advantage in the treatment of an obese person in providing a new set of behaviour patterns which, if they are pleasurable or satisfying in some way, at least have the chance of being retained over a long duration.

References

Barnard, D.L., Ford, J., Garnett, E.S., Mardell, R.J. & Whyman, A.E. (1969): *Metabolism* **18**, 564.

Brozek, J., Grande, F., Anderson, J.T. & Keys, A. (1963): *Ann. N.Y. Acad. Sci.* **110**, 113.

Burkinshaw, L., Jones, P.R.M. & Kaupowicz, D.W. (1973): *Human Biol.* **45**, 273.

Buskirk, E.R., Iampietro, P.F. & Welch, B.E. (1957): *US Army Med. Nutr.* Lab. Rep. No. 215.

Buskirk, E.R., Thompson, R.H., Lutwak, L. & Whedon, C.D. (1963): *Ann. N.Y. Acad. Sci.* **110**, Part 2, 918.

Durnin, J.V.G.A. & Womersley, J. (1973): *Br. J. Pharmacol.* **49**, 115.

Edwards, D.A.W., Hammond, W.H., Healy, M.J.R., Tanner, J.M. & Whitehouse, R.H. (1955): *Br. J. Nutr.* **9**, 133.

Entenman, C., Goldwater, W.H., Ayres, N.S., Nell, S. & Behnke, A.R. (1958): *J. Appl. Physiol.* **13**, 129.

Garrow, J.S. (1974): *Energy balance and obesity in man.* Amsterdam: North Holland Pub. Co.

Imbimbo, B., Fidanza, A.A., Caputo, V. & Moro, C.O. (1968): *Quad. Nutr.* **28**, 332.

Keys, A., Brozek, J., Henschel, A., Mickelsen, O. & Taylor, H.L. (1950): *The biology of human starvation.* Minneapolis: Univesity of Minnesota Press.

Lamb, D.R., Van Huss, W.D., Garrow, R.E., Heusner, W.W., Weber, J.C. & Kertzer, R. (1969): *Res. Quart.* **40**, 123.

Parizkova, J. (1969): *Biochemistry of exercise: medicine and sport,* Vol. 3, p.137. Basel: Karger.

Southgate, D.A.T. & Durnin, J.V.G.A. (1970): *Br. J. Nutr.* **24**, 517.

Womersley, J. & Durnin, J.V.G.A. (1973): *Human Biol.* **45**, 281.

25
Exercise in the treatment of obesity

R.A. NELSON
Mayo Medical School, Mayo Clinic and Mayo Foundation, Rochester, MN 55901, USA.

In practice, obesity remains one of the most difficult diseases to treat despite the fact that theoretically, both the cause and treatment of it are known. A calorie controlled diet designed to meet nutrient requirements, yet produce a daily deficit, is the best form of therapy. The lack of success of this program is attested to by other treatment programs for obesity such as starvation, hypnosis, injection of human gonadotropin, diet pills, excessive water drinking, and eating large quantities of bulking agents. Unfortunately, all of these programs have met with little success and we still have an obese population.

The purpose of this paper is to define the role of exercise in treatment of obesity. The concept of treatment in this paper is broadened to include both production of weight loss in obese people and prevention of the development of obesity in individuals at risk. Prevention may well be the most important single means by which obesity can be controlled. The results of diet therapy alone have been generally disappointing in producing lasting weight loss.

If exercise has a role in treatment of obesity, lack of exercise should be associated with its development. An inverse correlation between fatness and activity level can easily be seen in a comparison between individuals with the Prader-Willi syndrome and those with anorexia nervosa. Children with the Prader-Willi syndrome have hyperphagia and their total body fat, at times, exceeds 60 per cent of total body weight; they reach such an obese state that they can just barely exercise (Nelson *et al.*, 1970). On the other hand, preoccupation with physical exercise can be an obsession of patients with anorexia nervosa and can contribute materially to weight loss (Nelson, Hayles & Wahner, 1973*a*). However, in both of these extremes, degree of food intake (hyperphagia or hypophagia) is most important in producing the clinical syndromes. In the remaining portions of the spectrum of body size, data are sketchy as far as delineation of the role of activity in maintenance of a given body weight. However, in a study of 350 cases of obesity, Greene (1939) found that 67 per cent occurred simultaneously with inactivity; a history of increased food intake was obtained in only 3 per cent.

Chirico & Stunkard (1960) found that obese women were far less active than non-obese control subjects. Mean activity of obese women was 2 miles/day compared with 4.9 miles/day for non-obese women. Comparison of obese and non-obese men, however, showed much less difference in physical activity. Mean activity of obese men was 3.7 miles/day and that of non-obese men 6 miles/day. The results, however, were disproportionate because of the large quantity of exercise contributed to the series by the few non-obese men. In nine of the 25 cases, obese men walked further than their non-obese control. Obese women indicated that they were more passive than non-obese women in situations of despondency, boredom and social underaction. Obese men did not differ from non-obese men in their response to these situations. It seemed that physical activity was more a part of production of obesity in women than it was in men.

Studies by Johnson, Burke & Mayer (1956) and Stefanik, Heald & Mayer (1959) in young people have indicated that inactivity was more important than overeating in producing the obese state in both girls and boys. Besides these findings, they also noted that obese girls were found to be more advanced than similar girls of height, age and grade, in earlier deceleration of growth in height and earlier menarche (Johnson *et al.*, 1956).

In obese boys, eating more than average was not typical and although little difference was noted in the amount of time they scheduled for light, moderate and very active exercise, their degree of participation was generally less than for non-obese boys (Stefanik *et al.*, 1959). In more recent studies by Weidman and co-workers (1977), 104 students were randomly selected for a study of diet from a survey of school children. Diet studies were carried out two to six months following the initial screening studies. A 7-day diet diary was recorded under the supervision of a nutritionist by each child's mother. Validity was ascertained by subjective and objective methods. For instance, the subjective validity was determined by the nutritionist who reviewed the diet diary for accuracy with the mother. The objective method was measurement of urinary nitrogen excretion over a period of 12 hours. Urinary nitrogen excretion is constant and not related to periods of rest or activity, sleep or wakefulness, and overnight samples could be accurately collected, nitrogen determined, and total nitrogen excretion corrected to 24 hours. Although urinary nitrogen does not reflect intake of food that is predominantly composed of carbohydrate and fat, it is the only substance which can be used as an indirect but objective check on reliability of dietary data. Protein is found in so many foods that the accuracy of its recording should reflect the accuracy of recording fat and carbohydrate consumption as well (Huse *et al.*, 1974).

Of the 104 children chosen for detailed dietary studies, 17 were obese, 34 were muscular and 53 were thin. There was no significant difference in the average calorie intake between the three groups, when judged using all data or when judged using only the nitrogen-reliable data. Although these data confirm work of others that obesity in children is not apparently due to excessive intake of calories when judged by average calorie intake, it was obvious that the range of calorie intake of the obese, muscular and thin population groups described a spectrum; some children in each group ate very little, some ate average amounts, and some ate excessive amounts of calories (Nelson, Elveback, Hodgson & Ellefson, unpublished data).

Thus, inactivity apparently can produce obesity in an individual who does not overeat when judged by food intake of a matched, non-obese control person. Unfortunately, activity data are difficult to collect and quantify. Many times, the conclusion that inactivity is a cause of obesity is reached by exclusion, ie if calorie intake is similar in two population groups and one group is thin and the other fat, then the fat group must exercise less.

The sketchy data do not permit inferences about food intake and activity in normal individuals and those at-risk to develop obesity. The conclusion is, however, that the amount of daily exercise is important in governing body size. As an aside, but pertinent to the discussion, it is worthy to mention the bear who goes through the spectrum of hypophagia to hyperphagia, anorexia to obesity, yearly and is able to treat himself, so to speak, in an as yet unknown fashion (Nelson, 1977). Observation of behaviors of bears throughout the year demonstrates that when bears leave dens in springtime, they are anorectic but active. This phenomenon has been observed in the wild and in captive bears taken out of their hibernaculam. Caged animals, upon emergence from their dens, do not assume normal intake of food until 10 days to 2 weeks have elapsed, although not allowed normal rations during this time. After 2 weeks they eat normally throughout the summer. In fall, however, bears demonstrate hyperphagia, usually more than doubling summertime rations. Bears consuming 8000 kilocalories per day in summer will consume 15 000 to 20 000 kilocalories per day in the fall. Grizzly bears observed in the wild feed 20 hours per day in the late fall to prepare for hibernation and they too consume upwards to 20 000 kilocalories per day. Then, when the bear enters hibernation, it becomes anorectic, but physical activity at this time is reduced to almost nothing. This animal integrates food intake and physical activity such that controlled states of obesity and anorexia nervosa are produced. This unlikely animal thus becomes an excellent model to use towards a better understanding of the problems of human beings in regulating body size. The reason this hibernation is of special interest is that the bear's body temperature varies no more than 2°C throughout these extremes of body size.

Metabolic effects of exercise in the treatment of obesity

Physiologic and biochemical changes

Plasma insulin levels decrease while sensitivity to insulin increases in peripheral tissues. Plasma cortisol and triglycerides decrease, plasma glycerol increases (Björntorp *et al.*, 1970; Björntorp *et al.*, 1977). Muscle temperature increases and may reach levels as high as 109°F. There is a tendency towards blood clotting. Increased oxygen consumption by muscle occurs and fibrinolysis is increased. Blood flow through the kidney and gastrointestinal tract decreases. Prolonged physical training causes blood volume and stroke volume of the heart to increase, decreases response of heart rate to work load and increases capacity of the heart and tissues to extract oxygen from blood (Ellestad, 1975).

Beneficial effects of exercise

A decrease in adipose tissue mass occurs along with a slight decrease in average systolic and diastolic blood pressure (Björntorp *et al.*, 1970; Ellestad, 1975). There is a decreased response of the heart rate to work load, some 40 beats different in matched control subjects. Blood triglycerides decrease as well as body fat under some conditions of exercise in middle-aged people. Physically active people tolerate coronary atheromata better. In the Olympic games in Mexico City, severe exhaustion was common but there were no myocardial infarctions diagnosed (Björntorp *et al.*, 1977; Ellestad, 1975).

Lack of physical activity is associated with detrimental effects on body metabolism. Twenty days of bed-rest in trained men produced a decrease in red cell mass, plasma volume and intracellular fluid volume. Loss of body calcium occurred. There was replacement of loose connective tissue with dense tissue so that joint mobility was considerably restricted in less than one week. Heart rate increased and negative nitrogen balance was the rule. It took 55 days of intensive training to bring the men back to pre-test levels (Ellestad, 1975).

Disappointing changes associated with physical activity

There is no change in glucose tolerance. No weight loss was found in obese populations subjected to training without dietary restriction (Björntorp *et al.*, 1970). Increased mobilization of cholesterol occurs but physical activity and training do not lower blood cholesterol (Björntorp *et al.*, 1977). In the human being, no demonstrable change in coronary collateral circulation occurs as a result of training although peripheral blood flow is improved (Ellestad, 1975). Some feel it is easier to eat 350 calories per day less than to exercise an extra 350 calories per day.

Considering the sum total of the effects of lack of exercise as it relates to body size, and the beneficial, disappointing, and hazardous effects of exercise, the conclusion is reached that an increased level of exercise is beneficial in the treatment of obesity.

In obese adults, a calorie controlled diet must be prescribed. The exercise prescription for adults should use a form of exercise the subject does best; it should be a type that does not require an abrupt change of environment (eg, going to a gym, YM or YWCA) or a change of clothes into a uniform. The activity should be easily incorporated into the daily schedule. Walking satisfies these requirements. The obese are as skillful in this activity as are the non-obese. Roughly, one can calculate 0.5 liters of oxygen used per minute of walking. This amounts to 30 liters/hour; assuming roughly 5 kcal/liter of oxygen used, about 150 kcal are expended per hour. Although this is not great, walking will increase physical fitness. Later, reasonable advances in the level of activity and type, depending on the patient's wishes, can be made.

Increasing the level of exercise in non-obese adults will be beneficial in preventing obesity because there is a decrease in calorie requirements with age due to the decrease in metabolic rate which occurs with age (Nelson *et al.*, 1973). This means that all adults should be considered at-risk to develop obesity because appetite control cannot be counted upon to decrease food intake when needs become less. Attitudes towards the intake of food must consciously be changed so that less is eaten. Unfortunately, exercise tends to decrease with increasing age as well. Obviously, increasing the levels of calorie expenditure through exercise will help all adults to maintain a normal body weight.

In children, the importance of exercise in treating obesity is heightened by findings which show that lack of proper amounts of exercise is an etiologic factor in producing the state.

That treatment is important cannot be argued; if a child enters adolescence obese, the chances are one to four that he or she will ever achieve a normal body weight. If a child leaves adolescence obese, the chances increase to about 28 to one against ever achieving a normal body weight (Stunkard & Burt, 1967).

A treatment program for children was defined by Huse and associates (1977) identifying those children with obesity and then proceeding to modify their habits and attitudes towards food and exercise through an individualized supportive program of nutrition and physical education. The program, in general terms, was as follows: (1) Each child was made aware of his daily food intake, (2) Each child became aware of his daily pattern of activity, (3) The need of the body for nutrients and how these nutrient requirements may be satisfactorily met, together with the nutrient contents of foods, were taught to the children, and (4) The relationship between physical activity and calorie expenditure was explained.

Using this approach it was found that six of eight obese children lost between 1.2 and 5.3 kg in 12 weeks and seven of eight decreased their relative weight index towards normal. All parents agreed not to criticize the eating habits of their children; that counselling and advice was given by a nutritionist.

This approach may be the only good technique for treating obese children. It develops attitudes and habits about food and exercise which hopefully formulate lifelong habits enabling the child to control body weight and minimize the occurrence of obesity. The child, however, must be motivated to want to learn how to regulate food intake, energy expenditure and maintain a normal body weight. We have instituted such individually designed programs for children in a public school system only on a short-term basis. Such a program could not be made immediately applicable to the mass of children at-risk to develop obesity, because of its expense.

Use of exercise as a first step towards developing a program to prevent obesity in children

Estimate of number of children at risk to develop obesity

In more recent studies at the Mayo Clinic (Weidman *et al.*, 1977) we surveyed 1918 school children age six to 15 selected randomly from a total sample of 4020 subjects. The children with rare exception were Caucasian, living in the mid-west and coming from families of middle and upper socioeconomic brackets. Less than 10 per cent lived on farms. Heights and weights were measured on each child and he or she was judged thin, muscular, or obese by an attending physician. Blood was drawn after an overnight fast for measurements of serum cholesterol and triglycerides. Children with conditions which might secondarily affect blood lipids were excluded from the study. Each child's relative weight, ie the actual weight divided by the ideal weight, was calculated. The ideal weight was judged at the 50th percentile for height, age and sex of the individual.

Overweight was diagnosed if the relative weight index was between 1.1 and 1.2; obesity if the relative weight index was 1.2 or greater. About 31 per cent of the 1918 school children studied were either overweight or obese. About 18 per cent had relative weight indices between 1.1 and 1.2 and these children were considered to be at risk to develop obesity.

Role of and requirements for a successful program of exercise as a preventative measure against developing obesity

Our data showed and our experience confirmed that nutrition counselling would be different in a quantitative sense for obese and overweight children. Would this be true as far as exercise is concerned? The most likely answer is, no: any obese or overweight child would benefit from any increase in calorie expenditure through exercise. A preliminary study supported this conclusion (Keane, Huse, Palumbo & Nelson, unpublished data). Nine obese children, eating between 10 000 and 20 000 calories per week showed a decrease in their relative weight index over 4 weeks of study when they participated in a jogging program before classes each day and these children did not receive any nutritional counselling. From the results of these studies, I propose that the first step which should be taken towards prevention of obesity in children would be to develop a successful exercise program for all school children. Despite the fact that physical education is taught as a required subject in our grammar and junior high schools, it has not been effective in preventing development of obesity in children at-risk to develop obesity, nor are its goals directed towards this end. Physical education as taught now does not appear to instill into all children a desire to keep active as they grow older. Their physical skills do not seem to develop to a maximum, even though they may be taught to enjoy forms of physical activity. A desire to keep active and physically fit the rest of their lives is a must for the exercise program to succeed.

Under our current system of physical education there is too little time for instructors to develop physical fitness. Games played tend to be monopolized by natural athletes; even to a point where positions on teams tend to be played by the same players who have the best physical skills. Unfortunately, games require good eye and muscular coordination and this selects the natural athlete and excludes most students from participation. When teams are chosen by the children themselves, non-gifted athletes and/or obese children, are usually last to be chosen and play the least. Varsity athletic teams are too large. There is a tendency to use only a few children who have athletic potential, but who are still one year away from entering high school, to play on senior high teams to the exclusion of senior high students. Sometimes decisions are made by coaches to develop winning teams by playing only sophomores so that by the time these students are seniors they will win regularly; this excludes the current juniors and seniors from playing. At first, athletic programs for women appeared directed towards preventing the development of these deficiencies in our physical education system. The current situation is that coaches for women's teams make similar decisions as coaches for male athletes, ie decisions calculated to win.

Our current physical education system, therefore, is not doing the job of creating physically fit children who have a natural interest in keeping fit through daily exercise for the rest of their lives. Such a program would be beneficial not only for their physical and mental health, it would predictably help in preventing obesity in at-risk children as they mature. Physical education, therefore, should develop individual physical skills which stimulate in each child a desire to be physically active on their own terms and perform skills they can carry out best. Such a program would be predicted to fail if introduced to all school children at the present time; new concepts towards mass participation in physical activity, however, could be achieved if they were introduced to all children when they first receive their physical education. Such a development could be made as natural as required education in reading, writing and other subjects.

References

Björntorp, P., de-Jounge, K., Sjöström, L. & Sullivan, L. (1970): *Metabolism* **19**, 631.
Björntorp, P., Holm, G., Jacobsson, B. & Schiller-deJounge, K. *et al.* (1977): *Metabolism* **26**, 319.
Chirico, A.M. & Stunkard, A.J. (1960): *New Engl. J. Med.* **263**, 935.

Ellestad, M.H. (1975): *Stress testing: principles and practice*, p. 197. Philadelphia: F.A. Davis.
Greene, J.A. (1939): *Ann. Intern. Med.* 12, 1797.
Huse, D.M., Nelson, R.A., Briones, E.R. & Hodgson, P.A. (1974): *Am. J. Clin. Nutr.* 27, 771.
Huse, D.M., Palumbo, P.J., Nelson, R.A. & Hick, J.F. (1978): Abstr. Second International Congress on Obesity 1977. *Int. J. Obesity* 2, (in press).
Johnson, J.L., Burke, B.S. & Mayer, J. (1956): *J. Clin. Nutr.* **4**, 37.
Nelson, R.A. (1977): *Kidney International* (in press).
Nelson, R.A., Hayles, A.B., Novak, L.P., Margie, J.D. & Vernet, J. (1970): *Am. J. Clin. Nutr.* 23, 667.
Nelson, R.A., Anderson, L.F., Gastineau, C.F., Hayles, A.B. & Stamnes, C.L. (1973): *J. Am. Med. Ass.* 223, 627.
Nelson, R.A., Hayles, A.B. & Wahner, H.W. (1973*a*): *Proc. Mayo Clin.* **48**, 549.
Stefanik, P.A., Heald, F.P. & Mayer, J. (1959): *Amer. J. Clin. Nutr.* 7, 55.
Stunkard, A. & Burt, V. (1967): *Am. J. Psychiatry* 123, 1433.
Weidman, W.A., Hodgson, P.A., Nelson, R.A. & Elveback, L.R. (1977): *Pediatrics* (in press).

26
TO TREAT OR NOT TO TREAT – THAT IS THE QUESTION?

G.A. BRAY
Department of Medicine, UCLA School of Medicine, Harbor General Hospital Campus, Torrance, California 90509, USA.

To treat, or not to treat: that is the question:
Whether 'tis nobler in the doctor's mind to let the patient suffer
The slings and arrows of obesity,
Or to take arms against the sea of adiposity,
And by treating end it? To treat: to lose weight and regain no more;
And through a loss of weight to end
The heart-ache and the thousand natural shocks
That the corpulent are heir to, 'tis a consummation
Devoutly to be wish'd. To treat, to lose weight;
To lose weight? Perchance to regain. Ay, there's the rub;
For in this struggle with fatness, what depression may come,
When we have shoveled off those mortal pounds,
Must give us pause. There's the respect
That makes obesity of such long life;
For who would bear the whips and scorns of disapproval,
The employer's wrong, the thin man's contumely,
The pangs of dispriz'd love, the law's delay,
The insolence of office, and the spurns
That patient merit of the obese takes,
If he himself might thinness achieve
With a good diet? Who would curses bear,
To grunt and sweat under the heavy load,
But that the dread of something after weight loss,
The undiscover'd misery from whose bourn
The overweight returns, puzzles the doctor,
And makes us rather bear the fat we have
Than fly to dangerous cures we know not of?
Thus obesity doth make cowards of us all;
And thus the native hue of resolution
Is sicklied o'er with the pale cast of fat
And diets of great pitch and moment
With this regard their currents turn awry,
And lose the name of weight loss....

This adaptation of the famous soliloquy from Hamlet indicates the dilemma confronting both overweight individuals and those who would treat them. The decision about the desirability and appropriateness of therapy involves an assessment of medical, social, and economic risks of obesity, which must be balanced against the costs of potential benefits of treatment.

In the following paragraphs, we will examine several aspects of this decision-making process. First, we will review the effects of obesity on morbidity and mortality. With this discussion of relative risk as a background, the risk-benefit ratio for various therapies will be assessed. Third, reasons for failure of the standard methods of treatment will be evaluated.

Finally, a classification and proposal for new approaches to treatment of obesity will be examined in terms of mechanisms of production of various experimental forms of obesity.

Risks of obesity

Increased mortality in overweight individuals has been suggested by all of the insurance company studies which have looked at the relationship between body weight and excess mortality. The most recent and convincing of these is the Society of Actuaries Build and Blood Pressure Study of 1959 (Society of Actuaries, 1959). The data from part of this study are summarized in Fig. 1 (Bray, 1976). These are the results of individuals who were identified as overweight and followed for a period of 16-25 years. The excess mortality is the mortality ratio of the individuals, at each body mass index, compared to the mortality ratio of the total group of insured individuals. It is clear that as body mass index (an index relating body weight and height) increases, there is a rise in excess mortality which becomes clinically important at 30 per cent overweight (ie a body mass index of 30) and increases progressively thereafter. The causes of this excess mortality were ascribed to cardiovascular diseases, diabetes mellitus, renal disease, and gall-bladder disease (Marks, 1960).

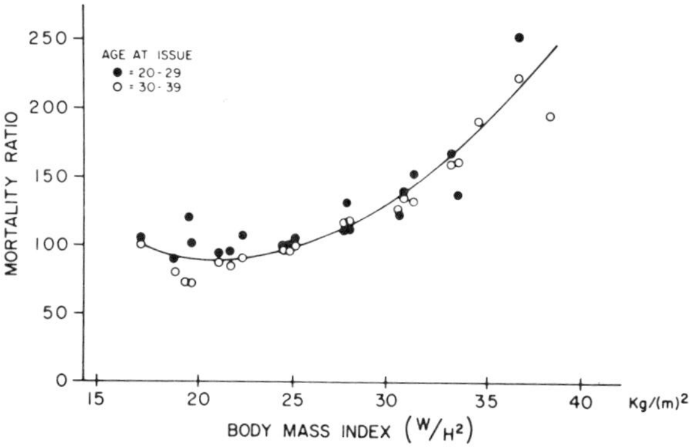

Fig. 1. Relation of body mass index to mortality. Data from the Build and Blood Pressure Study (Society of Actuaries, 1959) have been plotted using the body mass index and the mortality ratio. It can be seen that until the body mass index passes 25, there is no rise in mortality of overweight, relative to normal weight, subjects. But, as body mass index, an index of excess weight, rises further, there is a progressive increase in the excess mortality of overweight individuals compared to normal weight ones

The risks of cardiovascular disease

The relationship between overweight and cardiovascular disease has been difficult to quantify. In some studies, there is an increase in the risk of morbidity and mortality but in others there is not (Bray, 1976). Table 1 summarizes several of these studies. It shows that with long-term follow-up, there is an association between obesity and cardiovascular disease, particularly when obesity is present in men under 40 years of age. In the Cooperative International Study in Seven Countries (Keys *et al.*, 1972), all of the associated risk from overweight could be ascribed to the presence of hypertension. In most other studies, however, there was a significant effect of excess weight on morbidity and mortality from cardiovascular disease when individuals were followed long enough and when the study included younger men (Abraham, Collins & Nordsieck, 1971; Salel *et al.*, 1974).

From the information at hand, one can identify a pathogenic sequence which might produce the increased cardiovascular risk. It has been established that obese individuals have an increased blood volume, increased cardiac output, and increased heart size (Alexander, 1975). There is also convincing evidence that obesity is associated with an increase in blood pressure (Chaing, Perlman & Epstein, 1969) and, in one study, the increased risk of overweight on cardiovascular disease could be attributed entirely to the effects of hypertension (Keys *et al.*, 1972). Although obesity results in increased cumulative long-term risk, this increased risk is small and has not been detected in studies which have identified overweight after age 40 or 50.

Table 1. Obesity and overweight as factors for cardiovascular disease in prospective studies

Study	Author	Year	*n*	Criterion for obesity	Findings
Dupont	Pell & D'Alonzo	1963	86 570	Body wt. >20% above ideal	Myocardial infarct +150% in men < 45 yo. No excess risk in men > 45
Tecumseh	Epstein *et al.*	1965	8 641	Relative wt. from regression - 80th percentile	Risk of CHD +170% in men. No effect in women
Chicago Gas Co.	Stamler *et al.*	1968	1 329	Relative wt. >15%	Risk of MI slightly increased
Former college students	Paffenberger & Wing	1969	3 438	Ponderal index	Fatal MI +170% in men <45 yo, + 140% in men 45-54, + zero in men >54 yo
Health Insurance Plan of N.Y.	Shapiro *et al.*	1969	110 000	Body wt. >15% above av. wt./ht.	MI +50% in overweight
Los Angeles County civil servants	Chapman *et al.*	1971	1 859	Ponderal index	Increased MI in men 30-39; increased angina pectoris also noted
Evans County	Heyden *et al.*	1971	3 102	Body mass index (wt/ht^2)	Overwt. smokers +200% over non-obese smokers; cerebrovascular accidents increased in those gaining weight age >20
Seven Country	Keys *et al.*	1972	11 400	Body mass index (wt/ht^2)	Overwt. associated with hypertension, no independent effect of overwt. on heart disease in men >40
Framingham	Kannel & Gordon	1974	5 209	Relative wt. >20% above av. or ideal	Increase in sudden death and angina pectoris
Manitoba	Rabkin, Mathewson & Hsu	1977	3 983	Body mass index (wt/ht^2)	Wt. related to increase in heart disease in men <35; to sudden death in men < 39; no effects of wt. on heart disease in men >40 yo

MI = myocardial infarct
yo = years old

Gall-bladder disease

The relationship between obesity and gall-bladder disease can be given a more mechanistic basis (Bray, 1976). There is convincing evidence that increased cholesterol production is associated with increased body fat stores (Miettinen, 1974; Bennion & Grundy, 1975). For each kilogram of additional body fat, approximately 20 mg more cholesterol is synthesized each day by the body. Since the major excretory route for cholesterol is through the biliary tree, obese individuals have increased cholesterol excretion in the bile. This enhances the likelihood for development of cholesterol gall-stones since high cholesterol concentrations in the bile make precipitation of cholesterol stones more likely. That gall-bladder disease and obesity are clinically associated has been observed in several studies (Bernstein, Werner & Rimm, 1973). Sturdevant, Pearce & Dayton (1973) showed a significant increase in the frequency of gall-stones during a dietary study conducted at the Wadsworth Veterans Administration Hospital. Rimm & his colleagues (1975), in a retrospective study, showed an increase in gall-bladder disease in relation to both age and weight status. Thus the risk of developing gall-bladder disease, as well as the risk of surgery from gall-bladder disease, would both appear to be increased in obesity.

Diabetes mellitus

The relationship between obesity and diabetes mellitus was noted most recently in the findings of the National Commission on Diabetes (1975). They found that, for each 20 per cent increase in body weight, there is a doubling of the risk in developing diabetes. This relationship of obesity and diabetes mellitus has been known for many years, however. In 1935, Joslin and his colleagues observed that over two-thirds of the adult onset diabetics at their clinic were significantly overweight. Hundley (1956) found an important relationship between the degree of excess weight and mortality from diabetes in several populations. More recently, West & Kalbfleisch (1971) showed an association in large populations between the prevalence of diabetes mellitus and the relative weight status of the population. That is, the higher the average weight of a population, the greater the prevalence of diabetes. Obesity is also an important factor in the development of diabetes in offspring of families where diabetes is present. The risk of developing diabetes is increased two and one-half fold in the obese members of a family with a diabetic, when compared to the normal weight family members (Baird, 1973). A rationale for the increased risk of diabetes in obese individuals can be developed from the fact that, in obesity, there is an increased secretion of insulin and an increased resistance to its action (Bagdade, Bierman & Porte, 1967; Olefsky & Reaven, 1977). This in turn leads to further secretion of insulin by the pancreas since this hormone is essential for storage of calories as triglyceride in adipose tissue. With increasing demands on the pancreas, this organ may become more sensitive to injurious agents or to the presence of genetic factors which may lead to its failure (Inoue & Bray, 1977). Diabetes develops when insulin secretion can no longer be maintained at the levels required by the excess body weight.

Hyperlipidemia

Hyperlipidemia, particularly hypertriglyceridemia, and obesity have often been associated (Albrink & Meigs, 1964; Garcia-Palmieri *et al.*, 1972; Nichols *et al.*, 1976), but the correlation coefficients are low ($r = 0.20$ to $r = 0.35$). The hyperinsulinemia of obesity has been suggested as one mechanism for this association (Olefsky, Reaven & Farquhar, 1974; Bagdade *et al.*, 1967). Hypertriglyceridemia is an additional risk factor for cardiovascular disease (Salel *et al.*, 1974) in those individuals with a susceptibility to this problem. Since weight reduction can reduce serum triglyceride (Olefsky *et al.*, 1974), this is the appropriate first step in treatment.

Endometrial carcinoma

Although the overall risk of cancer is not increased in obesity, obesity does increase the risk for certain forms of cancer. Risk for developing endometrial cancer is increased in obese women (Lucas, 1974). Recent studies provide new understanding of this relationship. Adipose tissue has been shown to metabolize steroids and can convert androstenedione to estrone (Schindler, Ebert & Friederick, 1972). Increased production of estrone raises its concentration in the plasma, and there is positive correlation between estrone and estradiol levels and body weight and/or body fat (Rizkallah, Tovell & Kelly, 1975; Judd, Lucas & Yen, 1976). Although estrone is a biologically weak estrogen, increased concentrations may nonetheless act as a carcinogenic agent for the development of endometrial carcinoma in overweight women.

Summary of risks

Figure 2 shows the relationship between excess mortality and body mass index, and superimposes the cumulative percentage of males aged 40 - 54 with a body mass index above any given value. For a body mass index less than 27, there is no medically proven risk of obesity *per se*. With body mass index between 27 and 30, there is a low level of risk; between 30 and 42,

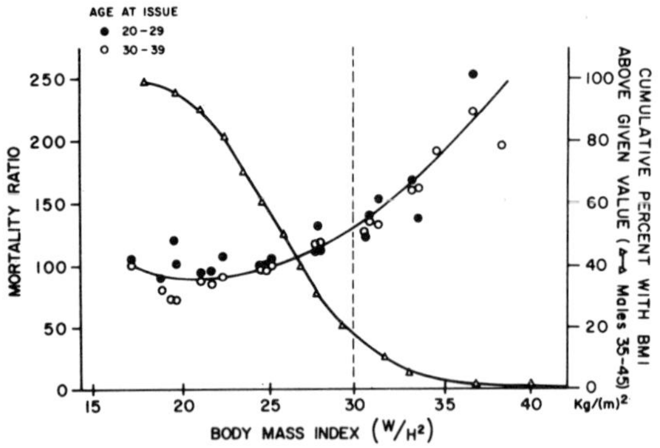

Fig. 2. Relationship of cumulative percentage of males aged 35 to 45 above a given body mass index with the mortality ratio for the same body mass index. It can be seen that approx. 20 per cent of males in this age group, according to the National Center for Health Statistics data from 1960-62, are above the body mass index where excess mortality becomes medically significant (a BMI of 30)

the risk is high; and above 42, very high. The number of individuals at risk with a body mass index above 30 is less than 20 per cent and declines with higher body mass index. The high risk groups are summarized in Table 2, along with an assessment of relative risk for men and

Table 2. High risks of obesity

1. Males BMI >27; age <39 years
2. Diabetics and their relatives
3. Massively obese (BMI >42)

women in relation to body mass index. The risk associated with progressive and morbid obesity may be equivalent to that seen with hypercholesterolemia or heavy cigarette smoking. These data are aptly summarized in the words of Shakespeare:

> Leave gormandising; Know the grave doth gape
> For thee thrice wider than for other men.
> SHAKESPEARE, *2 Henry IV*, v.v., *54-55.*

Treatment of obesity: risk versus benefit

> The human body is composed
> Of head and limbs and torso,
> Kept slim by gents
> At great expense,
> By ladies, even more so.
> OGDEN NASH

Obesity is a ten-billion-dollar-a-year industry. Do consumers get their money's worth? How beneficial is this expenditure of money? In an attempt to give a partial answer to this question, I will evaluate many of the individual treatments.

Since obesity results from an imbalance between caloric intake and expenditure, any treatment must strive to redress this imbalance. Approaches to treatment can be divided into those which reduce energy intake or absorption, treatments which increase energy expenditure, and treatments which modify the metabolic machinery with subsequent shifts in energy balance.

Treatments which reduce energy intake

There are numerous techniques for this purpose. They vary both in relative safety and efficacy as well as expense. At one end of the spectrum are the diets available in diet books. These have a relatively low cost (a trip to the library) and, with diligent application, can result in weight loss. At the other end of the spectrum are techniques such as starvation in the hospital and intestinal bypass which are highly expensive and which may carry substantial risk. In the ensuing sections, we will consider each of the techniques in some detail. These are summarized in Table 3.

Table 3. Treatments to reduce energy absorption

Treatment	Risk	Efficacy	
		Short-term	Long-term
Diets			
Zero calorie	Moderate	Very good	Low
Low calorie	Low	Fair	Low
Low carbohydrate	Low	Good	Low
Protein supplemented fast	Moderate	Good	?
Behavioral engineering	Low	Good	Low
Groups	Low	Good	Low
Drugs			
Appetite-suppressants	Intermediate	Good	Low
Invasive			
Acupuncture	Intermediate	Low	Low
Bypass	High	Very good	Many complications

Dietary treatments.

(a): Starvation

For the past 20 years, starvation in the hospital has been used with varying frequency as a treatment for overweight individuals (Bray, 1976; Garrow, 1974). Starvation for as long as 300 days has been reported but there have been several deaths. Other problems have also been reported with starvation, including attacks of acute gouty arthritis, uric acid renal stones, thiamin deficiency, magnesium deficiency, and symptoms of hypotension (Drenick, 1975). Because this technique requires hospitalization it may cost in excess of $400 per pound, and should be limited to special cases under a doctor's supervision.

(b): Diets

Diet has been one of the cornerstones of all therapeutic approaches for obesity for more than 200 years. Among the most famous and widely popularized of these diets is the one introduced by William Banting (1863). Let me quote from the diet which he published over 100 years ago in a small pamphlet entitled 'A letter on Corpulence Addressed to the Public' : 'Of all the parasites that affect humanity, I do not know of, nor can I imagine any more distressing than that of obesity' (Banting, 1863, p. 7). After years of trying and failing, Mr Banting was placed on a low carbohydrate diet by Dr William Harvey. On this diet, his weight declined from 202 pounds on 26 August 1862, to 156 pounds one year later. A modification of the low carbohydrate diet has since been published intermittently and has been espoused as an important dietary principle by Professor Yudkin in London (1968).

The balanced low calorie diet has been an alternative which has been promulgated widely. Among the most famous balanced low calorie diets is the Prudent Diet of Dr Jolliffe of the New York City Health Department (1963). This diet and its modifications have served as the dietary programs for some commercial and non-commercial groups.

The ever enlarging list of diets are an affirmation of the fact that no diet yet described is by itself a solution to the problem of obesity. The truth of this statement is reflected in the fact that new diets appear yearly each claiming to be the 'ultimate solution'. Yet, there is no argument with the statement that 'calories do count' (Kinsell *et al.*, 1964). Diet, properly used, is a mainstay in the medical management of obesity. Unless caloric intake is reduced below caloric needs, the extra calories which have been stored in adipose tissue cannot be catabolized. There is a large and convincing body of clinical information which shows that if caloric restriction is sufficiently severe and is maintained for a sufficiently long period of time, body weight will decline.

Whether the composition of the diet is important in determining the rate or amount of weight lost has long been debated. One claim which is often made for the low carbohydrate diet is that 3000 kcal/day or more can be eaten and the patient will still lose weight if the carbohydrate intake is restricted. There are no convincing studies to support this claim. On the contrary, several investigators have concluded, after careful investigations, that when fat is added as a caloric supplement to a weight-maintaining diet, body weight will increase in proportion to the added calories (Goldman *et al.,* 1976; Olesen & Quaade, 1960; Sims *et al.* 1973).

Short-term fluctuations in body weight which frequently accompany changes in the content of dietary carbohydrate, protein and fat can usually be attributed to rapid changes in water balance (Russell, 1962). It is now well-established that a low carbohydrate diet is followed by the excretion of water and that carbohydrate ingestion leads to retention of both salt and water (Bloom, 1967). However, when a rigid diet is maintained for a sufficiently long time, these transient effects on water balance are reduced or eliminated; thereafter, the weight loss can be attributed to the metabolism of calories stored as fat (Yang & Van Itallie, 1976).

One modification of the hypothesis that 'calories do count' is required; the ingested calories must be absorbed. Indigestible fats, for example, would be unavailable to the body and the ingested calories would not be usable calories (Fallat *et al.,* 1976). With this exception, however, it is fair to say that 'calories do count' in weight loss and that it is the total caloric intake, not the form in which those calories are ingested, that is important.

The use of diets in the treatment of obesity has been summarized in a very readable book by Berland (1974). Although calorically restricted diets should theoretically be highly successful, their success has been far from uniform. All diets will work for some patients, but no diet works for all patients unless they are confined to a hospital where there is no access to extra food. Most important is the fact that many patients who have lost weight while adhering to a diet will regain the weight later when dietary control becomes lax. Figure 3

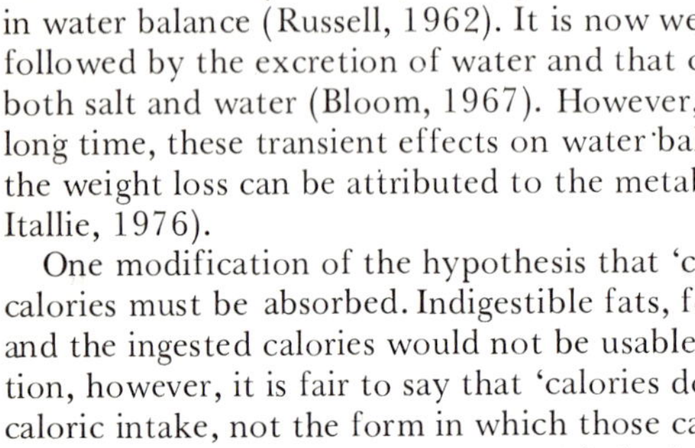

Fig. 3. Weight loss with various treatments. Percentage of patients entering a treatment program who lose 20 pounds (9 kg) or 40 pounds (18 kg) are shown. The three treatments on the left hand side are the low cost-low risk treatments, whose effectiveness is lower than two of the treatments on the right hand side, which are both more expensive and more risky. These data indicate the relatively low success rate found with treatments of low risks and lower costs, and that higher success rates are generally observed with treatments costing more and carrying a greater risk to the patient. (Copyright George A. Bray, 1977)

compares dietary treatment with the results o many other forms of therapy. The percentage of patients treated for obesity by diet, and who lost 20 or 40 pounds (9 or 18 kg), is shown on the left hand pair of bars (Stunkard & McLaren-Hume, 1959; Bray, 1970). Only 5 per cent lost 40 pounds (18 kg) or more (cross-hatched bars), while 25 per cent achieved a weight loss of 20 pounds (9 kg) or more (open bars). Because standard programs of dietary treatment are often unsuccessful, many other approaches have been evaluated.

(c). Protein-supplemented fasting

The high cost of in-patient fasting has led to exploration of out-patient fasting in which protein is also given. Several different programs have been developed that use different sources of protein (Table 4). The goal is to ingest 1.0 - 1.5 g of protein (or equivalent amino acids) per kg of desirable body weight.

Table 4. Protein supplements

1. Casein (milk protein)
2. Egg albumin
3. Complete amino acid mixtures
4. Lean meat
5. Digested collagen

One out-patient program of protein-supplemented fasting has shown a high success rate as compared to more orthodox methods (Fig. 3). The adherence to this program was fair, with 63 per cent of the patients achieving a weight loss averaging more than 16 pounds in eight weeks. Sixty per cent of these patients lost more than 40 pounds, and 70 per cent more than 20 pounds. Side effects of cold intolerance, dry skin, and loss of hair were occasionally troublesome and several deaths have occurred (Genuth, Castro & Vertes, 1974). Although more studies are needed, it would appear that, in highly motivated patients who have significant risk associated with their obesity, a protein-supplemented fast may have a significant advantage over the use of standard dietary programs in short-term therapy. Data on the long-term effectiveness of protein-supplemented starvation are not yet available, but two other groups of investigators have also reported encouraging results with this method (Baird, Parsons & Howard, 1974; Lindner & Blackburn, 1976). The liquid (pre-digested) protein diets may pose a particular hazard. The high concentration of proline, hydroxyproline, hydroxylysine and glycine can lead to excess loss of potassium to cover the excretion of these amino acid anions. Recently more than ten deaths have been associated with this treatment making it one of moderate risk.

(d): Self-help groups

Self-help groups are now widespread in the United States. Weight Watchers is the largest of these with an enrollment in excess of one million. The TOPS Club (which stands for Take Off Pounds Sensibly) is the second largest, with Overeaters Anonymous, Diet Kitchen, Diet Workshop and others being smaller. In one study group, Stunkard (1975) observed that some groups were considerably more successful than others. The major difference in success appeared to be how long the group had been in operation. Newly formed groups were generally more successful than the older, more established ones. The overall success rate appears to be slightly better than that of the dietary programs alone. Since membership in these groups can be quite low cost and there are few, if any, undesirable side effects,they may have some advantages over nutrition clinics which utilize the time of expensive professional personnel.

Data on the effectiveness of most commercial self-help groups are almost non-existent. During a program to evaluate medical risks associated with obesity conducted at the Harbor General Hospital, Torrance, California we examined 267 obese patients. Of these, 118 (44 per cent) had belonged to a Weight Watchers group at one time or another. During the average of 24 weeks participation in the Weight Watchers' program, these individuals had lost an average of 21 pounds, but by the time they came to our clinic, essentially all had regained their weight. Garrow compared three weight control groups in Great Britain (Garrow, 1975) and his data are similar to ours. Average length of membership ranged from 23.6 weeks in one group to 29.5 weeks in Weight Watchers. Average weight loss of those belonging to Weight Watchers was 25.6 pounds (11.8 kg) compared to 16.2 and 18.8 pounds (7.5 and 8.5 kg) for the other groups. Although these commercial groups serve a useful function, and have a low risk, they do not appear to be significantly more effective than the TOPS Club or nutrition clinics.

(e): Behavioral engineering (Behavior modification)

The use of psychological techniques to help patients control their eating has spread widely in recent years. My preference for the term 'behavioral engineering' results from the fact that 'behavior modification' includes a variety of techniques. Aversive techniques, such as associating food with a bad smell or a feeling of nausea have, in general, met with little long-term success and have produced considerable patient resistance (Ley *et al.,* 1974). By 'behavioral engineering' we mean a series of techniques for analysis and alteration in the environment which can reduce the likelihood that problematic foods, and problematic situations for eating, will arise. These techniques of positive reinforcement and environmental manipulation, pioneered by Stuart (1967), have proven considerably more successful. Although in their infancy, these techniques may be widely applicable (Stuart, 1976). There is now one five-year study on the effects of behavioral engineering (Stunkard, 1976). In this study, both behavioral engineering and standard dietary management were compared. At three and 12 months, the effectiveness of behavioral engineering was greater than dietary management, but at five years, the effectiveness of both methods seemed to decline. One must also express some other reservations about the effectiveness of techniques of behavioral engineering. Most studies of these techniques have been applied to groups on university campuses where a fee-for-service has been collected. Attempts to utilize behavior modification with the lower income groups in which obesity is more prevalent are few in number (Atkinson *et al.,* 1977; Dahms *et al.,* 1978). In our experience, both the drop-out rate and the success rate were lower in patients from lower socioeconomic groups treated in identical settings than with individuals from the higher social class. We thus feel that the currently available techniques offer important approaches for the overweight individual who is economically able to commit himself to this treatment but that their application to lower social and economic groups is limited.

Pharmologic agents

(a): Appetite-suppressing drugs

There are a variety of appetite-suppressing drugs on the market (Bray, 1976; Samuel & Burland, 1975; Scoville, 1975) and in the last few years, three additional drugs have been marketed in the United States. All of these agents are effective in enhancing weight loss (Scoville, 1975). They appear to produce this effect by suppressing the appetite, although the intricacies of the way they work are not fully understood. All of these drugs appear to be equal as appetite suppressants in producing weight loss (Samuel & Burland, 1975). The data from one study on the weight loss of patients treated with thyroid and appetite-suppressing drugs are summarized in Fig. 3 (Asher & Dietz, 1972). The overall results are only a little better than those obtained with diet, or self-help groups, and appear less effective than the one study of environmental engineering (behavior modification). Three of the appetite-suppressing drugs (methamphetamine, amphetamine and phenmetrazine) appear to have a higher frequency for drug abuse than others. When treatment with an anorexigenic drug is indicated, it would appear reasonable to choose from the group with lower potential for drug abuse (fenfluramine, phentermine, diethlypropion, chlorphentermine, clortermine, mazindol and benzphetamine).

We have recently been interested in the relative merits of environmental engineering as compared to pharmacologic agents. We have assessed these merits in two studies. In the first study, we evaluated two components of the therapeutic situation (Dahms *et al.,* 1978). The first was whether we could predict those patients who would drop out of treatment or fail to lose weight while remaining in treatment based on a series of questionnaires given at the beginning of therapy (Rodin *et al.,* 1977). As a second goal, we wanted to compare our early approaches at environmental engineering with the drop-out rate and success rate of a drug-treated group. In this study, we evaluated 120 patients, 30 of whom received placebo, 30 diethylpropion, 30 mazindol, and 30 our program of environmental engineering. This latter group received neither placebo nor drug. All patients were given the same diet and they were followed for a 14-week period. The drop-out rate and weight loss (Fig. 4) were essentially

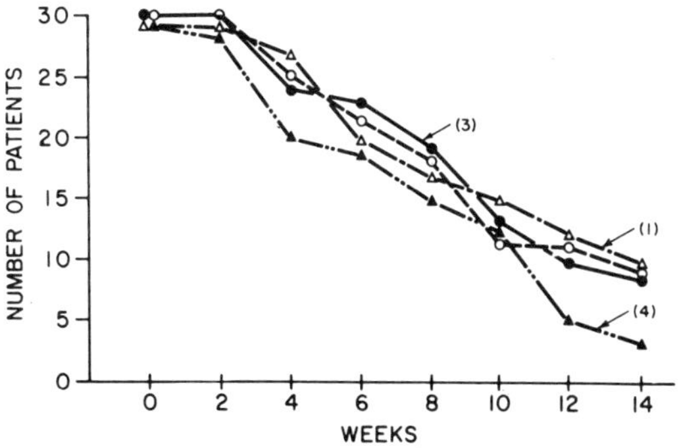

Fig. 4. Drop-out rate for patients in a behavioral and drug treatment program. Placebo-treated patients (open triangle), diethylpropion-treated patients (open circle), mazindol-treated patients (solid circle) and patients treated by behavioral approaches (solid triangle) show comparable drop-out rates after induction into a 14-week treatment period in which patients incurred no expenses

identical for all four groups. The half-time of patients remaining in the study was approximately eight weeks. Although we tested a large number of hypotheses about reasons why individuals might fail to return for therapy or fail to lose weight, few withstood the rigor of objective assessment. Success was related to social conformity and desire for social acceptance but not to self-esteem or locus of control. Individuals who believed that poor eating habits caused their obesity, and those who were less responsive to environmental cues which trigger feeding, were also more successful. In the setting of our County hospital, the program of behavioral engineering was as good as treatment with placebo or active pharmacologic agent.

A second drug trial gave us the opportunity to expand these findings (Atkinson *et al.*, 1977). In this study, a placebo and two active agents were part of a study which was conducted in four different hospitals (Walker, Ballard & Gold, 1977). In our hospital, a manual for behaviorai engineering was designed by five therapists. Each therapist treated 12 patients,

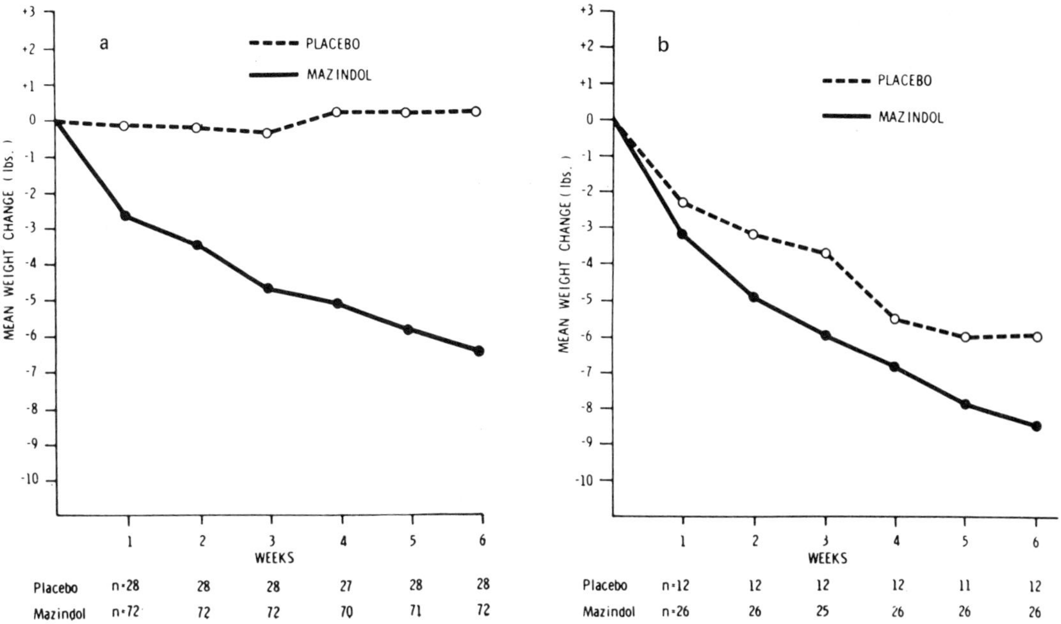

Fig. 5. Comparison of weight loss in a clinic at the Harbor General Hospital (a: right hand panel) **versus weight loss in a comparable treatment program at three other medical centers** (b: left hand panel). The placebo-treated patients in our clinic who, along with the drug-treated patients, had a behavioral program superimposed as part of their treatment, lost as much weight as the drug-treated patients in three clinics where patients did not receive a behavioral program

one-third of whom received placebo and two-thirds mazindol. This gave us the opportunity to evaluate our behavioral program, with or without drug treatment, against comparable groups run in three other hospitals which received no behavioral program. We also had the opportunity to examine the effectiveness of different therapists, since two were physicians and three were non-physicians. The results from the other three studies are shown in Fig. 5*a*. During the course of this drug trial, the drug-treated patients lost an average of seven pounds while the placebo-treated group lost no weight. This is contrasted with our patients shown in Fig. 5*b*. The placebo-treated patients in our group lost weight as rapidly as the drug-treated patients in the other three studies, and the patients treated with drugs in our institution lost weight no faster than those treated with placebo. Of equal interest to us was the finding that physicians were no more effective than our non-physicians in this therapeutic setting (Fig. 6). These studies suggested two things. First, that an effective program of

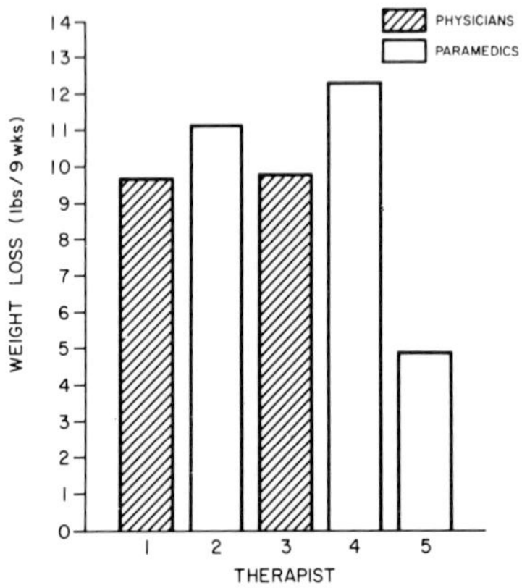

Fig. 6. Comparison of weight loss in patients treated by five different therapists. Physicians were no more successful than two non-physicians in the weight loss achieved by patients under their care. One paramedical therapist was significantly less effective. Whether this was the result of the therapist or the particular group of patients assigned to that therapist could not be determined from the data at hand

environmental engineering, conducted by either a physician or non-physician, could be as effective as an active appetite-suppressing drug over the duration of this study. Second, it suggested that non-physicians could be just as effective as physicians. Since physician manpower is limited and of high cost, these observations have led us to develop and continually improve our program of environmental and nutritional engineering, so that it can be applied in physician's offices by non-physician personnel who have been appropriately trained. This is currently a major effort of our research program because we believe this kind of therapy should precede therapies with protein-sparing fasts or drug therapy. Since pharmacological agents have more potential risks than the approaches which do not use drugs, the appetite-suppressants should be reserved for special situations.

(b): Human chorionic gonadotropin (HCG)

Injections of human chorionic gonadotropin, an extract of pregnant human urine, were introduced as a treatment of obesity by Simeons (1954). Since then, it has been widely used. Three recent careful clinical trials have indicated that this agent is no more effective than injections of inactive materials (Stein *et al.*, 1976; Young *et al.*, 1976; Greenway & Bray, 1977). In an early study, Carne (1961) concluded that HCG was no more effective than a placebo, but he also found that patients receiving injections lost more weight than was achieved by the group of patients receiving no injections. This effect may be attributed to the 'motivation' provided by returning to the doctor's office each day. Human chorionic gonadotropin, in the doses used in treating obese patients, would appear to be safe, but ineffective in treating the obese patient. Recent studies failed to demonstrate any effectiveness of this agent on appetite, on localized spot reducing, or on overall weight loss. There is thus no basis for its continued use as a therapeutic agent for obese individuals (Crout, 1974).

3. Invasive treatments

(a): Acupuncture

Treatment of disease by acupuncture involves inserting needles into various sites on the body. Some acupuncture therapists have suggested that there may be 'active' sites on the pina of the ear which can reduce appetite. In a controlled study of acupuncture using 'active' and 'inactive' sites, we were unable to demonstrate any difference in weight loss between the active and inactive sites or between unilateral and bilateral acupuncture (Mok *et al.*, 1976).

(b): Jaw-wiring

Mandibular fixation (jaw-wiring) restricts intake of foods to liquids (Garrow, 1974). In one series of 13 patients, jaws have remained fixed for periods of four to eight months. However, this procedure has the potential risk of permanent damage to teeth and risk of asphixiation should vomiting occur. Weight loss has been substantial (Rodgers *et al.*, 1977), but the published data is too sparse to allow comparison with other methods.

(c): Intestinal bypass and gastric bypass

The intestinal and gastric bypass have been used with a measured degree of success on a large number of patients, but there are major complications of the treatment, including a mortality which averages 3 per cent. As shown in Fig. 3, the percentage of successful patients using criteria of 9 kg (20 pounds) or 18 kg (40 pounds) of weight loss is greater than with any other therapy, but this higher success rate is accomplished at a high economic and human cost. When done under proper circumstances and on the appropriate patient, however, it can be helpful and, indeed, a life-saving procedure (Buchwald *et al.*, 1975; Bray, 1976; Bray *et al.*, 1977; Faloon, 1977). Surgery is only indicated when patients are at least 100 pounds over-weight and have long-standing obesity. Moreover, it should only be performed in hospitals where appropriate pre-operative and post-operative management are available. Even under these conditions, the appearance of significant complications have been reported in up to 50 per cent of the patients who have had this operation. These complications include operative difficulties, liver failure, malnutrition, oxalate kidney stones and migratory polyarthritis (Bray *et al.*, 1977). These metabolic problems with intestinal bypass appear to be reduced after gastric bypass (Mason & Ito, 1969; Mason *et al.*, 1978). However, this latter operation suffers from the types of syndromes associated with peptic ulcer operations.

Treatments which increase energy expenditure

An increase in caloric expenditure has been used as part of the effort to redress the imbalance between caloric intake and expenditure which produces obesity (Table 5).

Table 5. Treatments to enhance energy utilization

Treatment	Risk	Efficacy Short-term	Efficacy Long-term
Increase activity	Variable	Fair	?
Stimulate metabolic rate	Intermediate	Good	Low

Exercise

Increased exercise and the associated enhanced energy expenditure would provide one effective approach for dealing with this problem. The President's Council on Physical Fitness has urged all Americans to increase their exercise. Reduced physical activity is a risk factor for obesity and for cardiovascular disease (Shapiro *et al.*, 1969). However, it is clear that an exercise program for which the individual has not been appropriately screened, and evaluated, may be associated with severe stress. In appropriate hands, however, the use of an exercise program tailored to meet an individual's needs is a desirable adjunct to the treatment of obesity. There are only a few studies showing a beneficial effect of exercise in overweight individuals (Boileau *et al.*, 1971; Kenrick, Ball & Canary, 1972; Moody *et al.*, 1972; Gwinup,

1975; Björntorp, 1975). In the study by Gwinup (1975), individuals were brought into a weight loss program and given exercise as their total means of treatment. Approximately two-thirds of the patients dropped out of the study and, of those who remained, only the group who walked 30 minutes or more per day achieved a significant weight loss. It is interesting that bicycle riding, swimming, and playing tennis did not significantly modify body weight, while walking did. Thus an exercise program which involves walking may be an effective adjunct to the treatment of obesity.

Drugs

Thyroid hormone is the only drug currently used for increasing energy expenditure. It was introduced more than 80 years ago and has been widely used since that time. Because pharmacologic doses of hormone are required, there is a serious question about whether the risks of this form of therapy are appropriate for the degree of risk that affects most overweight individuals. Moreover, there is nothing to show that treatment with thyroid has produced long-term reduction in body weight any more than other measures (Bray & Greenway, 1976). This is summarized in Fig. 3 in which drug treatments (including appetite-suppressants and thyroid) are compared with other treatments. The results with techniques of behavioral engineering in our own experience are equal to that with drug therapy. When the cost factors involved in medical care, in writing a prescription or dispensing the drug, are entered into the equation, there is little doubt that pharmacologic techniques should be reserved as a second line of therapy and for individuals in the high risk category (Table 2).

Evaluation of the effectiveness of therapies for obesity

There is ample evidence that, in the short run, any regime in which total energy intake is sufficiently reduced will be associated with weight loss. This has been summarized for several therapeutic approaches by comparing the percentage of patients entering the treatment program who lost 9 or 18 kg (20 or 40 pounds) (Fig. 3). The treatments on the left half of this figure are associated with lower success rates, less professional time, and involve lower risk to the patient. Those treatments with higher success rates are on the right hand side of this figure, but they also have higher costs and higher intrinsic risk to the patient. The duration of the treatments summarized in Fig. 3 are short term. What can be said of the long-term effectiveness of weight control techniques? Unfortunately, only a few long-term studies exist. One of the earliest was the evaluation of employees in the Metropolitan Life Insurance Company who were treated, and whose results were reevaluated at one year later (Fellow, 1931). Of 294 patients 53 per cent lost more than 4.5 kg (10 pounds). With follow-up of 224 individuals at one year, 32 per cent of patients had continued to lose weight. Glennon (1966) had evaluated the effects on body weight of an in-hospital program two years following hospitalization. He found that only one patient had achieved 'ideal' body weight, but that 12 per cent had maintained or increased the degree of weight loss achieved at the beginning of the program. A similar assessment of long-term effectiveness was published by Sohar & Sneh (1973). In this study, 27 out of the original 33 individuals were reevaluated 14 years after an initial dietary program which consisted of a 550 calorie diet. Five (approximately one-fifth) of the patients lost and maintained their weight loss, 60 per cent lost weight, but regained all of the weight that they had lost, while the remaining five initially lost more weight but had regained all of this weight plus an average additional 20 kg (44 pounds). Finally, Stunkard (1976*b)* has provided data at three, 12, and 60 months after initiating two programs, one involving nutritional treatment and the other psychological techniques (Fig. 7). The groups treated with 'psychological' treatment had a higher percentage of successful individuals losing 9 or 18 kg at each reevaluation, as compared to the nutritionally treated individuals. However, at 60 months follow-up, the figures for the nutritional group ranged between 10 and 20 per cent and for the behavioral group between 10 and 30 per cent. These are considerably higher

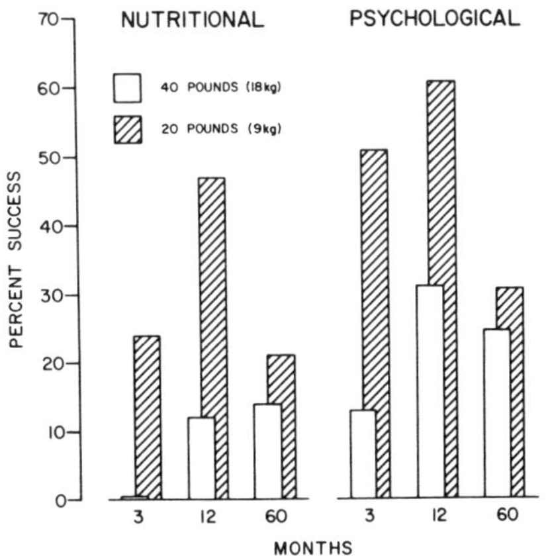

Fig. 7. Comparison of nutritional and psychological treatments on weight loss during the five-year period. In a format similar to that of Fig. 3, the percentage of patients losing 9 kg (20 lb) is compared with that losing 18 kg (40 lb). Success rate at 12 months was significantly greater by both criteria with both treatments, but seemed to be even greater in the patients receiving psychological behavioral engineering as compared to the straight, simple, nutritional approach. A five-year follow-up showed that both groups were considerably more successful than the average patient in the nutritional program shown in Fig. 3. Also, note where the patients participated in the behavioral engineering program were more successful after five years than those receiving only the nutritional program

figures than noted in Fig. 3 for a large number of nutritional programs, and suggests that nutritional treatment may have improved.

The observation that between 10 and 30 per cent of the patients will achieve and maintain a long-term weight loss, and that the percentage with 9 and 18 kg (20 and 40 pounds) weight loss groups has increased, is a cause for some satisfaction but no complacency. Progress toward future success in this field requires an assessment of factors influencing long-term success of weight control methods. The failure of the low risk approaches to obesity, and the ineffectiveness of many of the pharmacologic agents, is a cause for concern since we have documented the increased risk of obesity and indicated that this risk operates over many years. It should thus be clear that we need new low risk programs which can improve our long-term effectiveness in dealing with obesity, particularly for those individuals at high risk for cardiovascular-hypertensive disease, and for diabetes mellitus.

It has now been amply demonstrated that obesity develops in a social environment (Goldblatt, Moore & Stunkard, 1964; Silverstone, Gordon & Stunkard, 1969; Stunkard *et al.*, 1972). That is, there are important social correlates in the prevalence of obesity. In most cultures, obesity has a higher prevalence in the lower socioeconomic groups and is more prevalent among women than men (Christakis, 1975). In addition, religious, ethnic, and geographic backgrounds are all of importance in determining the prevalence of obesity in a given culture. Because of these differences in cultural factors involved in the development of obesity, it would seem clear that therapeutic programs must be tailored to meet the social and cultural markets for which the treatment is needed. This concept of using social marketing techniques to focus the most effective techniques on a given group has received little application up to the present time.

A second problem in dealing with obesity is the generally held assumption that it is a single entity. More appropriately, it should be considered as a group of syndromes with obesity as one manifestation (Bray, 1976). This would mean that obesity should be considered a sign of disease, not a disease in itself. Several approaches to classification have been developed. These include an anatomic classification based on the distribution and number of fat cells, a classification based on the age at which obesity begins, an approach based on etiologic factors which underly obesity, and an engineering or cybernetic approach to the developmental sequence of obesity (Bray, 1978). The role of the number of fat cells in predicting the response to dietary treatment has been noted recently in the observations of Björntorp and his colleagues (Krotkiewski *et al.*, 1977). They evaluated the degree of weight loss and duration of maintenance of a reduced weight in relation to numbers of fat cells. Individuals with an increased number of fat cells weighed more at the start of treatment and had a much shorter duration during which they maintained a lower body weight. Thus, more vigorous forms of therapy may be needed for individuals with so called 'hypercellular' obesity than for individuals whose obesity is associated with a normal number of fat cells.

Etiologic factors can also be used to classify obesity and have been helpful in differentiating different forms of obesity (Bray, 1976). Table 6 shows etiologic classification, along with those

Table 6. An etiologic classification of the mechanisms and treatments for experimental obesity

Classification Clinical/ Experimental	**Pathology**	**Mechanisms**	**Treatment** Work	Don't work
1. Hypothalamic	Trauma Chemicals	Vagal-mediated hyperinsulinemia	Vagotomy Intestinal bypass Quinine Islet transplant	Hypophysectomy Adrenalectomy
2. Endocrine				
Hypercorticism	Exogenous/ endogenous	Excess glucocorticoids	Reduce steroids	
Hyperinsulinism		Excess insulin	Reduce insulin	
Ovariectomy	Surgical/ menopause	Relative excess progesterone/ estrogen	Estrogen Adrenalectomy	Vagotomy
3. Nutritional				
High fat diet		?	Low fat diet	
'Supermarket diet'		?	Monotonous diet	
4. Physical inactivity		?	Physical activity	
5. Genetic				
Recessive	*ob/ob; db/db*	No thyroid - dependent $(Na^{+} + K^{+})$-ATPase	Hypophysectomy Adrenalectomy	Low fat diet Vagotomy
	fa/fa	?		
Dominant	A^{Y}; Ad		Intestinal bypass	Hypophysectomy

forms of treatment which have worked, and those which have not worked, to relieve the experimental situation. The syndrome of hypothalamic obesity in man and animals appears to be related to an exaggerated release of insulin in response to ingestion of food (Powley, 1977; Inoue, Bray & Mullen, 1977). Maneuvers which reduce insulin will reverse or control this syndrome (Powley & Opsahl, 1974; Inoue & Bray, 1977). In contrast, genetic obesities, although associated with marked elevation in insulin, do not seem to be dependent on insulin for their expression. Some of the genetic forms of obesity appear to be due to loss of a critical enzyme involved in controlling heat production in response to thyroid hormone (York, Bray & Yukimura, 1978). These contrasts between hypothalamic and genetic syndromes of obesity provide potential tools for evaluating this problem.

As we understand the underlying mechanisms for each of these exprimental types of obesity, we will be better equipped to design new pharmacological, nutritional, and behavioral interventions which may be useful in dealing with each of these forms. In the interval before new developments are available, it is particularly important to provide a broad based approach to the treatment of obesity, using all of the techniques which are now available. The rapid increase in our knowledge about obesity has led to the need for the First and Second International Congresses on Obesity as a ground for exchange of ideas. Similarly, this groundswell of new ideas and development has led to the publication of an 'International Journal of Obesity'. These important developments, and our rapidly expanding understanding of the mechanisms for several types of obesity, lead me to feel that we are at a point of great excitement in this field. This excitement has been amply captured in the following quotation:

There is a tide in the affairs of men,
Which, taken at the flood, leads on to fortune....
On such a full sea are we now afloat;
And we must take the current when it serves
Or lose our ventures.

SHAKESPEARE, *Julius Caeser,* IV, ii.

References

Abraham, S., Collins, G. & Nordsieck, M. (1971): *HSMHA Hlth Rep.* **86**, 273.

Albrink, M.H. & Meigs, J.W. (1964): *Am. J. Clin. Nutr.* **15**, 255.

Alexander, J.K. (1975): Effects of weight reduction on the cardiovascular system. In *Obesity in perspective,* Pt 2, ed G.A. Bray, p. 233. Washington DC: Govt. Ptg. Office.

Asher, W.L. & Dietz, R.E. (1972): *Curr. Ther. Res.* **14**, 510.

Atkinson, R.L., Greenway, F.L., Bray, G.A., Dahms, W.T., Molitch, M.E., Hamilton, K. & Rodin, J. (1977): *Int. J. Obesity* **1**, 113.

Bagdade, J.D., Bierman, E.L. & Porte, D. Jr. (1967): *J. Clin. Invest.* **46**, 1549.

Baird, J.D. (1973): *Proc. Nutr. Soc.* **32**, 199.

Baird, I.M., Parsons, R.L. & Howard, A.N. (1974): *Metabolism* **23**, 645.

Banting, W. (1863): *Letter on corpulence addressed to the public.* London: Harrison.

Bennion, L.J. & Grundy, S.M. (1975): *J. Clin. Invest.* **56**, 996.

Berland, T. (1974): In *Consumer guide: rating the diets.* London: Publications International Ltd.

Bernstein, R.A., Werner, L.H. & Rimm, A.A. (1973): *Hlth Serv. Rep.* **88**, 925.

Björntorp, P. (1975): Effects of physical conditioning in obesity. In *Obesity in perspective,* Pt 2, ed G.A. Bray, p. 397. Washington DC: US Govt. Ptg. Office.

Bloom, W.L. (1967): *Am. J. Clin. Nutr.* **20**, 157.

Boileau, R.A., Buskirk, E.R., Horstman, D.H., Mendez, J. & Nicholas, W.C. (1971): *Med. Sci. Sports* **3**, 183.

Bray, G.A. (1970): *Am. J. Clin. Nutr.* **23**, 1141.

Bray, G.A. (1976): *The obese patient.* Philadelphia: W.B. Saunders.

Bray, G.A. & Greenway, F.L. (1976): *Clins Endocrinol. Metab.* **5**, 455.

Bray, G.A., Greenway, F.L., Barry, R.E., Benfield, J.R., Fiser, R.L., Dahms, W.T., Atkinson, R.L. & Schwartz, A.A. (1977): *Int. J. Obesity* **1**, 331.

Bray, G.A. (1978): *Int. J. Obesity (in press).*

Buchwald, H., Varco, R.L., Moore, R.B. & Schwartz, M.Z. (1975): Intestinal bypass procedures. Partial ileal bypass for hyperlipidemia and jejunoileal bypass for obesity. In *Current problems in surgery,* ed M.M. Ravitch, p. 1. Chicago: Year Book.

Carne, S. (1961): *Lancet* 2, 1282.

Chaing, B.N., Perlman, L.V. & Epstein, F.H. (1969): *Circulation* **39**, 403.

Chapman, J.M., Coulson, A.H., Clark, V.A. & Boran, E.R. (1971): *J. Chron. Dis.* **23**, 631.

Christakis, G. (1975): The prevalence of adult obesity. In *Obesity in perspective* Pt 2, ed G.A. Bray, p. 209. Washington DC: US Govt. Ptg. Office.

Crout, J.R. (1974): *Federal Register* **39**, 42397.

Dahms, W.T., Molitch, M., Bray, G.A., Greenway, F.L., Atkinson, R.L. & Hamilton, K. (1978): *Am. J. Clin. Nutr.* (in press).

Drenick, E.J. (1975): Weight reduction by prolonged fasting. In *Obesity in perspective* Pt. 2, ed G.A. Bray, p. 341. Washington DC: US Govt. Ptg. Office.

Epstein, F.H., Ostrander, L.D., Johnson, B.C., Payne, M.W., Hayner, N.S., Keller, J.B. & Francis, T. jr. (1965): *Ann. Intern. Med.* **62**, 1170.

Fallat, R.W., Glueck, C.J., Lutmer, R. & Mattson, F.H. (1976): *Am. J. Clin. Nutr.* **29**, 1204.

Faloon, W.W. (1977): *Am. J. Clin. Nutr.* **30**, 1.

Fellows, H.H. (1931): *Am. J. Med. Sci.* **181**, 301.

Garcia-Palmieri, M.R., Costos, R. jr., Schiffman, J., Colon, A.A., Torres, R. & Nazasio, E. (1972): *Circulation* **45**, 829.

Garrow, J.S. (1974): *Proc. Nutr. Soc.* **33**, A29.

Garrow, J.S. (1975): A survey of three slimming and weight control organizations in the UK. In *Recent advances in obesity research:* I, ed A.N. Howard, p. 301. London: Newman.

Genuth, S.M., Castro, J.H. & Vertes, V. (1974): *J. Am. Med. Ass.* **230**, 987.

Glennon, J.A. (1966): *Archs Intern. Med.* **118**, 1.

Goldblatt, P.B., Moore, M.E. & Stunkard, A.J. (1964): *J. Am. Med. Ass.* **192**, 1039.

Goldman, R.F., Haisman, M.F., Bynum, G., Horton, E.S. & Sims, E.A.H. (1975): Experimental obesity in man. Metabolic rate in relation to dietary intake. In *Obesity in perspective*, Pt 2, ed G.A. Bray, p. 165. Washington DC: US Govt. Ptg. Office.

Greenway, F.L. & Bray, G.A. (1977): *West J. Med.* **127**, 461.
Gwinup, G. (1975): *Archs Intern. Med.* **135**, 676.
Heyden, S., Cassel, J.C., Bartel, A., Tyroler, H.A., Hames, C.G. & Cornoni, J.C. (1971): *Archs Intern. Med.* **128**, 915.
Hundley, J.M. (1956): *J. Am. Diet. Ass.* **32**, 417.
Inoue, S. & Bray, G.A. (1977): *Endocrinology* **100**, 108.
Inoue, S., Bray, G.A. & Mullen, Y. (1977): *Nature* **266**, 742.
Jolliffe, N. (1963): *Reduce and stay reduced on the prudent diet.* New York: Simon & Schuster.
Joslin, E.P., Dublin, L.I. & Marks, H.H. (1935): *Archs Intern. Med.* **189**, 163.
Judd, H.L., Lucas, W.E. & Yen, S.S.C. (1976): *J. Clin. Endocrinol. Metab.* **43**, 272.
Kannel, W.B. & Gordon, T. (1974): Obesity and cardiovascular disease: the Framingham Study. In *Obesity: Medical and social aspects,* ed W.L. Burland, J. Yudkin & P. Samuel, p. 24. London: Churchill Livingstone.
Kenrick, M.M., Ball, M.F. & Canary, J.J. (1972): *Archs Phys. Med. Rehab.* **53**, 323.
Keys, A., Fidanza, F., Karvonen, M.J., Kimura, N. & Taylor, H.L. (1972): *J. Chron. Dis.* **25**, 329.
Kinsell, L.W., Gunning, B., Michaels, G.D., Richardson, J., Cox, S.E. & Lemon, C. (1964): *Metabolism* **13**, 195.
Krotkiewski, M., Sjöström, L., Björntorp, P., Carlgren, G., Garellick, G. & Smith, U. (1977): *Int. J. Obesity* **1**, 395.
Ley, P., Bradshaw, P.W., Kincey, J.A., Couper-Smartt, J. & Wilson, M. (1974): Psychological variables in the control of obesity. In *Obesity: Medical and social aspects* ed W.L. Burland, J. Yudkin & P. Samuel, p. 316. London: Churchill Livingstone.
Lindner, P.G. & Blackburn, G.L. (1976): *Obesity Bariatric Med.* **5**, 198.
Lucas, W.E. (1974): *Obstet. Gynecol. Surv.* **29**, 507.
Marks, H.H. (1960): *Bull. N.Y. Acad. Sci.* **36**, 296.
Mason, E.E. & Ito, C. (1969): *Ann. Surg.* **170**, 329.
Mason, E.E., Printon, K.J., Blommers, T.J. & Scott, D.H. (1978): *Int. J. Obesity* (in press).
Miettinen, T.A. (1974): *Horm. Metab. Res.* **14**, 37.
Mok, M.S., Parker, L.N., Voina, S. & Bray, G.A. (1976): *Am. J. Clin. Nutr.* **29**, 832.
Moody, D.L., Wilmore, J.H., Girandola, R.N. & Royce, J.P. (1972): *Med. Sci. Sports* **4**, 210.
National Commission on Diabetes (1975): USDEW Publication No. 76-1018.
Nichols, A.B., Ravenscroft, C., Lamphiear, D.E. & Ostrander, L.D., jr. (1976): *J. Am. Med. Ass.* **236**, 1948.
Olefsky, J., Reaven, G.M. & Farquhar, J.W. (1974): *J. Clin. Invest.* **53**, 64.
Olefsky, J.M. & Reaven, G.M. (1977): *Diabetes* **26**, 680.
Olesen, E.S. & Quaade, F. (1960): *Lancet* **1**, 1048.
Paffenberger, R.S. & Wing, A.L. (1969): *Am. J. Epidemiol.* **90**, 527.
Pell, S. & D'Alonzo, C.A. (1963): *J. Am. Med. Ass.* **185**, 831.
Powley, T.L. & Opsahl, C.A. (1974): *Am. J. Physiol.* **226**, 25.
Powley, T.L. (1977): *Psychol. Rev.* **84**, 89.
Rabkin, S.W., Mathewson, F.A.L. & Hsu P-H. (1977): *Am. J. Cardiol.* **39**, 452.
Rimm, A.A., Werner, L.H., Van Iserloo, B. & Bernstein, R.A. (1975): *Publ. Hlth Rep.* **90**, 44.
Rizkallah, T.H., Tovell, H.M.M. & Kelly, W.G. (1975): *J. Clin. Endocrinol. Metab.* **40**, 1045.
Rodin, J., Bray, G.A., Atkinson, R.L., Dahms, W.T., Greenway, F.L., Hamilton, K. & Molitch, M. (1977): *Int. J. Obesity* **1**, 40.
Rodgers, S., Goss, A., Goldney, R., Thomas, D., Burnet, R., Phillips, P., Kimber, C. & Harding, P. (1977): *Lancet* **1**, 1221.
Russell, G.F.M. (1962): *Clin. Sci.* **22**, 269.
Salel, A.F., Riggs, K., Mason, D.T., Amsterdam, E.A. & Zelis, R. (1974): *Am. J. Med.* **57**, 897.
Samuel, P.D. & Burland, W.L. (1975): Drug treatment of obesity. In *Obesity in perspective* Pt 2, ed G.A. Bray, p. 419. Washington DC: US Govt. Ptg. Office.
Schindler, A.E., Ebert, A. & Friederick, E. (1972): *J. Clin. Endocrinol. Metab.* **35**, 627.
Scoville, B. (1975): Review of amphetamine-like drugs by the Food and Drug Administration. In *Obesity in perspective*, Pt 2, ed G.A. Bray, p. 441. Washington DC: US Govt. Ptg. Office.
Shapiro, S., Weinblatt, E., Frank, C.W. & Sager, R.V. (1969): *Am. J. Publ. Hlth* **59**, 1.
Silverstone, J.T., Gordon, R.P. & Stunkard, A.J. (1969): *Practitioner* **202**, 682.
Simeons, A.T.W. (1954): *Lancet* **2**, 946.
Sims, E.A.H., Danforth, E. jr., Horton, E.S., Bray, G.A., Glennon, J.A. & Salans, L.B. (1973): *Rec. Prog. Horm. Res.* **29**, 457.
Society of Actuaries (1959): Build and blood pressure study. Chicago: Society of Actuaries.
Sohar, E., Scapa, E. & Ravid, M. (1973): *Archs Dis. Childh.* **48**, 389.
Sohar, E. & Sneh, E. (1973): *Am. J. Clin. Nutr.* **26**, 845.
Stamler, J., Berkson, D.M., Morjonner, L., Lindberg, H.A., Hall, Y., Levinson, M., Barkey, F., Miller, W., Epstein, M.B. & Andelman, S.L. (1968): *Prog. Biochem. Pharmacol.* **4**, 30.

Stein, M.R., Julis, R.E., Peck, C.C., Hinshaw, W., Sawicki, J.E. & Deller, J.J. (1976): *Am. J. Clin. Nutr.* **29**, 940.
Stuart, R.B. (1967): *Behav. Res. Ther.* **5**, 357.
Stuart, R.B. (1975): Behavioral control of overeating: a status report. In *Obesity in perspective* Pt 2, ed. G.A. Bray, p. 367. Washington DC: US Govt. Ptg. Office.
Stunkard, A.J. & McLaren-Hume, M. (1959): *Archs Intern. Med.* **103**, 79.
Stunkard, A.J., D'Aquili, E., Fox, S. & Filion, R.D.L. (1972): *J. Am. Med. Ass.* **221**, 579.
Stunkard, A.J. (1975): Studies on TOPS: a self-help group for obesity. In *Obesity in perspective,* Pt 2, ed G.A. Bray, p. 387. Washington DC: US Govt. Ptg. Office.
Stunkard, A.J. (1976): Nutrition, aging and obesity. In *Longevity and aging,* ed M. Rockstein & M.L. Sussman, p. 253. New York: Academic Press.
Sturdevant, R.A.L., Pearce, M.L. & Dayton, S. (1973): *N. Engl. J. Med.* **288**, 24.
Walker, B.R., Ballard, I.M. & Gold, J.A. (1977): *J. Int. Med. Res.* **5**, 85.
West, K.M. & Kalbfleisch, J.M. (1971): *Diabetes* **20**, 99.
Yang, M-U. & Van Itallie, T.B. (1976): *J. Clin. Invest.* **58**, 722.
York, D.A. & Bray, G.A. (1972): *Endocrinology* **90**, 885.
York, D.A., Bray, G.A. & Yukimura, Y. (1978): *Proc. Natn. Acad. Sci.* In press.
Yudkin, J. (1968): *Practitioner* **201**, 330.
Young, R.L., Fuchs, R.J. & Wolfjen, M.J. (1976): *J. Am. Med. Ass.* **236**, 2495.

27
Commercial weight loss groups*

M. ASHWELL
Clinical Research Centre, Watford Road, Harrow, Middlesex, England.

Summary
This paper reviews the contribution that commercial weight loss groups have made to the treatment of obesity. The groups which are discussed are TOPS, Weight Watchers, Slimming Magazine Clubs and Silhouette Slimming Clubs. Surveys on these groups in America, Australia and the United Kingdom by independent researchers have enabled the methods used by the groups and the results obtained by them to be compared.

TOPS are the cheapest group to join; members tend to stay longer and lose less weight than members of the more expensive groups. In the UK, members of Weight Watchers lose more weight and stay longer with the group than those from Slimming Magazine or Silhouette.

Drop-out frequency has been investigated in several of the groups. It is usually increased by previous exposure to group treatment and is decreased by a high initial weight and a good weight loss.

Weight losses achieved during group membership show a wide range of individual variation and also vary greatly between the different classes in the same group. Considering all the groups together, the average weight loss per member is 8.5 kg.

Although all the groups run schemes to aid weight maintenance after recommended weight has been reached, members who reach this goal do not always maintain their weight loss and members who do not reach it invariably gain weight when they leave the group.

The weight losses achieved by commercial groups are certainly as good as those achieved by medical practitioners. However, these groups have still to overcome their main problems of high drop-out rate and poor maintenance of weight loss. The new techniques of behaviour modification which are being introduced into some of the groups might help to overcome these problems to some extent.

Introduction
The emergence of several commercial weight loss groups during recent years has given a new approach to the treatment of obesity. Since the standard treatment of obesity by the medical profession is acknowledged by most to have such poor results (Garrow, 1974), an analysis of the results of treatment by commercial groups should not only prove an interesting comparison, but might point to the aspects of treatment which are the most successful and from which the medical profession could learn.

The theoretical treatment of obesity is simple enough: energy intake must be reduced to a level sufficiently below that of energy output to cause mobilisation of fat stores. However,

**In this review I have taken the definition of Commercial Weight Loss Groups to refer to any group which is not directly run under the auspices of a Medical Practitioner. 'Commercial' does not necessarily imply profit-making.*

problems arise when the obese patient puts this theoretical solution into practice, mainly because of the lack of willpower. One of the ways in which willpower can be strengthened is for the patient to feel that his or her progress is continually being monitored by others. Family doctors do not always have the time to spend in counselling their obese patients. In fact, the obese patients who are most dissatisfied with the way their doctors treat them are those who were not asked to report back to him at regular intervals (Ashwell, 1973). The recent Department of Health & Social Security Medical Research Council report, *'Research on obesity'* (1976), also concluded that 'Success appears to be greater if there is some interested, well informed and reasonably sympathetic person to weigh the subject not less than once a month and preferably weekly'. The great advantage of commercial groups is that they can provide regular meetings for the monitoring of progress and strengthening of willpower. This review will attempt to report the results achieved by these groups, as seen in data collected by independent researchers.

Independent surveys of commercial weight loss groups

Published data from independent researchers on the results achieved by commercial groups are rare. Garb & Stunkard (1974) summarised two separate surveys of 21 Philadelphian chapters of Take Off Pounds Sensibly (TOPS), one conducted in 1968 and one in 1970. Information was obtained each time from questionnaires filled in by the chapter leaders. Data were obtained for 485 women in 1968 and 560 women in 1970. Since the results from the two surveys were very similar in terms of weight loss by members and drop-out frequency, I have calculated and presented an average of the data in the two surveys.

In the survey of commercial groups in UK (Ashwell & Garrow, 1975) questionnaires were sent to a randomly selected sample of individual members from the three major UK groups who had joined their group exactly one year previous to the time of survey (ie they had joined in 1973). The groups studied were Weight Watchers, Slimming Magazine Slimming Clubs, and Silhouette Slimming Club. The number of completed questionnaires received from members was respectively 119, 107 and 115. The overall response rate was 56.8 per cent.

Williams & Duncan (1976) reported a statistical analysis of the complete records of Weight Watchers International in Adelaide, S. Australia (1971-1974). Their total sample of 5558 subjects included 112 men.

Stuart & Jacobson (1978) have compared the characteristics and experiences in a randomised sample of 72 men and 941 women who joined Weight Watchers classes in North America in 1975.

Stuart & Guire (1978) have collected data from 721 members of American Weight Watchers classes some 15 months after they reached their recommended weights. These members were selected at random from lists of those who had reached their recommended weight in blocks of six states including all 48 continental states. Questionnaires were distributed either by post or via the class leader.

Stuart (1977) also conducted a survey of American Weight Watchers in which several counties in one state were selected as a test site because their populations were adequate to generate samples of 2000 or more members which were comparably varied. In this survey, one area was selected randomly to continue using the traditional Weight Watchers programme (n=2856) during the same 12 weeks that another area was selected for the introduction of a new module programme (n=2219).

One further survey mentioned in this review is that by Nash (1977) who studied a group of Weight Watchers in the USA. This survey concentrates on the factors affecting drop-out rate. Questionnaires were sent to over 1000 individuals on joining the group; and, from these, 100 people who had been previous members of a group and 100 people who had not joined a group before, were randomly selected.

Some details about the groups in the surveys

TOPS (Take Off Pounds Sensibly)

TOPS was started in 1948 by a Milwaukee housewife, Esther Manz. There are 345 000

TOPS members organised in over 12 000 chapters throughout the world. These chapters delight in names such as the Taperettes, Shrinking Violets, Pound Pushers and Tummy Tuckers. TOPS is non-profit making. Their current annual fee is $9.00 decreasing to $7.00 after 2 years (equivalent to £5.17 and £4.02). No set weekly fee is charged. TOPS likes to work closely with the medical profession and for this reason relies on members getting not only their recommended weight from their doctor but also their dietary advice. There is no standard TOPS diet.

TOPS meetings are held weekly and last from 1.5 to 2 hours. They are under the direction of a TOPS leader who is a non-paid volunteer, elected for a one-year period. The meetings usually start with a song followed by the weigh-in. The announced weight changes are applauded or booed, depending whether they are up or down. The best loser of the week might be designated the 'Queen' and have a crown placed on her head. The less fortunate lady who has gained the most weight may be called 'Pig of the week' and might have to wear a toy pig around her neck and be banished to a symbolic 'pig pen'. The rest of the meeting is devoted to discussion and playing games about dieting. Successive steps in weight reduction are rewarded by bracelet charms and competition between members is strongly encouraged. Members who reach their recommended weight are rewarded with a special ceremony; if they maintain this weight for 90 days they are awarded a special membership called KOPS (Keep off pounds sensibly). KOPS members continue as full paying members of the original group. Further details about TOPS meetings are described by Wyden (1965).

Weight Watchers

Weight Watchers was started in the USA in 1961 by Jean Nidetch and came to the United Kingdom in 1967. The UK Founder-Director was a lawyer, Bernice Weston, who had slimmed successfully with the American Weight Watchers. There are now over 800 weekly classes of Weight Watchers in the United Kingdom. At the time of the 1974 survey, the membership fee for this group was £1.30 and the weekly fee £1.00. These fees are currently £1.50 and £1.30 respectively.

The start of the weekly meetings resembles TOPS meetings, but they do not have any communal singing and do not select a Queen or Pig of the Week. In order to join Weight Watchers (UK) a potential member must be at least 4.5 kg (10 lb) above her ideal weight. (The ideal weights used are slightly higher than those given by the Metropolitan Life Insurance Tables). In order to achieve her 'goal weight' the member is given a Reduction Programme which is basically a low fat, high protein regime, working out at about 4.99 to 6.24 mJ (1200 to 1500 kcal daily). Once a member has got to within 4.5 kg (10 lb) of her 'goal weight' she is given a levelling plan which represents a slightly greater energy reduction and is designed to shift the last few pounds above goal. At 'goal weight' the member is given an 8-week maintenance plan during which time some of the previously 'forbidden foods' are put back into the programme. At the end of these 8 weeks, the member is given a special brooch and the reward of free lifetime membership which means that she can attend one meeting a month free providing she maintains her 'goal weight' within 0.9 kg (2 lb).

Weight Watchers International (Australia)

The Australian branch was formed in 1969. The meetings, programmes and rules are essentially the same as those outlined above. In 1974, the membership fee was seven Australian dollars and the weekly fee was three Australian dollars (equivalent to £4.40 and £1.90 respectively).

Silhouette Slimming Club

This organisation was started in 1968 by a housewife, Thelma Brown. There are now over 1000 classes throughout the United Kingdom. At the time of the 1974 survey, the membership fee was £1.10 and the weekly fee was £0.33. These fees are currently £1.20 and £0.70 respectively.

Meetings run along broadly similar lines to those of Weight Watchers (UK). The dietary advice is actually based on a daily allowance of 4.82 mJ (1000 kcal) although a points system (1 point = 25 kcal) is used. To join, a potential member must be at least 3.2 kg (7 lb) overweight. A 'gold star weight' is set with reference to Life Insurance Tables, but, at the leader's discretion, the 'gold star weight' may be set above the ideal. If a member is very overweight, she might be given a 'silver weight', possibly at the half-way mark. Successive weight losses are rewarded with coloured discs and a presentation brooch is given at 'silver weight' and 'gold star weight'. Once a member has attained her 'gold star weight' she is allowed to attend a class free once a month providing she is within 1.4 kg (3 lb) of her 'gold star weight'.

Slimming Magazine Slimming Clubs

Slimming Magazine set up slimming clubs in 1971. There are now more than 420 classes. At the time of the 1974 survey, the membership fee was £1.15 and the weekly fee was £0.55. These fees are currently £1.60 and £0.80 respectively.

Members of this group have to be at least 3.2 kg (7 lb) overweight to join and recommended weight is referred to as 'target weight'. New members fill in a comprehensive questionnaire and on the basis of this, they are assigned one of the 16 possible recommended diets. On reaching 'target weight', the member is rewarded with free lifetime membership providing she maintains her 'target weight' within 3.2 kg (7 lb). Meetings are run on broadly similar lines to the other UK groups.

Table 1. Characteristics of group members (female): WW = Weight Watchers, SM = Slimming Magazine Slimming Clubs, SIL = Silhouette Slimming Club

	UK			USA	USA	AUS
	WW	SM	SIL	TOPS	WW	WW
Age (yr)						
mean	35.8	39.4	35.0	41.8	36.2	–
s.d.	12.2	13.2	11.3	12.1	–	–
Starting wt. (kg)						
mean	80.3	78.9	74.4	85.0	80.0	78.0
s.d.	16.0	13.6	16.6	16.9	–	–
Referral by medical practitioner (% Sample)	1.7	2.9	0	3	–	7.3

Results of independent surveys

Characteristics of group members

Table 1 shows some of the characteristics of the group members in the British, Australian and American surveys. There is a general similarity about age and starting weight of the members of groups in all three countries, the typical member being in her thirties or forties and weighing about 70 to 80 kg. The social class of members of the UK groups was similar, the majority of members (77.2 per cent) of all three groups belonging to Social Class II or III. Table 1 also shows how few group members had been referred to the group via the medical profession.

Length of membership of group

Figure 1 compares the drop-out rate of all the groups surveyed during the first year of membership; the USA survey only covered a period of 24 weeks. The drop-out frequency for TOPS was much lower than most of the other groups, in fact the average length of membership was 18.5 months (s.d. = 17.4). The highest frequency of drop-out was shown by Weight Watchers of Australia & USA. Of the UK groups, Weight Watchers showed the lowest drop-out rate.

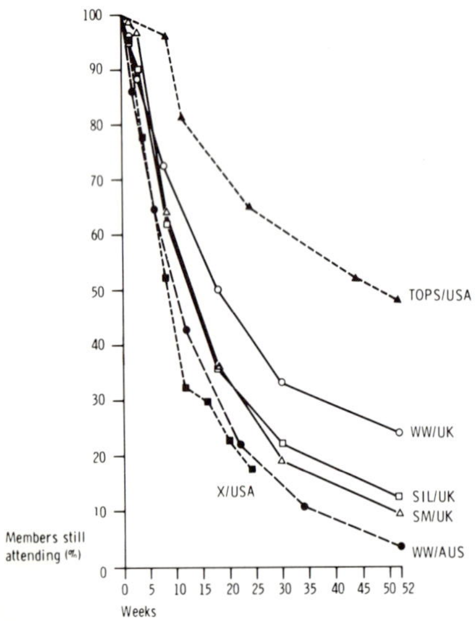

Fig. 1. Drop-out rates during first year of membership. This graph shows the proportion of members still attending commercial weight loss groups at intervals of up to one year after first joining. **TOPS/USA:** The drop-out rate has been calculated as the mean of the overall drop-out rate reported by Garb & Stunkard (1974). Only the first year's drop-out rate has been shown here. At 100 per cent, *n*=560. **ALL UK groups:** The drop-out rate has been calculated from the stated length of membership of the respondents in the survey of Ashwell & Garrow (1975). At 100 per cent, *n*=119(WW/UK), *n*=107(SM/UK), *n*=115(SIL/UK). **WW/AUS:** The drop-out rate has been calculated from the data given for all members by Williams & Duncan (1976). At 100 per cent *n*=5558. **WW/USA:** The drop-out rate has been calculated from the data given by Nash (1977) for all members staying in treatment during a period of 24 weeks. At 100 per cent, *n*=187

Factors affecting drop-out rate

For the purpose of this review, I reanalysed some of the original data on the UK groups to give further information about the factors affecting drop-out rate.

Drop-out rates were assessed from the stated average length of membership. Younger women tended to drop out sooner than older women and members with small weight losses tended to drop out sooner than those with greater weight losses. The drop-out rate was slightly higher for members who were least overweight initially. Members who had belonged to another club previously tended to drop out sooner than those who were at their first club. There was no difference in drop-out rate between women of different social class groups or between the child onset obese and the adult onset obese. The two commonest reasons given by members for leaving the group were that it was inconvenient to attend regularly or that it was too expensive to attend regularly. The first reason was the most common with members of Slimming Magazine and Silhouette groups and the second reason was most common with members of Weight Watchers (UK).

In the TOPS survey (Garb & Stunkard, 1974) the drop-out rate was highest for those members who were least overweight initially. Members with smaller weight losses were also more likely to drop out than those with greater weight losses.

Nash (1977) studied this drop-out problem in greater depth. The most important factor affecting drop-out rate was previous exposure to group treatment, ie members who rejoined the group were more likely to drop out before members who joined the group for the very first time. Age of onset of obesity and initial degree of overweight did not influence drop-out rate. Also, early drop-outs tended to rate emotions and eating habits as more importantly involved in their weight problem than did the late drop-outs.

Weight losses

Figure 2 shows the comparative results of the different groups when they are expressed as the proportion of women in each sample who achieved a total weight loss of more than 9.1 kg (20 lb) and the proportion who achieved a total weight loss of more than 18.2 kg (40 lb). On this criterion, Weight Watchers (UK) achieved the best results, with 52 per cent of members losing more than 9.1 kg and 14 per cent of members losing more than 18.2 kg. As a comparison, in reports of treatment of obesity by specialist doctors, the proportion of patients losing more than 9.1 kg ranges from 58 per cent to 8 per cent (Stunkard, Levine & Fox, 1970).

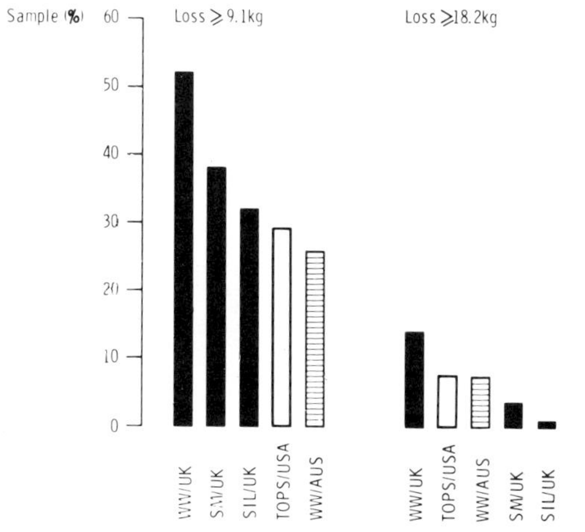

Fig. 2. Weight losses equal to or in excess of 9.1 kg & 18.2 kg. The data has been derived from the same references as Figure 1. (No data on weight losses were reported for WW/USA). **TOPS/USA & WW/AUS:** the figures which refer to the average weight loss of all classes have been shown. **WW/AUS:** only the weight losses of female subjects (n = 5446) have been used. **UK groups:** the proportion of respondents who had lost more than 9.1 kg (20 lb) and 18.2 kg (40 lb) had to be estimated* because the questionnaire had only asked respondents to state their weight loss to the nearest stone (= 14 lb, 6.35 kg). **All groups**: weight losses refer to total weight losses attained during membership of the group, ie weight on joining group – weight on leaving group or weight at time of survey.

*Number losing more than 20 lb = No. losing ≥2 stone (28 lb) + ½ (No. of respondents losing between 14 & 27 lb). Number losing more than 40 lb = No. losing ≥3 stone (42 lb)

Table 2 gives further information about the weight losses achieved by the different groups. Of the UK groups, Weight Watchers (UK) achieved the greatest average weight loss and also the greatest rate of weight loss (average weight loss divided by length of membership). Weight Watchers (Australia) did not achieve such high average weight losses as Weight Watchers (UK) but their rate of weight loss was greater because their length of membership was shorter. Members of TOPS achieved the smallest average weight loss and since their length of membership was so much longer than the UK or Australian groups, their rate of weight loss was by far the slowest.

It has been possible to make a rough assessment of the cost of weight loss with commercial groups. TOPS turned out to be the cheapest way of losing weight and Weight Watchers (Australia) the most expensive. It is interesting to note that the cost of losing a kilogram with Weight Watchers (UK) is about the same as losing the same amount of weight with Weight Watchers (Australia) when the difference in the cost of living between the two countries is taken into account. It can also be seen that losing weight with Weight Watchers (UK) is more expensive than losing weight with either of the other UK groups. It was not only the fees which were more expensive for members of Weight Watchers (UK); they were also more likely than members of the other groups to rate their diet as more expensive than normal ($P<0.001$).

Table 2 also shows the proportion of members who reached their recommended weight. The data for Weight Watchers (UK and Australia) cannot be directly compared since the figures for Australia refer to the proportion of free lifetime members, ie those who reach recommended weight and stay in contact with the club, whereas the figures from the UK refer to all those who attained their recommended weight even if they subsequently left the group. In fact, only 14.7 per cent of the Weight Watchers (UK) sample were free lifetime members which implies that 13.3 per cent of them had reached 'goal weight' but were not free lifetime members at the time of the survey.

It is also difficult to compare the proportions of members of the three UK groups who reached recommended weight because of the different methods used by the groups to set this goal. The group which sets this goal using Life Insurance Tables (Slimming Magazine, UK) did, however, have the smallest proportion of members achieving it and the group which allowed most flexibility in setting this goal (Silhouette, UK) had the highest proportion of members achieving it.

Table 2. Weight losses achieved

	UK			USA	AUS
	WW	SM	SIL	TOPS	WW
Average wt. loss (kg)	11.8	8.6	7.3	6.6	8.2
s.d.	7.9	5.4	4.6	7.2	6.4
Average length of membership (weeks)	29.5	23.5	23.6	74	17
Average rate of wt. loss (kg/weeks)	0.40	0.36	0.31	0.09	0.48
Cost of wt. loss per kg* (£ sterling)	2.61	1.64	1.21	1.46† (≡ £0.61)	7.1 (≡ £4.40)
Attainment of recommended weight (% sample)	28.2	19.8	30.7	–	21.7‡

* Calculated from [membership fee + (*n* x weekly fee)] ÷ wt lost (kg) where *n* = average length of membership (week). (Fees refer to fees at time of survey)
† Annual fee to TOPS taken to be $7 at time of 1968/1970 survey since 1965 fee was $6 and 1977 fee is $9.
‡ Refers to 'free lifetime members'.
– Not reported

Factors affecting weight losses

Reanalysis of the original data from the UK groups showed that the greatest weight losses (expressed either in absolute terms or as a percentage of initial weight) were more likely to be achieved by women over 30 compared with women under 30, women who were married rather than single, women with high initial weights and women who had not previously belonged to a group. Not surprisingly, women who attended the group regularly and stuck strictly to their diet instructions lost more weight than those who did neither of these things. The age of onset of obesity and the social class of the member did not affect the weight loss achieved. The factors which determined whether a member would reach her recommended weight were almost the same as those which determined her weight loss, except that women who had low initial weights were more likely to reach this goal than those with high initial weights.

Stuart (1977) has compared the average weekly weight losses of Weight Watchers members who participated in his 12-week survey. He showed that men (n=555) lost significantly more weight than women (n=6499); that members under 21 and over 51 were slightly less successful than those in the middle age groups and that those who worked outside their homes scored better results than those who did not.

No data are reported for the factors affecting weight loss for Weight Watchers (Australia) members and TOPS members except that weight loss in both groups was positively related to length of membership.

On leaving the group

Available data on what happens to the weights of members after they have left a group is even more scanty than that of weight changes during group membership. Williams & Duncan (1976) sent questionnaires to the first 150 free lifetime members of Weight Watchers in Adelaide, all of whom had attained their recommended weight between 28 and 24 months previously. Of the 37 replies received, one member had died, 18 had kept within 1 kg of recommended weight and 18 had gained weight. The mean weight gain was 6.0 kg and since the mean weight loss of all members of this group was 11.8 kg, these results could be interpreted to show an average improvement of 5.8 kg. However, it is very likely that the majority of the 113 women who did not reply to the questionnaire had not maintained their recommended weight and so this interpretation is probably somewhat over-optimistic.

Ashwell & Garrow (1975) sent letters to the 136 women who had lost at least 6.35 kg (14 lb) with the UK groups but were no longer members of the club. (Free lifetime members were not included.) Ninety-two replies were received to this follow-up letter and these showed that only 13.1 per cent had maintained or improved their weight loss. Sixty-three per cent of members had gained some, but not all, of the weight they lost and 23.9 per cent had regained all their lost weight. Overall, members of Silhouette (UK) and Slimming Magazine (UK) had fared better than members of Weight Watchers (UK). Assuming that the 44 members who did not reply to the follow-up letter had probably regained weight, these figures show that the majority of people who lose weight with commercial groups regain it when they leave the club.

A recent appeal survey (Consumers' Association, unpublished) has shown that members who reach recommended weight in UK groups maintain their weight losses better than members who do not reach this goal. Two-thirds of members who reached their recommended weight had not gained any weight, compared with less than one-quarter of the members who did not reach this goal.

Stuart & Guire's (1978) survey of Weight Watchers members in the USA who had reached their recommended weight showed that 15 months later, 24.6 per cent were below recommended weight, 46.4 per cent were within 10 per cent of this goal, and 28.9 per cent were 11 or more per cent above it. Those who maintained their recommended weight, as opposed to those who regained weight, tended to have several things in common; they attended classes after reaching recommended weight in the same locations and with the same teachers that assisted their weight loss; they had lower initial weights; they had improved self-concepts; they made more life-style changes supporting weight maintenance; and they continued to use many of the techniques that had helped them reach recommended weight.

Comparative effectiveness of different classes of the same group

Williams & Duncan (1976) examined the records of 40 different classes of Weight Watchers (Australia). The largest had 121 current members and the smallest had 16, the average being 45. The mean weight loss varied from 4.8 kg in the least successful class to 14.1 kg in the most successful class. The factors influencing this difference between classes were not reported.

The comparative effectiveness of the 21 different TOPS chapters was studied in detail by Garb & Stunkard (1974). In their 1968 survey, they showed that the proportion of members in the different chapters losing more than 9.1 kg (20 lb) varied between 4.5 per cent and 62.5 per cent with a mean weight loss between 3.9 kg (8.5 lb) and 10.7 kg (23.5 lb). However, the 1970 survey produced strong evidence that the observed differences in weight loss were not due to real differences in the effectiveness of the chapters. First, the variance of the weight loss of individual chapters was very large. Secondly, there was a marked variability of the weight losses of chapters from 1968 to 1970; the rank order changing dramatically. Thirdly, there was an apparent regression towards the mean in the results of the individual chapters (ie the least successful became more successful and the most successful became less successful). Garb & Stunkard (1974) concluded that 'Chapters seem to have no intrinsic effectiveness, and stability in weight loss is largely a function of the stability of individual members who remain in the chapter'.

Subjective assessment of groups

Since Ashwell & Garrow's survey (1975) was conducted via questionnaires to individual members rather than by taking data from record cards, they were able to obtain a subjective assessment of the groups by those with first hand experience of them. Of the UK group members, 55.4 per cent thought that group slimming was a successful way of losing weight permanently; current members and free lifetime members were particularly likely to hold this view. The constant encouragement given by the leader and being part of a group with similar problems were the most successful factors. Only 10.2 per cent of members thought that group slimming was an unsuccessful way of losing weight; most of these people had left the group completely.

Behaviour therapy

Convinced of the effectiveness of behaviour modification in the treatment of obesity (Stunkard & Mahoney, 1970), Levitz & Stunkard (1974) tried to discover whether behaviour modification could increase the effectiveness of commercial groups. Sixteen chapters of TOPS (234 members) received either behaviour modification or a control treatment for 12 weeks and were then followed up at 9 months. During the 3-month treatment period, behaviour modification produced significantly lower drop-out rates and significantly greater weight losses than did the control methods of treatment (nutrition education or continuation of usual TOPS programme). At the 9-month follow-up the difference among treatments were even greater. It is worth noting that the average weight loss in the group receiving behaviour modification from a professional therapist was only 2.63 kg at the end of a year, which although an improvement on the average weight *gain* of 1.81 kg and 1.27 kg in the control groups was less than the amount of weight lost in other studies using behaviour modification techniques (Stuart, 1967) and also less than the weight losses achieved by other CWLG.

Weight Watchers have been the first group to introduce the techniques of behaviour modification by giving the Weight Watchers 'personal action plan' modules to its members.

Stuart's (1977) comparison of the traditional Weight Watchers method with the new module programme over a 12-week study showed that members of traditional classes lost less weight than members of module classes (1.19 lb/week compared with 1.34 lb/week, $P<0.01$). Further analysis of the data showed that members who were better at self-monitoring their own behaviour lost more weight than those who were not so good at self-monitoring.

General comparison of groups

In comparing the different groups with respect to the results they achieve, it is obvious that TOPS are different from the other groups which is not altogether surprising since they operate on a very different basis. Their members stay much longer but lose less weight than the members of other groups. This is probably explained partly by the fact that they pay no regular weekly fee and, therefore, are not tempted to leave because of the expense. TOPS do not have a standard diet and this might be another factor which causes members to stay longer (they do not leave because they cannot tolerate the set diet). This absence of a standard diet might be one of the reasons why TOPS members lose less weight since they have less opportunity to discuss their diet with other group members. Also, the many different diets being used by chapter members could lead to confusion between members and thus impede weight loss.

It is extremely difficult to make a direct comparison between Weight Watchers in Australia and Weight Watchers in the UK. The size of the Australian sample was much larger because information was obtained directly from record cards whereas the UK survey was conducted via questionnaires sent to a random sample of individual members. Members of Weight Watchers (UK) appear to stay with the group longer and lose more weight than members of Weight Watchers (Australia), but this could be due to the fact that it was the more successful members in the UK who returned their questionnaires.

Of the UK groups, members of Weight Watchers stay the longest and lose most weight. Unfortunately, they have to pay more for this privilege and also have to be prepared for much stricter dietary control than members of the other groups. The principle of having a reduction programme followed by a levelling plan is a very good one and is based on a sound scientific principle (ie energy requirements decrease with prolonged dietary restriction). It is unfortunate that Weight Watchers set so much importance by the nutrient balance of their various programmes rather than explaining the simple principles of energy balance to their members. This is possibly why members of Weight Watchers fare less well on leaving the group than the members of other groups.

As far as choosing a group is concerned, the choice of the overweight individual will depend mainly on which groups operate in her locality and to a lesser extent on her own character. In the hypothetical situation of her having the choice of all the groups discussed here, she would probably do best to join Weight Watchers if she wanted to lose most weight in a reasonably short time, provided she was able to afford the cost and tolerate the authoritarian approach. On the other hand, if she was prepared to lose less weight but wanted to enjoy a more social atmosphere, she should join TOPS. In the case of a doctor advising his patient, he should recommend TOPS if he insists on setting her weight goal and providing the dietary advice himself, but should send her to one of the other groups if he knew she could afford it and he was prepared to accept the dietary system of the group in return for a greater chance of a successful weight loss.

Conclusions

There is no doubt that commercial groups achieve weight losses from their members which are comparable with other groups treated either in general practice or at hospital out-patient clinics. An average weight loss of all members of all groups of 8.5 kg is certainly a worthwhile amount and *if* this weight loss could be maintained, then commercial groups could do a lot to solve the problem of obesity which exists today.

However, the results concerning the maintenance of weight loss are as poor for commercial groups as they are for the medical profession. All groups have schemes to encourage members who reach their recommended weight to maintain their weight loss and these schemes are sensible. The trouble is that no more than one-third of all members reach their goal and, therefore, more than two-thirds of the members have no opportunity of benefiting from the maintenance schemes.

It is surely true that a weight loss which is maintained is better than a weight loss of twice the magnitude which is not maintained; therefore, one must question the reasons why commercial groups have not yet devised any schemes to encourage the maintenance of their lesser weight losses. Perhaps the groups only like to recognise two types of members: those who are currently losing weight and are potential successes, and those who have reached and maintained weight goals and are, therefore, complete successes. I would like to urge them to devise schemes to cater for their partial successes - otherwise these members will almost certainly end up as total failures.

Finally, I must stress that the commercial groups will only be a successful method of treating those overweight patients who are willing to be treated in a group situation in the first place. However many groups become established in the future and whatever success rate they show, they will only assist that proportion of the population who like the general idea of being a member of a group with a common aim.

Acknowledgement – I would like to thank the organisers of all groups for supplying me with information about the size of their organisation, their methods and fees.

References

Ashwell, M. (1973): *Practitioner* 211, 653.
Ashwell, M. & Garrow, J.S. (1975): *Nutrition* 29, 347.
Department of Health & Social Security/Medical Research Council (1976): *Research on Obesity*. London: HMSO.
Garb, J.R. & Stunkard, A.J. (1974): *Archs Intern. Med.* 134, 716.
Garrow, J.S. (1974): In *Energy balance and obesity in man*, p. 249. Amsterdam: North Holland.
Levitz, L.S. & Stunkard, A.J. (1974): *Am. J. Psychiatry* 131, 423.
Nash, J.D. (1977): Paper presented at Association for the Advancement of Behaviour Therapy, New York, 1976.
Stuart, R.B. (1967): *Behav. Res. Therapy* 5, 357.
Stuart, R.B. (1977): Self-help group approach to self-management, In *Behavioural self-management. Strategies, techniques and outcome,* ed R.B. Stuart, p. 278. New York: Bruner-Mazel.
Stuart, R.B. & Jacobson, B. (1978): Sex differences in obesity. In *Gender and psychopathology: sex differences in disordered behaviour.* New York: Bruner-Mazel (in press).
Stuart, R.B. & Guire, K. (1978): *Int. J. Obesity* 2, (in press).
Stunkard, A., Levine, H. & Fox, S. (1970): *Archs Intern. Med.* 125, 1067.
Stunkard, A.J. & Mahoney, M.J. (1970): Behavioural treatment of the eating disorders. In *Handbook of behaviour modification,* ed H. Leitenberg. New York: Appleton-Century-Crofts.
Williams, A.E. & Duncan, B. (1976): *Med. J. Aust.* 1, 781.
Wyden, P. (1965): *The overweight society,* p. 79. New York: William Morrow.

28
Battling the bulge: a continuing struggle. Two-year follow-up of successful losers in a commercial dieting concern

J.T. DWYER and E.M. BERMAN

Departments of Medicine and Community Health, Tufts University Medical School, and Frances Stern Nutrition Center, New England Medical Center Hospital, 185 Harrison Avenue, Boston, Massachusetts 02111, USA; Graduate Student, Massachusetts School of Professional Psychology, Newton, Massachusetts, USA.

Introduction

Self-help groups have become increasingly popular in the past decade for treating obesity. They employ not only diets but group pressure, group support, emphasis on exercise, and behavior modification and may thus be more powerful modes of treatment than conventional dietary therapy based on reducing diets alone (Allon, 1971; Dwyer, Feldman & Mayer, 1970; Stunkard, 1976; Stunkard, Levine & Fox, 1970; Wagonfeld & Wolowitz, 1968).

Commercial dieting groups are companies run for profit which use these techniques to assist their customers. Allon (1971) described the function of one such group. Stunkard (1977) has emphasized the promise of such groups in helping to control obesity.

It is well known with all methods developed to date for treating obesity that over the long term, at least, 'most obese persons will not stay in treatment for obesity. Of those who stay in treatment, most will not lose weight, and of those who do lose weight, most will regain it' (Garrow, 1974; Stunkard & McLaren-Hume, 1959). If the commercial dieting groups represent an exception to this rule, it is important to document the fact. Since so many Americans buy such services, in any event, it is legitimate to raise the question of exactly how effective they are.

In the United States, data for either short-term outcome (eg, at completion of treatment) or long-term (eg, one to five years post-treatment) success in weight loss from such companies is not available. Ashwell (1974) reported preliminary data of the effectiveness of commercial dieting groups in England and found that, among 2000 persons surveyed, dieting with the help of such a group was a better method of losing weight than self-imposed diets, physician-generated diets, or exercise alone. It is high time that hard data on short and long-term outcomes of weight reduction efforts replaced anecdotal reports of success on such commercial dieting endeavors. This paper is a first, albeit unsatisfactory, step in that direction. While the data we obtained is subject to a catalogue of legitimate scientific criticisms, perhaps the description of the process of attempting to collaborate with one such group will serve as a helpful guide to other investigators and encourage the groups themselves to better record-keeping.

Purpose of the study

The purpose of the study was to investigate present (mid-1977) weight status and opinions by mail survey of the total population of persons registered with 'Trim Down'- the pseudonym of a dieting company - in two cities between 1 January 1975 and 31 December 1975.

The hypothesis was that outcomes with respect to changes in eating behavior and life style, as well as changes in weight, would be evident among those who had participated in a commercial dieting company's program in 1975 on follow-up almost two years later.

A large city in the Middle Atlantic States was chosen as the survey site for the follow-up study of women following the 'regular' program of the company. The 'regular' program of this company has been described in detail by Allon (1971) and Berman (1975). In brief, it consists of weekly meetings held in locations convenient to the participants. After obtaining their physicians' permission, members were given a diet plan which averaged 1200 kcal (5000 kJ) per day, meeting the recommended dietary allowances for all individual nutrients, but not for energy, a weight target to aim for, and a card on which to list their weight each week. The weight target is usually determined jointly by the group inspector and the individual unless the physician specifies a goal. Lacking calipers, or other more scientific means, they examine wrist size and other aspects of build. A member may request a higher or lower goal if it falls within the range of average weights for height for different frame sizes used. This is done since otherwise successful completion or 'graduation' from the program would be more arbitrary and not fair financially to those who picked the lower goal.

In 1975 the company ran 25 classes in the city, with an average size of 24 members each. Competition between this and other dieting companies was sharp. Instructors were lay people who had successfully lost weight in the company's program, thus instructors served as a model to motivate members. They were provided with a ten-week instructor's guide which outlined material to be covered, possible problems and how to deal with them, protocols for isotonic exercises, and listed instructors' tasks and duties. They were also given a nutrition manual which discussed some common questions and answers about diet which members might ask. Each week instructors were given low calorie recipes to provide to the members.

Regular program members in 1975 were expected to pay $2.00 per meeting attended in addition to a $3.00 entrance fee. During the meetings each member was weighed at the door as he came in. After a brief time for chatter, while others were being weighed-in, a lay instructor lectured on some aspect of weight control, motivation to lose weight, and problems common in obesity and dieting, answered questions, provided low calorie recipes in line with the diet, read off the weight gain or loss of each member, led the group in exercises, and closed the meeting. Those who had joined were strongly encouraged to come each week. A ten-week 'package' was sold to those who wished it. Economic sanctions for non-attendance involved paying for each missed meeting.

A second large city, in the New England region, was chosen for the survey of women in the special 'diet seminar' program of the Trim Down Company. Seminars were designed for those who needed additional support for their dieting efforts after difficulties following the regular program. In general, these persons were heavier, and had higher educational and income levels, than regular program members. They often were attracted to the seminars by the greater flexibility and individual attention this approached involved (Berman, 1975).

The seminars were smaller in size, limited to 12 members. Greater emphasis was placed on individual responsibility for planning diets, and members kept detailed food records. Small commitments to the regime were asked for each week, rather than an 'all out dieting' approach, to encourage and reward desirable behaviors. A greater degree of group commitment and personal attention, including personal consultation and diets adjusted for individual situations, was possible. A discussion format rather than a lecture was employed in seminar meetings. In contrast to fierçe competition with other dieting companies in the regular program, there was no other company offering a seminar type approach. The seminars were less structured and smaller than non-commercial self-help groups, such as Over-eaters Anonymous and TOPS ('Take Off Pounds Sensibly').

In diet seminars, weight goals were set by each individual, and interim goals with progressive approximations downward were encouraged, because of the greater amounts of weight which needed to be lost, and the lack of financial pressures on most participants.

Population surveyed

'Regular' program

The study of the regular program was carried out in a large city in the Middle Atlantic States. A supposedly complete list of registrants was obtained from the district manager of the organization in that city during the Spring of 1977. A 13-page survey questionnaire was sent to all persons on the mailing list in August 1977, and a reminder postcard sent in early September 1977. In early October of 1977, as results were being analyzed, we were informed that the total population of registrants had not after all been provided. Instead, only the addresses of those who were successful in their weight losses were released. Therefore, *pari-passu,* the study's objective became one of evaluating the later progress of the unknown proportion of the total population seen that year who were 'graduates', ie successful in losing weight to the company's weight for height goals, and who responded to the questionnaire.

'Seminar' program

Similar procedures were followed for surveying all the participants of the seminar program. In contradistinction to difficulties encountered in the survey of the regular program participants, all persons in the original population, and not just those who were successful, were surveyed who had registered through 1975.

Methods

The 13-page questionnaire was designed to survey the former participants of these commercial dieting organizations in the following regards:

1. Past experience with weight reduction efforts, including the company's programs
2. Weight changes after leaving company's program
3. Personal and company weight goals
4. Changes in life style affected by weight
5. Effects of weight on life events
6. Demographic and social characteristics of participants

This questionnaire was sent to all persons who had successfully lost weight to the company's weight-for-height goals in one city where participants in the 'regular' program were surveyed, and to all persons registered in the special 'seminar' program in another city regardless of whether they had lost weight or not. Anonymity was assured, and names were not requested. Approximately one month after the initial mailing, a follow-up mailing to all persons was done to remind them to return their questionnaires.

Questionnaires were coded and transferred to IBM cards and processed on data processing equipment.

Results

Response rates

The response rates for the two groups are given in Table 1.

Response rates were 28 per cent among the successful losers who were re-surveyed. In contrast, the total population of seminar participants yielded a response rate of only 13 per cent. Results from the seminar respondents were not analyzed further because of the low response rate. Of this small number of respondents, 19 per cent had maintained their previous weights, 65 per cent had increased, 10 per cent had decreased and 5 per cent were still enrolled in the program.

There is no way of telling if either group of respondents was representative of the total populations since records from 1975 were unavailable in the first instance and found to be unretrievable in the second instance after the study started.

Reported weights at follow-up of 'regular' program 'graduates'

Weights reported at follow-up are presented in Table 2. It should be noted that these are

Table 1. Response rates for populations surveyed in two-year follow-up study

	'Trim Down' regular program female 'graduates' who lost weight to goal in 1975		'Trim Down' seminar program: all registrants prior to 1975	
	n	(%)	*n*	(%)
Total registrants	?		?	
Population surveyed	448		561	
– Responded	122	(28)	63	(13)
– No response	307		426	
Lost to follow-up	19		72	

reported weights, and thus are likely to be substantially lower than actual weights (Dwyer *et al.*, 1970). Also presented on the chart are the 'recommended' or 'goal' weights for height suggested by the company to customers with medium frames, and the average 'desirable' weights for heights developed from actual statistics which are the most commonly used medical criteria (Bray, 1975). Note that the company goal weights are based on tables of average weights for medium frames of adult women at age 30, and are substantially higher than desirable weights. For example, the medium framed woman of 5′ 5″ has a goal weight of 139 lb (63 kg), with a range of 130-148 lb (59-67 kg). The Fogarty Conference on Obesity 1973 published a 'Table on Recommended Weight' in relation to height (Bray, 1975) which suggests a mean of 123 lb (56 kg) (some 16 lb or 7.25 kg lower) and a range of 111-142 lb (50-65 kg). Since the goal weights were already considerably higher than recommended weights, and known under-reporting of actual weights is very common among the obese (Dwyer *et al.*, 1970) persons who exceeded their previously achieved goal weights at follow-up were deemed to be 'unsuccessful' with respect to weight maintenance at follow-up. For purposes of the study, those whose weights at follow-up were equal to, or lower than, company goals were regarded as 'successes'. The 32 respondents who were successful at follow-up had lost a mean of 23 ± 14 s.d. lb (10.5 ± 6.4 kg) in the dieting company's program. Those who were unsuccessful at follow-up and were now 1-10 lb (0.45-4.5 kg) above their goals had previously lost 24 ± 10 lb (11 ± 4.5 kg) (n=40). Those unsuccessful who were 11 lb (5 kg) over previous goals, had lost 22 ± 11 lb (10 ± 5 kg) (n=31). Table 3 presents outcomes using these criteria for the respondents to the survey. Of the respondents 35 (29 per cent) were presently at, or below their goal weights, while 84 were above their goal weights. Of those above their goal weights, seven persons were only 2 lb (0.9 kg) above their reported Trim Down weight goal at present and were eligible to attend meetings free, since this was regarded as close enough to goals to be evidence of continued success.

Table 2. Mean reported present weights (lb) by height at two-year follow-up of women who had reached their goal weights. Recommended weights are from the Fogarty Conference Table of recommended weights (Bray, 1975 p. 7) and are without clothing. The company's weight charts are with indoor clothing which can be up to 3-5 lb

Height	Present reported weight			Dieting company's weight chart goal weights		Recommended weights	
	n	Mean ± s.d.	Range	Medium frame	Range for other frames	Mean	Range
5′1″	23	131±22	106-208	124	116-132	110	99-128
5′2″	18	132±10	114-160	128	120-136	113	102-131
5′3″	16	139±15	114-170	132	123-140	116	105-134
5′4″	22	137±10	120-153	136	127-144	120	108-138
5′5″	15	137±10	112-150	139	130-148	123	111-142
5′6″	9	142±15	120-168	142	134-152	128	114-146
5′7″	9	144±10	123-158	146	138-156	132	118-150
5′8″	7	148±10	130-157	150	142-160	136	122-154

Table 3. Reported weights (lb) at two-year follow-up of 'graduates' of the regular program. Persons who had reached the Diet Company's Goal Weight. Such goals are approximately 10 pounds higher than the Fogarty International Center Conference on Obesity's average recommended weights in relation to height

Difference between present and goal weights at successful completion of program	Outcome with respect to dieting company's goals: Successful: at or below goal		Unsuccessful: above goal: 1-10 lb over goal		11 or more lb over goal		Total	
	n	(%)	*n*	(%)	*n*	(%)	*n*	(%)
No Difference	7	(20)	—	—			7	(6)
Higher								
1-10 lb			46	(100)			46	(39)
11-20 lb					25	(65)	25	(21)
21 + lb					8	(21)	8	(7)
Lower								
1-10 lb	25	(71)					25	(21)
11-20 lb	3	(9)					3	(2)
21 + lb	0							
No Response					5	(14)	5	(4)
Total	35	(100)	46	(100)	38	(100)	119	(100)

Maintainers, gainers, and losers

Table 4 describes two general patterns with respect to weight over the two year interim between graduation and follow-up. The minority of the population, the maintainers, reported that they maintained a stable weight with little deviation from it. The majority of the respondents reported that their weights had crept up again - for purposes of description we will refer to them as 'gainers'. A fortunate few had continued to lose even after reaching their goals. Maintainers were more common among those successful at follow-up.

Table 4. Gains and losses at two-year follow-up of 'graduates' of dieting company regular program

	Status with respect to goal at follow-up: Successful: at or below goal		Unsuccessful: 1-10 lb above goal		11-20 lb above goal		Total	
	n	(%)	*n*	(%)	*n*	(%)	*n*	(%)
Maintainers	18	(48)	10	(22)	2	(5)	30	(25)
Changers	14	(38)	30	(65)	36	(95)	80	(66)
Gainers*	(11)		(28)		(34)			
Losers†	(3)		(2)		(2)			
Preservers - still enrolled	4	(11)	6	(13)	—	—	10	(8)
No response	1	(3)					1	(1)
Total	37		46		38		121	

*Means were 12 lb gained for successes, 11 lb for those 1-10 lb above goal, and 29 lb for those 11+ lb above goal

†Means were 32 lb lost for successes, 9 lb for those 1-10 lb above goal, and 10 lb for those 11 + lb above goal

The yo-yo pattern

Fluctuations in weight patterns were even more complicated than the classification in Table 4 might suggest. A yo-yo type pattern was also evident; that is, most respondents' weights had both risen and fallen in the two year interim, with gains followed by losses. Table 5 shows the dimensions of this yo-yo phenomenon.

Table 5 also shows that maintenance of weight was more common, and repeated cycles of gain were less so, among the successes on follow up. They were four times more likely never to have gained weight back and also less likely to experience repeated cycles of gain than were those who had been unsuccessful.

Table 5. The yo-yo phenomenon: 'graduates' of the diet company who reported that they had regained weight on two-year follow-up. 'Have you ever been close to your "Trim Down" goal weight and then gained a significant amount of weight back again?'

	Classification at follow-up							
Pattern with respect to weight gain	**Successful:** at or below goal *n*		**Unsuccessful:** 1-10 lb over goal		11+ lb over goal		**Total** *n*	
Maintainers (Never gained weight back)	19	(51%)	9	(20%)	–	(0%)	28	(23%)
Gainers	14	(38%)	31	(67%)	36	(95%)	81	(67%)
Regained once	7	(19%)	18	(38%)	18	(47%)	43	(36%)
Regained twice	3	(8%)	9	(20%)	14	(37%)	26	(21%)
Regained thrice or more	4	(11%)	4	(9%)	4	(11%)	12	(10%)
Never close to goal	–	(0%)	1	(2%)	–	(0%)	1	(1%)
No response	4	(11%)	5	(11%)	2	(5%)	11	(9%)
Total *n*	37		46		38		121	

The constant struggle: repeated efforts to control weight

Further analysis of the data suggested a reason why a large proportion of those who were successful also exhibited the yo-yo pattern of repeated gain and yet this did not spell the end of weight stabilization. The 1975 graduates had continued their weight control efforts in the succeeding two years, taking action on gains. Sixty-two per cent of the respondents had participated in the dieting company's programs or other weight control efforts in subsequent years, and 67 per cent were engaging in them on the day of the survey. Differences between successes and failures in these efforts will shortly become evident.

Types of weight control efforts employed

Interesting differences emerged when the subsequent and current weight control efforts of those who had been successful and unsuccessful at follow-up were analyzed. Table 6 presents these findings. Successes at follow-up were somewhat more likely never to have attempted to engage in weight control prior to the program in 1975. In the years between 1975 and 1977, both groups increasingly adopted group self-help commercial type efforts and abandoned approaches involving diet pills and the more bizarre of the miracle diets. Sixty-two per cent of the respondents had engaged in some weight reduction effort since they had left the Trim Down program. On the day the survey questionnaire was answered, 81 per cent of the successes and 61 per cent of those unsuccessful at follow up were engaged in some weight reduction effort. Group methods accounted for at least half of all efforts. Thus, successes were more likely to have done nothing to control their weights prior to 1975, and since that time they were more likely to make efforts, particularly group-related efforts coupled with additional calorie-counting or other private efforts, than were those who were unsuccessful at follow-up. Further questioning revealed that they had apparently been weaned from more individualistic efforts to loyalty to Trim Down because of their greater satisfaction with its dieting program.

Table 6. Types of programs reported for weight control by respondents who had 'graduated' successfully from dieting company program and who were successful (n=37) and unsuccessful (n=84) at two-year follow-up (see Table 4)

Weight control efforts used	Percentage of respondents using*					
	Prior to entering dieting company's program		Weight control efforts in interim		Currently used at two-year follow-up	
	Successful	Unsuccessful	Successful	Unsuccessful	Successful	Unsuccessful
Nothing	32	18	35	39	19	39
Physician prescribed diets, dietitians	14	20	3	1	5	0
Spas/exercise	8	10	—	7	—	2
Diet pills and medication	59	67	—	—	0	0
Miracle and Magazine Diets	27	31	11	7	0	0
Groups	24	27	38	26	65	35
Calorie counting	49	54	19	15	22	12

*Responses do not total 100% because several choices were allowed

Characteristics of successes

Other demographic and social characteristics of the total population of the 'graduates' who were successful and unsuccessful in still being at their goal weight two years later are presented in Table 7. This analysis revealed few differences between the two groups. The most

Table 7. Characteristics of female respondents at two-year follow-up

Characteristic	Maintenance of company goal weights			
	Successful: at or below goal (n=37)		Unsuccessful: *above goal* (n=84)	
	(mean±s.e.)	(%)	(mean±s.e.)	(%)
Overweight persons in household	0.6±0.2		1.5±0.2	
Total persons in household	3.6±0.3		3.8±0.3	
Types of weight reduction measures before joining dieting company	2.1±0.2		2.5±0.3	
Types used in two year interim	1.2±0.1		1.3±0.1	
Types used presently	1.3±0.1		1.1±0.0	
Married		92		85
Education beyond high school		48		57
Weight lost in 'Trim Down' program to 'graduate' (lb)	23±2.5		23±1.3	
Onset of obesity in childhood or adolescence		32		40

striking finding was that there was almost one fewer overweight person in the household of the successes, as might be expected if they had indeed lost weight. Successes were more likely to be enrolled in programs aimed at weight reduction at the present time than were those who were unsuccessful, but no other significant differences were apparent.

Comparisons between personal weight goals and comfortable ranges of weights: constant aspirations

Table 8 shows that mean personal weight goals for height closely approximated the dieting company's goals. The midpoint of the comfortable range which subjects reported also was very close to company goals. Those unsuccessful at follow-up (whose weights no longer approximated company goals) had apparently not resolved the cognitive dissonance of possessing higher weights by altering their aspirations with respect to weight goals.

Table 8. Mean personal weight goals at two-year follow-up midpoint of 'comfy range' and dieting company's goals for medium frame by height

Height	Personal weight goal		Median of 'comfy range'		Dieting company's goals	
	n	mean	*n*	mean	Mean goal reported	Actual chart for medium frame
5′1″	21	119	23	123	123	124
5′2″	17	120	18	124	124	128
5′3″	16	124	16	126	127	132
5′4″	23	127	23	129	133	136
5′5″	14	129	15	132	135	139
5′6″	9	134	9	135	137	142
5′7″	8	135	9	136	137	146
5′8″	7	139	7	141	142	150

A favorable net effect: differences between highest and present weights

In spite of the fact that many of these formerly successful weight losers had subsequently gained back considerable amounts of weight, Table 9 shows that they were still better off than they had been at previous times in their lives. Only 3 per cent of the respondents were currently at their highest adult weights. Among those who were at their goals at follow-up, the difference between highest adult weights and present weights was over 20 lb (9 kg). Those who were no longer at their 'graduation' weights at follow-up were some 10 lb (4.5 kg) leaner than they had been at some other point in their adult life. Moreover, subjects reported having lost a mean of 23 ± 12 lb (10.5 ± 5.5 kg) (n=103) during their enrollment in the program, while the mean gain since the program had ended had been only 7 ± 3 lb (3.2 ± 1.4 kg) (n=98).

Table 9. Mean reported highest adult weights by height and present weights at two year follow-up of dieting company 'graduates'

Height	Highest adult weights		Present weights	
	n	mean ± s.d.	*n*	mean ± s.d.
5′1″	22	151±24	23	133±22
5′2″	19	158±18	18	132±10
5′3″	15	156±28	16	139±15
5′4″	23	160±15	22	137±10
5′5″	13	160±11	15	137±10
5′6″	10	163±23	9	142±15
5′7″	9	163±19	9	144±10
5′8″	7	170±15	7	148±10
5′9″	—	—	—	—
Total	118	160±22	119	138±14

Factors associated with continuing weight control problems
We then attempted to document some of the difficulties listed by respondents which led to their continuing struggles to control their weights, even after the battle of shedding excess pounds had seemingly been won and they had 'graduated' from the company's program.

Most common situations triggering overeating
Table 10 summarizes the most common situations in the subjects' opinion which triggered overeating. Social events related to food represented a great temptation to most respondents, regardless of success at follow-up. Emotional difficulties and events were the next most likely to trigger overeating.

Table 10. Most common situations triggering overeating listed by respondents

Type of situation	Percentage of respondents reporting (n=122)
Social and food related events	
Holiday meals	88
Going to a party	82
Restaurant eating	76
Having a party	73
Emotional states	
Happiness and celebration	68
Boredom and loneliness	68
Tension, worry, pressure	63
Frustration	61
Food itself	
Sight and smell of food	65

The double bind - a vicious cycle
A number of events were thought both to cause and be the effects of weight gain. Table 11 shows the most common aspects of life style affected by weight gain and loss. Effects of weight gain in the subjects opinions were decreased physical activity, decreased social life, decreased outside interests and hobbies, and deteriorating relationships with their partners.

Table 11. Most common life styles affected by weight reported at follow-up by respondents (n=122). 'Some people find their life style is affected by change in their weight. Others find that changes in their weight affect life style. Please indicate how each of the following changes in your weight affect your life style.'

Situation	More likely to occur when weight less (% of respondents)	More likely to occur when weight more (% of respondents)
Fostered by weight gain		
Decrease in physical activity	7	52
Decrease in outside interests, hobbies	5	48
Less active social life	2	47
Deteriorating relationship with partner	1	25
Fostered by weight loss		
Increase in physical activity	57	8
More active social life	51	2
Increase in outside interests, hobbies	50	2
Better relationship with partner	48	2

Situations leading to weight gain or loss
Table 12 shows situations respondents believed to be associated with weight gain which were also examined. Decreased physical activity, decreased outside interests and hobbies, decreased social life, birth of a child, and deteriorating relationships with their partner led to weight gain. A more active social life was thought to have the same effects by a considerable proportion of subjects. Breaking habits such as smoking were also believed by a sizeable proportion of the respondents to lead to weight gain.

Table 12. Most common situations 'graduates' reported at follow-up which made them gain or lose weight (n = 122). 'Some people find their life style is affected by change in their weight. Others find that changes in their weight affect life style. Please indicate how each of the following situations affect changes in your weight.'

Situation	Leads to weight gain (% of respondents)	Leads to weight loss (% of respondents)
Fosters gain		
Decrease in physical activity	65	—
Decrease in outside interests/hobbies	53	2
Less active social life	44	10
Birth of a child	31	15
More active social life	26	36
Deteriorating relationship with partner	23	11
Breaking a habit such as smoking	23	—
Fosters loss		
Increase in physical activity	3	63
Increased outside interests	1	52
More active social life	26	36
Death of someone close	11	33
Better relationship with partner	25	11
Increased job responsibility	14	23
Begin job	9	23

Discussion

Response rates in this survey were low. This was a not unexpected finding in view of the length of the questionnaire, the sensitive nature of information from participants, the time after involvement in the program, and the high mobility of the population. Even more damaging to efforts to replicate the study, or relate results to the population surveyed, is the fact that baseline data on the demographic, social and anthropometric characteristics of the parent population are unavailable. Therefore results must be interpreted with caution, since the respondent population may not be at all representative. Jeffrey (1977) admirably summarizes the difficulties such defects in study design create for data analysis and interpretation of results with respect to the efficacy of weight reduction.

In spite of similar survey techniques, response rates were higher from the successful 'graduates' of the 'regular' program than they were among former 'seminar' participants. There are several possible explanations for this finding. First, the probability that they were less obese when they entered the program and the very success implied by definition in graduating from the program made it more likely that they would be more likely to be able to control their weights in the future and to report positive results. Continued success is something to boast about; continued failure is not. Second, graduates of the Trim Down regular program are encouraged to continue as non-paying group members in a weight maintenance program as long as their weights do not deviate upward by more than 2 lb (0.9 kg) from their goal. The continued involvement of many of these members, some as company employees such as group leaders or assistants, no doubt made them sympathetic and receptive to the survey. In contrast the seminar participants did not represent a population selected on the basis of previous success in weight reduction, were heavier than participants in the regular program, and had turned to the special seminars after experiencing difficulty in the regular program. Thus they were perhaps more sensitive about their progress and less likely to have positive results to report than the graduates of the regular program. Additionally, one of the authors of this paper (EMB) had directed the seminar program and lived in the same city as the participants. It is possible that, despite our assurances, fears of lack of anonymity or being checked also militated against compliance with the survey. From the medical standpoint, one measure of success in adult dieting efforts is weight reduction to desirable weight levels maintained over time; usually five years being taken as evidence of long-term success. Therefore, weight outcomes remain of crucial importance for any program which purports to impact favorably on obesity as a health hazard.

Weights at follow-up revealed that even those who are successful at short-term weight loss continue in active combat fighting the battle of the bulge, if these results are valid. Maintenance of weight in almost two years after successful completion of a weight control program was reportedly achieved by roughly a third of a group of successful graduates of the regular program who responded to a questionnaire. Unfortunately, the respondents only represented a quarter of all short-term successful losers surveyed. There was no means available for ascertaining the representativeness of the respondent population. Moreover, reported weights are notoriously unreliable, particularly among the obese. No means of checking the responses for validity were available.

The criteria for company goals are based on average weights rather than desirable weights from actuarial data, so the criteria for success in this study were quite liberal by medical standards. A much lesser proportion of respondents would be considered successful if desirable weight standards were used (Table 13). More generous goals than desirable weights can

Table 13. Classification of respondents by reported weight status using Fogarty International Obesity Conference criteria at two-year follow-up (Bray, 1975)

	n	(%)
Below mean	12	(10)
At mean	3	(2)
Above mean	107	(88)
Total	122	(100)

perhaps be justified in view of the dubious validity of the data upon which desirable weights are based (Bray, 1975; Seltzer, 1968) and the fact that, in a sense, all estimates of fatness based on overweight are arbitrary (Bray, 1975). In the experience of both authors, from a practical standpoint, realistic goals depend upon age, life style, and degree of deprivation required to maintain a desired weight. Persons who set their goals too low often gain back more than they originally lost. On the other hand, while the medical risks may be less with lower goal weights, for non-health related reasons these considerations must be tempered with practical realities. For example, a 60-year-old grandmother who started weight reduction from size 26 1/2 and 225 lb (102 kg) may be comfortable and healthy when she loses enough weight to fit into size 14 clothes. This goal may be the best one for her, rather than the size 10 her fashion model neighbor may choose at the same height, which may be more in line with actuarial data. This dieting company's goal thus represents a compromise between the practical and possible with that thought to be the most desirable from the actuarial standpoint. But they thus possess the disadvantage for studies of this sort of not being standard for all persons of a given height, weight and frame. However, goals are clearly in the desirable direction and in this sense are appropriate targets to aim for. Whether they are appropriate for other purposes, such as lowest actuarial risk, or are best for comparative studies, is not so clear.

A wag once said that dieting companies and therapists were profitable because they had an enormous repeat business. Indeed, if our respondents are any indication, most of the respondents find it necessary to continue to be constantly vigilant to keep weight from going up.

The minority pattern after graduation apparently involves constant address to the problem by continued participation in the dieting company's program. Graduates of the Trim Down regular program who stay within 2 lb (1 kg) of their goal weights are allowed to come free to group meetings and are provided with weight maintenance diets which are slightly higher in energy than the reducing diets. Such persons are called 'maintainers'. However, in spite of the lack of financial barriers, it appears that few persons do this. The majority pattern followed by graduates was that of the gainers. This involved greater upward rebound of weight, with re-entry into the regular program on a fee paying basis or adoption of other measures to lose what had become accumulated. This gain-then-loss cycle was apparently common among many graduates. The major factors which distinguished those who reported they were at their goal two years after graduation, from those who were not, was that seemingly a greater proportion of the former became maintainers in the regular program, and that the gainers among the successes were less likely to have experiences repeated cycles of gain which then necessitated corrective action.

It is interesting to note that most of the respondents had turned increasingly to dieting companies, and the more moderate weight reduction regimes they advocate for weight control efforts after graduation, rather than 'miracle' diets, and diet pills. Successful loss in such a dieting company's program apparently generates a good deal of customer loyalty and satisfaction with their approach thereafter.

In spite of the relatively poor maintenance of previously attained goal weights among this population, it is important to note that the respondents' weights were somewhat below the highest weights they had already achieved as adults. In this sense these previously successful weight losers were still ahead of where they had been in the past. It is not possible to determine whether this is a result of highest adult weights including pregnancy weight gain, self-selection or response bias, or a true effect of the program. However, success in maintenance of weight loss some two years later was associated with continuing use of the dieting company's program, or other weight control regimes, rather than demographic or social characteristics. And the original amounts lost in the program were 23 lb (10.5 kg), while weight changes averaged only 7 lb (3.2 kg) overall. Thus, it is likely that the program did have positive effects.

The respondents apparently were most likely to be triggered to over-eat by social and emotional situations. Weight gain was seen as having powerful social effects. For such persons, a dieting regime which stresses group dynamics, environmental and behavioral modification, social support and social pressure, might very well be helpful to them in their continuing efforts to keep weight in line. At least, they reported that it was. We have apparently identified a group of relatively satisfied users of the dieting company's techniques and, for such persons, this may be their single best weight control option, even if it is by no means foolproof.

Problems with the study

The major flaws in the study involve the failure to define the sampling population or the more general total population of successful short-term weight losers by any objective means. The proportion of the total population who lost weight over the short run is unknown; the direction of bias with respect to the survey as opposed to the overall population of short-term weight losers, and the accuracy of reported as opposed to actual weights, are all unknown. Low response rates exacerbate the sampling and representativeness problems. In view of these damning limitations, the study should be viewed as an exploratory exercise for both investigators rather than as a serious scientific effort.

In the Trim Down Company, several steps have already been taken to improve record-keeping. One of the owners (EMB) has requested all area directors to provide year as well as dates on all weight record cards and to preserve cards of all persons entering the program, and to deposit them in a central record office at the end of each year. While area directors have a good deal of latitude and are free to refuse this request, this is a step in the right direction.

The research gap

We must address the more important questions of the short and long-term weight outcomes of the populations serviced by dieting company programs. These are public health issues of great significance. Until more such studies of self-help programs of the dieting companies and other new treatments are forthcoming, there is no evidence to assume that these programs are any more successful than other treatment modalities. The need for data on effectiveness and outcome of all obesity prevention treatment programs has been stressed again and again over the past several decades. Particular attention was given to the paucity of short and long-term outcome data from newer treatment methods at the 1973 Fogarty Conference on Obesity (Bray, 1975). Indeed, since that time, numerous reports have appeared in the literature on outcomes of behavior modification therapies and group methods of treatment conducted by non-profit groups such as foundations, out-patient nutrition clinics, and so forth. But with the exception of a few reports, the literature is nearly devoid of studies involving outcome data from dieting companies. Therefore, why is it that the advisors and owners of such companies have not risen to the challenge? Difficulties may be attributed to the companies, the customers, and researchers.

Difficulties related to the dieting companies

1. *There is ignorance about, or lack of motivation to obtain, the data needed to resolve questions on the short or long-term effectiveness of weight loss.* Surely the medical advisors and nutritionists employed by these companies are well aware of the importance of such data since, for the most part, they are competent professionals. In contrast to these health professional advisors, it may be that company management is not aware of these requirements.

2. *Extra expense is involved in such studies.* While such studies do cost money, at least some companies finance obesity research through foundations, and it would seem that this question would deserve high priority. Also, enlightened management may see the additional utility of such data in streamlining and improving programs.

Behavior modification protocols have been incorporated into most dieting company programs over the past few years and have involved great development costs, for example the hiring of consultants. Yet it would seem that the companies have no way of measuring whether these modifications have been beneficial by any measures other than marketing criteria. Similarly, dieting companies may be unable to develop targeted messages or programs for subgroups of the obese, because they lack information on the types of programs best suited to these various groups, not only for initial purchase of services but, more importantly, for repeat purchases of the program package. The vast majority of dieting company drop-outs are not people who have lost weight to their goals and therefore no longer need the program. Some are customers to whom the program has failed to deliver enough satisfaction to engender repeat purchase. Others are people who believe it to be their own fault that they have not lost weight in spite of satisfactory service. Better programs need to be developed for both groups. One way to do this is through better record-keeping.

3. *Record-keeping systems are poor.* Record-keeping is done in such a manner as to make it extremely difficult to conduct long-term follow-up studies in an appropriate manner. For example, one company studied by the investigator does not record the year of the record on weight record cards, so there is no way to ascertain the total population of registrants during a given time period. Instructors in the groups keep the weight loss cards and distribute them

to other instructors if the customer changes groups. Record cards are discarded if the registrant drops out or fails to return to the group after a period of time. Only names and addresses of registrants are kept permanently on file by regional officials. That particular company is now initiating steps to improve this system.

These types of record-keeping systems are of course unacceptable for any programs whose purpose is positively to benefit health. They are also useless for program management purposes. The problem in hospitals and health centers is that data on nutrition encounters exist and are well documented, but are buried in a mass of other data, making it difficult and costly to obtain non-duplicating records of a patient's encounters, and longitudinal records of a person's experience rather than visits. Such records either do not exist or are not available for objective scrutiny within dieting companies. Obviously such records make audits impossible and would seemingly preclude the possibility of third party reimbursement from federal or other sources, which require documentation of services rendered and their appropriateness.

4. *There may be concealment for business reasons.* Both short and long-term effectiveness in weight loss may be seen as actually being harmful, rather than simply non-beneficial, to the company's program. Indeed, the existence of such data might inhibit claims which could be made in advertising.

5. *Data on outcome may be seen as irrelevant to profitability.* After all, profitability is the major objective of such concerns. Profits depend primarily on volume, but relatively low operating costs, and customer satisfaction, are also factors which are considered. Customer satisfaction is engendered primarily by low price, success in weight loss over the short run, and other program-related benefits obtained (such as feelings that the company cares about them as human beings, group support and friendships resulting from meetings). Long-term success in weight loss may be somewhat useful in recruiting new members, and thus related to profitability, since a formerly overweight person who is now slim is the best possible walking advertisment for the program, but this is a more remote consideration. Thus financial pressures may lead to an overemphasis on volume, new gimmicks, short-term satisfaction in program planning, marketing, and market research. Long-term outcomes are thus of greatest interest to investigators interested in preventive medicine and cost-effectiveness, but of less direct relevance to those more concerned with the companies from the business standpoint.

6. *There may be insufficient social, physical and demographic data on the populations served by the dieting companies to ascertain if they are similar or different from overweight persons seen in other settings.* Because we lack data on these characteristics, particularly on degree of overweight and related health of customers problems, it is unclear if populations are similar to patient populations seen in out-pateint clinics and other health care settings. The companies market their services; the latter group do not. This as well as differences in price and health focus suggest that characteristics might well be different.

Insofar as such characteristics impact upon the likelihood of successful outcomes, it is difficult to make comparisons between programs without them. Since the health related characteristics are extremely important in the associated benefits or risks accruing to weight loss, it complicates further the problem of assessing health effects of such programs.

7. *Intra-company pressures may be involved.* Owners have a responsibility to their franchisees not to do anything to harm their business. Therefore, if owners or franchisees believe that such data might be detrimental to business, such data might not be produced.

8. *At present, government regulations do not insist that such statistics be kept.* Therefore, there is little reason for diet companies to feel that they must do so.

9. *Standard of success are different from those recommended for research purposes.* The major dieting companies suggest weight goals higher than desirable weights usually used in the scientific literature which are based on actuarial data. They may object to comparisons with these latter standards, as persons classified as 'successful' by their criteria might not be so if more stringent criteria were used. Indeed, for some persons, 'graduation' and goal weights

are not meaningful either, since these persons have in fact lost considerable amounts of weight in any event. Moreover, other factors, such as greater social acceptability, positive body image, new friends, thought to result from the program may be regarded as equally or more important than weight reduction to both company management and customers alike. Thus, there is a justifiable objection to the exclusive use of weight criteria. Clearly these programs deserve careful evaluation on all of these criteria.

10. Companies and researchers may disagree about issues of identifying the company upon which the research was based.

11. Diet companies may be threatened with law suits by irate researchers.

Customer related difficulties

1. Customers are more likely to enroll in these programs for social, emotional and cosmetic rather than for health reasons and are thus not enthused about participation in follow-up studies concentrating on weight loss. Older persons are more likely to be concerned about health, younger persons for cosmetic reasons (Berman, 1975).

2. Weight is a sensitive and embarrassing topic to most customers.

3. Response to follow-up surveys is almost always incomplete because of the high mobility of the population, the extreme reticence of failures to report, and no doubt a variety of other factors.

4. Customers may not agree to actually being weighed at follow-up.

5. The 'repeater' and yo-yo phenomena make it difficult to assign positive effects to a given treatment period. Many dieting company customers join, drop out, and rejoin the company or other similar companies, as well as using a variety of additional helps to supplement these services. Weight outcomes at follow-up therefore represent not only the services period which is documented, but additional services or efforts which may subsequently be obtained, and other, concomitant treatments which may or may not be documented.

6. Dieting companies cater to mass markets, group norms and values, and employ standardized procedures. Group norms with respect to weight may not be synonymous with health related norms. Standardized 1200 kcal (5000 kJ) diets are bound to generate fastest weight losses in persons who were eating the most to begin with if all other factors are held constant. Approaches which are successful and helpful to persons who are 20-30 lb (9.5 - 13.75 kg) overweight may not be so for the very obese. Thus some customers must conform to standardized prodecures which are unsuitable to their special needs. In some instances, these may militate against short or long-term success.

Researcher related problems

1. Researchers may not be aware of the effects of negative findings on the image or market for the company's programs.

2. Researchers may require procedures or client interviews which are thought to increase business costs or bother members.

3. Researchers publish their findings in journals which are available to the competitors.

4. Health professionals, particularly those specializing in weight control, may be regarded as competitors.

5. Health professionals often refuse to lend their names to marketing efforts or endorsements of the programs although they are willing to receive fees as consultants.

6. Health professionals may be interested in research topics which are of little importance and/or direct interest to the proprietors of the dieting companies. One such example is outcomes of pregnancy among persons who enrolled in dieting companies during pregnancy.

7. Researchers are constantly changing their minds as to the most effective types of programs for the treatment of obesity. For example, the previous furor about behavior modification has now lessened, and is being replaced by an interest in modified fasts.

8. Health professionals look primarily at objective benefits of groups. Positive subjective outcomes, other than weight-related, such as supportive milieu for economically disadvantaged persons with emotional problems, the group meeting as a 'night out', etc., also deserve study.

9. The researchers sometimes distort facts to support a theoretical position or magnify facts to fit hypothesis. This is regarded as a special problem of social scientists with respect to the social dimensions of the programs, and of nutritionists and physicians with respect to the diet and health-related aspects of the programs.

10. Researchers may be threatened by law suits by irate dieting company officials.

11. Researchers are loath to use data supplied. It may not be complete. Unless there are ways to check on its completeness (as is the case in prospective studies), they may not wish to become involved in retrospective studies.

Conclusion

Health professionals who refer obese patients to these companies might do well to query the owners as to outcome data, so as to place their patients in the most cost-effective programs.

In view of the enormous popularity of such self-help groups, and the substantial amounts of money consumers spent engaging in such programs, consumer organizations might do well to encourage the dieting companies to furnish fuller information on short and long-term outcomes of treatment. Dieting companies are not yet convinced that they are socially accountable for providing information and documenting outcomes with respect to weight or other possible benefits and detriments of the services they provide. Just as consumer pressure, and not the law, forced the automobile manufacturers to greater disclosure of information to consumers, so it may be that a coalition of health professionals and consumers may be able to stimulate these companies to more full and objective reporting of outcomes. Legislative efforts may be necessary if such voluntary efforts fail.*

But weight outcomes are only one of the many effects which need to be studied. The other possible effects of participation in the dieting company programs are also worthy of investigation.

Self-help groups and commercial dieting companies use voluntary participation in groups, group support and group pressure primarily to achieve their ends with respect to weight loss, but it is entirely possible that changes in customer attitudes or life style not related to weight may also result from participation. For example, the groups might supply social support with positive benefits such as friendship, increased self-esteem, feelings of solidarity with others with similar problems, more positive outlooks toward life. Participants may find that positive acceptance in such a group is reinforcing and helps them to become more outgoing, confident, organized, assertive, and goal-oriented in their approaches to other problems in life. On the other hand, it may be that group approaches reinforce feelings of dependency and inability to help oneself in some persons. Those who do not succeed in weight loss may feel more inadequate as a result of membership and failure to achieve expectations, their body images may be increasingly undesirable after group meetings extolling the values of leanness, and their life styles, especially with respect to eating, may seem to be increasingly unsatisfactory to them in spite of the fact that they fail to change. These alterations also deserve careful investigation.

Summary

The programs and methods employed by a large commerical dieting company utilizing group weight reduction methods were studied. Two follow-up surveys of all registrants during the calendar year 1975 were planned in conjunction with a company owner; one of the 'regular' weekly program in a city of the Middle Atlantic States, and one in a New England city of a more intensive and expensive 'seminar' series for persons with more severe obesity and/or serious emotional social problems were undertaken. The surveys were apparently

**From 'The research gap', on page 289, to this point this paper represents the personal position of the senior author only.*

perceived as threatening by other company officials. After a series of misadventures and persistent questioning on the part of the authors, it became evident that only the names of those who had been successful losers attaining the company's weight goals in the regular program had been furnished for follow-up, and that all objective data on heights and weights, either at admission to the program or at completion were unavailable. All objective data on seminar participants were unretrievable while the study was in progress.

Response rates from the successful short-term losers in the regular program were low, 28 per cent. No checks were possible on the representativeness of the respondent population of the total population of 'graduates' who had lost weight in the program. Among the group of persons who did respond, approximately one-third of the population reported weights at or below those at the company's goal. However, for most of these persons, their weights had fluctuated in the two year interim, and the majority of 'successes' who were at or below dieting company goals at follow-up reported that they had gained weight back. Only after additional weight control efforts, either by rejoining the group or by adoption of other regimes, had the successes been able to keep weight in line. Failures at follow-up had also gained weight, but apparently failed to lose as much in the interim, and hence were now above previous weight levels. It is highly likely that reported weights at follow-up were grossly underestimated. The dieting company's goals are at least ten pounds above mean desirable weights for height. But if these limitations are accepted, it is likely that some proportion of these persons actually did find that an ongoing or episodic membership in the dieting company was helpful in controlling their weight. Indeed, mean reported weights at present were still lower than the highest weights these respondents has achieved in the majority of cases. Therefore, at least for this undefined group of respondents, such companies may provide help in long-term maintenance of lower weights, furnish social support these persons need for other reasons, and have other positive effects. But long-term outcomes, for either those whose short-term weight loss was successful, or, more important, for all of those who entered such programs in a given year, could not be ascertained.

Some of the reasons why studies of commercial dieting groups are so difficult to mount are discussed, and the weaknesses of the present study are enumerated. Health professionals, consumers, social scientists and government regulatory officials all have a role to play in encouraging more adequate studies of this type in the future.

Acknowledgement – Dr Dwyer is grateful for the support furnished by Research Career Development Award, K 04 A M 0027201, National Institutes of Health which permitted her to carry out this research. The Research and Development Section of the Diet Workshop, Inc. is thanked for funds it made available for the design, execution and computer data analysis of this survey. Ms Sonja Strong and Ms Ellen Ruppert designed the computer programs for data analysis. Dr Dwyer is not nor has she ever been a paid consultant to the company.

References

Alton, N. (1971): Group dieting interaction. Unpublished dissertation. Brandeis University.
Ashwell, M. (1974): In *Obesity: medical and social aspects,* ed W.L. Burland, P.D. Samuel & J. Yudkin, p. 239. Edinburgh: Churchill Livingstone.
Ashwell, M. & Garrow, J.S. (1975): *Nutrition* 29, 347.
Berman, E.M. (1975): *J. Nutr. Educ.* 7, 155.
Bray, G.A. ed (1975): *Obesity in perspective,* Pt 1, p.7. Washington DC: US Govt. Ptg. Office.
Dwyer, J.T., Feldman, J. & Mayer, J. (1970): *J. Hlth Soc. Behav.* 11, 269.
Garrow, J.S. (1974): In *Energy balance and obesity in man.* Amsterdam: North Holland.
Jeffrey, D.B. (1976): Treatment outcome issues in obesity research. In *Obesity: behavioral approaches to dietary management,* ed B.J. Williams, M. Sander & J.P. Forey. New York : Brunner Mazel.
Seltzer, C.C. (1967): *J. Am. Med. Ass.* 201, 221.
Stunkard, A.J. (1975): Studies in Tops: a self-help group for obesity. In *Obesity in perspective,* Pt 2. p. 3 & 7. Washington DC: US Govt. Ptg. Office.

Stunkard, A.J. (1977): In *Diet related to killer diseases,* II, p. 81. Obesity hearings before the Select Committee on Nutrition and Human Needs of the US Senate, Feb. 1,2, 1977. Washington DC: US Govt. Ptg. Office.
Stunkard, A.J., Levine, H. & Fox, S. (1970): *Archs Intern. Med.* 125, 1067.
Stunkard, A.J. & McLaren-Hume, M. (1959): *Archs Intern. Med.* 103, 79.
Wagonfeld, S. & Wolowitz, H. (1960): *Am. J. Psychiat.* 125, 249.

29
Behavioral treatment of obesity: the first ten years

A. J. STUNKARD
Department of Psychiatry, University of Pennsylvania, 205 Piersol Building, Philadelphia, Pennsylvania 19104, USA.

Ten years ago the appearance of a small article in a little-known journal devoted to behavior therapy (Stuart, 1967) sparked unprecedented activity in the psychological treatment of obesity and led to major advances in the scientific study of psychotherapy. Within 5 years of the publication of 'Behavioral control of overeating' (Stuart, 1967), this topic had achieved a popularity bordering on faddism and the next 5 years saw the appearance of 50 more or less well-controlled clinical trials and five review articles (Abramson, 1973; Jordan & Levitz, 1975; Stuart, 1975; Stunkard, 1975; Stunkard & Mahoney, 1976).

It is now possible to look back upon these 10 years of activity and to begin to sort out what has, and has not, been accomplished. From this perspective it seems clear that behavior therapy represents a significant improvement over traditional methods of treatment of mild and moderate obesity; a number of controlled clinical trials have established this as a fact. The weight losses, however, although consistent, have been only modest and of limited clinical significance. Furthermore, 10 years after its introduction, there has been no improvement upon the results of the first report of behavioral control of overeating.

It now appears that the major advances of the past 10 years in the behavioral treatment of obesity have been methodological rather than substantive. These advances have been important. A field which, despite its aspirations towards rigor, had had little experience with problems of research design and has faced and solved problems of considerable complexity, as we shall see. In the process, psychotherapy research has benefitted far beyond the treatment of obesity. It may be fair to say that research on the behavioral treatment of obesity has had as much impact upon psychotherapy research as has any other field of contemporary psychotherapeutic endeavor. The time is ripe for further improvement in the effectiveness of therapy. Three recent studies reviewed below suggest that this time may be at hand.

Methodological developments

The reasons for the current intense interest of behavior therapists in the treatment of obesity are not hard to find. Obesity offers a superb proving ground for measuring the effects of behavioral treatments and behavior therapists have a long-standing concern with measurement of treatment effects. But first, what is behavior therapy?

The distinguishing characteristic of the various methods called behavior therapy, or behavior modification, is the belief that behavior disorders of the most divergent type are learned responses and that modern theories of learning have much to teach us regarding both the acquisition and the extinction of these responses. Behavior therapy, thus, is distinguished more by its character as a *method* of solving problems than by the myriad of therapeutic techniques that are called 'behavioral'. Furthermore, behavior therapists have been distinguished by their explicit statements of methods and goals, and by their willingness to put their results on the line for comparison with different methods of treatment. They were thus quick to recognize the power, as a dependent variable in psychotherapy research, of weight change, and they have turned to the treatment of obesity in increasing numbers in order to utilize this measure. No other dependent variable in psychotherapy research approaches the sensitivity, reliability and validity of weight change.

One of the reasons for the strong impact of behavior therapy was the relative ease of assessing the effectiveness of outpatient treatment for obesity. The results of traditional treatment have been uniformly poor and the treatments obviously inadequate. (Inpatient treatment, with its potential for greater control over the patient has, of course, achieved greater weight losses. Its usefulness has been limited, however, by the almost invariable regaining of weight after discharge.) Some years ago a review of the medical literature revealed that only 25 per cent of persons entering conventional outpatient treatment for obesity lost as much as 20 lb (9.2 kg) and 5 per cent as much as 40 lb (18.4 kg) (Stunkard & McLaren-Hume, 1959). A more recent report suggests somewhat better results: 38 per cent lost 20 lb (9.2 kg) and 10 per cent lost 40 lb (18.4 kg) (Asher & Dietz, 1972).

Against this background, Stuart's report on 'Behavioral control of overeating' (1967) stands out. It describes the best results obtained up to that time in the outpatient treatment of obesity. Even the absence of a control group does not vitiate the significance of its findings. Figures 1 and 2 show that the eight patients who remained in treatment out of an original ten lost large amounts of weight: three more than 40 lb (18.4 kg) and six more than 30 lb (13.8 kg).

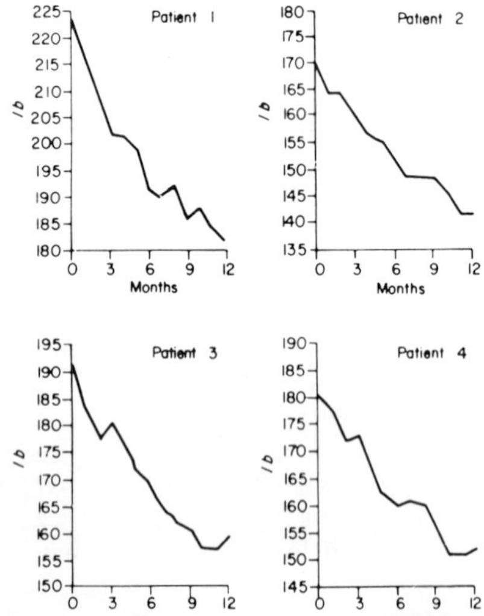

Fig.1. Weight profiles of four patients undergoing behavior therapy for obesity (Stuart, 1967)

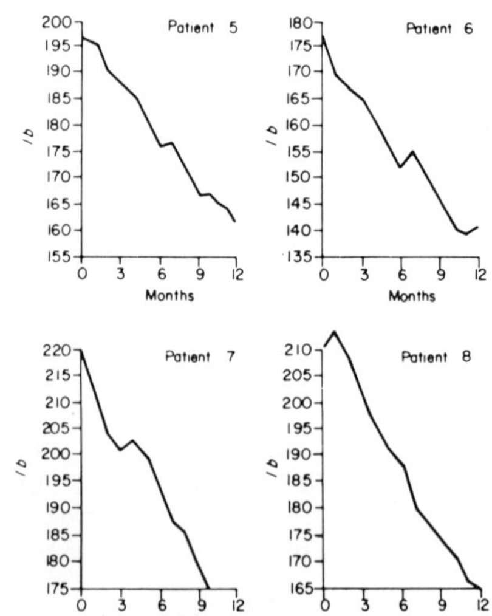

Fig.2. Weight profiles of four patients undergoing behavior therapy for obesity (Stuart, 1967)

Certain features of this report highlight its significance. First, the expenditure of time was not exorbitant. In fact, time spent in treatment was no greater than that of a number of other studies which achieved far poorer results. At the beginning of the treatment period, patients were seen in 20 minute sessions held three times a week for a total of 12 to 15 sessions. Thereafter, treatment sessions were scheduled as needed, usually at 2-week intervals for the next 3 months. Subsequently there were monthly sessions and finally 'maintenance' sessions as needed. Total number of visits during the year varied from 16 to 41.

There was no evidence of untoward responses to the program or of 'symptom substitution'. Seven of the eight patients reported that they had developed an increased range of social activities, and three of the six married patients reported more satisfying relationships with their husbands. Furthermore, three of the eight who were also smokers applied the principles they had learned to smoking and either substantially reduced or eliminated it.

A description of the essential elements of behavioral treatments for obesity is beyond the scope of this report and the interested reader is referred to the extended descriptions of Stuart & Davis (1972), Mahoney & Mahoney (1976*b*) and Stunkard & Mahoney (1976) and to the detailed manual of Ferguson (1975).

The behavioral approach, with its stress on rigid specification of each step in treatment and its strong experimental tradition, resulted in a large amount of research on the behavioral control of obesity. Soon after Stuart's report the first controlled outcome study of behavior modification of obesity was carried out. Mildly overweight women college students lost an average weight loss of 10.5 lb (4.8 kg) (Harris, 1969). Subjects in a no-treatment control group gained 3.6 lb (1.7 kg), yielding a difference significant at the 1 per cent level. Furthermore, patients continued to lose weight during a 16-week follow-up period, an unusual occurrence in the treatment of obesity at that time.

A no-treatment control group, such as that used by Harris, was quite acceptable in the psychotherapy research of 1969. Yet it has serious disadvantages. Postponing treatment for someone who has come seeking it is far from a neutral event. Deterioration in the condition of members of a control group, which has been disappointed in its expectation of treatment, could give the false impression that a treatment was effective. The problem calls for the use of a placebo control group to match the attention and interest received by patients in the active treatment program. An elaborate study by Wollersheim (1970) provided precisely such controls and opened up new vistas of research on psychological treatment.

Wollersheim's design contained four experimental conditions: (1) 'Focal' (behavioral) treatment; (2) 'Non-specific therapy', which explored psychological issues related to the patient's obesity but avoided specific behavioral considerations; (3) 'Social pressure', patterned after that of the self-help group TOPS (Take Off Pounds Sensibly) (Stunkard, Levine & Fox, 1970), and (4) A no-treatment weight control condition of persons promised treatment but receiving it later.

The study thus contained three treatment conditions (1, 2 and 3) and three control conditions (2, 3 and 4) for behavior modification. The 80 subjects were mildly (29 per cent) overweight female college students. Four therapists each treated one group of five subjects in each of the three treatment conditions for ten sessions over a 3-month period.

Figure 3 shows that at the end of treatment, and at 8-week follow-up, subjects in the behavioral treatment condition had lost more weight than those in the no-treatment condition. In addition, they had lost significantly more weight than those in the two placebo control conditions who had themselves both achieved significant weight losses. Clearly, the behavioral program had contributed something to the outcome which was over and above the usual effects of psychological treatment.

This contribution seems to have resulted from the specific effects of the behavioral intervention. A detailed eating patterns questionnaire revealed that subjects in the 'behavior' therapy condition showed major changes in their reports of their eating behavior. Statistically significant differences between the behavior therapy and the other three conditions were found in four of the six factors: 'emotional and uncontrolled eating', 'eating in isolation', 'eating as a reward', and 'between-meals eating'. Weight loss in the two placebo control conditions apparently occurred without affecting these behaviors; weight loss in the behavioral condition, on the other hand, apparently was a result of changes in these behaviors.

Wollersheim's study solved the problem of placebo controls, but, in the process, brought psychotherapy research face-to-face with a new problem: experimenter bias. Although the

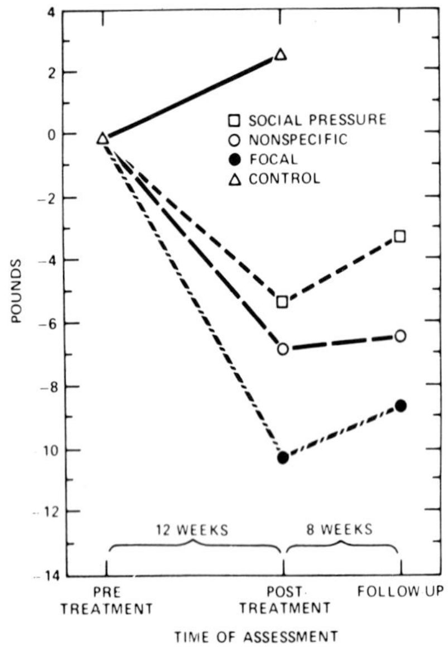

Fig.3. Mean weight loss of the focal (behavioral) treatment group, the two alternative treatment groups and the no-treatment control group (Wollersheim, 1970)

placebo therapy controlled for the patient's expectations of treatment, it did not control for the therapist's, and this is not a trivial matter. The double-blind experiment in psychopharmacology has shown how powerful this influence can be in dealing with drugs. It is surely more powerful in the more emotional case of the psychotherapies.

The problem of experimenter bias was approached in an ingenious manner in the study by Penick & co-workers (1971) which was also one of the very few to deal with severely (78 per cent) overweight persons. Penick biased the study against the behavioral approach by selecting as therapists for the control group himself, an internist with 10 years experience in the treatment of obesity, and by using the entire conventional therapeutic armamentarium including medication, diet, nutritional counselling and his prestige as an authority in the field. Behavior modification, on the other hand, was carried out by persons with no previous experience in treatment. Fifteen patients were treated with behavior modification and 17 by conventional therapy, both on a once-a-week basis for 2 hours over a period of 3 months.

The results of treatment favored the behavioral approach. Thus, weight losses of the control group were comparable to those in the medical literature: none lost 40 lb (18.4 kg) and only 24 per cent lost more than 20 lb (9.2 kg). By contrast, 13 per cent of the behavior modification group lost more than 40 lb (18.4 kg) and 53 per cent lost more than 20 lb (9.2 kg).

Variability in the weight losses of the behavior modification subjects was greater than that of the patients treated by traditional methods ($P < 0.05$). The five best performers were behavior modification patients, as was the single least effective one. Such greater variability has in other circumstances been explained by a greater specificity of treatment, and this explanation of the findings seems reasonable. For half of the patients it appears that behavior modification offered something specific that resulted in greater than usual weight loss. For another half, it was of considerably less value.

The most important implication of the Penick study lies in its promise of greater applicability of the behavioral therapies. For it showed that behavior modification, devised by a team with little experience in the modality, was more effective in the treatment of obesity than was the best alternative program that could be devised by a research team with long experience in treatment of this disorder. The inexperienced therapists achieved about a two-fold increase in the effectiveness of treatment over conventional measures. Lesser increases in effectiveness have brought about major changes in the management of other disorders.

Clearly, the period of methodological development has borne rich fruit. It has left us, however, with areas of ignorance and it has been dominated by one methodology – analysis of variance designs. This ignorance is in part attributable to the exclusive use of these designs and the time has come for new experimental approaches. The analysis of variance designs have tended to use standardized treatments administered to groups of patients. Data have been collected on only a few variables (and on few behavioral ones), typically only at the onset and end of treatment, and the results have been reported in terms of mean values. The sources of the great variance in outcome have thus been obscured and we have not learned vital information about how individual patients learn, and fail to learn, to change individual behaviors.

A methodology which has gained increasing acceptance in recent years seems made to order for these problems. The intensive single-case design focusses upon precisely these areas, attempting to isolate the influence of specific measures for changing behavior (Hersen & Barlow, 1976). It is possible that such efforts may prove more useful in advancing our knowledge at this particular time than a large number of additional parametric studies. A very recent report by Coates (Coates, 1977; Coates & Thoresen, in press) illustrates the potential of the method.

Coates carried out an intensive study of the effects of a variety of behavioral change measures upon two obese 16-year-old girls over a period of 3 months, while keeping a third girl as a placebo control. The study was characterized by the collection of large amounts of data, both by daily self-report (n=60) and by non-participant observers in the home (n=30), on such items as the quality and quantity of food in the home and consumed by the patients, exercise behavior and the places, times and activities associated with eating.

A key finding was that different patients were benefitted by different treatment techniques. The study documented for the first time, and in a convincing manner, a point that has been made by clinicians in the field: effective treatment requires matching of technique to specific behavioral deficits or excesses. In this study behavior changes occurred in those areas where the subjects were the most deviant. Thus, for one patient the primary behavioral problems fell into the category of stimulus control. Large amounts of food were available for frequent eating in her home, food at meals was plentiful and portions, served by the patient's mother, were large. Treatment directed at limiting the number, times and places of eating and increasing the availability of lower calorie foods was effective in helping this 286 lb (131.6 kg) girl to lose 21 lb (9.7 kg) in 10 weeks. By contrast, she ate at a moderate rate prior to treatment and made no change in rate.

The second patient, on the other hand, ate quite rapidly and in a number of different places. Treatment was focussed upon these behaviors with moderate success – 11.5 lb (5.3 kg) weight loss in a 194 lb (89 kg) girl. High calorie foods and large portions at meals were not characteristic of her family patterns and few changes were made in the category of stimulus control.

Substantive developments

The demonstration that behavior therapy is more effective than traditional methods, however well established, tells us little about its effectiveness as a practical measure for the control of obesity. How effective is it?

Several factors make it difficult to get a clear picture of the clinical impact of behavioral treatments for obesity. Sample sizes have been small, treatment restricted to short time periods and follow-up data negligible. All-too-often the constraints of a doctoral dissertation have taken precedence over the need for clinically meaningful results. Far too many of the subjects of studies have been mildly overweight college women and far too many of the studies have been content with ascertaining the relative effectiveness of small differences in techniques. The emphasis has been on analogue studies rather than on clinical efficacy. But some definitive findings have emerged from all of this effort. A review of 21 of the better reports and of the results of the more-or-less routine clinical treatment of the first 125 patients in a well-established clinical service gives a basis for some generalizations about the overall efficacy of behavioral treatments for obesity (Jeffery, Wing & Stunkard, in press).

(1) The first important finding is that great progress has been made in decreasing drop-outs from treatment. Whereas drop-outs from traditional outpatient treatment were as high as 25 to 75 per cent (Stunkard & McLaren-Hume, 1959), most behavioral programs report rates of 10 per cent or less, and these results have been obtained in both research and clinical programs. The use of contingency contracting, or the earning back of deposits made by the patients at the beginning of treatment, has played a major part in coping with the problem of drop-outs, but it appears that other aspects of the behavioral programs also play a part.

(2) The second major advance has been in reducing the untoward side effects of weight reduction regimens, a problem which has plagued routine medical office treatment of obesity. It appears that as many as half of all obese patients undergoing this treatment may suffer from such symptoms as anxiety, irritability and depression (Stunkard & Rush, 1974). By contrast, untoward reactions to behavioral programs are uncommon.

(3) The single most important measure of treatment efficacy is weight loss. Table 1 reviews 21 recent reports which provided sufficient detail to permit assessment of weight loss results. This assessment included assurance that the studies met basic criteria such as that the results were based upon all patients starting treatment and drop-outs were included. Table 1 shows that the weight losses of no more than half the programs exceeded 10 lb (4.6 kg) and those of only 20 per cent exceeded 15 lb (7 kg). There are many reasons for

Table 1. Results of behavioral treatments for obesity

Study	*n*	Initial weight (lb)	Mean weight loss* (lb)	Treatment length (weeks)
Abrams & Allen (1974)	23	182.5	11.9	9
Hagen (1974)	18	153.0	15.0	10
Hall (1972)	10	173.0	3.2	4
Hall *et al.* (1974)	40	–	11.1	10
Hall *et al.* (1975)	25	197.6	15.0**	12
Hanson (1976)	32	212.0	13.0**	10
Harris (1969)	7	171.1	6.9	10
Harris & Bruner (1971)	11	164.7	7.4	12
Harris & Bruner (1971)	6	143.7	1.8	16
Harris & Hallbauer (1973)	27	165.4	8.0	12
Jeffrey (1974)	34	183.8	6.0	7
Levitz & Stunkard (1974)	73	180.8	4.2	12
Mahoney (1974)	9	–	7.4	8
McReynolds (1976)	41	178.4	17.4	15
Penick *et al.* (1971)	15	251.0	22.3	12
Romanczyk (1974)	17	175.7	10.6	6
Romanczyk *et al.* (1973)	18	178.8	7.0	4
Romanczyk *et al.* (1973)	18	173.0	8.0	4
Stuart (1967)	8	183.6	37.8	52
Stuart (1971)	6	–	14.0	15
Wollersheim (1970)	18	154.1	10.4	12

* Data describe the most effective treatment combination only. Results from control groups and partial treatments are not included

** Extrapolated from weight reduction indices

these limitations - most of the programs were short-term, many involved patients who were only mildly overweight and a large number were carried out by inexperienced therapists. But the fact remains: the results are modest and, from the perspective of clinical utility, disappointing.

These results from the research literature are not dissimilar to those which have been reported recently from a program with a primarily clinical focus. Jeffery, Wing & Stunkard (in press) found a weight loss of no more than 11.0 lb (5 kg) for the first 125 patients in a behaviorally oriented obesity treatment program.

(4) There is great variability in weight changes during treatment, as first noted by Penick *et al.* (1971) and even greater variability following treatment. Very little is know about factors underlying this variability.

(5) Prediction of outcome of treatment has generally been unsuccessful whether the variables were demographic (Harris, 1969; Mahoney, 1974; Wollersheim, 1970), personality (Abrams & Allen, 1974; Balch & Ross, 1975; Mahoney, 1974; Penick *et al.,* 1971; Stuart, 1971; Wollersheim, 1970), behavioral.(Hagen, 1974; Mahoney, 1974; Wollersheim, 1970). Three predictors have, however, emerged. The first is the extent of weight loss early in treatment. Jeffery & co-workers (in press) report a correlation of 0.40 ($P<0.01$) between weight loss during the first week of treatment and that during the next 20 weeks, a finding that is particularly instructive since the patients' only assignment during the first week had been to record their eating behavior.

The second factor predicting outcome is percentage overweight (Murray, 1975), a robust finding which has also been found in non-behavioral treatments - intestinal by-pass surgery (Mills & Stunkard, 1976) and patient self-help groups (Garb & Stunkard, 1974). Percentage overweight is closely linked to what may be an even more powerful predictor of weight loss recently noted by Björntorp & colleagues (Sullivan *et al.,* 1977). An equation incorporating measurements of fat cell number, basal metabolic rate and cephalic insulin secretion has been able to predict 80 per cent of the variance in weight loss in a group of patients treated in Gothenburg, Sweden.

(6) Patients with onset of obesity early in life lose as much weight as those with onset in adult life (Jeffery *et al.,* in press). This finding appears somewhat at variance with predictions based upon expected fat cell size and number. There is no information on possible differences in the ability to maintain weight loss by juvenile- and adult-onset obese persons.

(7) Despite the fact that behavioral techniques can be adapted for use by less skilled therapists, skill of the therapist does have a positive effect upon the outcome of therapy. Two studies have shown that therapist experience was positively related to weight loss (Levitz & Stunkard, 1974; Jeffery *et al.,* in press).

(8) Patterns of weight loss do not accord with the theoretical basis for behavioral treatments. Such treatments are presumed to achieve their results through changes in behavior brought about by learning and such learning is presumed to be incremental. If this were the case, one would expect that initially, when few changes in behavior had been made, the rate of weight loss should be slow. Later, with the learning of additional skills, the rate of weight loss should increase. In fact, patterns of weight loss in behavioral therapy, as in other forms of treatment, tend to show a slowing over time.

(9) The question of maintenance of weight losses achieved during behavioral treatments has recently been reopened. It had been an article of faith that weight losses achieved by behavioral measures were more stable than those achieved by other means. A recent analysis has called this point into question and it now appears that maintenance of weight loss following behavioral treatment is no better than that following other treatments (Stunkard, in press).

The future: combined treatments

The challenge for the future of behavioral treatments is how to continue the development that has made them superior to many traditional therapies and to realize the promise that has remained latent during the past 10 years of methodological refinements. The limits to the effectiveness of current behavioral methodologies may well have been reached. To go beyond these limits will probably require new technologies or new combinations of technologies. A combination of behavioral technology with other measures would seem to offer great promise. Three recent studies support this view; each has for the first time achieved results which equal those of Stuart's. For the first time in 10 years substantive results match methodological ones.

Protein-sparing modified fast

The first study to match Stuart's results combined a behavioral therapy with the use of a protein-sparing modified fast (Lindner & Blackburn, 1976). The protein-sparing modified fast is a relatively recent development, designed to take advantage of some of the more impressive benefits of fasting, including rapid weight loss, relative freedom from hunger and simplicity while avoiding some of its disadvantages, notably loss of body protein. Bolinger & co-workers (1966) showed that an egg albumen supplement approached a restoration of nitrogen balance in the fasting state and Apfelbaum & colleagues (1970) later showed that this effect could be approached by as little as 55 g of casein daily. Blackburn and his associates (Blackburn, Bistrian & Flatt, 1975; Bistrian *et al.,* 1976) have subsequently developed protocols for rapid weight reduction based upon the ingestion of 1.4 g of protein per kg of ideal body weight per day which maintained 'true' nitrogen balance in outpatients engaging in a wide variety of occupations and life-styles.

The protein-sparing modified fast was integrated into a weight reduction program which relied heavily upon behavioral principles. Treatment took place according to very similar protocols at two sites: 67 patients were treated in a private weight reduction clinic, another 100 were treated in a university medical center. Composition of the patient samples in the two clinics were quite similar. Twenty-one were men, 146 were women, average age was 43 years and percentage overweight ranged between 50 and 80.

The first phase of the program consisted of a period of evaluation during which patients ate their usual foods, recorded them on a food diary, measured physical activity with a pedometer, and were introduced to behavioral techniques in a classroom setting. The protein-sparing modified fast was introduced after patients had demonstrated satisfactory progress in the first phase. It consisted of three meals a day containing from 270 to 700 kcal, either in the form of protein hydrolysate or protein - lean meat, fish or fowl. Intake was calculated from estimated lean body mass to yield 1.4 g of protein per kg of lean body mass. Vitamin and mineral supplements were used.

Patients were seen as often as five times a week for the first 2 weeks of the program and then with a frequency which decreased to once a week for the remainder of the treatment. An effort was made to reduce patients to their desirable weight and treatment averaged 48 weeks in duration. Patients were encouraged to continue their normal physical activities and to increase them with the aid of feed-back from the pedometer. When they reached desirable weight, or if they were unable to continue weight loss, they began to eat first vegetables, then fruit and then returned to a balanced diet which restricted only refined carbohydrates. During this termination phase, group sessions emphasized more detailed behavioral techniques and an effort was made to shift responsibility from staff management to self-management.

Figure 4 shows the results of treatment as compared with those reported for two series from the medical literature. About half of the patients lost 40 lb (18.4 kg) and over 80 per cent lost 20 lb (9.2 kg). The mean pretreatment weight of patients at one of the clinics was 206 lb (94.8 kg), falling to 161 lb (74 kg) at the end of treatment. The majority of patients in this clinic maintained their weight loss. The results in the other clinic, although not presented in the same detail seemed similar, as measured by one criterion of success in weight reduction - that of Trulson, Walsh & Caso (1947).

Use of couples training program

A second method of increasing the effectiveness of the usual behavioral measures has been

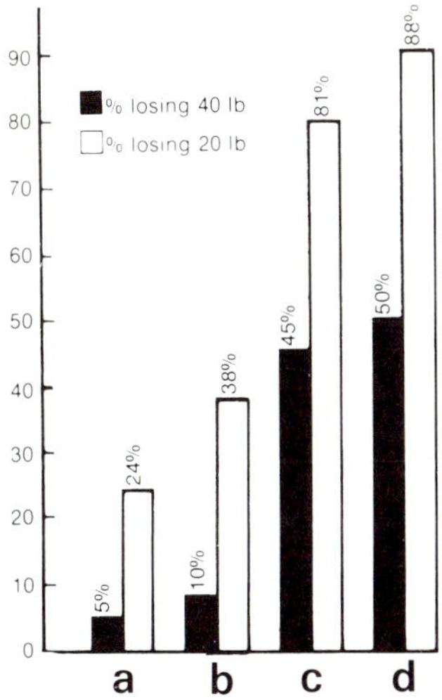

Fig.4. Percentages of patients losing 20 lb (9.2 kg) and 40 lb (18.4 kg). The first bar graphs represent the results of a literature review, the second those of a group of practising physicians and the latter two sets of bar graphs those of the patients undergoing the protein-sparing modified fast (Lindner & Blackburn, 1976) a: Literature group n = 979, 40 lb (18.4 kg); n = 1269, 20 lb (9.2 kg). b: Bariatric group, n=1409. c: PSMF – group 1 n = 67. d: PSMF – group 2 n = 100

their incorporation into a couples training program. Here the emphasis was upon maintenance of weight loss rather than increasing the speed of initial weight loss, and again the results of the first efforts have been most promising. Earlier studies had suggested that such an approach might be fruitful. Stuart & Davis (1972) had reported that an analysis of mealtime interactions between spouses revealed that husbands may exert either a negative or a positive influence on their wives' effort to lose weight. And the Mahoneys (1976*b*) had reported a high correlation between indices of 'social support' within the family and weight loss during treatment.

Brownell (1977) compared the results of a standard behavioral program with those of a program to which was added a couples training program which included modelling, mutual monitoring techniques, cooperative efforts at stimulus control and reinforcement of the couple rather than the subject, for habit change. For each part of the patient's program there was a corresponding part for the spouse, and spouses attended each training session. Here they were instructed to model appropriate eating behaviors such as putting the fork down between bites to 'set a good example'. Similarly they learned specific ways of engaging the patient in activities incompatible with eating during times of temptation. Each member of the couples monitored the partner's behavior as well as his/her own. The program emphasized that mutual effort was critical to success.

Three treatments were assessed: (1) 'cooperative-spouse-couples training'; (2) 'cooperative-spouse-patient-alone training, using patients who attended meetings alone even though their spouse had agreed to enter treatment, and (3) 'non-cooperative-spouse-patient-alone training' of patients whose spouses had refused to enter treatment. Treatment occurred once weekly for 1.5 hr over a period of 10 weeks, with once monthly treatments for the next 6 months. A $50 deposit which was returned contingent upon attendance, not weight loss, helped to eliminate drop-outs. Patients consisted of ten men and 19 women who averaged 56 per cent overweight.

All groups lost weight. Figure 5 shows that at the end of the 10-week treatment program losses in the three groups were 19.5, 14.8 and 11.5 lb (9, 6.8 and 5.3 kg) for the couples training and the cooperative-spouse-patient-alone and uncooperative-spouse-patient-alone treatments, respectively. Those differences did not quite reach statistical significance, but 6 months later weight loss of the couples training group had reached 29.6 lb (13.6 kg), which was significantly greater than that of the two patient-alone groups which had lost 19.4 lb (9 kg) and 15.1 lb (6.9 kg) each. At the end of treatment 44 per cent of the couples treatment patients had lost over 20 lb (9.2 kg) and none had lost more than 40 lb (18.4 kg).

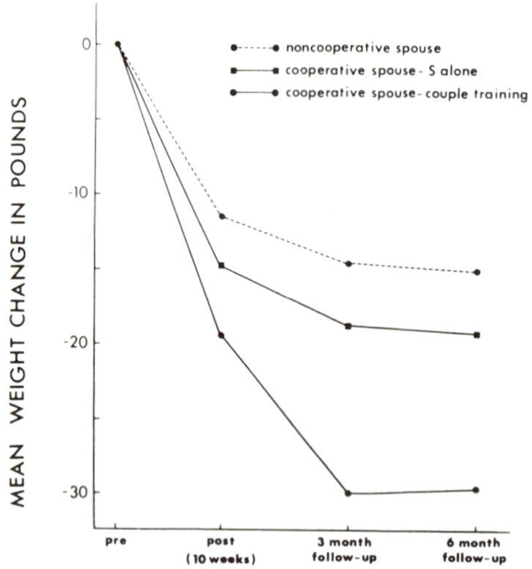

Fig. 5. Weight losses of patients receiving spouse training and of two groups receiving individual treatment, one consisting of 'cooperative' spouses and one 'uncooperative' spouses (Brownell, 1977)

These figures had risen to 67 per cent and 22 per cent 6 months after the end of active treatment, again considerably better performance than that of the patient-alone conditions.

Pharmacotherapy plus behavior therapy

The third method of increasing the effectiveness of behavioral measures has been through combining them with pharmacotherapy. It is a curious aspect of modern therapy that the behavioral and pharmacological therapies have developed in isolation from each other. With the exceptions of Marks' (1976) efforts, largely in the treatment of phobias, we are not aware of any behavioral treatment program which has involved the systematic use of pharmacological agents. And the development of the drug therapies, notably psychopharmaceuticals, has made little use of findings which are emerging from the rapidly developing fields of behavioral science. In particular, dosage schedules of medication have continued to be determined by reputed durations of action or, at best, by drug levels. The possibility of increasing the effectiveness of drug therapies by the contingent use of medication is unexplored territory.

The first attempt to combine behavioral and pharmacological measures in the treatment of obesity reaffirmed the promise of this approach. Craighead, O'Brien & Stunkard (in preparation) conducted a randomized clinical trial of four treatments with a sample of 140 moderately to severely obese (80 per cent overweight) men and women. The treatments consisted of: (1) routine individual medical treatment in the doctor's office using a common antiobesity medication - fenfluramine; (2) behavior modification carried out in groups of ten according to a standard protocol (Ferguson, 1975); (3) fenfluramine combined with Rogerian non-directive therapy in groups, and (4) fenfluramine combined with behavior modification in groups (Ferguson, 1975). Weight losses over a period of 6 months for the four treatments were 14, 24, 30 and 32 lb (6.4, 10.9, 13.6 and 14.5 kg) respectively. An unusually low drop-out rate (18 per cent) contributes to the assurance with which these figures can be regarded.

This study has significance far beyond the behavioral control of obesity. First, it is apparent that the effectiveness of medication can be greatly increased by the way in which it is delivered - from a mean weight loss of 15 lb (6.4 kg) in the doctor's office to 30 lb (13.6 kg) in the group format. This finding has been previously reported (London & Schreiber, 1965) but not to this degree. By itself it brings into question the conventional wisdom that medication is of only slight and transient benefit in the treatment of obesity. Second, the major effectiveness of the medication appears to be exerted in the first 2 months of treatment when the rates of weight loss of patients on medication greatly exceeded those of patients receiving behavior modification alone. The rate of weight loss of the subjects receiving medication and Rogerian therapy slowed later in treatment, at a time when patients receiving behavior modification (with and without medication) were continuing a steady weight loss.

Third, although this study has been concerned so far with increasing the rate of weight loss early in the program, it is also evaluating maintenance of weight loss by means of 'booster sessions' of decreasing frequency.

Acknowledgement – The work in this paper was supported in part by Grant MH28124 from the National Institue of Mental Health.

References

Abrahms, J.L. & Allen, G.J. (1974): *Behav. Ther.* **5**, 391.
Abramson, E.E. (1973): *Behav. Res. Ther.* **11**, 547.
Apfelbaum, M., Boudon, P., Lacatis, D. *et al.* (1970): *Presse. Med.* **78**, 1917.
Asher, W.L. & Dietz, R.E. (1972): *Curr. Ther. Res.* **15**, 510.
Balch, P. & Ross, A.W. (1975): *J. Consult. Clin. Psychol.* **43**, 119.
Bistrian, B.R., Blackburn, G.L., Flatt, J.P., Sizer, J., Scrimshaw, N.S. & Sherman, M. (1976): *Diabetes* **25**, 494.
Blackburn, G.L., Bistrian, B.R. & Flatt, J.P. (1975): Role of a protein sparing fast in a comprehensive weight reduction program. In *Recent advances in obesity research:* I, ed A. Howard, pp. 279-281. London: Newman.
Bolinger, R.E., Lukert, B.P. & Brown, R.W. *et al.* (1966): *Archs Int. Med.* **118**, 3.
Brownell, K. (1977): The effect of spouse training and partner cooperativeness in the behavioral treatment of obesity. Unpublished doctoral dissertation, Rutgers University.
Coates, T.J. (1977): The efficacy of a multicomponent self-control program in modifying the eating habits and weight of three obese adolescents. Unpublished doctoral dissertation, Stanford University.
Coates, T.J. & Thoresen, C.E. (in press): Treating obesity in adolescents: a behavioral approach. In *Advances in behavioral medicine,* ed J.M. Ferguson. New York: Academic Press.
Craighead, L., O'Brien, R. & Stunkard, A.J. (in preparation): New treatments for obesity. *Psychosom. Med.*
Ferguson, J.M. (1975): *Learning to eat. Behavior modification for weight control.* Palo Alto, CA: Bull Publishing Co.
Garb, J.R. & Stunkard, A.J. (1974): *Archs Int. Med.* **134**, 716.
Hagen, R.L. (1974): *Behav. Ther.* **5**, 224.
Hall, S.M. (1972): *Behav. Res. Ther.* **10**, 59.
Hall, S.M., Hall, R.G., Hanson, R.W. & Borden, B.L. (1974): *J. Consult. Clin. Psychol.* **42**, 781.
Hall, S.M., Hall, R.G., Borden, B.L. & Hanson, R.W. (1975): *Behav. Res. Ther.* **13**, 167.
Hanson, R.W., Borden, B.L., Hall, S.M. & Hall, R.G. (1976): *Behav. Ther.* **7**, 366.
Harris, M.B. (1969): *J. Abnorm. Psychol.* **74**, 263.
Harris, M.B. & Bruner, C.G. (1971): *Behav. Res. Ther.* **9**, 347.
Harris, M.B. & Hallbauer, E.S. (1973): *Behav. Res. Ther.* **11**, 523.
Hersen, M. & Barlow, D.H. (1976): *Single-case experimental designs: strategies for studying behavior change.* New York: Pergamon.
Jeffery, D.B. (1974): *J. Abnorm. Psychol.* **83**, 404.
Jeffery, R.W., Wing, R.R. & Stunkard, A.J. (in press): Behavioral treatment of obesity: the state of the art in 1976. *Behav. Ther.* **9**, 189.
Jordan, H.A. & Levitz, L.S. (1975): *Obesity Bar. Med.* **4**, 58.
Levitz, L. & Stunkard, A.J. (1974): *Am. J. Psychiat.* **131**, 423.
Lindner, P.G. & Blackburn, G.L. (1976): *Obesity Bar. Med.* **5**, 198.
London, A.M. & Schrieber, E.C. (1966): *Ann. Int. Med.* **65**, 80.
Mahoney, M.J. (1974): *Behav. Ther.* **5**, 48.
Mahoney, M.J. & Mahoney, K. (1976*a*); Treatment of obesity: a clinical exploration. In *Obesity: behavioral approaches to dietary management,* ed B.J. Williams, S. Martin & J.P. Foreyt. New York: Brunner-Mazel.
Mahoney, M.J. & Mahoney, K. (1976*b*): *Permanent weight control: a total solution to the dieters dilemma.* New York: Norton.
Marks, I.M. (1976): *Am. J. Psychiat.* **133**, 253..

McReynolds, W.T. & Lutz, R.N. (1976): *Behav. Ther.* 7, 283.
Mills, M.J. & Stunkard, A.J. (1976): *Am. J. Psychiat.* 133, 527.
Murray, D.C. (1975): *Psychol. Rep.* 37, 243.
Penick, S.B., Filion, R., Fox, S. & Stunkard, A.J. (1971): *Psychosom. Med.* 33, 49.
Romanczyk, R.G. (1974): *Behav. Ther.* 5, 531.
Romanczyk, R.G., Tracey, D.A., Wilson, G.T. & Thorpe, G.L. (1973): *Beh. Res. Ther.* 11, 629.
Stuart, R.B. (1967): *Behav. Res. Ther.* 5, 357.
Stuart, R.B. (1971): *Behav. Res. Ther.* 9, 177.
Stuart, R.B. (1975): Behavioral control of overeating: a status report. In *Obesity in perspective,* ed G.A. Bray. Washington DC: US Govt. Ptg. Office.
Stuart, R.B. & Davis, B. (1972): *Slim chance in a fat world: behavioral control of obesity.* Champaign, Illinois: Research Press.
Stunkard, A.J. (1975): *Psychosom. Med.* 37, 195.
Stunkard, A.J. (in press): Behavioral treatment for obesity: failure to maintain weight loss. In *Behavioral self-control,* ed R.B. Stuart.
Stunkard, A.J., Levine, H. & Fox, S. (1970): *Archs Int. Med.* 125, 1067.
Stunkard, A.J. & Mahoney, M.J. (1976): Behavioral treatment of the eating disorders. In *Handbook of behavior modification and behavior therapy,* ed H. Leitenberg, pp. 45-73. Englewood Cliffs: Prentice-Hall.
Stunkard, A.J. & McLaren-Hume, M. (1959): *Archs Int. Med.* 103, 79.
Stunkard, A.J. & Rush, J. (1974): *Ann. Int. Med.* 81, 526.
Sullivan, L., Bjurö, T., Garellick, G., Krotkiewski, M., Perrson, G. & Sjöström, L. (1978): Abstr. Second Int. Congress on Obesity 1977, *Int. J. Obesity,* 2, (in press).
Trulson, M., Walsh, E.D. & Caso, E.K. (1947): *J. Am. Diet. Ass.* 23, 941.
Wollersheim, J.P. (1970): *J. Abnorm. Psychol.* 76, 562.

30
Myths and realities in the treatment of obesity

P.L. WHITE
Department of Foods and Nutrition, American Medical Association, 535 North Dearborn Street, Chicago, Illinois 60610, USA.

Obesity pervades our society. Preoccupation with the threat, the fact and the consequences of obesity is present in every walk of life and in the institutions that define society. Millions of people are afflicted with it and many millions more struggle to prevent it. Too often they give up and let nature take its course if, indeed, obesity is 'nature's course'. The treatment of obesity is so difficult that relatively few physicians care to attempt treatment and those who do may find themselves 100 per cent devoted to bariatric practice. This international congress is devoted to the understanding of the obese state and how to treat and prevent the problem. The complexity of the program topics illustrates quite well the complexities of the problem itself.

Unlike the relatively quiescent wait for the cure of an infectious disease during which the public stands by until it is found, in the case of obesity the public takes matters into its own hands. Often with disastrous results and seldom with a cure. Business stands ready to capitalize on public impatience and provides one scheme after another to oblige. The result is a drama as American as 'baseball, hot dogs, apple pie and Chevrolet'. Let us take a look at the present environment in the United States that produces both a fantasy to be thin and the proclivity to be fat.

As if the States were a stage, reflect on the scene in which the majority of players lead a style of life known to be conducive to obesity. The life-style reflects: efficiency of motion and work, freedom from heat as well as cold, observing rather than doing. The stage is one on which 50 000 people in person and 80 million more at home will watch on their TV sets while 22 superbly conditioned athletes perform when it would be better if the 22 athletes watched the 80 million people perform. It is a stage where 80 million riding to work curse 20 000 others who jog, bicycle, roller-skate or walk to work. The 80 million curse because the exercisers are in their way. It is a stage where discussion of dieting, diet books and spas is conversation at calorie-laden cocktail parties and heavy dinners. Where to talk about weight loss while gaining weight is acceptable social behavior. It is a stage where social and financial status have more influence on body composition than does the medical profession.

In the United States, according to Garn, Clark & Guire (1975), fatness in children as measured by skinfold thickness correlates with the level of family income or occupations of the parents. Utilizing cross-sectional data from many thousands of subjects, including the ethnic lines found in the United States, Garn & co-workers found that poverty results in thin children. The males become thin adults and the females become fat adults. In contrast, affluence results in heavier children, the females of which become thin adults while the male members retain their heavier weights as adults. Affluence yields heavier adult males and thinner adult females no matter what the economic level of the family was when the subjects were children. At highest income levels, the thin male predominates. There is at present an inverse relationship between socioeconomic status and obesity (Stunkard, 1975).

The scene is America where automobiles are designed to be larger on the inside than on the outside in order to accommodate broad-beamed occupants while meeting required standards for smaller, more fuel efficient automobiles.

Yes, this is America where more money is spent on worthless 'cures' for obesity than is spent on all of medical research. And the nation grows fatter. America where the dimensions of medical ignorance about the causes, consequences, and cures of obesity are surpassed by the dimensions of the public knowledge of the very latest fad diet - whatever it may be at the time. This is not surprising since the authors of the last four best-sellers on dieting presented their schemes to the public without bothering with appropriate publication in professional journals. The library of the public becomes newspapers, magazines, television and paperback books. Advertising creates the authority.

This, then, is the stage upon which we play out our roles. This is the stage and the script is yours to edit as best you can. When editing, be aware that it is most difficult to separate realities from myths and that those who exploit the obesity market often fabricate apparent realities from myths, forever confusing the issues.

Somehow the notion (myth) persists that specific foods are fattening and that sugar and carbohydrates make one fat and that fat and protein are effective in weight loss. To be sure, fatty foods are also said to produce obesity. The solution, then, appears to be to decrease sugar and fat intake in order to lose weight. This approach, including justification and proposed solution, is exemplified in Dietary Goals for the United States (Select Committee on Nutrition and Human Needs, United States Senate, 1977). A brief review of that document should serve to illustrate the point - or the myth.

The major premise of the report is found in its introductory statement: '...our diets have changed radically within the last 50 years, with great and often very harmful effects on our health. These dietary changes represent as great a threat to public health as smoking. Too much fat, too much sugar or salt, can be and are linked directly to heart disease, cancer, obesity, and stroke, among other killer diseases. In all, six of the ten leading causes of death in the United States have been linked to our diet.' The report suggests that the incidence of heart disease, cancer, hypertension, diabetes, obesity and tooth decay could be reduced by making qualitative and quantitative changes in 'the American diet'.

The changes or goals are given as follows:

(1) Increase carbohydrate consumption to account for 55 per cent to 60 per cent of energy (caloric) intake.
(2) Reduce over-all fat consumption from approximately 40 per cent to 30 per cent of energy intake.
(3) Reduce saturated fat consumption to account for about 10 per cent of total energy intake, and balance that with polyunsaturated and monunsaturated fats, which should account for about 10 per cent of energy intake each.
(4) Reduce cholesterol consumption to about 300 mg/day.
(5) Reduce sugar consumption by about 40 per cent to account for about 15 per cent total energy intake.
(6) Reduce salt consumption by 50 per cent to 85 per cent to approximately 3 g/day

Specific recommendations follow for educational and regulatory intervention to help accomplish the dietary goals.

The Senate Select Committee correctly pointed out that the style of life in the United States is conducive to obesity, and may be conducive to early developement of coronary heart disease and cancer, but failed to appropriately point out the known associations between obesity and those diseases.

The problem according to the American Medical Association (Sammons, 1977 unpublished), is that the specific goals bear little resemblance to reality and that it is inappropriate for the Government to adopt national goals that specify such matters as the amount and proportions of total fat, type of fat, sugar, cholesterol, or salt content in the diets of the general public.

The Association believes that individual programs to prevent or to treat obesity through decreased caloric intake along with the programs aimed at improving physical fitness would be the most effective means of improving the health of our American citizens.

To reiterate the myths of the Senate Select Committee's approach: specific foods cause disease and obesity; the proportion of the macronutrients relate to disease and the greatest of all - the myth that there is an 'American diet'. There is no such thing as a typical American diet; dietary patterns are as varied in this country as are our ethnic origins.

The thought that sugar causes obesity has preoccupied consumer interest groups for years. These groups in turn have applied pressure for rules and regulations to control labels, advertising and use of sugar and foods containing sugar. These actions, in my opinion, divert public attention away from the real problem, the overall understanding of obesity and fitness. It is diverting because the proposed actions are against the symptoms of a medical disorder rather than toward the major problem.

There is another myth that needs attention and that is the myth that calorie-reduced foods are useful in general weight control programs. This myth is nearly as intriguing as the one that states: 'If you know the caloric value of foods you can successfully select a weight reducing diet'. Some of the best advertisements on television are for calorie reduced beer: one-third fewer calories than our regular beer, have another!

The US Food and Drug Administration has published proposed regulations establishing definitions for foods altered or designed to be reduced in caloric value or low calorie foods (Federal Register, 1977). By definition, low calorie foods will not have more than 40 kcal/serving and have a calorie density of no more than 0.4 kcal. Claims, names and label requirements are proposed. Whether such foods have real merit other than in the strictly controlled, institutionalized setting is highly debatable. The proposals did bring out a fascinating suggestion from one who believes that portion control, not special foods, is a reasonable approach to the dietary management of weight. He reasoned that provision of the calorie value and nutritive value of reduced serving sizes on the label of conventional foods would be more informative than would calling attention to reduced calorie foods. No doubt some compromise can be reached, but before long we will have the fattest food labels in existence. There is the option of publishing nutritive information for both one serving and one-half serving or the option of instructing dieters to learn how to divide by two.

A number of myths in the treatment of obesity have already been dealt with. Realities? The following realities can form a basis for the treatment of obesity:

(1) The probability of successful weight reduction decreases in proportion to the degree of obesity.
(2) The longer the time that obesity has been established, the lower the probability that successful weight reduction will be achieved, particularly if the obesity is of childhood onset.
(3) The probability of success decreases in any given patient as the number of his previous failures increases.
(4) Significant weight loss carries with it the potential for physiological and psychological harm that may place the patient in greater jeopardy than would perpetuation of the obese state.
(5) There being as yet no public health measure to cure obesity, more emphasis must be given to its prevention.

The end product of weight control should be the achievement of a 'desirable weight' and long time retention of that new weight. No weight reduction effort that 'allows' participants to regain weight can be considered to be successful. Briefly, this means that weight loss without rehabilitation of the life-style that produced obesity is essentially fruitless. The probability of retention of desirable weight should be entered into the risk-benefit ratio used in assessing the desirability of initiating a weight reduction program. The physician can do this. However, while individuals on self-prescribed regimens may successfully lose weight, the probability of successful retention of the new body weight is assumed to be very small. As an illustration, not long ago I received the following request: 'Please tell me of some warm place where I can lose 70 pounds regained after having lost weight on the Duke University program. They make you walk a great deal and it is too cold in North Carolina in the winter time'.

The risk-benefit ratio can not be assessed by individuals who undertake self-prescribed, non-supervised, non-supportive regimens, the regimens that one finds in all too many popular books on weight control.

Thus, it seems reasonable to counsel against self-prescribed, non-supervised regimens that carry some attendant medical risks eg, fasting and starvation, the protein-sparing modified fast and ketogenic diets. It does not, however, seem reasonable to take a stand on self-prescribed regimens on the basis that emotional or psychological problems may arise during the course of the programs. Admittedly, this is a nebulous issue.

I would like to leave you with a final reality. Obesity is cause by some deviation from normalcy: thus, there are causes and unless the causes of the deviation are understood and corrected (or compensated), no permanent relief can be expected. Finally, if when you look into a mirror and see the myth of what you would like to be instead of the reality of what you are, you will never lose weight.

References

Federal Register (1977): 42, 138, p. 37166.

Garn, S.M., Clark, D.C. & Guire, K.E. (1975): Growth, body composition, and development of obese and lean children. In *Childhood obesity,* ed M. Winick, p.23. New York: John Wiley.

Select Committee on Nutrition and Human Needs, United States Senate (1977): *Dietary goals for the United States.* Washington DC: US Govt. Ptg. Office.

Stunkard, A.J. (1975): *Psychosomatic Medicine* 37, 195.

31
The Stanford Three-Community Study: health education for cardiovascular risk prevention

J.W. FARQUHAR
Stanford Heart Disease Prevention Program, Stanford University Department of Medicine, Stanford, California 94305, USA.

Summary
Community based multifactorial health education involving mass media and some face to face instruction designed to reduce cardiovascular disease risk factors was carried out intensively for two years in two small northern California communities. Random samples of adults were surveyed at baseline and yearly for knowledge, for dietary intake and smoking rate and for various cardiovascular risk factors. Considerable stable change on net cardiovascular risk occurred in treatment samples as compared to controls. Changes in body weight were seen only in individuals given supplementary face to face instruction. Changes in smoking were also greater in the cohort that received face to face instruction. However, net cardiovascular risk reduction that resulted from mediated instruction was considerable and this suggests that cost-effective methods for delivery of preventive health services can be devised.

Introduction
In this paper I will describe the background, design, methods, and results of the first two years of a public health education campaign carried out in two moderate sized Californian communities with a third untreated community as a control. Education and skills training to achieve control of obesity was imbedded in a broad multifactorial campaign designed to reduce all cardiovascular disease risk factors. Our reasoning was that obesity was linked to sedentary life-styles, to hypertension and to elevated levels of plasma lipids.

The Study: background, design and methods
The background suppositions of the Stanford Three-Community Study
The background of the Stanford Three-Community Study stems from the convictions of a group at Stanford that the widespread changes in life-style that will be necessary for an effective public health attack on cardiovascular disease will require methods directed at large groups of individuals, and that the cost of these efforts is likely to be reduced if prolonged educational efforts are directed at communities rather than at individuals.

The suppositions that led to the design of the Stanford Three-Community Study are as follows:

(1) The ability to generalize from any success in single or multifactorial risk reduction trials on highly selected volunteers ultimately requires testing in free-living populations in their natural communities.

(2) The inherent natural reinforcers and opportunities for diffusion in such communities offer theoretical advantages, in both total effect and in economic efficiency, over the classical medical model, if widespread and prolonged health education is applied through all available channels for prolonged periods.

(3) Cost-effectiveness will be enhanced if the primary educational effort is exerted through mediated rather than face to face techniques.

(4) Past educational efforts in which mass media have been the principal method of education have generally been successful (Bauer, 1964; Cartwright, 1951; Griffiths & Nutson, 1960; Robertson *et al.*, 1974); however, our group believed that a successful program could be created in which mass media were the principal ingredients by drawing on principles derived from recent advances in communication research and in social learning theory. These principles include the following: (a) the educational material should consider the special characteristics of subgroups within the audience, (b) the material should be pretested, (c) all available channels should be used for its delivery, (d) the campaign strategy should provide the following components and in this sequence: information, motivation, skills training, and maintenance, (e) fear arousal should be avoided, and (f) source credibility should be provided.

(5) Our last supposition was that important degrees of stable behavioral change in risk factors might require additional educational input beyond extensive and prolonged mass media of a supplementary face to face intensive instruction directed toward high risk individuals.

Steps in campaign planning

I will describe the steps used in planning the Stanford Three-Community project and trust that many of these steps will be applicable to the needs of other groups who wish to begin research projects of this type. The sequence may be summarized as follows:

(1) Define the general program goals. These goals follow naturally from one's hypotheses, assumptions, interests, and resources.

(2) Assemble the professional talents needed. The initial program planning involved the medical and epidemiological talents of Drs Michael Stern, William Haskell, Peter Wood, and John Farquhar of Stanford's Department of Medicine and a team of social scientists led by Dr Nathan Maccoby of Stanford's Department of Communication. The latter group, Drs Henry Breitrose, Anthony Meyer, and Ms Janet Alexander supplied the needed skills in surveying methodology, communication research, social psychology, and media development and production.

(3) Program planning of specific goals. This requires close collaboration between medical and behavioral scientists.

(4) Community selection and recruitment. Data from the 1970 census, data on the nature of media channels available in communities (newspapers, radio and television stations) and geographical factors were used to pick 24 communities whose size and distance from Stanford University indicated their suitability for inclusion in the project. A final set of three communities was selected on the basis of independence of the three communities from domination by neighboring larger urban centers, similarity of demographic characteristics and proximity to Stanford University. Contacts were then made with the following groups: leaders of the health professionals serving the community; community leaders, including representatives of significant minority groups, and the owners and managers of newspapers, radio and television stations that serve the communities. Agreement was sought and received from these groups for the specific goals of the research project. Agreement was sought and received for participation of the major media outlets in the project's media plans. The project was explained to the local community physicians through hospital staff meetings.

(5) The instructional methods for mediated instruction and for face to face intensive instruction were developed and pretested in small groups. (See Meyer & Henderson, 1974, for a description of the research project that provided this pretest.)

(6) The final form of the instructional materials was prepared, the survey instruments were developed and pretested, and the final forms and questionnaires for these instruments

were prepared. Approximately one year was required to prepare for the start of formal field operations.

The design and time sequence of the Three-Community Study
Figure 1 outlines the structure, content, and sequence of the Three-Community study.

	1972	1973		1974		1975	
Watsonville	Baseline Survey (S1)	Media campaign Intensive instruction (II) (2/3 of high risk participants)	Second Survey (S2)	Media campaign Intensive instruction (II) Summer follow-up	Third Survey (S3)	Maintenance (low-level) Media campaign	Fourth Survey (S4)
Gilroy	Baseline Survey (S1)	Media campaign	Second Survey (S2)	Media campaign	Third Survey (S3)	Maintenance (low-level) Media campaign	Fourth Survey (S4)
Tracy	Baseline Survey (S1)		Second Survey (S2)		Third Survey (S3)		Fourth Survey (S4)

Fig. 1. Study design and timeline for Three-Community Study

The communities were all semi-rural marketing towns of approximately 15 000 population. They were reasonably similar in demographic characteristics, with approximately 15 per cent of adults preferring Spanish as their language rather than English. Tracy was the control community; Watsonville and Gilroy the treatment communities. In the Fall of 1972 a random sample of 500 to 600 adults in the age range of 35 to 59 was surveyed for health attitudes, knowledge, and risk factors. Surveys of the original cohort were repeated at the end of the first and second years of campaigning. In addition, at the end of year one, an additional 'after-only' sample of individuals was surveyed as a measure of the impact of surveying as an educational or sensitizing influence. Watsonville and Gilroy were subjected to a symmetrical mass media campaign involving radio, television, newspapers and direct mail during a nine-month campaign, a high risk subset of individuals within Watsonville were subjected to a ten-week duration intensive instruction program which will be desribed below. The media campaigns were of lesser intensity during the second year and the intensive instruction program was markedly decreased in intensity in the second year.

The media campaign
For the mass media campaign a broad range of materials was produced. The media campaign began two months after the initial survey, was continued for nine months in 1973, stopped during the second survey, and continued for nine more months in 1974. Because of the sizeable Spanish speaking population in the communities, the campaign was presented in both English and Spanish. Over the two years, about three hours of television programming, 50 television spots, 100 radio spots, several hours of radio programming, weekly newspaper columns, and newspaper advertisements and stories were produced. Printed material of a variety of sorts was mailed directly to participants and posters in public places such as in buses were also used. The mass media campaign was intended to produce awareness of the probable causes of coronary disease and of the specific behaviors which may reduce risk. The campaigns were designed to provide not only knowledge and skills to achieve recommended changes, but were designed to help the individuals become self-

sufficient in maintenance of new health habits and skills. All participants were advised to follow dietary habits that would lead to a reduction in body weight through calorie restriction and increased physical activity was advised for those who were overweight, and cigarette smokers were educated in the need and methods for ceasing or reducing their daily rate of cigarette consumption. Methods for self-scoring of risk factors and of risk related habits were presented through many media channels. The mass media campaign was monitored during its administration and revised in accordance with knowledge gained on the success in reaching goals. The instructional content, development, pretesting, application, and reformulations were done by closely coordinating the various professional skills within our organization. Media development was, therefore, done by a combination of individuals skilled in behavioral science, media production, and cardiovascular epidemiology.

Figure 2 shows the mix of types of media used in the English and Spanish language campaigns.

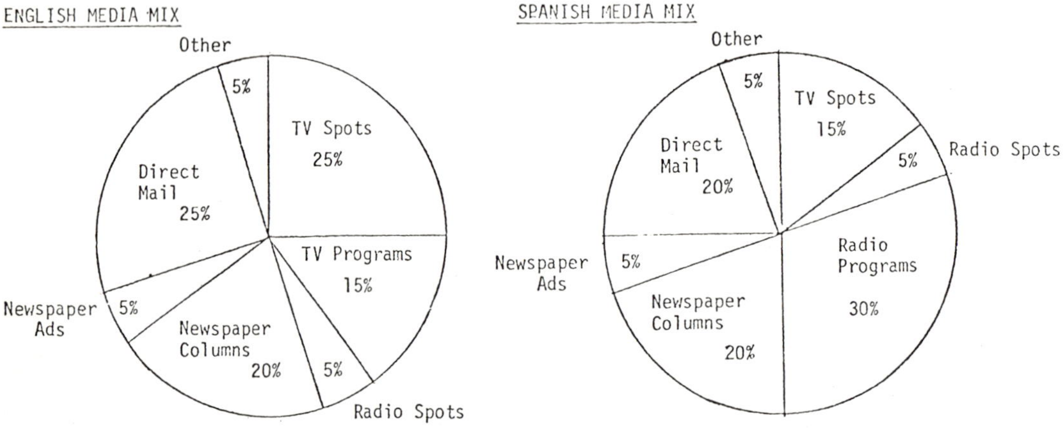

Fig. 2. Media mix for English and Spanish language campaigns

It can be seen in Fig. 2 that the major difference between the English and Spanish media campaigns was the relatively greater proportion of radio programming in the Spanish language campaign. This difference was built into our campaign because of our knowledge that the Spanish language section of the community had received much of their information from radio. It was due in addition to the fact that numerous radio stations split up the available audience such that the most popular English language radio station could reach only 10 per cent of the available audience and that to reach even 20 per cent of this audience we would have required six radio stations to cooperate in our program. On the other hand, we were able to reach fully half of the Spanish speaking audience by using only three of seven available Spanish language radio stations. It is, therefore, important to make clear that the choice of media channels is dependent on both their accessibility to the investigators and the proportion of a potential audience that they serve.

The intensive instruction program

The purpose of the intensive instruction program was twofold. First, it was designed to determine whether the addition of face to face intensive instruction to high risk individuals (who of course received the mass media campaign) would be superior to the mass media treatment alone. Our assumption was that this combination would be more efficacious.

Secondly, we hoped to learn from our experience with intensive instruction how better to build future mediated instruction that might contain the ingredients discovered to be effective in the inherently more costly face to face instruction.

Participants for the intensive instruction program were selected as a random two-third subset of men and women ages 35 to 59 who were in the top quartile of the Truett-Cornfield multiple logistic of risk (Truett, Cornfield & Kannel, 1967). This high risk cohort was comprised of 107 subjects out of 113 assigned to treatment and they were drawn from a random sample of approximately 500 adults in that age group that represented the cohort on whom baseline and posttreatment evaluations were done. These 107 individuals and spouses were treated over a ten-week period with first weekly and then biweekly three-hour sessions. The treatment was administered either in groups of 12 to 15, or for approximately one-third of the group, in single treatment sessions in the individuals' homes. The treatments were administered under the guidance of behavioral scientists and dietitians. The majority of the therapists were individuals with college degrees in the liberal arts who were trained for one week at Stanford in methods of counselling. Two of the therapists were graduate students in the Department of Communication at Stanford who were well versed in the behavioral science and communication theory needed for carrying out these interventions. In its early phases, the bulk of the education was informational instruction. However, the content of the intensive instruction program was one of behavior modification, representing a field application of the principles of social learning theory as outlined by Albert Bandura (1969). The behavior modification principles in the intensive instruction program follow five general steps: (1) Analysis of target behavior, (2) modelling of new behaviors, (3) guided practice in the new behaviors, (4) artificial reinforcement from instructors, and (5) maintenance without artificial reinforcement. Individuals were given instructions that were specific to their own particular risk factors. For example, smokers who were lean and had what were considered to be normal plasma cholesterol or triglyceride values, were given supplemental instruction only in how to stop smoking. Individuals with raised blood pressure were given special instruction in salt restriction and weight loss, whereas individuals with elevated plasma lipids were given supplemental instruction in qualitative dietary change.

Results

Changes in knowledge

Knowledge about risk factors and associated risk-producing habits changed dramatically in all treatment groups by the end of the first year of campaigning. The extent of knowledge of dietary risk factors corresponded quite well with the estimated magnitude of the intensity of educational treatment administered to various study groups.

We were pleased to note the surprisingly good correspondence between our estimate of the educational input and the magnitude of change in knowledge that occurred. Participants in the control community who were only examined and interviewed (Tracy total participants) showed very little apparent change in knowledge, whereas mass media plus intensive instruction (Watsonville-intensive instruction) had considerable effect on knowledge gained. The participants exposed to mass media only had intermediate changes. Of interest is that the 'after-only' groups had lesser changes, indicating that the antecedent surveying procedures experienced by the 'Gilroy-total participants' and 'Watsonville-reconstituted' groups enhanced the effects of the subsequent mass media campaign. The increase in knowledge was greater among Watsonville participants who not only were exposed to mass media, but lived in a community with individuals who had received face to face instruction (Watsonville-reconstituted), than among Gilroy participants who were exposed only to mass media (Gilroy-total participants). It is our view that a potential cause for this difference was related to diffusion of information from the intensive instruction participants to the other Watsonville participants. Evidence for such diffusion has been obtained (Meyer, Maccoby & Farquhar, in press).

Measurements of changes in knowledge were made of dietary risk factors at the end of one year and at the end of two years of health education comparing the English language and the Spanish language groups. It is clear that impressive gains occurred in knowledge in both groups.

We found that whereas the English language group began with approximately twice the amount of knowledge of these issues, at the end of two years the rate of gain among the Spanish language group had decreased the knowledge gap to a considerable degree. Our view of this finding is that it is attributable in large part to the care that was taken in tailoring the Spanish language campaign to the information seeking habits of the Spanish language community. We were very pleased to find that an educationally disadvantaged group did so well, particularly since this is counter to the usual experience reported in the literature.

Changes in dietary habits

Changes in food habits were determined by use of a precoded abbreviated dietary questionnaire requiring about ten minutes to administer, and fully suited to field work in epidemiology. Our questionnaire yielded correlation of approximately 0.6 for both dietary cholesterol and for dietary saturated fat when applied one year apart by different observers to individuals within our control community. More extensive in-depth interviews requiring about one hour to administer, and applied to individuals by the same highly trained professional, typically yield correlations between 0.6 and 0.9. Thus we feel our abbreviated questionnaire furnished an adequate degree of reproducibility. Validity of our dietary index, applied for groups, was obtained by our finding a correlation for eight different cohorts within our communities of 0.7 ($P = 0.02$) between self-reported dietary change and observed plasma cholesterol concentration change (Stern *et al.*, 1976). It was of interest that the degree of cholesterol change that occurred was approximately half that predicted from the formula developed by Keys & co-workers (Stern *et al.*, 1976). We are, of course, unable to determine whether the attenuation of our results is due to defects in the original formula, conscious overreporting of adherence to dietary change by participants, or to unknown factors that dilute the effectiveness of dietary changes when they occur in individuals in the free-living state rather than in subjects in the more tightly controlled environments of clinical research projects. Nonetheless, the changes in self-reported dietary patterns were extensive within all treatment groups and the degree of change correlated rather closely to the degree of educational input. As an example of the extensive changes observed in self-reported diet change, we observed an impressively large reduction in egg intake of 61 per cent in the intensively instructed group compared to a 40 per cent reduction in the group receiving mass media alone. The comparable control group in the untreated community reported only slight changes.

Figure 3 shows that decreases of a similar degree occurred in self-reported saturated fat consumption after the end of two years of campaigning in both men and women in all treatment groups, with essentially no change occurring in the control.

It can be seen that the largest changes occurred in the Watsonville intensive instruction group. This was an expected finding since this group received both mass media and supplemental face to face instruction. The next largest changes occurred in the Watsonville sample that is called the reconstituted sample. This sample is obtained by removal of the intensively instructed individuals from the total Watsonville participants with reconstitution of these individuals by expansion of the values of the randomized high risk individuals who did not receive intensive instruction. The reconstituted sample, therefore, tells us what the residents of this community, exposed to mass media alone, experienced in risk factor changes. The Gilroy sample, also exposed only to mass media, changed slightly less than did

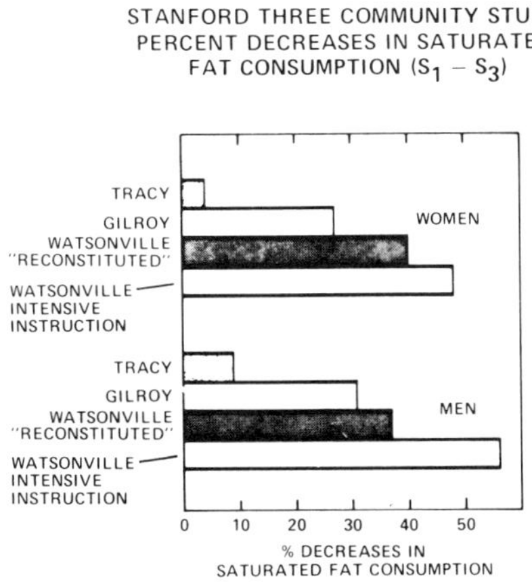

Fig. 3. Changes in saturated fat consumption among various participant groups in the three communities after two years of campaigning

the Watsonville sample and the Tracy control changes were very slight. The difference between the Watsonville reconstituted and Gilroy samples may be related to the effectiveness of the campaigns in the two communities or to the presence within Watsonville of the high risk individuals who enhanced the total educational effect on their townsmen through diffusion.

Changes in plasma cholesterol moved in the directions predicted by changes in our dietary index as mentioned above. Table 1 shows changes that occurred in the high risk groups at the end of one year of campaigning.

Table 1. Plasma cholesterol changes (S1-S2) in high risk participants

Group	% Change
Tracy	+ 1.4
Gilroy	–0.2
Watsonville R.C.	–3.5*
Watsonville I.I.	–5.0*

R.C. = Randomized control, I.I. = intensive instruction
* Differences significant at $P<0.01$, one-tailed test

As can be seen, the Tracy participants experienced a modest increase in cholesterol after the end of one year; a not unexpected finding for a control group. The Gilroy sample experienced a slight fall in cholesterol. This, however, was not significantly different from the Tracy value and indicated that the media only group did not experience a significant difference at the end of one year. The 'Watsonville R.C.' sample was the randomized control for the intensively instructed individuals. These people received only mass media and did experience a 3.5 per cent fall in plasma cholesterol concentration. The difference between this and the Tracy sample is approximately 5 per cent. This difference was significant at the $P<0.01$ level. The 'Watsonville I.I.' sample, which represented those who received intensive instruction, experienced a greater decline in cholesterol of 5 per cent, for a net difference of 6.4 per cent at the end of one year from the control group. This too was significant at the $P<0.01$ level.

Differences in cholesterol level between the control and treatment communities were also present after the second year of campaigning despite a considerable decrease in the intensity of the campaigning during the second year. Table 2 shows that a statistically decrease in plasma cholesterol was present in all three communities in all three treatment conditions following the second year of campaigning. These changes are expressed as

Table 2. Percentage net change in risk factors after two years of health education (relative to control = no change)

Risk factors	Gilroy (M.M.)	Watsonville (M.M.)	Watsonville (M.M. & I.I.)
Plasma cholesterol	–3.8*	–2.3*	–3.6*
Systolic blood pressure	–8.6*	–5.9*	–5.8*
Smoking:			
cigs/day	–4.2	–11.2*	–25.1*
smokers	–5.8	–2.6	–31.6*
Relative weight	–0.6	+0.2	–0.5
Multiple logistic function of risk	–23.8*	–22.7*	–30.3*

M.M. = mass media, I.I. = intensive instruction
*$P < 0.05$, one-tailed test

percentage net change in cholesterol relative to the control considered as no change. It can be seen that the mass media only participants in Gilroy increased their degree of cholesterol change from the first year results and that these are now statistically significant. However, slight recidivism occurred in both of the Watsonville samples, such that the difference between treatment and control was only 3.6 per cent compared to 6.4 per cent at the end of one year for the intensively instructed group. The difference for both the Watsonville media only sample and the intensive instruction sample in Watsonville remained statistically significant.

Changes in cigarette smoking continued to be impressive following the second year of campaigning for the group that received intensive instruction. A drop of 25 per cent in number of cigarettes per day and a 32 per cent drop in smokers was noted in this group that had supplemental face to face instruction. In contrast, the mass media treatment was relatively ineffective: the Watsonville sample that received mass media only was unique in that the drop in cigarette smoking reached statistical significance there as compared to the control community. These findings indicate that personal face to face instruction when supplemented with mass media seems to be more effective than mass media alone in changing smoking habits.

Statistically significant and surprisingly large drops occurred in blood pressure in the treatment communities in all major treatment cohorts. There was a modest rise in blood pressure after the first and second years in the control community. Table 2 shows that the participants in the mass media treatment in Gilroy were found to have a mean systolic blood pressure 8.6 per cent lower than that in the control at the end of two years. The comparable media only group in Watsonville was 5.9 per cent lower than its control and the Watsonville intensively instructed sample was 5.8 per cent lower. The degree of these changes was surprising in that there was no attempt in the three-community study to become personally involved in blood pressure management. However, all individuals were instructed to restrict their salt intake. A second reason for blood pressure change may have lain in greater compliance to preexisting medications as a result of a raised level of health consciousness on the part of the residents of the treatment communities. This supposition was borne out by evidence that an interaction effect was noted between being a resident of the treatment communities, weight loss, and a history of being on anti-hypertensive medications.

The net effect of the changes in smoking, plasma cholesterol, and blood pressure was to create a rather surprisingly large degree of reduction in the multiple logistic of risk. Table 2 shows that this change, as compared to control, was approximately 30 per cent for the intensively instructed group in Watsonville and 23 and 24 per cent respectively, for the media only participants in Watsonville and Gilroy. It is relevant to point out that the changes in blood pressure occurred to a larger extent in individuals in the upper ranges of blood pressure. Some of the improvement in cardiovascular risk may, therefore, be attributed to this alteration in the distribution in risk factors in the upper ranges of their distribution.

Changes in body weight of a significant degree occurred only in the group of high risk individuals who were given the supplementary intensive instructions in addition to the mass media campaign. Not all of this group was advised to lose weight since risk was determined from a composite of smoking rates, plasma cholesterol, and blood pressure. However, among those whose weights were above the group mean, a statistically significant 8.5 lb (3.8kg) loss occurred at the end of the first year. Since these individuals were drawn from a random sample we were gratified at these results. By the end of year two, some recidivism in weight occurred and there was no longer a significant difference between treatment and control. However, the blood pressure changes in the treatment communities were maintained and multivariate analysis indicated that weight loss was an important contributor to the blood pressure change.

We found that increases in risk appeared in the control groups despite the cohort having yearly examinations in which their risk factors were reported to them and to their physicians. Despite this potential 'treatment' the examined cohorts in the control community showed modest increases in blood pressure and cholesterol. We have, therefore, shown a lack of a treatment effect despite this yearly screening and notification. This finding was not unexpected and is quite analogous to the experience of many prospective epidemiological studies which have regularly shown an age-related increase in risk factors to occur despite yearly or biannual survey examinations. In contrast to the increase in risk in the control groups, reductions in risk occurred during the first year in the two treatment groups. These changes were not only maintained but improved further during the second year. It was also evident that groups in Watsonville in which some direct face to face instruction was provided, show a greater decrease than the media only groups at the end of the first year. However, by the end of the second year the groups exposed only to media show substantial further gains and the difference between media and media plus face to face instruction was diminished and no longer was statistically significant. There was a close parallel relationship of the two media groups in Gilroy and Watsonville. This provides evidence for the similarity of the media campaigns and for their effects on risk in the two treatment communities.

Conclusions

Community based health education can succeed, given prolonged application of information supplied through multiple channels, including print media. Smoking cessation and weight reduction were most successfully managed through a combination of mass media and supplementary face to face instruction. However, we have considerable hope and some early evidence that even those recalcitrant problems can be managed through programs that are predominantly delivered through mediated methods.

Two recent publications of the Stanford Heart Disease Prevention Program contain more extensive descriptions of the results of the three-community study (Farquhar *et al.*, 1977; Maccoby *et al.*, 1977). Our group believes that the impact of community based intervention methods is magnified by the extra power obtained by informal discussion of information within the community system and by generation of networks of social support within the community. Given equal inputs of educational effort we, therefore, believe community based efforts to be inherently superior to efforts devoted to screening, detection, referral, and treatments delivered through more traditional medical institutions. Clearly an interaction between broadly based educational efforts and the efforts of medical practitioners would be anticipated. However, cost-effectiveness would be enhanced were a reasonably large proportion of educational effort directed to the community at large. Cost-effectiveness would also be served in future efforts at obesity control if such efforts are carried out as part of a broad cardiovascular disease prevention program.

References

Bandura, A. (1969): *Principles of behavior modification.* New York: Holt, Rinehart & Winston.
Bauer, R.A. (1964): *Am. Psychologist* 19, 310.
Cartwright, D. (1951): *Human Relations* 4, 381.
Farquhar, J.W., Maccoby, N., Wood, P.D. *et al.* (1977): *Lancet* 1, 1192.
Griffiths, W. & Nutson, A. (1960): *Am. J. Pub. Hlth* 50, 515.
Maccoby, N., Farquhar, J.W. & Wood, P.D. *et al.* (1977): *J. Comm. Hlth* 3, 100.
Meyer, A.J. & Henderson, J.B. (1974): *Prev. Med.* 13, 225.
Meyer, A.J., Maccoby, N. & Farquhar, J.W. (in press): Generating opinion leadership and the diffusion of innovations in a cardiovascular health education campaign. *Communication Yearbook.*
Robertson, I.S., Kelley, A.B., O'Neill, B. *et al.* (1974): *Am. J. Pub. Hlth* 64, 1071.
Stern, M.P., Farquhar, J.W. & Maccoby, N. *et al.* (1976): *Circulation* 54, 826.
Truett, J., Cornfield, J. & Kannel, W. (1967): *J. Chron. Dis.* 20, 511.

32
Relation of lipoprotein and cholesterol abnormalities to obesity

P.NESTEL
Cardiovascular Metabolism and Nutrition Research Unit, Baker Medical Research Institute, Commercial Road, Prahran, Victoria 3181, Australia.

Obesity and plasma lipids

Hyperlipidemia is commonly associated with overweight. The incidence of hypertriglyceridemia, in particular, is high, the frequency depending on the definitions of normal values for body weight and serum triglyceride. The corollary of this is that overweight is very common in patients with hyperlipidemia, especially those with hypertriglyceridemia (Blacket *et al.*, 1975). A recent survey of a healthy Swedish population showed that the mean body weights of men and women with Type 4 hyperlipoproteinemia were 6 and 8 kg higher than those with normal levels of triglyceride (Olsson, 1975). The excess lipid is transported predominantly as very low density lipoproteins (VLDL), which also contain increased amounts of cholesterol, even when the cholesterol concentration in whole plasma is normal (Wilson & Lees, 1972; Carlson & Ericsson, 1975). The cholesterol content in other lipoproteins, notably the high density class (HDL), may be reduced (Carlson & Ericsson, 1975) and may return to normal levels with weight reduction. Other varieties of hyperlipoproteinemia are also influenced by overweight. Weight loss lowers the lipoprotein levels in Types 3, 5 and 2b (also known as combined hyperlipidemia) (Fredrickson, 1972). Type 3 hyperlipoproteinemia is particularly sensitive to relatively small changes in body weight and the response to drug therapy is enhanced by weight reduction in at least those forms of hyperlipoproteinemia in which hypertriglyceridemia is a significant factor. The relationship between overweight and the plasma cholesterol concentration is more controversial. Two recent studies of large populations have, however, shown marginally significant correlations, at least in some age groups. Montoye, Epstein & Kjelsberg (1966) found that fatness raises the serum cholesterol concentration between the ages of 15 and 45 years, while Rifkind & Begg (1966) reported a similar association in men aged 40 to 59 years.

The effect of weight reduction has not established an unequivocal relationship between obesity and plasma cholesterol levels (Bierenbaum *et al.*, 1973). Two recent studies have, however, shown that weight reduction may be useful in patients with hypercholesterolemia, though in neither study were variables other than weight completely controlled (Leelarthaepin *et al.*, 1974; Olefsky, Reaven & Farquhar, 1974). When weight loss is rapid, the fall in serum cholesterol concentration can be great (Galbraith, Connor & Stone, 1966).

Obesity presumably accentuates some of the metabolic disorders that give rise to hypertriglyceridemia, such as an increased transport of VLDL through plasma. Obese diabetics are more likely to have raised serum triglyceride than lean patients and most patients with Type 5 hyperlipoproteinemia are overweight (Fredrickson, Levy & Lees, 1967). Brunzell (Brunzell *et al.*, 1974) has pointed out that in families having the trait for combined hyperlipidemia, more obese members show excess levels of VLDL while the non-obese show elevated levels of low density lipoproteins (LDL).

The hyperlipidemia of obesity can be reproduced in normal subjects by overfeeding, but the response to excess energy intake depends on its nature. The increase in plasma triglyceride is greater than that in plasma cholesterol, especially if the excess energy is mainly derived from carbohydrate (Sims & Horton, 1968; Nestel, Carroll & Havenstein, 1969; Goldrick, Havenstein, Carroll & Reardon, 1972). However, these changes may be short-lived (Olefsky *et al.*, 1975).

Obesity and cholesterol metabolism

Fatness is closely related to several parameters of cholesterol metabolism. In a study of 22 unselected subjects, Nestel, Whyte & Goodman (1969) found a highly significant correlation between body weight and the daily production rate of cholesterol. As measured by compartmental analysis of the plasma cholesterol specific radioactivity-time curve, each kg of excess weight increased the turnover of cholesterol by 22 mg. The body's exchangeable cholesterol was also increased in proportion to the degree of adiposity. Interestingly, the amount of cholesterol in the very slowly exchanging pool does correlate with the serum cholesterol concentration (Smith *et al.*, 1976). Miettinen (1971), who measured cholesterol turnover from the rates of excretion of cholesterol and bile acids, also found that cholesterol production in fat people amounted to 20 mg/kg adipose tissue compared to 12 mg/kg of body weight in subjects of normal weight. In a study of extremely obese people, a correlation has been found between cholesterol synthesis and adipose cellularity (Nestel, Schreibman & Ahrens, 1973), suggesting that cholesterol is stored in adipocytes together with triglyceride and released from adipocytes during lipolysis of triglyceride. This supported by the very high correlation between the cholesterol content and fat cell size (Schreibman & Dell, 1975).

Cholesterol is rapidly mobilized into plasma when weight is lost and high density lipoprotein (HDL) may be the plasma acceptor for this cholesterol (Fig. 1). Cholesterol synthesis

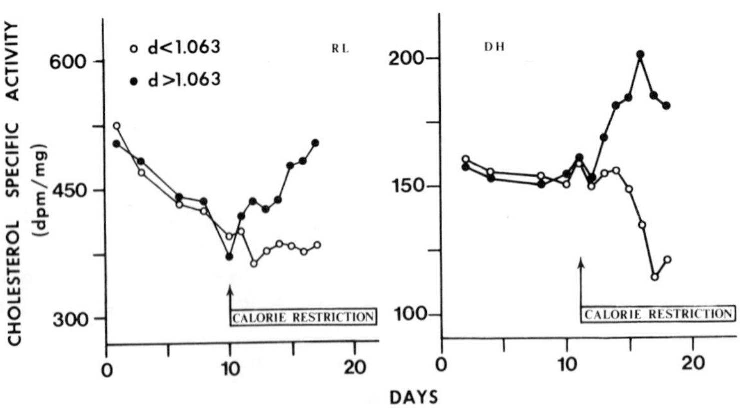

Fig. 1. Rise in HDL cholesterol specific radioactivity during weight reduction. Shows that cholesterol leaving adipocytes is transferred predominantly to HDL

in the expanding adipose mass is unlikely, but has not been ruled out. The kinetic analysis of cholesterol turnover in the adipose tissue of fat people seems to exclude significant synthesis in that organ (Schreibman & Dell, 1975). Direct *in vitro* measurement of cholesterol synthesis in human adipose tissue has shown only low rates of conversion of labelled precursors into sterols, although this may be due to dilution of label in later cholesterol precursors. Schreibman & Dell (1975) have calculated that the synthesis of cholesterol was unlikely to be greater than 1 mg/day/kg fat tissue, which is slight in relation to the turnover of cholesterol in fat people (20 mg/kg/day). This suggests that 95 per cent of cholesterol in adipose tissue is derived from plasma.

If the increased turnover of cholesterol that occurs in obesity does not derive from synthesis in adipose tissue, then the liver and possibly the intestine may be responsible for the over-production. The increased hepatic secretion of VLDL in obesity could account for the higher turnover of cholesterol. An additional 500 mg cholesterol/day could be secreted if the excess output of VLDL was equivalent to 2.5 g of triglyceride. The daily triglyceride turnover in obese subjects, even in those with normal plasma lipids, exceeds that in lean subjects by considerably more than this amount (Grundy *et al.*, 1976). The production of VLDL by the liver is closely linked to the turnover of plasma FFA which is increased in obesity. The high turnover of FFA may also contribute to cholesterol synthesis by enriching the supply of 2-carbon fragments in the liver. If FFA turnover is 900 μmol/min and all 16 carbons of palmitic acid are incorporated into cholesterol (27 carbons), then this would approximate 693 mmol cholesterol/day or 268 g/day. Less than 0.5 per cent of FFA turn-over would, therefore, provide the substrate for the amounts of cholesterol that are synthe-sized in obese subjects.

Sodhi & Kudchodkar (1973) have also noted the association of increased cholesterol production, overweight and hypertriglyceridemia. Multivariate analysis of their data shows that, in overweight subjects, the primary correlation is between plasma triglyceride concentration and cholesterol synthesis. Einarsson, Hellström & Kallner (1974) found that bile acid production was increased in hypertriglyceridemic subjects and was related to body weight. The origin of the excess bile acid may be from increased cholesterol synthesis in the liver or from the increased turnover of circulating lipoprotein cholesterol. Weight loss results in a marked reduction in bile acid turnover and in cholesterol synthesis (Miettinen, 1968; Liu *et al.*, 1974).

The increased turnover of cholesterol in obesity may be responsible for the high incidence of cholesterol gall-stones in fat people (Grundy, Metzger & Adler, 1972). This predisposition to gall-stone formation can be reversed by weight reduction. However, a lower secretion of biliary cholesterol is achieved only after the establishment of weight maintenance at a lower level (Bennion & Grundy, 1975). In fact, the lithogenicity of bile actually rises during rapid weight loss (Schreibman *et al.*, 1974), reflecting the mobilisation of cholesterol from adipose tissue and the reduction of bile acid synthesis.

Other indices of cholesterol metabolism also increase with overweight. One of these is the concentration of plasma squalene, a precursor of cholesterol, which is raised in obese people (Liu *et al.*, 1974) and in overweight hypertriglyceridemic subjects (Nestel & Kudchodkar, 1975). The turnover of plasma esterified cholesterol also increases with fatness (Nestel & Monger, 1967; Nestel, 1970; Akanuma *et al.*, 1973) and appears to be related to the increased transport of VLDL.

Obesity and triglyceride metabolism

Raised levels of plasma free fatty acids (FFA) have been consistently observed in obese subjects (Opie & Walfish, 1963; Gordon, 1970). They also have increased turnover of plasma FFA which is significantly correlated with excess weight (Miller, Bortz & Durham, 1968; Nestel & Whyte, 1968; Birkenhäger & Tjabbes, 1969). This results from enhanced lipolysis which is augmented by the increased size of fat cells (Goldrick & McLoughlin, 1970). A second major factor is the regulation of lipolysis and esterification in adipocytes which appears to be disturbed in obese subjects. This was measured during prolonged constant infusions of radiopalmitate towards the end of sustained glucose ingestion, and again 6 to 8 hours after stopping glucose. Net transport of FFA was suppressed to equally low levels in obese and lean subjects though at the expense of higher insulin concentrations in the obese (Fig. 2). In the lean, the clearance of FFA was significantly stimulated with glucose, but in the obese, low clearance rates were observed both during and after stopping glucose (Fig. 3). The diminished clearance of FFA from plasma in the obese suggests impaired esterification of FFA in muscle and adipose tissue.

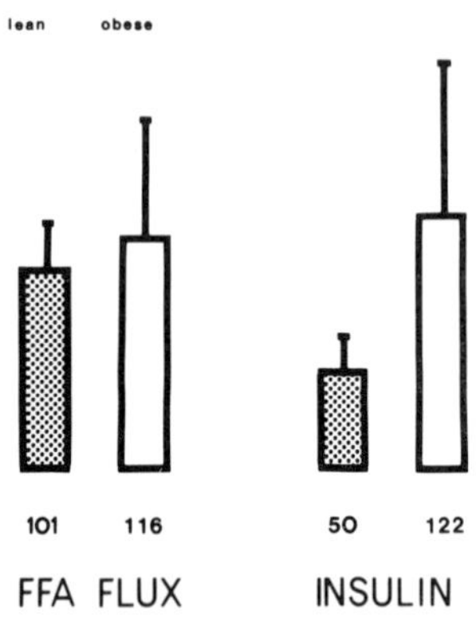

Fig. 2. Suppression of FFA flux (or net lipolysis) by glucose. Shows equal suppression in lean and obese subjects but requiring greater secretion of insulin in the obese

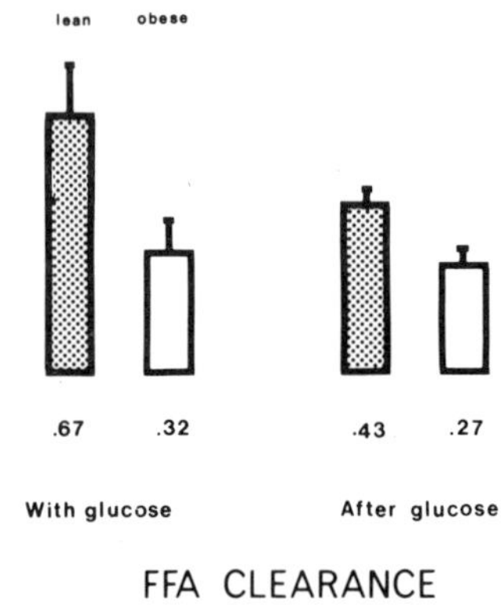

Fig. 3. Reduced fractional removal of FFA (or esterification) in obese compared to lean subjects

This may reflect the profound resistance to the action of insulin that develops in obesity (Assimacopoulos & Jeanrenaud, 1976). The evidence for adipose tissue is less convincing and, in fact, enlarged fat cells are metabolically overactive and the rate of utilization of glucose for esterification of FFA increases in proportion to the enlargement of the cell (Smith, 1971). In the liver, the extraction of FFA from the splanchnic circulation is increased in obese subjects in direct proportion to the increased FFA transport (Felig *et al.*, 1974).

The relevance of these findings to the hypertriglyceridemia of obesity lies in the close relationship between the hepatic uptake of plasma FFA and the secretory rate of triglyceride (Havel *et al.*, 1970). Greater availability of plasma FFA stimulates triglyceride formation. Increased conversion of FFA to VLDL triglyceride has been demonstrated in several studies of obese subjects (Nestel & Whyte, 1968; Olefsky *et al.*, 1974) and a reduction in triglyceride turnover has been shown to parallel weight loss (Olefsky *et al.*, 1974).

There may be additional sources for the excess plasma triglyceride. In obese subjects, as much as 80 per cent of newly secreted triglyceride fatty acid is derived from sources other than circulating FFA (Barter & Nestel, 1973). Havel & co-workers (1970) have suggested that the large mass of splanchnic adipose tissue might provide fatty acids via the portal circulation. It is also possible that lipogenesis from carbohydrate in the liver is greater and more persistent in obese than in lean subjects (Wolfe & Ahuja, 1972). Even in the absence of a high carbohydrate intake, the liver of an obese subject may have available for lipogenesis a greater than normal supply of glucose, since the hepatic extraction of glucose precursors (lactate, glycerol and alanine) is twice as great in obese as in lean subjects (Felig *et al.*, 1974). By contrast, lipogenesis from glucose in adipose tissue is of little quantitative importance even in obesity (Sjöström, 1973).

Hypertriglyceridemia in obesity does not appear to reflect diminished removal of plasma triglyceride. Removal mechanisms have been studied by measuring the activity of lipoprotein lipase, the enzyme that regulates the hydrolysis of circulating triglyceride. Pykälistö, Smith & Brunzell (1975) have found a direct correlation between the size and the lipoprotein lipase content of isolated adipocytes; the total enzyme capacity in adipose tissue would, therefore, be increased in obesity and would not be expected to lead to hypertriglyceridemia.

Summary

Hyperlipidemia is common in obesity. Plasma triglyceride levels are closely linked to overweight. The plasma cholesterol level is only weakly associated with excess weight, but weight reduction may effectively lower the cholesterol as well as the triglyceride concentration.

The exchangeable cholesterol in the body is strongly influenced by overweight and by weight change. Cholesterol production is directly related to excess body mass and adipose cellularity. The amount of cholesterol in the body increases with increasing weight. The high flux of cholesterol through the biliary system predisposes to gall-stone formation. Adipocyte cholesterol is readily mobilized during weight loss and may exacerbate the lithogenicity of the bile.

Hypertriglyceridemia is the result of several factors. Plasma free fatty acid transport is increased due to an increase in total lipolysis in the expanded adipose mass. The production of triglyceride in the liver both from plasma FFA and from glucose is increased. Triglyceride is also released from expanded triglyceride stores in the liver. The capacity of adipocytes to remove plasma triglyceride is probably normal since lipoprotein lipase activity increases with cell size. Fatty acid synthesis in adipocytes is not increased. Enlarged adipocytes appear to be less responsive to glucose and insulin, in that esterification is not stimulated by glucose consumption in obese people, and although lipolysis is suppressible it appears to require excessive insulin secretion.

References

Akanuma, Y., Kuzuya, T., Hayashi, M., Ide, T. & Kuzuya, N. (1973): *Europ. J. Clin. Invest.* 3, 136.
Assimacopoulos, J.F. & Jeanrenaud, B. (1976): *Clins Endoc. Metab.* 5, 337.
Barter, P.J. & Nestel, P.J. (1973): *Metabolism* 22, 779.
Bennion, L.J. & Grundy, S.M. (1975): *J. Clin. Invest.* 56, 996.
Bierenbaum, M.L., Fleischman, A.I., Raichelson, R.I., Hayton, T. & Watson, P.B. (1973): *Lancet* 2, 1404.
Birkenhager, J.C. & Tjabbes, T. (1969): *Metabolism* 18, 18.
Blacket, R.B., Woodhill, J.M., Leelarthaepin, B. & Palmer, A.J. (1975): *Lancet* 1, 517.
Brunzell, J.D., Hazzard, W.R., Motulsky, A.G. & Bierman, E.L. (1974): *Clin. Res.* 22, 462*a*.
Carlson, L.A. & Ericsson, M. (1975): *Atherosclerosis* 21, 417.
Einarsson, K., Hellström, K. & Kallner, M. (1974): *J. Clin. Invest.* 54, 1301.
Felig, P., Wahren, J., Hendler, R. & Brundin, T. (1974): *J. Clin. Invest.* 53, 582.
Fredrickson, D.S. (1972): *Modern concepts of cardiovascular disease* 41, 31.
Fredrickson, D.S., Levy, R.I. & Lees, R.S. (1967): *New Engl. J. Med.* 248, 971.
Galbraith, W.B., Connor, W.E. & Stone, D.B. (1966): *Ann. Int. Med.* 64, 268.
Goldrick, R.B. & McLoughlin, G.M. (1970): *J. Clin. Invest,* 49, 1213.
Goldrick, R.B., Havenstein, N., Carroll, K.F. & Reardon. M. (1972): *Metabolism* 21, 761.
Gordon, E.S. (1970): *Advances in metabolic disorders* 4, 229.
Grundy, S.M., Metzger, A.L. & Adler, R.D. (1972): *J. Clin. Invest.* 51, 3026.
Grundy, S.M., Mok, H., von Bergmann, K., Zech, L., Berman, M. & Steinberg, D. (1976): *Circulation* 54, Suppl. 2, p. 2 (Abstr).
Havel, R.J., Kane, J.P., Balasse, E.O., Segel, N. & Basso, L.V. (1970): *J. Clin. Invest.* 49, 2017.
Leelarthaepin, B., Woodhill, J.M., Palmer, A.J. & Blacket, R.B. (1974): *Lancet* 2, 1217.
Liu, G.C.K., Schreibman, P.H., Samuel, P. & Ahrens, E.H., Jr. (1974): *J. Clin. Invest.* 53, 47*a*.
Miettinen, T.A. (1968): *Clin. Chim. Acta* 19, 341.
Miettinen, T.A. (1971): *Circulation* 44, 842.
Miller, H.I., Bortz, W.M. & Durham, B.C. (1968): *Metabolism* 17, 515.
Montoye, H.J., Epstein, F.H. & Kjelsberg, M.O. (1966): *Am. J. Clin. Nutr.* 18, 397.
Nestel, P.J. & Monger, E.A. (1967): *J. Clin. Invest.* 46, 967.
Nestel, P.J. & Whyte, H.M. (1968): *Metabolism* 17, 1122.
Nestel, P.J., Carroll, K.F. & Havenstein, N. (1969): *Metabolism* 19, 1.
Nestel, P.J., Whyte, H.M. & Goodman, DeW.S. (1969): *J. Clin. Invest.* 48, 982.
Nestel, P.J. (1970): *Clin. Sci.* 38, 593.
Nestel, P.J., Schreibman, P.H. & Ahrens, E.H. (1973): *J. Clin. Invest.* 52, 2389.
Nestel, P.J. & Kudchodkar, B. (1975): *Clin. Sci. Molec. Med.* 49, 621.
Olefsky, J., Reaven, G.M. & Farquhar, J.W. (1974): *J. Clin. Invest,* 53, 64.
Olefsky, J., Crapo, P.A., Ginsberg, H. & Reaven, G.M. (1975): *Metabolism* 24, 495.
Olsson, A.G. (1975): *Acta Med. Scand.* 197, 477.
Opie, L.H. & Walfish, P.G. (1963): *New Engl. J. Med.* 268, 757.

Pykälistö, O.J., Smith, P.H. & Brunzell, J.D. (1975): *J.Clin. Invest.* 56, 1108.
Rifkind, B.M. & Begg, T. (1966): *Br. Med. J.* 2, 208.
Schreibman, P.H., Pertsemlidis, D., Liu, G.C.K. & Ahrens, E.H. (1974): *J. Clin. Invest.* 53, 72a.
Schreibman, P.H. & Dell, R.B. (1975): *J. Clin. Invest.* 55, 986.
Sims, E.A.H. & Horton, E.S. (1968): *Am. J. Clin. Nutr.* 21, 1455.
Sjöström, L. (1973): *Scand. J. Clin. Lab. Invest.* 32, 339.
Smith, U. (1971): *J. Lipid. Res.* 12, 65.
Smith, F.R., Dell, R.B., Noble, R.P. & Goodman, DeW.S. (1976): *J. Clin. Invest.* 57, 137.
Sodhi, H.S. & Kudchodkar, B.J. (1973): *Metabolism* 22, 895.
Wilson, D. & Lees, R. (1972): *J. Clin. Invest.* 51, 1051.
Wolfe, B.M. & Ahuja, S.P. (1972) : *Clin. Res.* 20, 947.

33
Diet, muscle metabolism and capacity for exercise in obesity

E.S. HORTON
Department of Medicine, University of Vermont College of Medicine, Burlington, Vermont 05401, USA.

Diet, muscle metabolism and capacity for exercise in obesity

A decreased level of voluntary activity has been observed frequently in association with obesity (Bullen *et al.*, 1964; Johnson *et al.*, 1959; Bloom & Eidex, 1967; Lutwak & Coulston, 1975) and numerous studies have been made of the various factors possibly contributing to a decreased capacity for physical exercise in the obese (Buskirk & Bartlett, 1975; Alexander, 1975; Björntorp, 1975; Dempsey *et al.*, 1966*a*; Whipp *et al.*, 1975). These include studies of pulmonary, cardiac and circulatory function, muscle metabolism and both metabolic and mechanical efficiency of performing work. To date, no clear-cut abnormalities have been found in moderate obesity which can be considered inherent defects in the ability to perform physical work. Most, if not all, of the abnormalities can be overcome by weight reduction and physical conditioning.

In the treatment of obesity, the primary goal is to achieve a significant decrease in the adipose tissue mass while minimizing the concomitant loss of lean body mass and preserving protein stores. Many consider the ideal program to achieve this goal to consist of a combination of caloric restriction and physical exercise. However, with severely restricted diets it is difficult to avoid large negative nitrogen balances and it has been commonly assumed that restriction of carbohydrate intake will significantly decrease the individual's capacity to perform sustained physical exercise of moderate to high intensity.

Attempts have been made to devise weight reduction diets which, by severely restricting calories, will result in maximal rates of utilization of the individual's adipose stores for energy without resulting in a concomitant decrease in lean body mass. Apfelbaum (1970, 1972) showed that nitrogen balance could be maintained over periods of up to 3 weeks by feeding as little as 55 gm of casein daily to otherwise fasting subjects. Blackburn & Flatt (1972) have modified this regimen to a diet consisting primarily of lean meat. They find this diet to be 'protein sparing' because in the absence of any significant carbohydrate content of the diet, plasma insulin concentrations fall to extremely low levels, lipolysis proceeds uninhibited and the body rapidly adapts to starvation. Bistrian *et al.* (1975) have found 1.2 to 1.4 g of protein/kg of ideal body weight to be sufficient for maintaining nitrogen balance and have suggested that the addition of physical exercise to the program may even result in a positive nitrogen balance.

Whether or not such a 'protein-sparing modified fast' will result in any greater weight reduction and better preservation of lean body mass than an equicaloric diet containing carbohydrate has not been determined over an extended period of time. In short-term experiments, Yang & Van Itallie (1976) found no difference in loss of adipose or lean body mass in subjects fed 800 kcal diets with or without carbohydrates. The greater rate of weight loss on the ketogenic diet observed during the first 10 days was due entirely to increased loss of body water.

With increasing use of diets severely restricted in calories in the treament of obesity, some with and others without carbohydrate included, it becomes important to assess the effect of these diets on the capacity to perform physical work. Do hypocaloric diets result in a decreased ability to perform either high intensity or endurance work and does adaptation occur with time on the diet? To approach these questions, the various factors influencing work capacity in obesity must be considered.

Factors affecting capacity for exercise in obesity

There have been many studies of pulmonary function in obesity, often with varying results depending on the severity and distribution of the obesity in those being studied. These have been reviewed by Buskirk & Barlett (1975). In the so-called 'Pickwickian Syndrome' of extreme obesity, hypoventilation is associated with a decreased expiratory reserve volume and less frequently with a decreased vital capacity. Compliance of the chest wall is decreased (Naimark & Cherniak, 1960; Sharp *et al.*, 1964), work of breathing is increased and ventilation-perfusion abnormalities exist. All of these abnormalities of pulmonary function are thought to be secondary to the increased adipose tissue mass in the thorax and abdomen and are reversible by weight reduction.

Such severe abnormalities are present in only about 10 per cent of severely obese subjects and in the moderately obese pulmonary function is usually normal. Buskirk & Barlett (1975) suggest that varying degrees of abnormality of pulmonary function occur in the obese population depending on both the amount and distribution of the excess adipose tissue. In the absence of underlying cardiopulmonary disease, abnormalities should be reversible by a combination of weight reduction and physical conditioning.

Obesity is also associated with changes in the cardiovascular system, most of which are reversible by weight reduction (Alexander, 1975). There is an increase in cardiac output and oxygen consumption at rest which roughly parallels the increase in body weight. Cardiac hypertrophy occurs and blood volume, stroke volume and cardiac work are all increased. Left ventricular function may be impaired, and in severe cases, congestive heart failure may be manifest.

With weight reduction there is a decrease in total body oxygen consumption, blood volume, cardiac output, stroke volume and cardiac work. Systemic vascular resistance is unchanged because of a proportional decrease in mean arterial pressure and cardiac output. Left ventricular and diastolic pressure remains elevated during exercise, suggesting that cardiac hypertrophy may not be reversed by weight reduction or at least not as rapidly as the other parameters.

Obesity is considered by most to be a significant risk factor for coronary artery disease (CAD), either alone or in association with other factors such as hypertension, hypercholesterolemia and impaired glucose tolerance. Mortality and morbidity rates for cardiovascular disease are significantly higher in obese populations. Thus, underlying CAD may be a limiting factor to exercise in obesity. On the other hand, physical conditioning may be of benefit in reducing the disability of CAD in obesity by increasing maximum work capacity and efficiency of performing a given work load (Saltin, 1969). Although it is not yet clear whether or not physical conditioning results in a decreased incidence of CAD, survival rates following myocardial infarction may be improved in the physically fit individual (Paffenberger & Hale, 1975).

One of the most striking metabolic abnormalities in obesity is the association of hyperinsulinemia and insulin resistance. Decreased responsiveness to insulin is manifest in adipose tissue (Salans, Knittle & Hirsch, 1968), muscle (Rabinowitz & Zierler, 1962) and liver (Felig *et al.*, 1974) and is frequently associated with impaired carbohydrate tolerance. Whether or not insulin deficiency (absolute or relative) plays a major role in the ability to perform physical exercise has been a topic of some interest. During prolonged work of moderate or high intensity, plasma insulin falls significantly despite an increase in glucose uptake and metabolism by the exercising muscles (Pruett, 1970*b*; Wahren *et al.*, 1971). In physically conditioned patients with well-regulated diabetes mellitus, energy metabolism during exercise on a bicycle ergometer was found by Pruett & Maehlum (1973) to be similar to that of trained non-diabetic subjects over a wide range of intensities (20 to 90 per cent $\dot{V}O_2$ max). Although endurance was generally somewhat less in the diabetics, blood glucose concentration decreased similarly in both groups of subjects and hypoglycemia was the principal cause for termination of exercise when working at 50 per cent $\dot{V}O_2$ max. At higher intensities, carbohydrates contributed a greater percentage of energy in the diabetics and hypoglycemia was not the limiting factor to endurance as often as it was in non-diabetics.

Recovery of muscle glycogen stores following exhaustive exercise has also been compared in normal and diabetic subjects with no significant differences between the two groups observed (Maehlum, Histmark & Hermansen, 1977).

Using a perfused hind-limb preparation in the rat, Berger, Hagg & Ruderman (1975) demonstrated that insulin has a permissive effect with respect to the stimulation of glucose uptake in muscle by muscular contraction. This observation was subsequently borne out in studies of metabolic and hormonal effects of exercise in insulin-dependent diabetics with or without withdrawal of insulin. In moderately controlled diabetics, exercise induced a marked fall in blood glucose and an increase in the concentrations of free fatty acids, ketone bodies and glucagon similar to that seen in non-diabetic controls. Diabetics with ketosis secondary to insulin withdrawal exhibited increased blood glucose concentrations during exercise and rapid acceleration of ketosis (Berger *et al.*, 1977). Thus, 'permissive' amounts of insulin appear to be necessary for normal muscle metabolism and metabolic fuel homeostasis during physical exercise.

A final area of concern regarding the capacity of obese individuals to perform strenuous physical work relates to the question of mechanical and metabolic efficiency. It is well known that the energy required to lift and move the body weight increases in a linear fashion as body weight increases (Mahadeva, Passmore & Woolf, 1953; Miller & Blyth, 1955; Passmore, 1956). Thus, the heavier an individual is, the greater the amount of energy which will be expended in performing weight-bearing tasks. There has been a question, however, whether or not obesity imposes a handicap during non-weight-bearing exercise. In studies of cardiopulmonary function, oxygen transport and the physiological cost of performing external work on the bicycle ergometer, Dempsey *et al.* (1966*a*) found that obese subjects expended significantly more energy per unit work load than did lean subjects. Oxygen consumption increased linearly with increasing work load and was parallel to but higher in the obese than it was in the lean subjects, resulting in a lower calculated mechanical efficiency. In these studies, however, the calculation of mechanical efficiency did not take into account the oxygen cost of unloaded pedalling. As shown by Whipp *et al.* (1975), the parallel shift of the oxygen consumption curve generated by a progressive increase in work load can be accounted for by the work required to move the additional mass during unloaded pedalling and when one corrects for this, there is no change in the calculated mechanical efficiency after gain in weight. Thus, it is concluded that the increased metabolic cost of exercise observed in obesity is not the result of a decrease in muscular efficiency but is secondary to the increased cost of performing a given amount of external work. This may be related to a combination of factors including increased body mass, decreased muscular coordination, a 'hobbling effect' imposed by obesity or increased energy expended to maintain posture.

In addition to a higher oxygen cost of performing external work, obese subjects have a decreased maximal oxygen uptake capacity when expressed per kg body weight, suggesting a lower level of physical conditioning. When expressed per kg lean body mass, $\dot{V}O_2$ max has been found to be normal or decreased (Dempsey *et al.* 1966*a*; Buskirk & Taylor, 1957). Thus, obese individuals expend more energy to perform a given task and have less total capacity for exercise than normals.

Both acute gain in weight and acute ingestion of food result in higher oxygen uptake during work than under control conditions (Whipp *et al.*, 1975; Bray, Whipp & Koyal,

1974). The increased oxygen consumption in the former circumstance can be related to the increased weight and the work efficiency remains normal. Hanson (1973) studied work efficiency in normal volunteers before and after overfeeding a mixed diet and a 19 per cent increase in body weight (Sims *et al.*, 1973) and did not find any decrease in work efficiency. In this study the increased cost of work correlated with increased body weight.

The increased oxygen consumption observed during exercise after food ingestion appears to be an exercise-induced potentiation of dietary-induced thermogenesis (Miller, Mumford & Stock, 1967) and can be explained largely but not entirely by the increased resting metabolic rate which occurs (Goldman *et al.*, 1975). Further study is needed to clarify this phenomenon. Other factors which could potentially affect work capacity in the obese include the added energy requirement imposed by decreased lung volumes and decreased efficiency of breathing (Dempsey, 1966*b*). Heat dissipation may also be a problem.

Role of exercise in weight reduction

Despite the several factors which contribute to a decreased capacity for physical exercise in obesity, there are several real and potential benefits of employing increased exercise and physical conditioning in its treatment. These include increased energy expenditure, decreased hunger, a change in body composition with decreased adipose tissue and increased lean body mass, cardiovascular conditioning, and metabolic and physiological effects (Horton, 1975).

Of greatest importance to the present discussion are the effects of physical training on the cardiovascular system and on the metabolic abnormalities associated with obesity. Training results in an increased maximal work capacity and increased physiological efficiency of performing a given work load (Saltin, 1969), two functions which are usually decreased in obesity. Cardiovascular responses include a decreased pulse rate, both at rest and during exercise, an increased cardiac stroke volume and decreased peripheral vascular resistance. These result in a net decrease in cardiac work and a decrease in blood pressure (Hanson & Nedde, 1970). With training, a given work load is performed at a lower percentage of the individual's maximum aerobic capacity, oxidation of fatty acids provides a greater proportion of the energy for muscular metabolism (and carbohydrate less) and endurance is increased.

Physical training in obese subjects results in a decrease in both fasting and post-glucose plasma insulin concentration without any change in glucose tolerance (Björntorp *et al.*, 1970). This effect appears to be the result of improved tissue sensitivity to insulin. Plasma lipids are also decreased significantly, particularly triglyceride concentrations (Björntorp, 1972).

Numerous effects of physical training on muscle histology, composition and metabolism are now known (Pernow & Saltin, 1971). There is an increase in both the size and number of mitochondria (Gollnick, Ianuzzo & King, 1971; Morgan *et al.*, 1971) and a variety of biochemical adaptations occur in response to repeated endurance exercise. These have been reviewed recently by Holloszy & Booth (1976). Enzymes involved in the activation, transport and oxidation of long-chain fatty acids are increased as are mitochondrial enzymes of the citric acid cycle and respiratory enzymes involved in the oxidation of NADPH and succinate. The concentrations of myoglobin and cytochrome C are also increased. In addition, enzymes involved in glucose uptake and storage by muscle are increased. These include increased activity of hexokinase, glycogen synthetase and glycogen branching enzymes.

There is very little effect, however, on enzymes of the glycolytic pathway and, in fact, the rate of glycolysis is slower in trained muscle than in untrained muscle at the same rate of oxygen utilization. Thus, the major features of the adaptation of muscle to endurance training are an increase in the capacity for aerobic metabolism of both fatty acids and glucose, an increase in enzymes for glycogen storage, but no increase in the capacity for glycolysis. The result is that at a given submaximal intensity of work and oxygen consumption there is a relative increase in the rate of fatty acid oxidation and a decrease in glucose oxidation.

These findings agree with physiological observations in man that the mixture of metabolic fuels utilized at a given work intensity are affected by physical training. There is an increase in maximum oxygen uptake ($\dot{V}O_2$ max), the respiratory quotient (RQ) at the same work load is reduced, indicating that a greater percentage of energy production is derived from fatty acid oxidation, and the rate of muscle glycogen depletion is reduced. This is associated with an increase in endurance (Pernow & Saltin, 1971).

Metabolic fuels and dietary effects

The two primary fuels which provide energy for muscular work are fats and carbohydrates. The proportion of each which is metabolized depends on both the intensity and duration of the work performed (Felig & Wahren, 1975). At low levels of intensity, the major source of energy is derived from oxidation of fatty acids, and as the work level increases a greater proportion of energy is contributed by glucose oxidation. At or near the maximal aerobic capacity, a level of exercise which can be maintained for only a relatively short time, glucose derived from either muscle glycogen stores or from the circulation, becomes virtually the exclusive fuel for muscle metabolism.

During the first 5 to 10 minutes of exercise the rate of glycogenolysis in muscle is rapid and muscle glycogen is the major source of the glucose oxidized (Hultman, 1967). As exercise continues, muscle blood flow increases as does the uptake of glucose and free fatty acids. The former requires permissive concentrations of insulin and is possibly dependent on other, as yet unidentified, circulating factors whereas the uptake of fatty acids is proportional to their concentration.

After approximately 40 minutes of exercise, circulating glucose, derived from hepatic glycogenolysis and gluconeogenesis provides the majority of carbohydrate fuel (75 to 90 per cent) consumed by muscle (Wahren *et al.*, 1971). Glucose utilization continues to increase until exercise has continued for approximately 3 hours and then it declines slightly, presumably due to depletion of muscle and liver glycogen stores and the inability of gluconeogenesis to keep pace with the demand. Concomitantly, there is a progressive increase in uptake of fatty acids by muscle so that during prolonged exercise, energy derived from fatty acid oxidation may be twice that derived from glucose (Ahlborg *et al.*, 1974).

In association with increased metabolism in exercising muscle, there is an increase in the release of both pyruvate and alanine (Felig & Wahren, 1971). The branched-chain amino acids (valine and iso-leucine) are released from the splanchnic bed (Ahlborg *et al.*, 1974) and are preferentially taken up and oxidized by muscle, providing energy for muscle contraction and serving as amino-group donors for synthesis of alanine from pyruvate.

As hepatic glycogen stores diminish, gluconeogenesis increases approximately threefold and is associated with increased hepatic extraction of gluconeogenic substrates including alanine, lactate, pyruvate and glycerol.

At submaximal work loads (eg, 65 to 75 per cent max $\dot{V}O_2$) endurance may be limited by either local muscle fatigue (as in bicycle pedalling by untrained individuals) or by subjective exhaustion. Although the mechanism of the latter phenomenon is not fully understood, it is probably due to a failure to provide adequate glucose supplies to muscle to meet the requirements for energy production or to the development of systemic hypoglycemia (Knuttgen, 1969; Havel, 1971). Hermansen, Hultman & Saltin (1967) found that the possible duration of exercise prior to exhaustion is dependent on the initial muscle glycogen content and that exhaustion occurs when this reaches a critical low level. One may achieve the highest values of muscle glycogen content by exhausting exercises, which deplete muscle glycogen stores, followed by refeeding with a diet high in carbohydrate.

The mixture of metabolic fuels utilized at a given work intensity is affected by the level of physical training. In the trained individual there is an increase in maximum aerobic power ($\dot{V}O_2$ max) and compared to an untrained individual a given task is performed at a lower percentage of maximum working capacity. This is associated with a lower respiratory quotient, indicating that a greater percentage of energy production is from fatty acid oxidation and less from carbohydrate. There is a 'protective' effect on muscle glycogen stores, the rate of glycogen depletion being reduced and endurance increased (Pernow & Saltin, 1971).

On the basis of these observations one would predict that varying the composition of the diet would have measurable effects on muscular working capacity, particularly at high intensity where muscle glycogen stores and glucose availability via hepatic glycogenolysis and gluconeogenesis are not sufficient to meet the demands for energy production. In 1939, Christensen & Hansen first observed an effect of the antecedent diet on the capacity to perform endurance exercise. After 3 to 7 days of a high carbohydrate intake, subjects were able to work for 210 minutes at a fixed work load, whereas after an equal time on a high fat diet, they were able to perform the same work for only 80 minutes.

Bergstrom *et al.* (1967) studied the ability to exercise at 75 per cent of $\dot{V}O_2$ max after 3 days on either a high carbohydrate or a high protein-fat diet compared to an uncontrolled standard diet. The average work times to exhaustion were 189, 59 and 126 minutes respectively and endurance correlated well with the initial muscle glycogen content, total carbohydrate utilization and the decrease in muscle glycogen content during exercise. It was thus concluded that muscle glycogen content is affected by diet and is a major determinant of the capacity to perform long-term strenuous exercise.

In studies in which subjects were fed diets of varying compositions for 2 weeks, Pruett (1970*a*) found that at work loads of 70 per cent $\dot{V}O_2$ max, subjects living on a high fat diet had shorter work times than subjects eating either a standard or high carbohydrate diet. She postulated that at relatively high work levels, subjects taking a high fat diet may experience depletion of muscle glycogen before depletion of hepatic glycogen stores and that the rate of glucose transfer from blood to muscle is not high enough to maintain the required energy production. The critical work level at which this occurs is 65 to 75 per cent $\dot{V}O_2$ max.

More recent studies by Ahlborg *et al.* (1974) indicate that during exercise, the liver is the sole source of glucose delivered into the circulation and that the absolute rate of glucose release and the proportions which are derived from glycogenolysis and gluconeogenesis are dependent on both the duration and intensity of the exercise. During relatively mild, short-term exercise, total glucose output from the liver rises 25 to 100 per cent and the relative contribution from gluconeogenesis is approximately 15 to 25 per cent. During moderate to severe exercise, hepatic glucose output increases 100 to 400 per cent and the proportion derived from glycogenolysis increases to 90 to 95 per cent because of a failure of gluconeogenesis to keep up with the increased demand. Hepatic glycogen depletion during 10 minutes of severe exercise (800 to 1200 kg-m/min) amounts to approximately 18 grams.

On the basis of these studies, it seems reasonable that subjects fed isocaloric diets with very low carbohydrate content or hypocaloric diets, in which both total calories and carbohydrates are severely restricted, will experience decreased ability to perform high intensity exercise and will have less endurance at submaximal work loads. Bloom & Azar (1963) studied patients on 'carbohydrate-free diets' and found that they all complained of fatigue by the second day and did not have sufficient energy to continue normal activity after the third day of the diet. This is reminiscent of the studies by Kark, Johnson & Lewis (1945), in which Canadian troops were fed pemican (70 per cent fat, 30 per cent protein) while on field maneuvers in the subarctic in an attempt to determine if it would be a suitable emergency field ration for combat conditions. The experiment proved to be a disaster, since on the second day the ordinarily fit troops developed excessive fatigue and on the third day were too exhausted to complete ordinary operations. Examination on the fourth day 'revealed a group of listless, dehydrated men with drawn faces and sunken eyeballs whose breath smelled strongly of acetone'. In both of these studies, no period of adaptation to the low carbohydrate diet was allowed and it is not surprising that such dramatic changes in exercise tolerance were observed. It is possible, however, that such diets fed over a period of several weeks would result in adaptive changes in muscle metabolism which would allow a different mixture of fuels to be oxidized at a given work load. That this may be the case is suggested by the findings of Pruett (1970*a*) that subjects working at 50 per cent VO_2 max derived only 35 per cent of the energy produced from carbohydrate after 2 weeks on a high fat diet compared to 40 per cent on a standard diet and 50 per cent on a high carbohydrate diet.

Drenick *et al.* (1977) have recently studied energy consumption and metabolic substrates utilized during exercise in obese men fasted for 39 days. The work intensity was relatively low (25 to 30 per cent VO_2 max), but several subjects were able to maintain exercise for only 30 min. In contrast to the decrease in blood glucose normally seen during exercise in fed subjects, a moderate increase occurred in the fasted subjects suggesting that glucose production exceeded peripheral utilization. Arterial alanine concentration increased more than in fed subjects but urinary nitrogen excretion was unchanged. A relatively minor increase in free fatty acid concentration occurred despite a threefold increase in oxygen consumption during exercise and β-hydroxybutyrate concentration fell, consistent with increased utilization of fatty acids and ketones for energy production by muscle. Thus, it would appear that subjects adapted to fasting may utilize lipids more efficiently than fed subjects.

The studies reviewed above suggest that subjects fed isocaloric diets with very low carbohydrate content or hypocaloric diets, in which both total calories and carbohydrates are severely restricted, will experience decreased ability to perform high intensity exercise and will have less endurance at submaximal work loads. There is still a question, however, whether such diets fed over a period of several weeks will result in adaptive changes in muscle metabolism which will allow a different mixture of fuels to be oxidized at a given work load. Thus, a key question is whether or not muscle will adapt to derive a greater percentage of its energy from fatty acid oxidation during high intensity work. If such an adaptation does occur, the next question will be the nature of the mechanisms involved, either at the level of substrate availability, hormonal responses or adaptive changes within the muscle itself.

In order to determine the extent to which adaptation to a low carbohydrate diet can occur with respect to ability to perform submaximal endurance exercise, Drs Phinney, Hanson, Sims and I have recently studied a group of six moderately obese volunteers before and during treatment with a ketogenic diet providing 1.2 grams protein per kg ideal body weight fed as lean meat with supplements of potassium, calcium, vitamins and iron. The subjects were stabilized on a balanced, weight maintenance diet and maximum working capacity was determined on a treadmill. Endurance to the point of subjective exhaustion was measured at a work intensity of 57 to 74 per cent of maximum working capacity before starting the diet, after 1 week on the diet and again after 6 weeks on the diet. Steady state oxygen consumption and respiratory quotient were measured during each endurance test and glycogen content of the vastus lateralis muscle was determined before and immediately after exercise. Several substrate and hormone concentrations in blood were also measured.

The results of this study, which are still preliminary, can be summarized as follows: compared to the baseline study, there was a 20.5 per cent decrease in endurance after 1 week on the ketogenic diet. This was associated with a significantly lower pre-exercise blood glucose concentration and a greater decrease in glucose during exercise, although this did not reach hypoglycemic levels. The pre-exercise muscle glycogen content was also significantly decreased compared to the baseline study and fell significantly during exercise. The RQ during steady state exercise was unchanged, indicating no major shift in substrate utilization during exercise. After 6 weeks on the diet, however, a significant adaptation had occurred. Endurance was found to be 55 per cent greater than during the baseline study despite the fact that the subjects wore a backpack equivalent to the weight which had been lost. The RQ during exercise was significantly lower, blood glucose concentration fell only slightly during exercise, and muscle glycogen content, which was intermediate between the values observed at baseline and after 1 week on the diet, remained constant during the period of exercise. Thus, glucose homeostasis was maintained and the major source of energy for muscular work was derived from lipid oxidation.

Although these are preliminary results, they suggest that man can adapt to a ketogenic diet and retain the ability to perform endurance exercise of moderate intensity under such conditions.

Summary

Obviously, many questions remain to be answered regarding the ability of obese individuals to perform strenuous physical exercise and the role of physical exercise in weight reduction and weight maintenance programs. In studies to date, no inherent defects in energy metabolism have been discovered in obesity and several real and potential benefits of increased physical exercise for the obese have been identified. Much additional work needs to be done to clarify the changes in energy balance and metabolism, which accompany increased physical activity, and to determine the potential benefits and hazards of combining diet and exercise programs in the treatment of obesity. Additional studies on the ability of obese individuals to maintain normal or increased levels of physical activity while on diets severely restricted in carbohydrate or in total calories and the safety of such regimens are clearly needed.

Acknowledgement – This work was supported in part by USPHS grants RR109 (General Clinical Research Center) and AM10254 (Dr Sims).

References

Ahlborg, G., Felig, P., Habenfeldt, L., Hendler, R. & Wahren, J. (1974): *J. Clin. Invest.* **53**, 1080.
Alexander, J.K. (1975): Effects of weight reduction on the cardiovascular system. In *Obesity in perspective,* ed G.A. Bray, p. 233. Washington DC: US Govt. Ptg. Office.
Apfelbaum, M., Boudon, P., Lacatis, D. & Nillus, P. (1970): *Press Med.* **78**, 1917.
Apfelbaum, M., Bostasarron, J., Lacatis, D. & Duret, F. (1972): *Israel J. Med. Sci.* **8**, 867.
Berger, M., Berchtold, P., Cuppers, H.J., Drost, H., Kley, H.K., Muller, W.A., Viegelmann, W., Zimmermann-Telschow, H., Gries, F.A., Kruskemper, H.L. & Zimmerman, H. (1977): *Diabetologia* (in press).
Berger, M., Hagg, S. & Ruderman, N.B. (1975): *Biochem. J.* **146**, 231.
Bergstrom, J., Hermanse, L., Hultman, E. & Saltin, B. (1967): *Acta Physiol. Scand.* **71**, 140.
Bistrian, B.R., Blackburn, G.L., Flatt, J.P., Winterer, J., Cochran, D. & Young, V. (1975): *Clin. Res.* **23**, 315A.
Blackburn, G.L. & Flatt, J.P. (1972): Protein-sparing therapy in semi-starvation. Ph.D. Thesis, M.I.T., Cambridge, Mass.
Björntorp, P. (1975): Effects of physical conditioning in obesity. In *Obesity in perspective,* ed G.A. Bray, p. 397. Washington DC: US Govt. Ptg. Office.
Björntorp, P., deJounge, K., Sjöström, L. & Sullivan, L. (1970): *Metabolism* **19**, 631.
Björntorp, P., Fahlen, M., Grimsby, G., Gustafson, A., Holm, J., Renstrom, T. & Shersten, T. (1972): *Metabolism* **21**, 1037.
Bloom, W.L. & Azar, G.J. (1963): *Arch. Int. Med.* **112**, 333.
Bloom, W.L. & Eidex, M.F. (1967): *Metabolism* **26**, 679.
Bray, G.B., Whipp, B.J. & Koyal, S.N. (1974): *Am. J. Clin. Nutr.* **27**, 254.
Bullen, B.A., Reed, R.B. & Mayer, J. (1964): *Am. J. Clin. Nutr.* **14**, 211.
Buskirk, E.R. & Barlett, H.L. (1975): Obesity and pulmonary function. In *Obesity in perspective,* ed G.A. Bray, p. 225. Washington DC: US Govt. Ptg. Office.
Buskirk, E.R. & Taylor, H.L. (1957): *J. Appl. Physiol.* **11**, 72.
Christensen, E.H. & Hansen, O. (1939): *Scand. Arch. Physiol.* **81**, 160.
Dempsey, J.A., Reddan, W., Balke, B. & Rankin, J. (1966*a*): *J. Appl. Physiol.* **21**, 1815.
Dempsey, J.A., Reddan, W., Rankin, J. & Balke, B. (1966*b*): *J. Appl. Physiol.* **21**, 1807.
Drenick, E.J., Fisler, J.S., Johnson, D.G. & McGhee, G. (1977): *Int. J. Obesity* **1**, 49.
Felig, P. & Wahren, J. (1971): *J. Clin. Invest.* **50**, 2703.
Felig, P. & Wahren, J. (1975): *New Engl. J. Med.* **293**, 1078.
Felig, P., Wahren, J., Hendler, R. & Brundin, T. (1974): *J. Clin. Invest.* **53**, 582.
Goldman, R.F., Haisman, M.F., Bynum, G., Horton, E.S. & Sims, E.A.H. (1975): Experimental obesity in man. VII. Metabolic rate in relation to dietary intake. In *Obesity in perspective,* ed G.A. Bray. Washington DC: US Govt. Ptg. Office.
Gollnick, P.D., Ianuzzo, C.D. & King, D.W. (1971): Ultrastructural and enzyme changes in muscles with exercise. In *Muscle metabolism during exercise,* ed Pernow & Saltin, p. 69. New York: Plenum Press.
Hanson, J.S. (1973): *J. Appl. Physiol.* **35**, 587.
Hanson, J.S. & Nedde, W.H. (1970): *Circulation Research Suppl.* **1**, 26.

Havel, R.J. (1971): Influence of intensity and duration of exercise on supply and use of fuels. In *Muscle metabolism during exercise,* ed Pernow & Saltin, p. 315. New York: Plenum Press.
Hermansen, L., Hultman, E. & Saltin, B. (1967): *Acta Physiol. Scand.* 71, 129.
Holloszy, J.O. & Booth, F.W. (1976): *Ann. Rev. Physiol.* 273.
Horton, E.S. (1975): The role of exercise in the prevention and treatment of obesity. In *Obesity in perspective,* ed G.A. Bray, p. 62. Washington DC: US Govt. Ptg. Office.
Hultman, E. (1967): *Scand. J. Lab. Clin. Invest.* 19, (Suppl), 94, and 209.
Johnson, M.L., Burke, B.S. & Mayer, J. (1959): *Am. J. Clin. Nutr.* 4, 39.
Kark, R.M., Johnson, R.E. & Lewis, J.S. (1945): *War Medicine* 7, 345.
Knuttgen, H.G. (1969): *Medicine and science in sports* 1, 1.
Lutwak, L. & Coulston, A. (1975): Activity and obesity. In *Obesity in perspective,* ed G.A. Bray, p. 393. Washington DC: US Govt. Ptg. Office.
Maehlum, S., Histmark, A.T. & Hermansen, (1977): Synthesis of muscle glycogen during recovery after prolonged severe exercise in diabetic and non-diabetic subjects. *Scand. J. Clin. Lab. Invest.* (in press).
Mahadeva, K., Passmore, R. & Woolf, B. (1953): *Am. J. Physiol.* 28, 225.
Miller, A.T. & Blyth, C.S. (1955): *J. Appl. Physiol.* 8, 139.
Miller, D.S., Mumford, P. & Stock, M.J. (1967): *Am. J. Clin. Nutr.* 20, 1223.
Morgan, T.E., Cobb, L.A., Short, F.A., Ross, R. & Gunn, D.R. (1971): Effects of long term exercise on human muscle mitochondria. In *Muscle metabolism during exercise,* ed Pernow & Saltin, p. 87. New York: Plenum Press.
Naimark, A. & Cherniak, R.M. (1960): *J. Appl. Physiol.* 15, 377.
Paffenberger, R.S., Jr. & Hale, W.E. (1975): *New Engl. J. Med.* 292, 545.
Passmore, R. (1956): *Am. J. Clin. Nutr.* 4, 692.
Pernow, B. & Saltin, B. (1971): *Muscle metabolism during exercise,* ed Pernow & Saltin, New York-London: Plenum Press.
Pruett, E.D.R. (1970*a*): *J. Appl. Physiol.* 28, 199.
Pruett, E.D.R. (1970*b*): *J. Appl. Physiol.* 29, 155.
Pruett, E.D.R. & Maehlum, S. (1973): *Scand. J. Clin. Lab. Invest.* 32, 139.
Rabinowitz, D. & Zierler, K.L. (1962): 41, 2173.
Salans, L.B., Knittle, J.L. & Hirsch, J. (1968): *J. Clin. Invest.* 47, 153.
Saltin, B. (1969): *Med. and Sci. in Sports* 1, 50.
Sharp, J.T., Henry, J.P., Sweaney, S.K., Meadows, W.R. & Pietras, R.J. (1964): *J. Clin. Invest.* 43, 728.
Sims, E.A.H., Danforth, E., Jr., Horton, E.S., Bray, G.A., Glennon, J.A. & Salans, L.B. (1973): *Recent Prog. Horm. Res.* 29, 457.
Wahren, J., Felig, P., Ahlborg, G. & Jorfeldt, L. (1971): *J. Clin. Invest.* 50, 2715.
Whipp, B.J., Bray, G.A., Koyal, S.N. & Wasserman, K. (1975): Exercise energetics and respiratory control in man following acute and chronic elevation of caloric intake. In *Obesity in perspective,* ed G.A. Bray. p. 157. Washington DC: US Govt. Ptg. Office.
Yang, M.U. & Van Itallie, T.B. (1976): *J. Clin. Invest.* 58, 722.

34
Some psychiatric aspects of obesity

A.H. CRISP
Academic Department of Psychiatry, St. George's Hospital Medical School, London S.W.17, England.

The presumed origins of obesity in terms of disturbed energy balance, feeding behaviour and physical activity have usually been examined in the experimental laboratory. Can reductionist concepts developed in the laboratory ever be translated into human experience? Conversely, can such research as there is be dissected into its components of primary and secondary experiences of gain and/or loss (eg, pleasure, unpleasure) and be reexamined biologically, behaviorally and socially in respect of feeding, various kinds of related and specific activity (eg, foraging, sexual activity, rest), arousal, energy balance and fatness itself in the human. Certainly it is when such a variety of potential personal experience of the obese clash within the individual and produce the dissonance that precipitates a search for help or change, that we as clinicians are given the special chance to study the mechanisms involved.

From the laboratory standpoint, Mayer, after a lifetime's study of the subject, was still claiming in 1970 that the psychological effects of obesity were at least as important and probably more universal than were the psychological factors leading to it. He suggested for instance that obesity often caused depression in the young adult but was doubtful about depression causing obesity. Since then there has been a spate of new research into the area of energy balance and control of feeding by the central nervous system, including its perceptual and behavioural aspects in the human being. Workers such as Booth (1976) have dismissed the centralist/peripheralist controversy within the organism as being unproductive and irrelevant, but have insisted on the scientific need to retain mechanistic models for the purposes of research. Booth doubts whether the field is yet at a point of maturity wherein environmental approaches to appetite and research on food intake can be integrated with the organismic peripheral and central approaches. These comments, expressed at the Dahlem conference on appetite and food intake, can be set against the group report also presented at the meeting by those concerned with feeding behaviour and the central nervous system (Blundell *et al.*, 1976). In their proposals for further research they warn that feeding behaviour cannot be studied in isolation - satiety is associated with such effects as grooming behaviour and sedation, and is intimately related to sleep. Hervey (1973) too, has emphasised the role of inactivity in generating obesity through a delay in the shift in regulatory mechanisms in accommodating the former, which he claims is now often characteristic of our life-style. He contented himself with commenting on present day inactivity in our technological society associated with such areas as work and sedentary entertainment. It would seem that feeding and the obese state may also, in complex ways, contribute to such areas of human existence and experience as sexual activity and adjustment, and to the search for reduction of anxiety.

Meyer, Pudel and their group have been studying the hyperphagic response in humans for a number of years (Meyer & Pudel, 1977). Their populations have included both weight-disordered and normal weight subjects. Hyperphagia, of course, occurs commonly both amongst the adolescent incipiently obese (eg, 'compulsive eaters') and the massive obese seen in the medical clinic, often as a reported feature of their current lives and/or their earlier lives. Indeed, it is often the experience for which the decompensated obese attending the clinic are most urgently seeking help. They fear an endless cycle of impulsive overingestion and weight gain with progressive obesity, increasing humiliation and ever-diminishing self-esteem. In this group, overeating in childhood often seems at a clinical level to have been accentuated in association with the challenge of adolescence. Rapid biological growth as a byproduct of the childhood overnutrition, pubertal plumpness and initial low self-esteem have set the scene. Of course, the decompensated anorectic who has often previously been obese, with poor adolescent impulse control, and who has now relapsed into greater than ever hyperphagia, has, by vomiting and purging to excess, found one desperate solution to the problem of shape control in the face of overwhelming appetite, but at the price of continued high energy expenditure and its associated anticipatory sexual perils for them (Crisp, 1967, 1977; Garrow *et al.,* 1976). Thus, hyperphagia is not exclusive to the obese, nor do we know how common it is amongst the millions of uncomplaining obese.

Meanwhile the Meyer/Pudel group, using the food dispenser technique first developed by Stunkard (Rodin, 1976) have found hyperphagia to characterize not only obese patients but also potential or latent obese people (those with a history of weight disorder and including erstwhile anorectics). Moreover, they have advanced our thinking on the matter of externality as a characteristic of the obese, first put forward by Schacter (see Rodin, 1976). Thus obese adults often remain potentially hyperphagic. They often hyperrespond to palatable foods (Wooley *et al.,* 1976) and to the presence of available food, irrespective of time relationship to a previous meal and the level of anxiety (Abramson & Wunderlich, 1972). More recently many non-obese subjects, under certain conditions, have also been found to be very responsive to external signals in their eating behaviour. The Meyer/Pudel group conclude, endorsing Hilda Bruch's (1957) views, that 'the influence of cognitive factors on food intake is better defined (and more universally applicable) in terms of the size of the external/internal stimulus discrepancy.' They go on to claim 'normal subjects resolved this discrepancy in favour of the external cues only when the discrepancy was moderate, whilst obese subjects oriented themselves to the external cues in their eating behaviour especially when a large discrepancy existed between external and internal cues.' The respective concepts of externality and internality should not be exclusively associated with socially acquired habits on the one hand and genetico-biologically determined processes on the other. Both are aspects of the individual's present constitution and adaptations, shaped by genetic and past experiential influences.

This, then, is by way of preamble to the main theme of this paper - the experiential aspects of obesity itself. What are the experiences of the obese in respect of their obesity?

It is pertinent to start by reminding ourselves that many of us interested in the subject have a prejudice - we are opposed to obesity. We have been confronted by a tiny minority of the total obese population, mostly females, themselves dissatisfied by their state, and we have been able to convey the official medical view that obesity is associated with a higher than average morbidity. We have more often ignored the thin, except for the pathological condition of anorexia nervosa, forgetting that they too carry a high morbidity in relation to some conditions eg, peptic ulcer, schizophrenia and neurosis. In the last few years, researchers have begun to question such views. Obesity may be an epiphenomenon of a lifetime's programmed rapid growth, reproduction and decay, goes one argument (McCance & Widdowson, 1962; Crisp *et al.,* 1970). At least when present in relatively minor degree, obesity does not carry a higher than average morbidity after all, say others. Indeed, it causes a lower morbidity in the range 25 to 35 per cent above ideal weight. Only when it reaches the state where relative obesity is 160 per cent and above does increased morbidity and mortality characterize it, say Dyer and his colleagues (1975). Obesity in the general population is associated with less reported experience of anxiety and depression than average say others (Crisp & McGuinness, 1976). Moreover, Shakespeare's characters preferred their men fat and content rather than lean and grasping. Other ages have preferred and other cultures do prefer their women obese. In past times obesity has been seen as a sign of health - the opposite of wasting and disease; and as a sign of wealth. Perhaps we can pause to take stock once again of a few social and psychiatric factors possibly relevant to our own day and age and seen from a clinical and adaptational standpoint.

I will restrict myself to three areas of enquiry: (1) What do we know of the relationship between psychiatric morbidity and obesity? (2) Why is there such an excess of females amongst the clinic obese? (3) What may be some of the neurotic mechanisms operating amongst all those massively obese subjects, sometimes male as well as female, who reach our clinics?

Obesity and psychiatric morbidity

Hippocrates drew attention to the relationship between body build, shape, and temperament. More particularly Kretschmer (1936) claimed an association between the propensity for cyclothmyia and manic depressive psychosis and the pyknic habitus. The term pyknic was given by Kretschmer specifically to individuals with large visceral cavities and a tendency to fat on the trunk, especially its lower part, as well as slightly built shoulder girdle and slender extremities tapering to small hands and feet. This view, that a physique associated with obesity was more frequent in patients suffering with manic depressive illness than in the general population retained considerable support for some while (Mayer Gross, Slater & Roth, 1969). However, it has recently been challenged (Beck, 1967; Angst & Perris, 1972; Crisp, Stonehill & Koval, 1975; Crisp & McGuinness, 1976). A recent study of a psychiatric clinic population (Crisp & Stonehill, 1976) again showed no relationship between obesity and depressive illness but did reveal relationships between neurotic depression and tension states and thinness. In the same study approximately one-sixth of all patients were found to have gained a substantial amount of weight with their illness and one-sixth to have lost a substantial amount. Psychiatric patients showing such major fluctuations gave a history of having once been obese. A question arises: are the obese-unhappy the same population as the unhappy-obese? Certainly the linkage either way is not unduly common. Thus, in a general population study - the Mid-town Manhattan study (Moore *et al.*, 1962), only limited association was found between obesity and psychiatric status. Silverstone (1968) has reported that men who were 45 per cent or more above ideal weight reported less neuroticism than others, and Simon (1963) had earlier found much less depression amongst a group of obese service personnel than amongst their non-obese colleagues. More recently Crisp & McGuinness (1976) have found, in a general population study of middle-aged people, a significant relation between substantial obesity and low levels of anxiety (in men and women) and depression (in men), see Fig. 1. Moreover, there was no excess of neurotic avoidance or other defence mechanism amongst the obese population. In another general population survey (Crisp *et al.*, 1970), obese adolescents were found to be more assertive than their non-obese counterparts.

In summary, the majority of the evidence indicates that moderate degrees of obesity, say 20 to 50 per cent above ideal weight, are associated with low levels of dysphoria, at least in those aged 40 years and older. We do not know why this is so. Is the state of static obesity (ie this may imply that it is not associated with frequent hyperphagia) incompatible with or resistant to the experience of anxiety and depression? What might be the chemistry of this? Will our understanding of the chemistry one day illuminate for us such psychological concepts as denial, avoidance, sublimation? Is there a lower and fairly precise biological threshold of obesity below which experience of the self changes?

The large numbers of seemingly contented middle-aged moderately obese people presumably stem, in the main, from the populations of childhood and adolescent obese. How does the isolated, shy, inactive, excessively tense, obese child and the shape-conscious, plump female adolescent evolve into such an enviable middle-aged stereotype? We do not know. One could perhaps argue that, in revolutionary terms, and in line with Cahill's thesis (this volume), obese people have reason to be content, even smug. They have money in the bank, so to speak; they are well insulated. Only in terms of more modern social pressures, operating more on

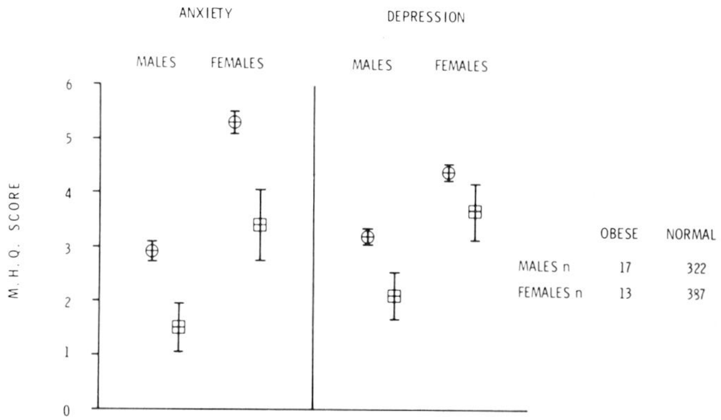

Fig. 1. A suburban general population study (subjects aged 40 to 65 years): mean (+ s.e.) MHQ scores for obese (□) and normal (○) groups (obesity defined from relative weight). There were 17 obese and 322 normal men and 13 obese and 387 normal women

young and mainly female people, might their contentedness sometimes now be challenged

If some psychiatric patients gain or lose a considerable amount of weight, during their illness, is this a simple function of altered food intake or activity, or does it have some more complex experiential significance? Has it to do with their attempts to resolve underlying emotional conflicts? Why and in what way and for what reason have their regulatory mechanisms changed? Can such a shift in basic metabolic rate and arousal be psychologically protective on a larger scale? Do some seek, experientially, through hyperphagia and weight gain, an increasing internal orientation consequent on the accompanying reduced arousal, together with increased basic metabolic rate; others the reverse? Such populations should be especially fruitful of study.

Finally, the findings suggest that the sub-populations of the obese who confront us in the clinic, at least those who are middle-aged, are very different from the mainstream of the obese. They are usually highly self-selected. They are strikingly characterized by being female and usually by being massively obese. Often their obesity is progressive, presumably due to long-term failure of regulation of energy balance or its more recent decompensation.

Sex ratios in the clinic obese

Why, then, such an excess of females? Firstly, obesity is more common amongst females than males in most present day Western societies and this is especially so in the lower social class segment of society. Indeed, it contrasts strikingly with anorexia nervosa in this latter respect. Such obesity is, of course, also superimposed on the basically greater amount of fat present in the normal weight adult female compared with her male counterpart.

For the female, fatness seems to be complexly bound up with her sexuality, both biological and social. Puberty is the time when this is first declared. Reaching puberty earlier than the male, she finds her shape beginning to change under the influence of hormones governing new fat deposition which confer upon her and those around her a sense of her biological ripeness and readiness for reproduction. Such fat, it has been argued, reflects, in evolutionary terms, a necessary foetal food reserve in the face of unpredictable food supplies during gestation. At the same time it commands the attention of the male. By the age of 17, whether in Europe or North America (Heunemann *et al.,* 1966; Nylander, 1971), the majority of young women are striving to reduce their fatness. Clearly not all of them are obese in a statistical or medical sense. Fashion is not a sufficient explanation. Fashion, I suggest, merely reflects the underlying needs and conflicts of people in society. Seemingly often rooted in such needs as conformity and the search for increased self-esteem, but probably more fundamentally related to the search for more general and personal impulse-control in our increasingly free, unstructured society, it can, if some weight is lost and shape changed to major egodystonic proportions, serve instead merely to deepen the female adolescent existential uncertainty. Order and control can them be salvaged without other resource for some, who find security in the avoidance behaviour through biological regression that is the essence of anorexia nervosa. The vast majority, however, continue to struggle on, changing little in shape and remaining sensitive about it. Not until the mid-twenties, after the die has been cast in terms of marriage, motherhood, and other life roles, do many cease to be concerned about their shape. However, shape may remain some kind of concern to be rekindled at times of crisis. Perhaps it survives more strongly in those middle-aged obese women who still hope to become thinner. In them it often seems to be that their main concern is their hyperphagia.

The majority of men, whilst sometimes admiring non-obese women in real life and/or in the girlie magazines, feel much less concerned about obesity in their own sex. Moreover, male fatness is not often condemned by the female. The adolescent male will often have been more preoccupied with increasing his bulk than with reducing it. The male with a hearty appetite is often admired.

Neurosis and obesity

Finally then, what may be some of the neurotic mechanisms operating amongst those hyperphagic and obese, usually massively obese subjects, sometimes male but usually female and middle-aged, who reach our clinics?

There is, of course, an extensive and conflicting literature, largely psychiatric, concerning the changes in mood following prolonged dietary restriction in the obese. Both Bruch (1957) and Stunkard (1957) in early papers, reported a high incidence of depression in obese clinic populations after prolonged dieting and weight loss. More recently Stunkard (1974), reviewing the literature, finds confirmation of this view.

Meanwhile, other investigators have studied a wider range of affective and behavioural characteristics in such populations. Thus Robinson & Winnik (1973) report a variety of psychotic reactions amongst obese patients losing substantial amounts of weight. Glucksman & Hirsch (1968) noted that body image disturbances persisted among the chronically obese despite major weight reductions. Other have reported increased sexual activity in their patients after major weight loss, which sometimes seemed to rekindle latent social problems. Indeed, our own group (Crisp, 1967; Crisp & Stonehill, 1970; Kalucy & Crisp, 1974) has emphasised the importance of massive obesity in some cases for the promotion of sexual inactivity and associated resolution of sexual conflict. Glucksman & Hirsch (1968) describe an increase in anxiety and depression during and after weight loss, while an initial increase in hostile aggressive behaviour disappeared once the subjects were stabilised at the lower weight and were again eating normally. They and Crisp (1967) suggest that there are both non-specific symptoms due to starvation and also specific symptoms which arise in the fat-reduced obese person and which are related to individual character structure and the pattern of personal relationships.

Meanwhile, others (Crisp & Stonehill 1970) have also found that obese patients, after major weight loss achieved by dieting combined with psychotherapy (with weight reductions of around 50 kg), were characterised not so much by depression as by a loss of the capacity to deny their inter-personal problems. When these were considerable, and personal relationships particularly barren, then relapse rapidly ensued. These workers thought that there was a critical weight threshold below which such denial was no longer achieved and that this was about 25 per cent or so above normal weight. They described patients whose biological and perhaps optimal psychosocial status appeared to be consonant with a moderate degree of obesity but who had 'decompensated'. This had often occurred in adolescence, in relation to such experiences as loss (provoking greater hyperphagia) or sexual conflict (for which the immobility of massive obesity became protective). Treatment, of a combined dietetic and psychotherapeutic kind, was aimed at restoring a moderate degree of obesity. The existence of such a weight threshold was also proposed by Glucksman & Hirsch (1968). In contrast to this, Solow, Silverfarb & Swift (1974), and Kalucy & Crisp (1974) in a preliminary study, found that massively obese people, losing weight after ileojejunal bypass, showed little tendency to develop depression, but there were often major changes in their life-styles which affected people living with them. They concluded that food deprivation, to which the bypass patients losing weight were apparently not exposed, might be an important factor generating depression in those losing weight through restriction of diet. Moreover, these patients remained moderately obese, above the threshold level described above.

This leads me finally to report briefly some findings from our latest study which have been salutary for us. Our study involved the psychosocial and psychobiological monitoring of 26 massively obese subjects (22 female, four male), inevitably highly self-selected as well as being considered suitable on medical and surgical grounds, who underwent ileojejunal bypass surgery. They were studied before operation and at four, 12, 24 & 48 months following surgery. This prospective study had been designed to succeed our first retrospective investigation in this area reported in 1974 (Kalucy & Crisp, 1974). This second population was studied with particular interest since the confident expectation now was that it would provide an opportunity to investigate the experiential accompaniments of major weight loss and shape change in the absence of dietary restriction. In the event, as we subsequently reported (Pilkington *et al.*, 1976), we were to learn that the majority of weight lost, which happens in the first six months post-opertaively, was due to reduced food intake. Thereafter, weight begins to level out in association with increasing food intake, and more normal eating patterns supervene. Some of our findings have already been reported in detail elsewhere (Kalucy *et al.*, 1975, 1976; Crisp *et al.*, 1977). Briefly, weight loss at two years was 44 ± 10 kg (range 18-84 kg), the population previously having been 2.06 ± 0.28 overweight (expressed in terms of ideal weight).

Pre-operatively, the psychoneurotic status of the population was similar to that of a psychoneurotically ill population with high levels of anxiety, depression, social avoidance mechanisms and somatic complaint. Such experience had not infrequently been the basis of the complaint to the doctor by the patient, who had often attributed it to her obesity. Frank psychiatric morbidity, when searched for carefully, was quite common in the histories of such patients.

The purpose of the study was twofold: (1) To identify any experiential and behavioural changes in the patients as they lost weight, and also in those most closely related to them. (2) To search for experiential, behavioural and social factors affecting outcome.

Behavioural/experiential changes in the patients and others

At the six-month follow-up, when it will be remembered that most patients were eating very little and losing weight rapidly, the majority were miserable and complaining, some bitterly, about their inability to eat because of the effect of various foods in either causing vomiting or diarrhoea.

However, at the one-year and again the two-year follow-up, the majority of patients were less anxious and less depressed, although still more so than the majority of normal weight people. However, they showed a more marked and statistically significant diminution in social avoidance behaviour and functional somatic complaint.

The majority now experienced a much more normal appetite. They were much less prone to hyperphagia and were able to eat once more with the rest of the family.

Other important changes seemed to be linked to this even more than to the weight loss and shape change. Thus their sense of self-esteem and of autonomy was much greater. They had frequently become more assertive and more demanding of those around them.

The importance of the bypass in all this seemed to have been : (a) To have prevented them eating much at all for six months, thus permitting weight loss. (b) Possibly to have contributed to the major change in their appetite experience in the long term, via radical modification of gastro-intestinal tract regulators (Smith & Gibbs, 1976). (c) To provide a continued significant degree of malabsorption.

Within this context, the psychological changes, when they occurred, could be said to have been forced. Rapid retreat from change back into hyperphagia and obesity was very difficult.

Most patients also became much more active and some became very active sexually. This behavioural change was mirrored in and probably to some extent based in a return towards normal of their gonadotrophic function and its biological concomitants (Fig. 2). Such changes sometimes threaten existing relationships - some marriages deteriorated. One patient in particular became panicky, guilty and depressed.

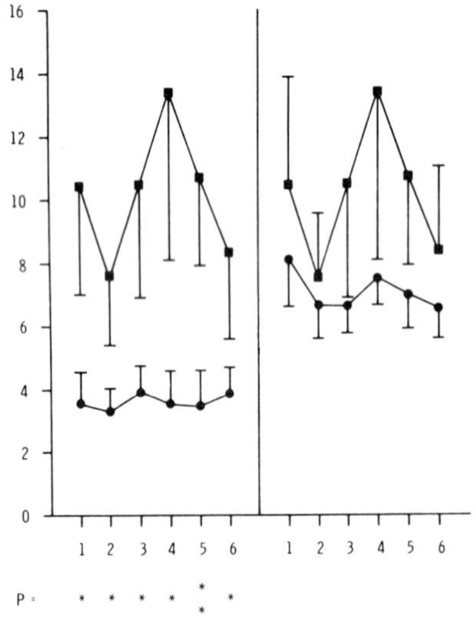

Figure 2. Nocturnal profiles of plasma LH levels in 14 patients: (a) with massive obesity compared with normal weight subjects(left hand side of figure).(*$p<0.05$;**$p<0.02$); (b) The same patients two years after ileojejunal bypass (right hand side of figure). Post-operatively the levels are significantly more normal. (Based on work reported elsewhere: Kalucy *et al.*, 1976)

These patients' attitudes to and experience of their shape changes were very variable in some respects. For some the change was not important or else only important for its convenience eg, buying clothes. For others it was as rewarding as the amelioration of their appetite disorder. A most striking finding now emerged concerning their reports of their body widths. They continued to grossly overestimate them but, as a group, came to identify an ideal shape for themselves that was larger than they now were. More moderate obesity in the absence of hyperphagia was no longer viewed negatively by the majority.

Only a few patients could not, it seemed, cope with their reduced size. They now felt more insignificant and even less effective. Two such female patients managed to gain substantial amounts of weight, overeating despite the discomfort. In one of them the bypass was abolished on her insistence. The few males in the series were less happy with their reduced shape. They tended to lose more weight than the females. Two older men felt much more frail and vulnerable and wished they had not lost so much weight. The two younger men became more sociopathic.

Our conclusion at this point was that for a minority of our patients at least, obesity had been an important and immutable aspect of their psychological adjustment, probably conferring both primary and secondary gain.

Predictors of outcome

Our search in this respect was not all that fruitful. It is possible to say that: (1) A history of psychiatric illness and current high levels of psychoneurotic disability are not contra-indications to treatment, except that current high levels of social avoidance behaviour were associated with poor outcome. (2) Such patterns and associated social isolation characterized some of the less obese amongst the population. They had been particularly insistent on having the operation despite our doubts. They appeared especially to be ascribing their sense of inferiority entirely to their fatness. The two female patients described above who did particularly badly fell into this category, both having lost substantial amounts of weight in the first instance.

(3) In contrast, a previous history on having been sociable and extrovert was associated with a good prognosis.

In summary then it can be said that at least some obese people become depressed if they do not eat for a prolonged period. This is not specific to the obese but it may happen more frequently amongst them; we do not know.

Hyperphagia characterizes massively obese females seeking help, and reduction of this is associated with greatly increased psychological well-being.

Most such patients welcome a reduction in their obesity but its elimination is not often crucial to their well-being. Indeed, many prefer to remain moderately obese.

We do not know how relevant these findings are to the majority of obese individuals in the general population who do not come to us seeking change.

Conclusions

In my view we still need to know more about the following: (1) The way that large numbers of contented middle-aged obese (25 to 40 per cent above ideal weight) are related to those teased, isolated, unhappy, obese children/young adolescent females. (2) The way that the massively, progressive, decompensated obese and those amongst them who complain bitterly about this, are related to the moderately obese population and the uncomplaining obese population. (3) When obesity is experienced as unwanted, what are its overall experimental and social correlates? (4) To what extent is hyperphagia also a feature of the contented obese population, and to what extent is the propensity for hyperphagia exclusive to the obese population overall? (5) What are the correlates and precipitants of hyperphagia, expressed both experientially and biochemically in the human? How are the latter related to the interaction between biological and social stimuli?

Two main areas of research will, therefore, continue to be important. They are: (1) Surveys of the general population, broken down by age, sex, social class, birth order, in respect of (a) obese status: past/present; (b) psychological status including personality structure; (c) hyperphagic status. (2) Studies in depth of small numbers of subjects; for example (a) psychiatric patients whose weights and fat status change markedly within the context of their illness, seeking for relationships in them between mood, activity and eating, including shifts in the direction and size of the internal/external stimulus discrepancy. What for instance, as I have discussed earlier, distinguishes those whose weight rises from those whose weight falls? (b) patients with anorexia nervosa. What for instance distinguishes those who maintain low weight control by abstaining from those who do so by hyperphagia and compensatory vomiting/purging.

References

Abramson, E.E. & Wunderlich, R.A. (1972): *J. Abnorm. Soc. Psychol.* 79, 317.

Angst, J. & Perris, C. (1972): *Int. J. Ment. Health* 1, 145.

Beck, A.T. (1967): *Depression*, p. 128. London: Staples Press.

Blundell, J.E. and many others (1976): The CNS and feeding Group Report 1. In *Appetite and food intake*, Dahlem Conference Proceedings, ed T. Silverstone, p. 109. Berlon: Abakon.

Booth, D.A. (1976): Approaches to feeding control. In *Appetite and food intake*, Dahlem Conference Proceedings, ed T. Silverstone, p. 417. Berlin: Abakon.

Bruch, H. (1957): *The importance of overweight.* New York: Norton.

Crisp, A.H. (1967): *J. Psychosom. Res.* 11, 117.

Crisp, A.H. (1977): *Proc. R. Soc. Med.* 70, 464.

Crisp, A.H., Douglas, J.W.R., Ross, J.M. & Stonehill, E. (1970): *J. Psychosom. Res.* 14, 313.

Crisp, A.H., Kalucy, R.S., Pilkington, T.R.E. & Gazet, J-C. (1977): *Am. J. Clin. Nutr.* 30, 109.

Crisp, A.H. & McGuinness, B. (1976): *Br. Med. J.* 1, 7.

Crisp, A.H. & Stonehill, E. (1970): *J. Psychosom. Res.* 14, 327.

Crisp, A.H. & Stonehill, E. (1976): *Sleep, nutrition and mood.* London: Wiley.

Crisp, A.H., Stonehill, E. & Koval, J. (1975): The pyknic habitus in psychiatric illness. In *Recent advances in obesity research: I*, ed A. Howard, p. 199. London: Newman.

Dyer, A.R., Stamler, J., Berkson, D.M. & Lindberg, H.A. (1975): *J. Chron. Dis.* **28**, 109.
Garrow, J.S. and many others (1976): Pathology of eating - Group Report 4. In *Appetite and food intake*, Dahlem Conference Proceedings, ed T. Silverstone, p. 405. Berlin: Abakon.
Glucksman, M.L. & Hirsch, J. (1968): *Psychosom. Med.* **30**, 1.
Hervey, G.R. (1973): Physiological mechanisms of energy balance. In *Symposium on anorexia nervosa and obesity*, p. 7. Royal College of Physicians, Edinburgh, Publication No. 42.
Huenemann, R.L., Shapiro, L.R., Hampton, M.C. & Mitchell, B.E. (1966): *Am. J. Clin. Nutr.* **18**, 325.
Kalucy, R.S. & Crisp, A.H. (1974): *J. Psychosom. Res.* **18**, 465.
Kalucy, R.S., Crisp, A.H., Chard, T., McNeilly, A., Chen, C.N. & Lacey, J.H. (1976): *J. Psychosom. Res.* **20**, 595.
Kalucy, R.S., Solow, C., Hartmann, M., Crisp, A.H., McGuinness, B. & Kalucy, E.C. (1975): Self-reports of estimated body widths in female obese subjects with major fat loss following ileojejunal bypass surgery. In *Recent advances in obesity research: I*, ed A. Howard, p. 331. London: Newman.
Kretschmer, E. (1936): *Physique and character*, 2nd edn. London: Kegan Paul.
Mayer, J. (1970): Some aspects of the problems of regulating food intake and obesity. In *Anorexia nervosa and obesity*, ed C.V. Rowland, p. 255. Boston: Little, Brown.
Mayer Gross, W., Slater, E. & Roth, M. (1969): *Clinical psychiatry*, 9th edn. London: Bailliere, Tindall & Cassel.
McCance, R.A. & Widdowson, E.M. (1962): *Proc. R. Soc. Med.* Series B, **156**, 326.
Meyer, J-E. & Pudel, V.E. (1977): *Psychosom. Med.* **39**, 153.
Moore, M.A., Stunkard, A.J. & Srole, L. (1962): *J. Am. Med. Ass.* **181**, 962.
Nylander, I. (1971): *Acta Sociomed. Scand.* **3**, 17.
Pilkington, T.R.E., Gazet, J-C., Ang, L., Kalucy, R.S., Crisp, A.H. & Day, S. (1976): *Br. Med. J.* **1**, 1504.
Robinson, S. & Winnik, H. (1973): *Archs Gen. Psychiat.* **29**, 559.
Rodin, J. (1976): The role of perception of internal and external signals on the regulation of feeding in overweight and nonobese individuals. In *Appetite and food intake*, Dahlem Conference Proceedings, ed T. Silverstone, p. 265. Berlin: Abakon.
Silverstone, J.T. (1968): *Proc. R. Soc. Med.* **61**, 371.
Simon, R.I. (1963): *J. Am. Med. Ass.* **183**, 208.
Smith, G.P. & Gibbs, J. (1976): What the gut tells the brain about feeding behaviour. In *Appetite and food intake*, Dahlem Conference Proceedings, ed T. Silverstone, p. 129. Berlin: Abakon.
Solow, C., Silverfarb, P.M. & Swift, K. (1974): *New Engl. J. Med.* **290**, 300.
Stunkard, A.J. (1957): *Am. J. Med.* **23**, 77.
Stunkard, A.J. (1974): *Ann. Int. Med.* **81**, 526.
Wooley, S.C. and many others (1976): Psychological aspects of feeding - Group Report 3. In *Appetite and food intake*, Dahlem Conference Proceedings, ed T. Silverstone, p. 331. Berlin: Abakon.

35
The physiology of fasting and semistarvation: roles of 'caloristat' and 'aminostat' mechanisms

E. B. MARLISS
Division of Endocrinology and Metabolism, Department of Medicine,
University of Toronto, Toronto, Ontario, M5S 1A8, Canada.

The intact organism has a system of precisely-regulated mechanisms which function to maintain equilibrium between fuel economy and protein metabolism. This homeostatic system assures that if a deficit in external supply of calories occurs, it is made up from endogenous stores. Conversely, caloric excesses are stored in the form of lipid. Protein homeostasis requires that exogenous protein be supplied. The amino acids required for protein synthesis are directed into these pathways, and any excess carbon skeletons are converted to carbohydrate and fat for storage. The nitrogen is excreted. No specific 'storage' form of protein appears to exist. Thus, there appears to be a mechanism for monitoring body protein status and signalling to the appropriate tissues that excesses or deficits exist.

The mechanisms of fuel homeostasis may operate through a 'caloristat', and those mediating protein homeostasis through an 'aminostat'. Their interrelationships are schematized in Fig. 1. The operation of such mechanisms is relevant to obesity in two ways. First

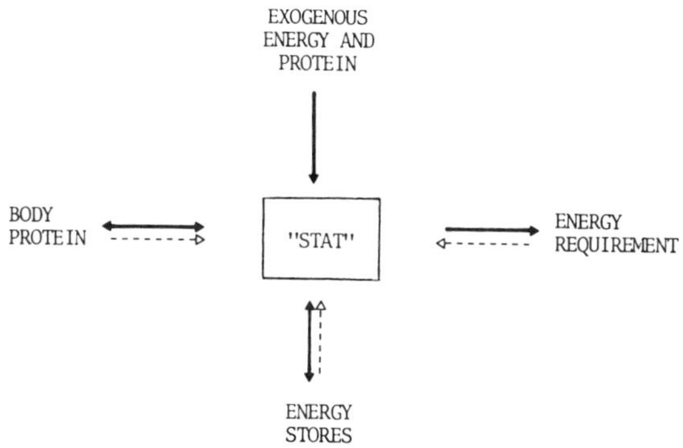

Fig. 1. The 'caloristat-aminostat'. Solid arrows represent direction of fluxes of energy and protein; broken arrows indicate the presence of mechanisms whereby the states of body protein, energy stores and energy requirement are communicated to the 'stat', which subsequently effects responses appropriate to exogenous input

there appears to be no limit to the storage of excess calories or protein as fat. Second in the treatment of obesity, the optimal modalities should remove the excess fat without loss of essential protein. Thus, understanding of the mechanisms of fuel and protein homeostasis is critical to improved comprehension of obesity and its treatment. This review attempts to identify and describe the operation of the postulated 'caloristat' and 'aminostat'. Since fuel homeostasis may be most simply summarized by reference to the fasted state, the responses to prolonged total fasting are described in detail. The fed state is considerably more complex, and is influenced both by the amounts of energy and protein delivered and their route of delivery. Therefore, these are reviewed under headings considered to represent variables contributing to the operation of the 'caloristat-aminostat'. These will be summarized under six headings: (1) protein, (2) calories, (3) hormones, (4) the patient, (5) vitamins, cofactors and trace metals, and (6) time (Table 1). Emphasis is placed upon the responses to protein when there is no other source of energy since this approach forms the basis of the currently popular 'protein-sparing modified fast' as a therapy for obesity. An analogous review in relation to metabolic responses to parenteral nutrition has been published recently (Marliss, 1977).

Table 1. Factors in energy and protein homeostasis

(1) Protein Amount Quality	(4) The patient Prior State Fuel Demand Concurrent Illness
(2) Calories Amount Type	(5) Trace substances Vitamins Cofactors Metals
(3) Hormones Insulin-glucagon Others	(6) Time

Metabolic responses to the fasted state

Figure 2 presents the principal fuel stores and the flux of energy substrates in a normal adult fasted 24 h. As reviewed elsewhere by Cahill (1970, 1971), the principal fuel stores are protein in muscle as the source of most readily mobilizable amino acids (6 kg, 24 000 kcal, in a 70 kg male); fat, as the adipose organ (15 kg, 140 000 kcal); and carbohydrate, principally as hepatic glycogen (0.15 kg, 600 kcal). Over 24 h of fasting, the caloric requirement has

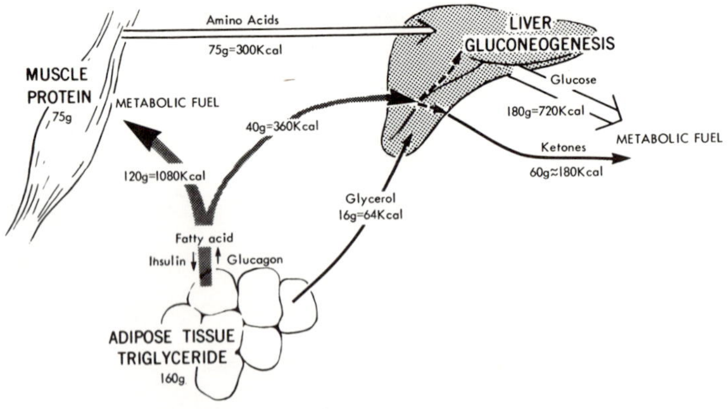

Fig. 2. Fuel fluxes during total fasting in normal man

been set at 1800 kcal for this idealized person. The fundamental requirement of the brain for 600 kcal, as glucose, has been interpreted as the major determinant of minimum glucose production (150 g) by the liver. Additional obligate glycolytic tissues require 40 g of glucose, recycled as lactate, pyruvate (and alanine) in the Cori cycle, with no net gain or loss of carbon atoms.

The sum of these metabolic processes sets the obligate lower limit of endogenous glucose production which must come from glycogenolysis and gluconeogenesis. The portion from glycogenolysis can only be estimated by the gap between glucose output and the sum of the uptake of individual gluconeogenic substrates (Chiasson *et al.*, 1975). Based upon estimates of regional substrate exchange and nitrogen excretion, the contribution of amino acids as gluconeogenic substrates would be about 75 g/24 h (Table 3, column 1). The 'alanine cycle' of glucose metabolism to pyruvate in muscle, transamination and return of alanine to liver has been reviewed (Felig, 1973). Branched chain amino acids have been shown to be a quantitatively important source of the amino groups (reviewed by Adibi, 1976). The remainder of the gluconeogenic substrate is provided as glycerol released during lipolysis in adipose tissue, amounting to 16 to 40 g/24 h depending upon the technique employed (summarized in Streja *et al.*, 1977).

During fasting, the major metabolic fuel is derived from adipose tissue triglyceride. Those tissues which can adapt to either fatty acid or ketone utilization then derive their energy primarily from fatty acids, which amounts to 120 g/24 h (1100 kcal). The liver also derives its energy from oxidation of fatty acids, and in doing so converts 60 g/24 h of FFA into 'ketone bodies', acetoacetate and 3-hydroxybutyrate. (Control of ketogenesis has been the subject of another recent review by McGarry & Foster, 1975). The ketone bodies form part of the available fuel, although a part is lost in the urine.

Control over the adaptation to fasting is exerted principally by insulin (Cahill, 1970, 1971), secondarily by the interaction of insulin and glucagon (Unger, 1971; Liljenquist *et al.*, 1977), and with 'permissive' effects by a wide variety of hormones whose levels may or may not change (see Table 2). In the absence of exogenous nutrients, circulating glucose levels decline, and combined with a variety of other influences result in lowering the insulin levels (Table 3). This decline results in augmented lipolysis in adipose tissue (reflected in increased circulating free fatty acids (FFA) and glycerol) and release of amino acids from muscle protein. The liver takes up more fatty acids and gluconeogenic substrate for energy supply, for ketogenesis and for gluconeogenesis, Glycogenolysis is activated and supplies the glucose not provided by gluconeogenesis. Glucose is utilized primarily by the central nervous system and obligate glycolytic tissues, and the rest of the organism utilizes fatty acids and to a lesser extent ketone bodies.

The role of glucagon in the regulation of energy flux during fasting has been largely based upon measurement of endogenous levels (Aguilar-Parada, Eisentraut & Unger, 1969; Marliss *et al.*, 1970), the effects of exogenous hormone (Marliss *et al.*, 1970; Liljenquist *et al.*, 1974; Felig, Wahren & Hendler, 1976), and influences based upon known metabolic effects. With the advent of somatostatin, experiments in which both insulin and glucagon could be selectively replaced after suppression of endogenous secretion have allowed for more direct dissection of the role of glucagon (Liljenquist *et al.*, 1974, 1977; Cherrington *et al.*, 1976; Gerich *et al.*, 1976; Vranic *et al.*, 1976). With this technique it has been shown that a fall in insulin alone will not cause the same increment in hepatic glucose output, and probably not the same degree of ketogenesis, as would occur physiologically with either basal or increased

Table 2. Humoral regulation of energy and protein homeostasis

A. Primary regulators

- Insulin
- Insulin-glucagon relationship

B. Modulators

Pituitary
- Growth Hormone
- ACTH, Prolactin, TSH

Adrenal
- Glucocorticoids
- Catecholamines

Reproductive Organs
- Estrogens
- Androgens
- Placental lactogen

Thyroid
- Throxine (T_4)
- Triiodothyronine (T_3)
- reverse triiodothyronine (rT_3)

Other
- Somatomedins
- Somatostatin
- Growth factors
- Gut hormones

Table 3. Typical hormone-substrate patterns and nitrogen balance in the fasted and fed states.

	Total fasting				Fed ('isocaloric')					Fed (hypocaloric)						
Column	1	2	3	4	5	6	7	8	9	10	11	12	13	14	15	16
Day	0	3	7	21	7	7	7	7	7	14	7 (Refed)	3	3	3	3	3
Nutrient input																
Protein (g/kg/d)							1	1	1	0.8	0.8		1	2	1	1
Glucose (kcal/kg/d)					20		40	7	20			10			10	
Lipid (kcal/kg/d)						30		33	20							10
Route					PO	PO	IV	IV	IV	PO	PO	IV	IV	IV	IV	IV
Substrates																
Glucose (mg/dl)	94	76	72	77	92	83	107	118	104	86	87	118	90	94	122	96
Lactate (mmol)	0.84	0.80	0.77	0.89	1.46	0.72	1.88	0.87	1.10	0.70	0.90	1.09	0.78	0.88	0.98	0.77
Pyruvate (mmol)	0.07	0.06	0.04	0.05	0.14	0.05	0.14	0.08	0.10	0.06	0.07	0.11	0.07	0.08	0.10	0.08
Alanine (μmol)	415	254	192	194	572	246	420	230		193	191					
Free Fatty Acids (μmol)	521	750	1216	1257	575	886	243	1322	490	747	866	341	618	570	428	759
Glycerol (μmol)	133	152	245	232	195	213	213	331	250	213	228	110	240	135	120	96
3-hydroxybutyrate (μmol)	192	1697	4223	4898	45	2731	43	726	180	2569	2919	122	1290	420	214	1405
Acetoacetate (μmol)	46	436	960	910	21	712	49	371	100	517	654	56	574	240	105	644
Urine 3 HB (mmol/d)	0	63	117	118	0.1	91				36	40					
Hormones																
Insulin (ng/ml)	1.2	0.51	0.35	0.58	0.84	0.62	2.07	0.50	0.65	0.51	0.58	1.30	0.66	0.62	1.67	0.71
Glucagon (pg/ml)	89	105	110	78	146	124	162	227	170	101	85	203	296	260	208	307
Nitrogen balance																
g/d	-14.5	-12.0	-9.4	-5.7	-4.7	-6.8	+2.4	+2.5	+2.6	-0.8	+2.3	-10.0	-4.8	+2.0	-5.0	-5.0
3-methylhistidine excretion (μmol/d)	174		139	117	172	159				249	254					
Data from reference No. *			6	3	6	6	1	1	2	3	3	4	4	5	4	4

* The data were obtained from the following references: 1. Jeejeebhoy *et al.*, 1975, 2. Jeejeebhoy *et al.*, 1976, 3. Marliss *et al.*, 1978, 4. Greenberg *et al.*, 1976, 5. Jeejeebhoy, 1977, and 6. Hanna *et al.*, 1978.

glucagon levels. In the presence of sustained or increased insulin, however, the responses to glucagon are different, and may be suppressed entirely (Felig *et al.*, 1976). Although pharmacologic amounts of glucagon exert a lipolytic effect on the liver and on the periphery (Lefebvre, 1972), a clear role in fat mobilization in man remains to be established.

The roles of other hormones in the adaptation to fasting have been the subject of detailed study, but exhaustive discussion is beyond the scope of this review. As listed in Table 2, a multitude of interacting humoral factors play a role. These are classified as 'modulators', a term which is employed in a fashion which might also be characterized as 'permissive'.

When fasting is prolonged beyond the first 24 h, a variety of additional adaptations occur (Table 3, columns 2 to 4). After 2 weeks of fasting, circulating FFA, glycerol and ketone bodies reach maximum levels, and the endogenous protein mobilization is minimized. This adaptation is due to the conversion of certain ordinarily obligate glucose-consuming tissues (notably the central nervous system) to the oxidation of ketone bodies (Owen *et al.*, 1967). The decreased requirement for glucose is translated into a decrease in the release of amino acids from protein stores, mainly muscle (Felig *et al.*, 1970; Cahill, 1970). This decrease occurs progressively even after hormone levels have reached a steady-state. Insulin falls to a nadir by day 5 and the transient elevation of glucagon has peaked by day 7. Despite this curtailed endogenous loss of protein, there appears to be an asymptote for the loss of nitrogen which is rarely less than -5 g daily (Table 3) (Owen *et al.*, 1969). This is partly due to the rate of hepatic gluconeogenesis (43 per cent of total), but also due to the augmented renal production of glucose and ammonia (30 per cent) associated with the chronic metabolic acidosis.

The contribution of muscle catabolism to this nitrogen loss in fasting obese subjects has been estimated by Young *et al.* (1973) using the excretion of 3-methylhistidine. They calculated that on the third day of fasting 26 g of nitrogen would be produced from muscle protein. This decreased to 17 g by day 20. However, only 12 g total nitrogen were excreted on day 3, and 5.6 g on day 20, suggesting that protein reutilization increases in prolonged fasting (67 per cent *vs* 53 per cent). This may be an important component of the mechanism of protein conservation in this state.

Thus in prolonged total fasting, the total energy requirement must be obtained by mobilization of endogenous fuels. At the outset, glycogen is mobilized and supplies are rapidly exhausted. Subsequently glucose is provided from gluconeogenic precursors by hepatic gluconeogenesis. Concurrently, mechanisms begin to develop for sparing protein. The tissues which can adapt to oxidize ketone bodies begin to do so, and thus the glucose requirement is decreased, and protein is spared. In operational terms, the 'caloristat' results in a set of adaptations to provide the requisite energy primarily from the expendable stores of fuel. Concurrently, the 'aminostat' operates to allow for the early mobilization of protein as requisite gluconeogenic substrate. Once the adaptation to ketone body utilization has occurred, curtailment of this protein loss supervenes.

Metabolic responses to the fed state

In principle, exogenous nutrients should provide substrates in amounts as least sufficient to sustain fluxes detailed above for the early fasted state, in order to maintain equilibrium of body constituents. During intake of exogenous nutrients the 'caloristat-aminostat' (Fig. 1) operates to integrate the status of body protein and the energy stores, to direct the incoming nutrients for oxidation, maintenance of protein mass, and restoration of any deficit in either protein or energy stores. Excess energy is processed for storage as lipid. The known determinants are considered in more detail below.

Protein input

By the turn of the century, it had become axiomatic that protein equilibrium could not be attained without exogenous protein (reviewed by Munro, 1964). The only possible exception is the recent demonstration that the alpha-keto derivatives of amino acids may spare protein (Sapir *et al.,* 1974). This observation indicates that the 'essential' nature of certain amino acids resides in the carbon skeleton, and that the alpha-amino group is not essential. Both the quantity and quality of protein are recognized as determinants of the responses. The 'quality' of protein which relates to its amino acid composition and availability will not be discussed here. The quantity of protein required has been the subject of extensive review (World Health Organization, 1973). In the presence of adequate caloric supplies, a value of 0.5 g/kg/d in normal adults is generally considered adequate. When subjects receive 40 kcal/kg/d of total energy parenterally they achieve protein equilibrium (Fig. 3). Increasing the protein progressively gives greater positive nitrogen balance in patients, in whom treatment followed prior protein depletion. Values for 1 g/kg/d are shown in columns 7 to 9 of Table 3.

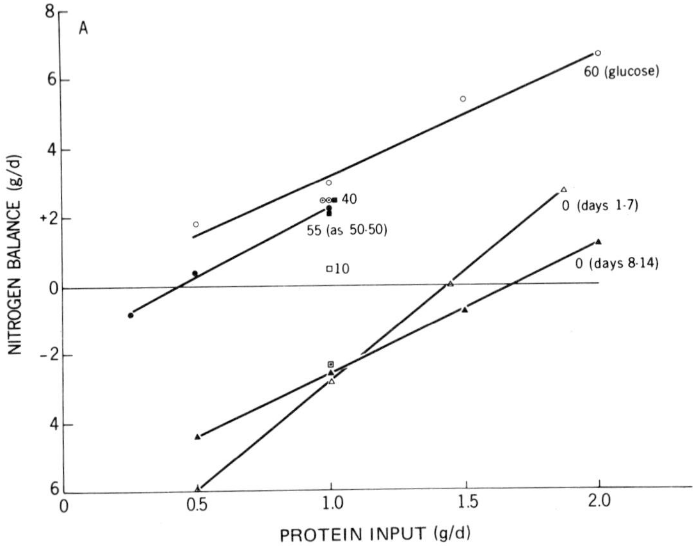

Fig. 3. Relationship of nitrogen balance to protein input in parenteral nutrition, at various levels of input of non-protein calories. Caloric input varies from 0 to 60 kcal/kg ideal body weight/d. The patients were not immediately postoperative except for one group ⊡ . The composition of the non-protein calories is as follows: 100 per cent glucose was given to the 10 □ and one 40 kcal group ⊙ ; 83 per cent Intralipid - 17 per cent glucose was given to one 40 kcal group ■ . The 55 kcal group ● received 50 per cent glucose - 50 per cent Intralipid, and the 60 kcal group ○ received 100 per cent glucose. Reproduced with the permission of Dr K. N. Jeejeebhoy

When exogenous energy is provided by protein alone, larger quantities of protein are required to achieve protein sparing. This was shown nearly 50 years ago by Strang, Evans & McCluggage (1930) and elaborated in detail during the past decade by several groups of workers (Apfelbaum, 1970; McLean Baird, Parsons & Howard, 1974; Genuth, 1973; Flatt & Blackburn, 1974; Blackburn *et al.,* 1975; Bistrian *et al.,* 1976; Howard & McLean Baird, 1977). It would appear that about 1 g/kg/d of high quality protein can produce nitrogen balance if given over a sufficient period of time (Table 3, column 10). With parenteral amino acid solutions alone, nitrogen balance is achieved after 7 d by about 1.7 g/kg/d with one commonly used formulation (Fig. 3 and reviewed by Jeejeebhoy, 1977). In protein-depleted patients, 2 g/kg/d produced sustained positive balance (Table 3, column 14).

The mechanism(s) whereby protein alone is able to result in body protein homeostasis remain unclear. Young *et al.* (1973) showed proportionally greater decreases in nitrogen than 3-methylhistidine excretion in fasting, providing evidence for concurrent decrease in catabolism and increase in reutilization of endogenous protein. Similar data are shown in

Table 3, columns 1 to 4, and in Fig. 4. For the constant protein input of 0.8 g/kg/d, data are presented in Table 3, column 10, and Fig. 4. The initial 3-methylhistidine excretion was twofold that of fasting, due to the protein consumed. (Mean day 1 excretion, without protein intake, is 170 to 230 μmol/day (Fig. 4). An increment in excretion of 1.4 μmol/g protein has been observed with differing protein intakes (Marliss, unpublished observations). After 7 d a progressive decrease of excretion was observed. The 50 per cent decrease by day 21, with

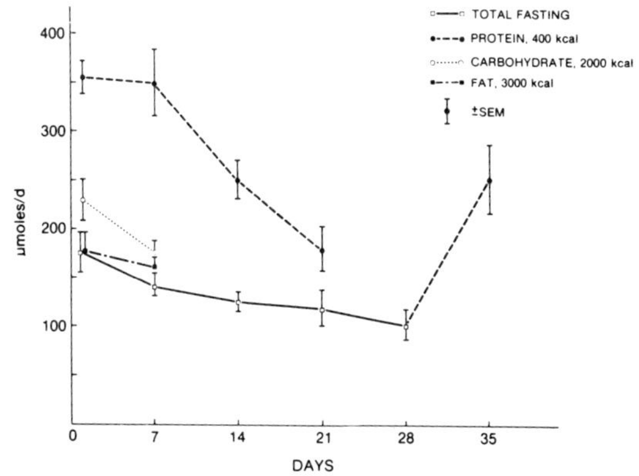

Fig. 4. 24-hour 3-methylhistidine excretion during prolonged total fasting and altered diets in obese, non-diabetic adults. Zero time is defined as the morning that each protocol began. The diets consisted of either protein alone (0.8 g/kg/d, 400 kcal/d, ●– – – – –●), carbohydrate as glucose (2000 kcal/d,O·········O, without protein), or fat (3000 kcal/d, X–·—·—·–X). In addition, the same protein diet was given as a refeeding regimen after 28 d of total fasting

constant exogenous input, is consistent with a considerably greater decrease in endogenous protein catabolism than in fasting (unless the absorption or excretion of dietary 3-methylhistidine were selectively altered). Such a decrease could account for the attainment of protein equilibrium, without increased reutilization, though the latter is not excluded. In both fasting and this diet, a concurrent decrease in the rate of protein synthesis must have occurred. When the same diet was given to 28-day fasted subjects for 7 d, positive nitrogen balance occurred, along with an increase in 3-methylhistidine excretion (Table 3, column 11 and Fig. 4). Since a greater catabolic rate existed prior to refeeding, and probably persisted (because the 3-methylhistidine excretion increased almost the amount predicted from the intake), the results suggest a greatly increased rate of reutilization.

Thus the data in both oral and parenteral nutrition with protein alone strongly support the notion of protein input being a major factor in determining protein homeostasis. Clearly, more direct measures of protein turnover in individual organs and the whole body are required (Waterlow, Garlick & Millward, 1977) for precise definition of the mechanisms involved. Both the techniques of nitrogen balance and 3-methylhistidine excretion give only indirect inferences as to the rates of these processes. The loss of body protein for energy production is reduced when energy (as either carbohydrate or fat) is provided at any given protein input, providing evidence for the close integration of 'aminostat' and 'caloristat' mechanisms.

Calorie input

The observation that carbohydrate spares protein dates back at least a century (Voit, 1869), but a systematic statement of the concept is most often credited to Gamble (1946-47). His data led to the use of solutions containing 5 per cent dextrose, in patients requiring intravenous nutrition. Protein sparing by glucose is demonstrated in Table 3. On day 3 of total fasting (column 3) the nitrogen balance is -12 g. Provision of glucose at 10 kcal/kg/d reduces this to -10 g (column 12) on day 3; 20 kcal/kg/d of glucose reduces this to -4.7 g (column 5) on day 7. Protein sparing by lipid alone, is also demonstrated. When 30 kcal/kg/d of triglyceride were given (column 6), unequivocal protein sparing occurred: -6.8 gN on day 7, as compared with -9.4 gN in fasting. Although more calories were given as lipid than as glucose (column 6 *vs* 5), better protein sparing was obtained with glucose. The difference of 2.1 gN on day 7 is precisely accounted for by the marked increase in ammonium nitrogen excretion associated with the ketoacidosis associated with lipid. These studies demonstrate that the 'caloristat' is capable of quantifying the energy input and responding to spare more protein when more calories are given. However, an obligate minimum daily protein loss persists, which varies between 4.7 and 6.8 gN. These values are not very different from the minimum of 5.7 gN for prolonged fasting (column 4). Somewhat lower minimum values have been reported with infusion of glucose during prolonged fasting (O'Connell *et al.,* 1974).

The mechanism of protein sparing by calories may be adduced in part from the 3-methylhistidine data (Fig. 4 and Table 3, columns 5 and 6). On the seventh day of fasting, 3-methylhistidine excretion was the same for fasting, carbohydrate and fat feeding. Although in each instance a modest fall occurred from values on day 1, the significantly lower nitrogen excretion in the fed subjects suggests that reutilization of endogenous protein was enhanced by energy provision.

The separate roles of dietary fat and carbohydrate given in the presence of exogenous protein have been studied in detail in both man and animals. Munro (1964) cites the studies of Rubner in 1903 and Neumann in 1919 as demonstrating that at a fixed nitrogen input, nitrogen balance becomes less negative or more positive by increasing the input of calories as either fat or carbohydrate. This interaction of protein and calories is dependent upon exogenous protein. Below a threshold supply of nitrogen, this dose-response effect of calories is less apparent, and analogous to the effects of energy supply without protein.

In comparing the effectiveness of fat and carbohydrate, it is clear that isocaloric amounts of fat are not as effective as carbohydrate, with a given protein intake, when energy is not limiting. An increase in nitrogen excretion of as much as 5 g/d occurs with a maximum at days 2 to 5 upon substituting fat for carbohydrate. When fat intake is continued for longer periods, however, equilibrium of nitrogen may be demonstrated. Studies of the interaction of carbohydrate and fat have shown a similar effect but of smaller magnitude. Interestingly, the effect of carbohydrate upon protein utilization is that carbohydrate must be available concurrently with the protein, or the energy-related benefit is not realized. This is not the case for fat (Munro, 1964). It is apparent from Fig. 3 and Table 3, columns 7 to 9, that significant differences between isocaloric glucose and lipid do not occur in parenteral nutrition. However, when lipid or glucose were substituted for each other sequentially, a transient (1 to 4 d) slight decrease in positive nitrogen balance was seen when lipid was given second. An equivalent transient increase in nitrogen balance was seen when glucose was second (Jeejeebhoy *et al.,* 1975). A transient increase in positive nitrogen balance was observed when a solution with 83 per cent lipid calories was followed by a solution of 50 per cent glucose and 50 per cent lipid, and a decrease in nitrogen retention when 100 per cent glucose preceded the 50/50 mixture (Jeejeebhoy *et al.,* 1976). The absence of larger differences between lipid and glucose may be related to the fact that a minimum of 17 per cent of calories were carbohydrate even when lipid was given.

Hormones

It has been classically taught that hormones are the central mediators of the responses to nutrients. Insulin has usually been assigned a prime role (Cahill 1970, 1971). The data in the following discussion confirm the responsiveness of insulin secretion to nutrients, but they also indicate that protein homeostasis can be achieved at widely divergent insulin and energy substrate levels.

The isocaloric fed state

After 7 d of oral glucose alone, the postabsorptive insulin levels decline, although plasma glucose levels do not decrease (Table 3, column 1 *vs* 5). Lactate, pyruvate and alanine levels are elevated, and free fatty acids are unchanged, although glycerol levels are moderately increased. Ketone body levels and excretion are suppressed. In contrast, feeding of fat is associated with fall in insulin and glucose, as well as alanine, and rise in FFA, glycerol and ketone bodies. The latter elevations are less than after 7 d of fasting (column 3). As already noted, nitrogen conservation is improved. In these two examples, protein sparing is associated with either no change or a fall in overnight-fasted insulin levels. Insulin levels following glucose feeding are considerably higher than in either fasting or feeding of fat.

With classical 'hyperalimentation' using hypertonic glucose as the sole energy source, extremely high insulin levels (fourfold postabsorptive) are observed in the presence of normal plasma glucose (column 7). Glucagon levels are unchanged from the postabsorptive state, perhaps reflecting the normal glucose levels, and suggesting that neither high rates of glucose infusion nor hyperinsulinemia are capable of suppressing glucagon secretion at normal glucose levels. Marked reduction of FFA and ketone body levels are apparent. The twofold elevation in lactate and pyruvate probably reflects the rate of glucose utilization perhaps combined with suppression of hepatic uptake.

The opposite extreme is seen with intravenous lipid (column 8). Insulin is maintained at postabsorptive levels; glucagon and plasma glucose are slightly elevated. FFA levels are equivalent to those after 7 and 21 d of total fasting (columns 3 and 4). Unlike fasting, however, there is only a modest increase in the levels of ketone bodies. The high levels of glycerol are presumably partly related to its presence in the infused intralipid^{R}. The mixture of 50 per cent lipid/50 per cent glucose produces hormone and substrate levels intermediate between the two extremes (column 9). A modestly elevated insulin and normal glucagon are associated with normal plasma glucose and postabsorptive levels of FFA and ketones. Glycerol is modestly elevated, and lactate levels are intermediate between the postabsorptive state and when glucose is given alone.

These data with isocaloric substitution of nutrients demonstrate that the hormonal response is determined by the input. Substrate levels in turn correspond in a predictable fashion to the input and resultant hormonal levels. We have demonstrated a significant negative correlation between nitrogen retention and insulin at levels of insulin between 0.1 to 0.5 ng/ml with calories primarily as lipid (Jeejeebhoy *et al.,* 1975). This correlation no longer existed at levels above 0.5 ng/ml, suggesting that a critical minimum insulin level exists for optimal nitrogen retention. In subjects receiving lipid, with insulin levels above 0.5 ng/ml, a significant positive correlation existed between FFA levels and nitrogen retention. This suggests that when optimal insulin levels are present, free fatty acid levels are the primary determinants of the magnitude of protein sparing. There is, thus, no clear 'anabolic' or 'catabolic' insulin/glucagon relationship. Although we have previously presented results of the 'insulin/glucagon molar ratios' these clearly do not have quantitative significance in assessing the metabolic state. For this reason, we consider the use of such ratios of qualitative interest only, except with rigorously defined experimental conditions (Unger, 1971).

The choice of the proportions of glucose and lipid for any given patient should be made in relation to his known or presumed ability to secrete insulin. Intravenous lipid would be preferable in known diabetics or individuals who have an impaired insulin secretion in response to glucose. The latter include patients with extensive injury or burns, or who are hypothermic. However, it is important to recognize the requirement for minimal levels of insulin even when lipid is the primary source of energy. Where there is any doubt, continuous infusion of insulin at about one unit per hour is desirable.

The roles of the 'modulator' hormones (Table 2) require detailed study in parenteral nutrition, although they have been quantified in a variety of models for oral feeding (Munro, 1964; Leathem, 1964). Of particular interest is the recent demonstration of dietary control of peripheral conversion of thyroxine, to triiodothyronine (T_3) or to inactivating pathways by conversion to reverse triiodothyronine (rT_3) (Chopra *et al.*, 1975). Altered thermogenesis in states where rT_3 is increased could well be of considerable importance in the response to nutrients (Danforth *et al.*, 1975). The advent of reliable assays for circulating catecholamines and their application to this area could also contribute important understanding of control of intermediary metabolism. Though listed in Table 2, the roles of somatomedins, somatostatin, growth factors, gut hormones, prostaglandins and other potential 'modulators' remain to be established (Munro, 1964; Leathem, 1964).

The hypocaloric fed state

The effect of infusing solutions of 5 per cent glucose for 3 d to postoperative patients is seen in Table 3, column 12 (Greenberg *et al.*, 1976). Plasma glucose is higher, and insulin levels are two to threefold greater than with fasting alone. This elevation in insulin is presumed to be the basis for the greater 'protein sparing' effect of this regimen than would be expected in fasted patients. This is also associated with a suppression in the levels of free fatty acids, glycerol and the ketone bodies (3-hydroxybutyrate, and acetoacetate).

Insulin levels in patients receiving 0.8 to 1.0 g/kg/d of protein alone remain below postabsorptive values after 3 d (column 13), and also after 14 d when without prior surgery or trauma (column 10). Plasma glucose is lower than with infusions of 5 per cent glucose. The combination of low insulin, and a relative or absolute increase in glucagon augment both hepatic gluconeogenesis and ketogenesis. With the small increases in FFA, ketone body levels also rise. This hormone-substrate milieu, combined with the exogenous protein, results in progressive curtailment of nitrogen loss and eventual nitrogen balance. The improved nitrogen balance is clearly the result of the supply of amino acids and corresponding availability of FFA and ketones. In patients receiving protein, the non-protein calories are provided primarily from endogenous fat, but at equal or higher insulin and lower FFA levels than during total fasting.

The comparison of these data on glucose and amino acid infusion suggests that rates of endogenous fat mobilization and utilization may not directly be estimated from circulating levels of FFA and ketones. This concept is contrary to the axiom that FFA uptake is concentration-dependent except in exercise.

Further evidence supporting this contention is presented in column 14. The administration of 2 g/kg/d of amino acids produces positive nitrogen balance on day 3 (and day 7, Jeejeebhoy, 1977) at glucose, insulin and glucagon levels that are not different from those in the patients receiving 1 g/kg/d. FFA levels are not elevated, and ketone bodies are only minimally increased above postabsorptive values. Because of the positive nitrogen balance, the caloric deficit must be met by endogenous mobilization of FFA. The prime determinant of nitrogen balance would appear to be the supply of amino acids. Although gluconeogenesis is undoubtedly stimulated (see nitrogen excretion data, Jeejeebhoy, 1977), the increase in ketogenesis which would ordinarily be expected is not apparent, at least as estimated by blood and urine levels.

The administration of 5 per cent glucose with 1 g/kg/d of amino acids (column 15) resulted in elevated levels of plasma glucose and insulin, and suppression of the levels of FFA and ketones. Not only do amino acids allow for protein sparing, but in spite of high levels of insulin, the caloric deficit (of 550 kcal) is provided from endogenous fat. If high levels of insulin are responsible for protein sparing, one must postulate a dissocation between inhibition of adipose tissue lipolysis, and inhibition of muscle proteolysis. Furthermore, it is a situation in which lipolysis and fat utilization occur at FFA levels below those observed in the postabsorptive state. Provision of lipid calories (column 16) in addition to amino acids results in higher FFA, and ketone body levels equivalent to those provided by amino acids alone. Nitrogen balance is similar to that with protein alone. The caloric deficit is made up once again from endogenous fat.

The patient

Many characteristics of the patient may be cited as factors in the response to protein and energy. Some are related to sex, age and anthropomorphic characteristics. Others are related to the generation of appropriate hormonal responses. For the sake of brevity, three groups of factors will be considered (Table 1).

Prior state

The state of depletion of body stores is a central determinant of the metabolic response. Whether one considers this as 'labile protein' or not (Munro, 1964), the presence of prior depletion renders the recipient more 'efficient' at retaining administered protein (Waterlow, 1969). Allison (1951) demonstrated that with a given level of protein intake, animals with prior depletion retained more than those which were normally fed. Many studies in humans have confirmed this finding, especially during recovery from chronic protein malnutrition. In Table 3, column 11, an input of 0.8 g/kg/d of protein caused a positive N balance of 2.3 g/d in previously fasted individuals, whereas equilibrium occurred without prior depletion (column 10). Therefore, it would be predicted that patients suffering acute or chronic malnutrition will respond quantitatively differently from obese or postoperative subjects without antecedent illness. Accordingly, it is essential in the assessment of any data, to evaluate prior nutritional state. Many of the controversies about the relative efficacies of lipid and carbohydrate can be accounted for in this fashion. The data from Table 3 are derived from patients with differing states of nutrition and it was explicitly indicated in which instances the presence of data on different subjects justify intergroup comparisons. Not only is the amount of amino acid important, but in depleted individuals, the amino acid composition is also critical. The requirement for specific amino acids in depleted adults is similar to that of the normal growing child (Anderson, Patel & Jeejeebhoy, 1973).

Fuel demand

The net energy balance may also be important.In depleted patients, more calories will be required to 'make up' for the loss of endogenous fuel stores, even in the absence of acute, ongoing disease. An increase in the day-to-day demand for calories occurs in any 'hypermetabolic' state, whether physiologic (eg, exercise, pregnancy) or pathologic. Such pathologic states include those with alterations in secretion of the hormones listed in Table 2; loss of nutrients via gastrointestinal fistulae or other diseases; extensive burns; and hyperthermia. Further complicating these states are the stress-related elevations of hormones which are either directly catabolic or which inhibit insulin secretion. The reported inefficiency of fat calories in nitrogen sparing in such patients, and apparent requirement for at least enough carbohydrate to account for resting metabolic rate remain unexplained (Long, 1976) and merit detailed study. It could be that by hormonal or specific drug intervention, such a failure of response could be corrected.

Concurrent illness

The presence of hepatic or renal disease may alter the response to administered nutrients. In addition, the use of drugs may directly or indirectly affect the metabolic response of specific target organs. Adrenergic agonists and antagonists are two such examples. Protein synthesis may be interfered with by antimicrobial agents such as tetracyclines and amphotericin B. Chemotherapeutic agents for cancer may also interact with nutrient supply. The presence of malignancy *per se* has long been recognized as affecting protein homeostasis. Undoubtedly, new insights into protein metabolism in malignant disease will come from controlled studies of affected recipients of parenteral nutrition.

Vitamins, cofactors and trace metals

Vitamins, other substrates or cofactors required in small amounts, and trace metals, may also affect protein metabolism. Since the water-soluble vitamins are usually included in therapeutic amounts in hypocaloric diets and during parenteral treatment, these do not ordinarily pose a significant problem. Of interest, however, is the requirement for essential amino acids as precursors for other metabolic intermediates. For example, metabolites of lysine have been shown to be important intermediates in carnitine biosynthesis. In the rat, it has been estimated that 0.1 per cent of dietary lysine is converted to carnitine which is required for intramitochondrial transport of fatty acids. Essential fatty acid deficiency in parenteral nutrition has been identified and recently reviewed in detail (Meng & Wilmore, 1976). The roles of certain of the trace metals in protein equilibrium are of established importance. Chromium deficiency caused a diabetic syndrome with normal insulin levels in a patient on long-term intravenous alimentation (Jeejeebhoy *et al.*, 1977). This was characterized by glucose intolerance, neuropathy, and failure to respond as before to the established therapeutic program. Addition of supplementary chromium corrected all aspects of this syndrome. Patients with significant loss of zinc, especially from upper gastrointestinal fistulae, respond with lower insulin and poorer nitrogen balance to the same nutrient intake as those without such losses. Adequate zinc replacement corrects this (Wolman *et al.*, 1978). Roles of other trace substances, including copper, manganese and iodide are the subject of reevaluation in parenteral nutrition, where input requires precise control.

Time

It has already been underscored above that a multitude of interacting variables determine nitrogen balance with different nutrient intake. When the input is isocaloric, the steady-state is achieved rapidly, that is, in several days to one week. This is not the case for hypocaloric regimens. In the studies shown in Table 3, column 10, a steady-state was only reached after 14 days: significant negative balance preceded nitrogen equilibrium (Fig. 5). The same

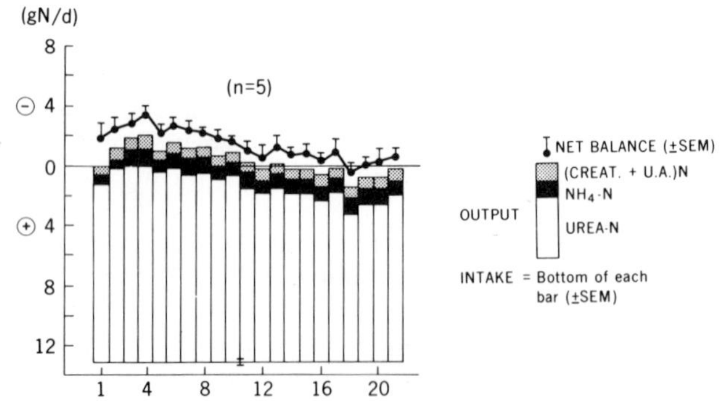

Fig. 5. Nitrogen balance with provision of 0.8 g/kg/d oral protein to obese subjects for 21 d. Nitrogen intake is plotted downward from the horizontal axis, and mean ± s.e.m. of intake is indicated at the base of the bars. Output components are plotted upward from the intake levels, and the net balance is indicated by the closed circles and solid line for each day

applies to intravenously administered amino acid solutions at a range of inputs of 0.5 to 1.0 g/kg/d (Fig. 2 and Table 3, columns 13 to 16). Since steady-state elevations of free fatty acids and ketone bodies are reached only gradually, it is probable that optimal utilization of the amino acids is only possible once endogenous fat mobilization is maximal. Accordingly, it should be considered that the true potential of specific regimens to improve nitrogen equilibrium must be demonstrated at a time when steady-state conditions obtain.

Summary

An homeostatic system responsible for energy and protein equilibrium has been postulated, and termed the 'caloristat-aminostat'. Its operation in fasting has been detailed. The close interaction between the 'caloristat' and 'aminostat' has been reviewed. Variables affecting the function of these mechanisms may be categorized as follows. Exogenous protein is required to achieve protein equilibrium and positive nitrogen balance, with both the amounts and the composition of protein being determinants. Energy supply alone spares protein. For a given protein input, the provision of energy improves the response. When that energy is provided as isocaloric glucose, lipid, or as equal parts of each, to prior depleted patients, equivalent positive balance is obtained. For both hypocaloric and isocaloric inputs, a finite though variable time is required to reach the optimal effect for that system. There is no absolute level of insulin which may be said to be universally 'anabolic', and there are no arbitrary 'anabolic' and 'catabolic' insulin-glucagon relationships.

Acknowledgements – The experimental results from parenteral nutrition are from studies performed under the direction of Dr K.N. Jeejeebhoy, and with the collaboration of Drs G.H. Anderson, G.R. Greenberg, A. Bruce-Robertson, and members of the Department of Surgery at the Toronto General Hospital. Substrate and hormone assays were performed by Hing-Luen Tang, Thelma Peregrino-Solomon and Katarina Thumm in the author's laboratory, to whom he expresses his continuing gratitude, and as well to Ms Diane Marliss for her excellent secretarial assistance. The studies were supported in part by the Ontario Ministry of Health (Health Research Grant PR 228, KNJ) by the Toronto General Hospital Foundation (Grant 616, KNJ and EBM), and by the Medical Research Council of Canada (EBM).

References

Adibi, S. (1976): *Metabolism* 25, 1287.
Aguilar-Parada, E., Eisentraut, A.M. & Unger, R.H. (1969): *Diabetes* 18, 717.
Allison, J.B. (1951): *Federation Proceedings* 10, 676.
Anderson, G.H , Patel, D.G. & Jeejeebhoy, K.N. (1973): *J. Clin. Invest.* 53, 904.
Apfelbaum, M. (1970): *Presse Med.* 78, 1917.
Bistrian, B.R., Blackburn, G.L., Flatt, J.P., Sizer, J., Scrimshaw, N. & Sherman, M. (1976): *Diabetes* 25, 494.
Blackburn, G.L., Bistrian, B.R., Flatt, J.P. & Sizer, J. (1975): In *Recent advances in obesity research:* I, ed A. Howard, p. 1. London: Newman.
Cahill, G.F., Jr. (1970): *New Engl. J. Med.* 282, 668.
Cahill, G.F., Jr. (1971): *Diabetes* 20, 785.
Cherrington, A.D., Chiasson, J.L., Liljenquist, J.E., Jennings, A.S., Keller, U. & Lacy, W.W. (1976): *J. Clin. Invest.* 58, 1407.
Chiasson, J.L., Liljenquist, J.E., Sinclair-Smith, B.C. & Lacy, W.W. (1975): *Diabetes* 24, 574.
Chopra, I.J., Chopra, U., Smith, S.R., Reza, M. & Solomon, D.H. (1975): *J. Clin. Endocrinol. Metab.* 41, 1975.
Danforth, E., Jr., Sims, E.A.H., Horton, E.S. & Goldman, R.S. (1975): *Diabetes* 24, 406.
Felig, P., Pozefsky, T., Marliss, E.B. & Cahill, G.F. Jr. (1970): *Science* 167, 1003.
Felig, P. (1973): *Metabolism* 22, 179.
Felig, P., Wahren, J. & Hendler, R. (1976): *J. Clin. Invest.* 58, 761.
Felig, P., Wahren, J., Sherwin, R. & Hendler, R. (1976): *Diabetes* 25, 1091.
Flatt, J.P. & Blackburn, G.L. (1974): *Am. J. Clin. Nutr.* 27, 175.
Howard, A.N. & McLean Baird, I.M. (1977): *Int. J. Obesity* 1, 63.
Gamble, J.L. (1946-47): *The Harvey Lectures, XLII,* p. 247.
Genuth, S.M. (1973): *Metabolism* 22, 927.
Gerich, J.E., Lorenzi, M., Bier, D.M., Tsalikian, E., Schneider, V., Karam, J.H. & Forsham, P.H. (1976): *J. Clin. Invest.* 57, 875.
Greenberg, G.R., Marliss, E.B., Anderson, G.H., Langer, B., Spence, W., Tovee, E.B. & Jeejeebhoy, K.N. (1976): *New Engl. J. Med.* 294, 1411.
Hanna, A., Nakhooda, A.F. & Marliss, E.B. (1978): *Clin. Res.* (in press).
Jeejeebhoy, K.N. (1977): In *AMA Symposium 'Clinical nutrition update: amino acids',* ed H.L. Greene, M.A. Holliday & H.N. Munro. Chicago: Am. Med. Assoc.
Jeejeebhoy, K.N., Anderson, G.H., Nakhooda, A.F., Greenberg, G.R., Sanderson, I. & Marliss, E.B. (1975): *J. Clin. Invest.* 57, 125.
Jeejeebhoy, K.N., Marliss, E.B., Anderson, G.H., Greenberg, G.R., Kuksis, A. & Breckenridge, C. (1976): In *Lipids in parenteral nutrition: studies of clinical and metabolic features,* ed H.C. Meng & D.W. Wilmore. Chicago: Am. Med. Assoc.

Jeejeebhoy, K.N., Chu, R.C., Marliss, E.B., Greenberg, G.R. & Bruce-Roberston, A. (1977): *Am. J. Clin. Nutr.* **30**, 531.
Leathem, J.H. (1964): In *Mammalian protein metabolism*, ed H.N. Munro & J.B. Allison. Vol. 1. New York: Academic Press.
Lefebvre, P. (1972): In *Glucagon*, ed P.J. Lefebvre & R.H. Unger. Oxford: Pergamon Press.
Liljenquist, J.E., Bomboy, J.D., Lewis, S.B., Sinclair-Smith, B.C., Felts, P.W., Lacy, W.W., Crofford, O.B. & Liddle, G.W. (1974): *J. Clin. Invest.* **53**, 198.
Liljenquist, J.C., Mueller, G.L., Cherrington, A.D., Keller, U., Chiasson, J.L., Perry, J.M., Lacy, W.W. & Rabinowitz, D. (1977): *J. Clin. Invest.* **59**, 369.
Long, J.M., III. (1976): In *Fat emulsions in parenteral nutrition*, ed H.C. Meng & D.W. Wilmore, Chicago: Am. Med. Ass.
Marliss, E.B. (1977): In *Clinical nutrition update: amino acids*, ed H.L. Greene, M.A. Holliday & H.N. Munro, pp. 34-45. Chicago: Am. Med. Assoc.
Marliss, E.B., Aoki, T.T., Unger, R.H., Soeldner, J.S. & Cahill, G.F., Jr. (1970): *J. Clin. Invest.* **49**, 2256.
Marliss, E.B., Murray, F.T. & Nakhooda, A.F. (1978): *J. Clin. Invest.* (in press).
McLean Baird, I.M., Parsons, R.L. & Howard, A.N. (1974): *Metabolism* **23**, 645.
McGarry, J.D. & Foster, D.W. (1975): *Am. J. Med.* **61**, 9.
Meng, H.C. & Wilmore, D.W. (1976): In *Fat emulsions in parenteral nutrition. Part 1: Metabolism and function of essential fatty acids.* Chicago: Am. Med. Assoc.
Munro, H.N. (1964): In *Mammalian protein metabolism*, ed H.N. Munro & J.B. Allison. New York: Academic Press.
O'Connell, R.C., Morgan, A.P., Aoki, T.T., Ball, M.R. & Moore, F.T. (1974): *J. Clin. Endocrinol. Metab.* **39**, 555.
Owen, O.E., Morgan, A.P., Kemp, H.G., Sullivan, J.M., Herrera, M.G. & Cahill, G.F. Jr., (1967): *J. Clin. Invest.* **46**, 1589.
Owen, O.E., Felig, P., Morgan, A.P., Wahren, J. & Cahill, G.F., Jr. (1969): *J. Clin. Invest.* **48**, 574.
Sapir, D.G., Owen, O.G., Pozefsky, T. & Walser, M. (1974): *J. Clin. Invest.* **54**, 974.
Strang, J.M., Evans, F.A. & McCluggage (1930): *Am. J. Med. Sci.* **179**, 687.
Streja, D., Steiner, G., Marliss, E.B. & Vranic, M. (1977): *Metabolism* (in press).
Unger, R.H., (1971): *Diabetes* **20**, 834.
Voit, C. (1869): *Z. Biol.* **5**, 431.
Vranic, M., Ross, G., Doi, K. & Lickley, L. (1976): *Metabolism* **25**, Suppl. 1, 1375.
Waterlow, J.C. (1969): In *Mammalian protein metabolism*, ed H.N. Munro & J.B. Allison. New York: Academic Press.
Waterlow, J.C., Garlick, P.J. & Millward, D.J. (1977): Amino acid supply and protein turnover. In *AMA Symposium 'Clinical nutrition update: amino acids'*, ed H.L. Greene, M.A. Holliday & H.N. Munro, pp. 1-9. Chicago: Am. Med. Assoc.
Wolman, S., Anderson, G.H., Marliss, E.B. & Jeejeebhoy, K.N. (1978): *J. Clin. Invest.* (in press).
World Health Organization (1973): Energy and protein requirements, joint FAO/WHO Expert Committee. WHO Tech. Rep. Series No. 522. Geneva.
Young, V.R., Haverberg, L.N., Bilmazes, C. & Munro, H.N. (1973): *Metab. Clin. Exp.* **22**, 1429.

36
Clinical results with starvation and semistarvation

F.A. GRIES, M. BERGER and P. BERCHTOLD
Diabetes Research Institute, University of Düsseldorf, Auf'm Hennekamp 65, 4000 Düsseldorf, W. Germany.

The mortality data of the life insurance companies have initiated a world wide medical campaign for the treatment of overweight in order to prevent increased mortality. The therapeutic eagerness of physicians has often evoked questions as to the necessity of therapy from patients who quoted ancestors who became old in spite of overweight. The doubts of patients seem to be justified in the light of the Chicago Peoples Gas Company study (Dyer *et al.*, 1975) and Seltzer's (1966) reevaluation of the build and blood pressure study (Society of Actuaries, 1959); they both showed a significant increase of mortality only when overweight surpassed 30 per cent of the ideal weight.

We differentiate preventive treatment of obesity in order to reduce the development of mortality risks and treatment of obesity for the cure of diseases associated with obesity. We induce preventive weight reduction in all cases of gross obesity, except after the sixth decade of life. A study in 500 grossly obese patients (Broca Index >1.25) has shown that 88 per cent exhibited coronary risk factors (Berchtold *et al.*, 1977). Only 12 per cent of them had no risk factors as compared with 34 per cent in a control population. Risk factors were absent only in younger patients with less overweight than patients with risk factors, which suggests, that almost all grossly obese subjects will develop risk factors when getting older. With respect to the correlations of overweight and risk factors (Fig. 1) we feel, therefore, that preventive therapy is indicated in younger subjects. However, independent of age, the presence of any risk factor associated with obesity is an indication to lower body weight.

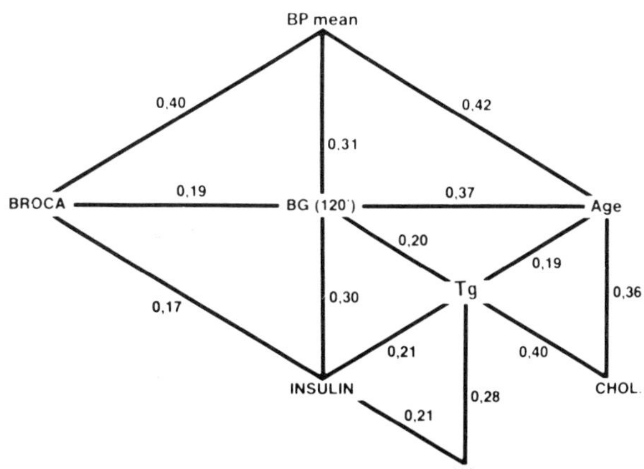

Fig. 1 Correlations between risk factors in obese patients (*n* = 397); all are significant, P $<$ 0.001
BP = blood pressure; UA = uric acid; Tg = triglycerides; Hb = hemoglobin; BG (120′) = blood glucose, 120 minutes after a 100g oral glucose load; Chol = cholesterol; Broca = Broca index; Insulin = basal insulin (Berchtold *et al.*, 1977)

The disappearance of risk factors is the final goal of therapy.

The following discussion will be concerned with the efficacy of therapy for weight reduction and with the effect of such a therapy on some metabolic risk factors.

Starvation

Side effects and complications

A negative energy balance, which is the basis for any weight loss, can be achieved by increasing energy consumption (which will not be discussed here) and/or by a restriction of energy supply. Apparently, total starvation is the most aggressive conservative approach to caloric restriction. It has been therapeutically used since Hippocrates.

The elaborate studies on the alterations of fuel homeostasis during starvation carried out by Benedict (1915) and Cahill and co-workers (1966) have demonstrated that fasting can be well tolerated by human beings even for prolonged periods of time. The most obvious limitation is the availability of mobilizable protein. Thus, the introduction of prolonged starvation as a routine therapeutic procedure in clinical medicine (Bloom, 1959) met, in general, with few difficulties. A variety of possible side effects has nevertheless been observed during therapeutic starvation of obese patients. A transitory rise of serum transaminases and bilirubin (Ditschuneit *et al.*, 1970; Barret, 1971) is frequently observed during prolonged starvation without its mechanism or significance being well understood. In addition, fasting is associated with the occurrence of hyperuricaemia mainly due to an impairment of its renal clearance (Lecocq & McPhaul, 1964). The precipitation of both gouty arthritis and renal uric acid calculi have been reported in obese subjects during starvation (Drenick, 1965). The most frequent side effects are hypotensive episodes early during total starvation and later transient phases of fluid retention, probably due to a hyperaldosteronism (Spark *et al.*, 1975). The management of both of these side effects rarely causes any significant problems. However, severe complications have been described during prolonged therapeutic starvation, such as cardiovascular disturbances (Duncan *et al.*, 1964; Lawlor, 1969; Sandhofer *et al.*, 1973), electrolyte imbalances (Runcie & Thomson, 1970; Lawlor, 1968; Drenick *et al.*, 1964; Birkenhager & Ackers, 1968), vitamin deficiencies (Drenick *et al.*, 1966; Lawlor & Wells, 1969), mental disorders such as depression (Farber, 1964), neutropenia (Drenick & Alvarez, 1971) and (keto-)acidosis (Ross *et al.*, 1971; Galton, 1974) and renal failure (Zürcher *et al.*, 1977). In fact, the literature contains several reports of deaths in patients on a starvation regimen (Norbury, 1964; Cubberley, Polster & Schulmann, 1965; Garnett *et al.*, 1969; Spencer, 1968).

Due to these complications a variety of contraindications to long-term fasting have been proposed (Table 1). In addition, it is important that patients be hospitalized during starvation. and subjected to close observation. A variety of bodily functions have to be monitored

Table 1. Contraindications to total starvation

1) consuming diseases (neoplasma, severe infections)

2) acute and chronic renal failure

3) liver diseases (except simple fatty liver) porphyria, anemia

4) juvenile type of diabetes mellitus

5) recent cardiovascular events (infarction, apoplexia, cardial insufficiency)

6) gout

7) psychoses

and sufficient amounts of fluids, electrolytes and vitamins have to be given (Gries, Berchtold & Berger, 1976). The importance of fluid supply was recently illustrated by Ditschuneit

(1976) in a 19-year-old patient, who for 4 days reduced drinking to 500 ml per day and promptly developed a severe acidosis which was readily reversed by sufficient supplies of fluid (Fig. 2).

When adhering to these precautions, we have not observed any significant side effects, except for the occasional orthostatic hypotension, which occurred in abour 80 cases of prolonged starvation carried out on inpatients over the last 6 years. Therefore, we think that in the hand of the experienced physician total starvation of inpatients must not be

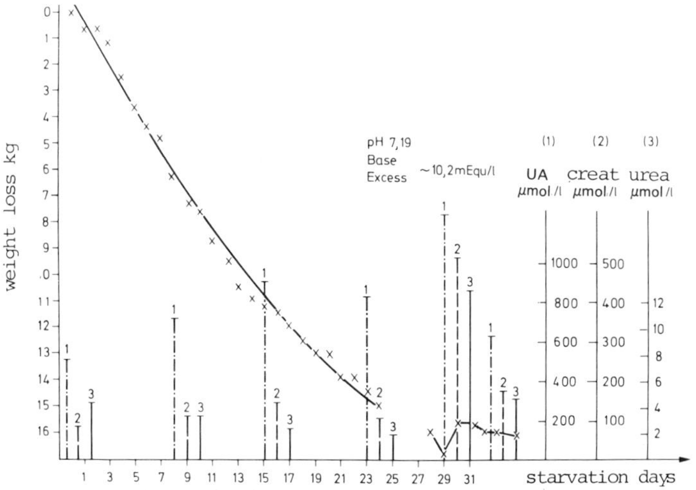

Fig. 2 Acidosis, elevation of uric acid (UA), creatinin (creat) and urea during total starvation of a 19-year-old patient (body weight 154 kg) after reduction of fluid supply to 500 ml for 4 days (Ditschuneit, 1976)

classified as a dangerous approach to treatment of obesity. Nevertheless, we do not recommend it as a routine therapeutic procedure (Berger *et al.*, 1976).

Results

After the initiation of starvation the loss of body weight usually is greater than can be ascribed to negative caloric balance. It is due to excessive losses of fluid and sodium chloride which have been attributed to the increased serum glucagon level (Kolanowski *et al.*, 1972). Prolonged starvation results in a continuous loss of body weight of 350 to 500 g per day. Metabolic as well as body compositional studies (Benedict, 1915; Owen *et al.*, 1969; Pozefsky *et al.*, 1976; Benoit, Martin & Watten, 1965; Ball, Canary & Kyle, 1967*a*; Yang & van Itallie, 1976) have shown that during early starvation weight loss is mainly due to a loss of fat free body mass, predominantly water and protein. Only later on do adipose stores meet a major part of energy needs. Therefore, short periods of total starvation as well as intermittent starvation should be avoided.

In our experience the adherence to starvation is good: less than 5 per cent of the patients that agreed to participate in a starvation program withdrew prior to 3 weeks of treatment. Although total starvation has in recent years become quite popular as a treatment for gross obesity, relatively few studies were performed to evaluate its long-term efficacy. Out of 42 patients reexamined in our department approximately 2 years following successful starvation lasting 25 (± 2 s.e.m.) days, 19 individuals had partly regained their weight loss and in nine patients the body weight was even higher than before the initiation of therapy (Berger *et al.*, 1976). This success rate of one-third is in accord with reports by several other groups (Harrison & Harden, 1966; Hunscher, 1966; Herman & Iversen, 1968; Swanson & Dinello, 1970; Innes *et al.*, 1974; Fisch & Reutter, 1976). The disappointing long-term effects are independent of age, sex, degree of original overweight, age of onset of obesity or apparent physical activity, but they can be improved by long-term close follow-up controls, dietary instruction and behavior therapy (Göschke *et al.*, 1976).

In the light of the immense cost of such treatment, which results from the necessity to hospitalize patients, and the fact that convincing long-term results can only be achieved when the initial starvation period is followed by a long conventional therapy with calorie restricted diet, we feel that the treatment of obesity by total starvation should not be a routine procedure but should be restricted to the rare, selected patient in whom long-term cooperation can be assumed or in whom a rapid weight loss appears to be vital.

The different situation that arose from the introduction of a protein supplemented very low calorie treatment is discussed by Dr Genuth in this volume.

Caloric restriction

Beginning with Banting (1864), dietary treatment of obesity by caloric restriction has been advocated with numerous modifications, which are intended to guarantee a predominant loss of body fat and to be acceptable to the patient for the long term. Being faced with the present epidemiological data, it is evident that none of these recommendations were able to solve the problem of obesity.

There has been a continuing discussion for nearly 100 years about possible differences in the efficacy of low carbohydrate diets versus carbohydrate rich diets. More effective weight loss with carbohydrate poor diets has been claimed, and shown repeatedly (Fig. 3) (for review see Rabast, Kaspar & Schöborn, 1976). However, the differences are apparently due

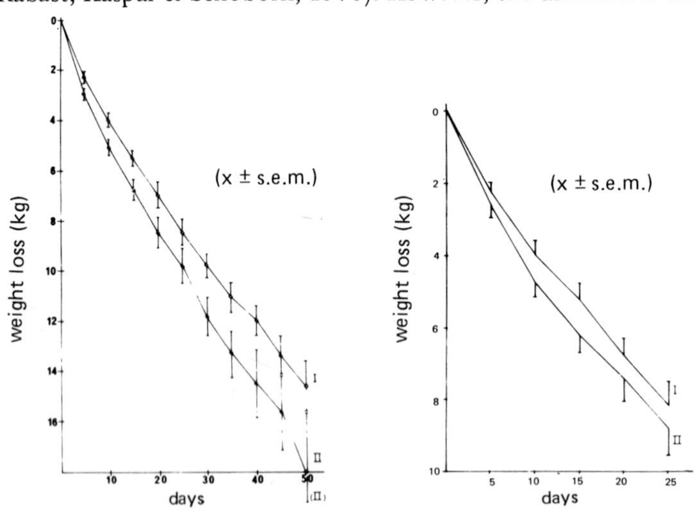

Fig. 3 Loss of body weight during treatment with carbohydrate rich or carbohydrate poor formula diet. Left: 45 patients, mean overweight 58 per cent Broca. Diet I = 170g carbohydrate, 11g fat, 46g protein (*n* = 20). Diet II = 25g carbohydrate, 75g fat, 46g protein (*n* = 25). **Right:** 28 patients, mean overweight 70 per cent Broca. Diet I = 355g carbohydrate, 22g fat, 50g protein (*n* = 13). Diet II = 48g carbohydrate, 158g fat, 50g protein (*n* = 15). (Rabast *et al.*, 1976)

to a greater loss of body water as we were able to demonstrate in two cases (Wessels *et al.*, 1970). This has recently been well documented in the elaborate study by Yang & van Itallie (1976) on sick patients (Fig. 4). A more detailed discussion of the pending controversy also requires an analysis of energy metabolism, which is beyond the topic of this review. It should be mentioned, however, that relatively higher blood levels of glycerol, free fatty acids and ketone bodies but lower levels of glucose during a ketogenic diet can be expected and have been described (Schonborn *et al.*, 1976).

We recommend a mixed low calorie diet relatively rich in protein (about 20 per cent of the calories) which is calculated and composed for each individual according to his food

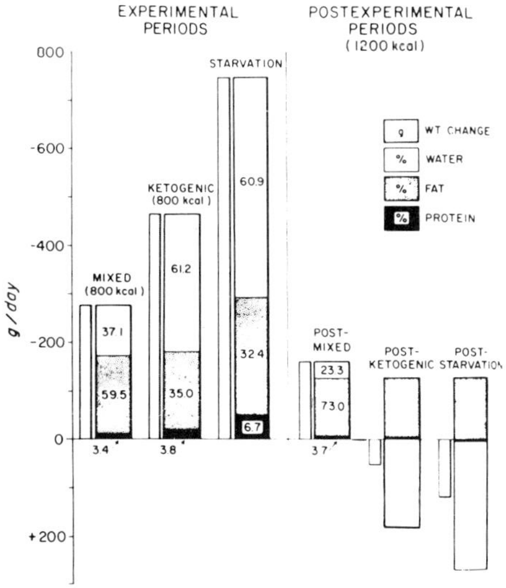

Fig. 4. **Mean daily rate and composition of weight change of obese subjects during and after 10-day periods of 800 calorie mixed or ketogenic diet or total starvation respectively** (Yang & van Itallie, 1976)

preferences. By calculation, such a diet provides all needs for essential components such as calcium, phosphorus, iron, thiamin, riboflavin, niacin and vitamins A and C.

Except for two patients, in which weight reduction had to be interrupted because of depression and the infrequent occurrence of orthostatic hypotension in initially normotensive patients, no side effects associated with the 1000 calorie mixed diet have been observed by us in approximately 3600 patients over a period of 15 years. This regimen is not associated with the development of hyperuricaemia, electrolyte or acid-base imbalances, significant disturbances of the cardiovascular system or deficiency syndromes. Thus this regimen can be prolonged without interruption or any supplementation until normal weight has been achieved.

Results

Valid assessments of long-term success rates are available for only a few treatments. In general, such evaluations have indicated that the adherence of patients was disappointingly poor.

Within the framework of the Obesity Clinic of the Department of Medicine at the University of Düsseldorf (Berger *et al.*, 1976) we have combined repeated dietary counselling (mixed 1000 caloric diet), and elements of group and behavior therapy. Since 1965, we have acheived a mean weight loss of 11 kg in 1610 patients; almost 20 per cent of the population, however, reached a weight loss of more than 20 kg. The success of therapy apparently depends on the duration of controlled treatment. From 1021 patients that attended the outpatient clinic for an average of 100 days, 50 per cent lost more than 9 kg body weight, 15 per cent more than 18 kg, while the 17 per cent of the patients, who remained under control for an average of 235 days, had a mean weight loss of 23.5 kg. A long-term follow-up in 96 patients, who had lost at least 60 per cent of their overweight, showed that the patients with the best long-term results were those with longest adherence to the treatment in the outpatient clinic (von Rekowsky, 1977) (Table 2).

Similarly, and in some cases, even worse, long-term results were reported by others (Fellows, 1931; Evans, 1931; Stunkard & McLaren-Hume, 1959; Liebermeister, 1971; McCuish, Munro & Duncan, 1968; Sohar & Sneh, 1973). Only recently Krotkiewski and co-workers (1977) reported, that adipose tissue cellularity has an apparent influence on prognosis which was relatively better in hypertrophic than in hyperplastic or combined forms of obesity. Overall, the long-term results from our outpatient treatment of obesity appear to be comparable to respective effects of the much more costly therapy of prolonged

Table 2. **Changes in body weight of patients exhibiting loss of >60 per cent overweight (Broca) during a 1000 calorie diet, at a reevaluation after 13 to 120 months – dependence on adherence to treatment in the outpatient clinic of Düsseldorf.** A = further weight loss or constant weight; B = weight gain less than weight loss during active treatment; C = weight gain greater than weight loss during active treatment. Mean values ± s.d. (von Rekowsky, 1977)

	n	Age years	Height cm	Weight before treatment kg	Weight at end of active treatment kg	Weight difference at reevaluation kg	Active treatment time months
A	18	42 ± 17	166 ± 10	98 ± 14	77 ± 13	–2 ± 2	19 ± 12
B	72	39 ± 12	171 ± 9	108 ± 24	79 ± 14	+10 ± 10	15 ± 13
C	6	37 ± 11	169 ± 5	96 ± 12	76 ± 8	+32 ± 14	8 ± 3

starvation. They are consistent with the general experience that it is apparently easier to lose weight than to keep reduced body weight over the long term. Clearly, any diet prescription alone is insufficient and supplementary efforts - education, motivation, conditioning - are needed for better long-term results.

Effects of weight loss on the endocrine metabolic syndrome

Numerous studies have shown that the endocrine metabolic syndrome of obesity is reversible by weight reduction. This has been shown for fat cell hypertrophy, basal, and stimulated hyperinsulinemia, decreased insulin sensitivity *in vivo* as well as of various tissues *in vitro,* impaired glucose tolerance, hyperlipoproteinemia, increased cortisol secretion, and other abnormalities (for review see Gries *et al.*, 1976). Observations during and immediately after caloric restriction have to be clearly differentiated from those subsequent to weight loss. The accumulated data can not be reviewed here, except for some changes in lipid and glucose metabolism.

During starvation and semistarvation plasma lipid concentrations decrease (Voight & Apostolakis, 1969; Hartl, 1976; Bayer, Flegel & Pointner, 1977). The fall of triglyceride levels is marked (Moore *et al.*, 1954; 1955; Liebermeister *et al.*, 1968*a*; Gries *et al.*, 1969), the decrease of cholesterol is less pronounced, sometimes even insignificant (Poindexter & Bruger, 1935; Joliffe, Rinzler & Archer, 1962; Ende, 1962; Caldwell *et al.*, 1963; Galbraith, Connor & Stone, 1966; Liebermeister *et al.*, 1968; Miettienen, 1971; Leelart-haepien *et al.*, 1974; Olefsky, Reaven & Farquhar, 1974; Groothof *et al.*, 1975; Angel, 1975; Kempner *et al.*, 1975). Starvation hyperlipemia is rarely seen and transient (Gries & Vogelberg, 1973). The lowering of fasting serum lipids during caloric restriction is mainly due to the decreased production of endogenous VLDL (Olefsky *et al.*, 1974; Farquhar *et al.*, 1975).

In a study on overweight patients with primary hyperlipoproteinemia Preiss (1970) analyzed 84 periods of weight loss, 20 periods of constant weight and 22 periods of weight gain. He observed remarkable correlations between changes in relative body weight and serum triglycerides (Fig. 5). Apparently, the relative body weight is less important as a regulator of circulating lipoprotein concentrations than the dynamic state of obesity, ie the actual state of nutrition.

The decrease of plasma triglycerides in obese subjects without overt diabetes during a calorically reduced diet of several weeks is independent of glucose tolerance (Liebermeister *et al.*, 1968).

Long-term studies on weight loss and serum triglycerides are rare. In earlier studies (Liebermeister *et al.*, 1968; Hewing *et al.*, 1973) we have seen no decrease of serum triglyceride levels in patients with stable weight several years after weight loss was terminated. However, at that time we did not follow an untreated group. In a recent prospective study on grossly obese subjects, 34 patients reduced their overweight from 78 to 48 per cent (Broca index) while 29 patients without weight loss maintained an overweight of 62 to 66 per cent (Broca index). After an observation period of 10 years there was no decrease of serum triglycerides in the patients with weight loss, but an increase in the patients without weight loss. Cholesterol levels remained unchanged (Toeller *et al.*, 1977, unpublished results).

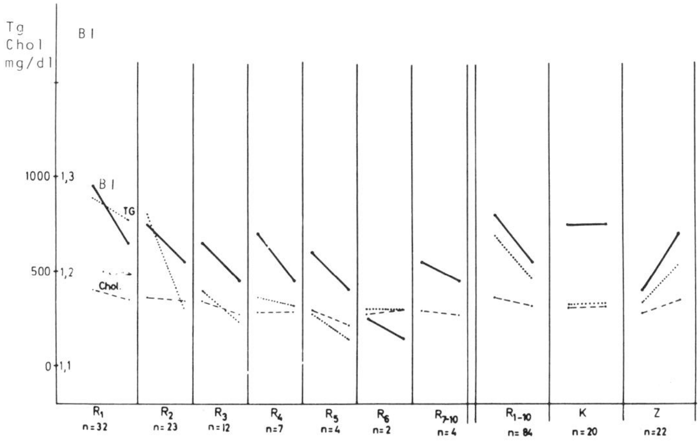

Fig. 5. Changes of relative body weight (Broca-index BI), serum levels of triglycerides (Tg) and Cholesterol (chol) during repeated periods of weight reduction (R_1 - R_{10}), constant body weight (K) and weight gain (Z) in 22 overweight hyperlipemic patients. (Preiss, 1970)

Hyperlipoproteinemia in obesity is due to overproduction of lipoproteins as a consequence of increased supply of substrates to the liver. Only a small amount of these substrates is derived from endogenous lipid stores and hence obesity dependent, while the major part stems from food. Therefore, recent food intake is a more important regulator of lipoprotein synthesis than is obesity *per se.* In fact, it is overnutrition that is responsible for the association of obesity and hyperlipoproteinemia as well as is caloric restriction for weight loss and lipid lowering respectively (for review see Gries, Koschinsky & Berchtold, 1977).

We shall arrive at similar conclusions when considering carbohydrate metabolism. It is well known that in normal subjects fasting may impair glucose tolerance. This phenomenon has been called starvation diabetes and also been observed in some obese patients with normal glucose tolerance (Hales & Randle, 1963; Arnould *et al.*, 1965; Genuth, 1966; Anderson & Herman, 1972). However, in the majority of obese subjects during starvation there is a striking improvement of glucose tolerance irrespective of whether it was normal or impaired (Yalow *et al.*, 1965; Schalch, 1966; Schless & Duncan, 1966). Apparently, this effect of fasting is associated with changes in insulin secretion and insulin sensitivity, which cannot be discussed in detail.

According to recent studies of Ebert *et al.* (1976), the change in insulin secretion seems to be modulated by the secretion of GIP (immunoreactive, gastric-inhibitory polypeptide; or glucose-dependent, insulin-releasing polypeptide). This group showed that in obese subjects there was an exaggerated GIP response to test meals or oral glucose, which decreased as early as 5 days after food deprivation and was restored by 3 days of refeeding. Since GIP is not released by i.v. glucose, the data are compatible with the contention that the exaggerated GIP response of obese subjects to oral glucose or a fat load is secondary to the increased food intake.

In contrast to the marked effects of starvation, caloric restriction to 500 calories or more does not change glucose tolerance in normal subjects (Anderson & Herman, 1972). However, it is well documented that caloric restriction decreases insulin release in obese subjects and improves glucose tolerance as well as carbohydrate metabolism in overt diabetics. More important are the long-term results after stabilisation of the reduced body weight. The beneficial effect of weight reduction on overt and chemical diabetes has often been quoted. Three to five years after the initiation of weight loss there is a correlation between weight loss and improvement of glucose tolerance. However, the beneficial effect is rather small and inconsistent (Fig. 6). It is absent in the extremely obese (overweight >100 per cent

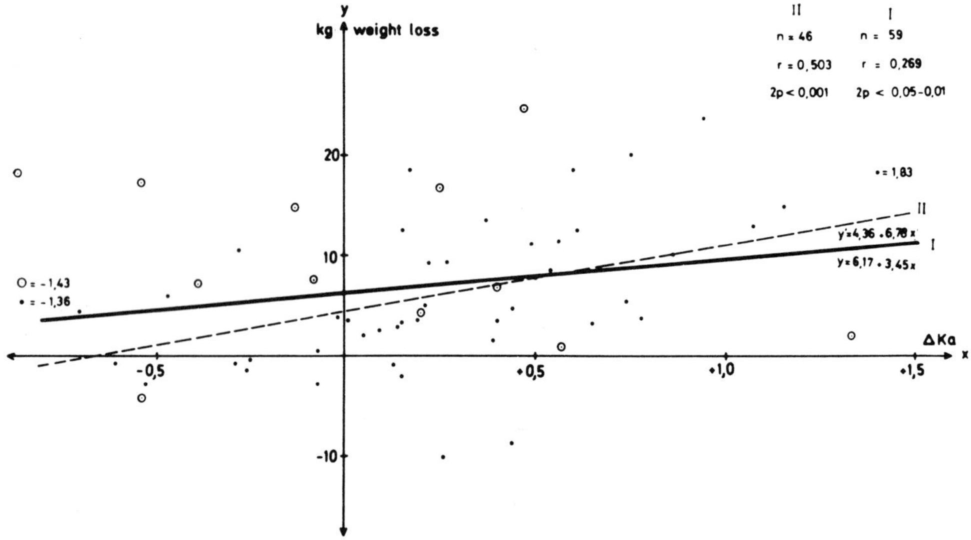

Fig. 6. Correlation between weight loss (kg) and improvement of glucose tolerance (ΔKa; Ka = area under the glucose curve after a 100 g oral glucose load). I: total group. II: after exclusion of 13 patients ⊙ with initial overweight > 100 per cent Broca (Berger *et al.*, 1976)

Broca) and seems to depend on age: younger patients, presumably with a shorter duration of obesity, having a greater chance to improve glucose tolerance (Berger *et al.*, 1975) (Table 3). The long-term results are even less encouraging. In a 10-year study on 63 patients

Table 3. Effect of age on the improvement of glucose tolerance by weight reduction. Reevaluation of data from Fig. 6 (Berger *et al.*, 1976)

	Age of patients: < 50 years	> 50 years
initial overweight	+68 ± 19 %	+69 ± 15 %
initial age (years)	38 ± 9	58 ± 6
n	12	12
r	0,8655	0,233
2 *P*		>0,1

with slightly impaired glucose tolerance (Toeller *et al.*, 1977 unpublished results), constant overweight resulted in an increasing deterioration of glucose tolerance, pointing to the importance of the duration of obesity. In fact, about one-third of these patients developed overt diabetes, although insulin secretion remained elevated over the normal range. For the clinician, it is of even greater importance that glucose tolerance deteriorated also in those patients, who had decreased their body weight by an average of 30 per cent. Consequently, it has to be concluded that it is of little benefit to reduce overweight only in part as long as gross obesity persists.

Summary

With respect to the strong correlation between obesity and mortality risk factors, weight reduction is indicated in younger patients with gross obesity. Overweight must be treated when obesity-induced diseases are present independent of age.

Total starvation should not be a routine procedure for the treatment of obesity. Because of frequent complications, high costs and unsatisfactory long-term results, it should be restricted to selected patients, in whom long-term poststarvation cooperation can be assumed or in whom rapid weight loss appears to be vital. Short-term and intermittent total starvation should be avoided since weight loss during early starvation is mainly due to a loss of fat free body mass.

As routine weight reducing therapy, a 1000 calorie mixed diet is recommended. This treatment is safe and low in cost. It lowers increased blood lipids, preferentially triglycerides, and improves impaired glucose tolerance. The longer the adherence to controlled therapy the better are the long-term results. With respect to blood lipids and glucose tolerance, partial weight loss is of little benefit for the long term as long as gross obesity persists.

References

Anderson, J.W. & Herman, R.H. (1972): *Amer. J. Clin. Nutr.* **25**, 41.
Angel, A. (1975): Cholesterol and obesity. In *Obesity in perspective,* ed G.A. Bray, p. 265. p. 265. Washington DC: US Govt. Ptg. Office.
Arnould, V., Balasse, E., Franckson, JR. M. & Bastenie, P.A. (1965): *Diabetologia* **1**, 136.
Ball, M.F., Canary, J.J. & Kyle, L.H. (1967*a*): *Am. Intern. Med.* **67**, 60.
Banting, W. (1864): Letter on corpulence. Addressed to the Public. London: Harrison.
Barrett, P.V.D. (1971): *J. Amer. Med. Ass.* **217**, 1349.
Bayer, P.M., Flegel, U. & Pointner, H. (1977): *Wien Klin. Wschr.* **89**, 222.
Benedict, F.G. (1915): A study of prolonged fasting. Carnegie Institution of Washington, Publication Nr. 203, Washington DC.
Benoit, F.L., Martin, R.L. & Watten, R.H. (1965): *Ann. Intern. Med.* **63**, 604.
Berchtold, P., Berger, M., Greiser, E., Dohse, M., Irmscher, K., Gries, F.A. & Zimmermann, H. (1977): *Int. J. Obesity* **1**, 219.
Berger, M., Baumhoff, E. & Gries, F.A. (1975): Effect of weight reduction upon glucose tolerance in obesity. A follow-up study of five years. In *Recent advances in obesity research:* I, ed A. Howard, p. 128. London: Newman.
Berger, M., Berchtold, P., Krüskemper. G.M. & Zimmermann, H. (1976*a*): *Internist* **17**, 494.
Birkenhäger, J.C., Haak, A. & Achers, J.G. (1968): *Metabolism* **17**, 391.
Bloom, W.L. (1959): *Metabolism* **8**, 214.
Cahill, G.F., Herrera, M.G., Morgan, A.P., Soeldner, J.S., Steinke, J., Levy, P.L., Reichard, B.A. & Kipnis, D.M. (1966): *J. Clin. Invest.* **45**, 1751.
Caldwell, A.B., Watson, P., Green, D.B., Florin, A., Braun, P. & Bierenbaum, M.L. (1963): *Amer. J. Clin. Nutr.* **12**, 401.
Cubberley, P.T., Polster, C.S.A. & Schulmann, C.L. (1965): *New Engl. J. Med.* **272**, 628.
Ditschuneit, H. (1976): *Internist* **17**, 622.
Ditschuneit, H., Faulhaber, J.-D., Beil, J. & Pfeiffer, E.F. (1970): *Internist* **11**, 176.
Drenick, E.J. (1965): *Arthritis Rheum.* **8**, 988.
Drenick, E.J. & Alvarez, L.C. (1971): *Am. J. Clin. Nutr.* **24**, 859.
Drenick, E.J., Joven, C.B. & Swenseid, M.E. (1966): *New Engl. J. Med.* **274**, 937.
Drenick, E.J., Swendseid, M.E., Bland, W.H. & Tuttle, S.G. (1964): *J. Am. Med. Ass.* **187**, 100.
Duncan, G.G., Duncan, T.G., Schless, G.L. & Cristofori, F.C. (1964): *Ann. N.Y. Acad. Sci.* **131**, 632.
Dyer, A.R., Stamler, J., Berkson, D.M. & Lindberg, H.A. (1975): *J. Chron. Dis.* **28**, 109.
Ebert, R., Willms, B., Brown, J.C. & Creutzfeld, W. (1976): *Europ. J. Clin. Invest.* **6**, 327.
Ende, N. (1962): *Amer. J. Clin. Nutr.* **11**, 270.
Evans, F.A. (1931): *J. Amer. Med. Ass.* **97**, 1063.
Farber, I.J. (1964): *J. Amer. Med. Ass.* **188**, 88.
Farquhar, J.W., Olefsky, J., Stern, M. & Reaven, G.M. (1975): Obesity, insulin and trigleycerides. In *Obesity in perspective,* ed G.A. Bray. Washington DC: US Govt. Ptg. Office.
Fellows, H.H. (1931): *Amer. J. Med. Sci.* **181**, 301.
Fisch, H.P. & Reutter, F.W. (1976): *Schweiz. Med. Wschr.* **106**, 339.
Galbraith, W.B., Connor, W.E. & Stone, D.B. (1966): *Ann. Int. Med.* **64**, 268.
Galton, D.J. (1974): Treatment of obesity. In *Obesity,* eds W.L. Burland, P.D. Samuel & J. Yudkin. Edinburgh, London, New York: Churchill Livingstone.

Garnett, E.S., Barnard, D.L., Ford, J., Goodbory, R.A. & Woodhouse, M.A. (1969): *Lancet* 1, 914.
Genuth, S.M. (1966): *Diabetes* 15, 798.
Göschke, H., Hausser, R., Lauffenburger, Th., Maier, I., Ott, S. & Vogel, M. (1976): *Schweiz. Med. Wschr.* **106**, 713.
Gries, F.A., Berchtold, P. & Berger, M. (1976): *Adipositas-Pathophysiologie, Klinik und Therapie.* Berlin, Heidelberg, New York: Springer.
Gries, F.A., Koschinsky, Th. & Berchtold, P. (1977): Obesity, diabetes and hyperlipoproteinemia. In *Atherosderosis Rev.* New York: Raven Press.
Gries, F.A., Jahnke, K., Preiss, H., Canzler, H. & Miss, H.D. (1969): *Dtsch. Med. Wschr.* 94, 2307.
Gries, F.A. & Vogelberg, K.H. (1973): Einfluss der Ernährung auf die Lipoproteine des Blutes. In *Die Lipoproteine des Blutes,* ed H. Ditschuneit, p. 152. Darmstadt: D. Steinkopff.
Groothof, G., Du Plessis, J.P., Versluis, E.E., Louw, M.W., Alberts, A., Visagie, M.E., Laubscher, N.F., Galpin, J.S. & Markham, R. (1975): *S. Afr. Med. J.* 49, 893.
Hales, C.N. & Randle, P.J. (1963): *Lancet* 1, 790.
Harrison, M.T. & Harden, R.M. (1966): *Lancet* 2, 1340.
Hartl, O. (1976): *Wien Klin. Wschr.* **88**, Suppl. 54.
Herman, L.S. & Iversen, M. (1968): *Lancet* 2, 217.
Hewing, R., Liebermeister, H., Daweke, H., Gries, F.A. & Grüneklee, D. (1973): *Diabetologia* 9, 197.
Hunscher, M.A. (1966): *Metabolism* 15, 383.
Innes, J.A., Campbell, J.W., Campbell, C.J., Needle, A.L. & Munro, J.F. (1974): *Brit. Med. J.* 2, 356.
Jolliffe, N., Rinzler, S.H. & Archer, M. (1962): *Arch. Intern. Med.* 109, 506.
Kempner, W., Newborg, C., Peschel, R.L. & Skyler, J.S. (1975): *Arch Intern. Med.* 135, 1575.
Kolanowski, J., de Gasparo, M., Desmecht, P. & Crabbe, J. (1972): *Europ. J. Clin. Invest.* 2, 493.
Krotkiewski, M., Sjöström, L., Björntorp, P., Carlgren, G., Garellick, G. & Smith, U. (1977): *Int. J. Obesity* 1, 395.
Lawlor, T., (1968): *Lancet* 2, 44.
Lawlor, T. (1969): *Lancet* 1, 1051.
Lawlor, T. & Wells, D.G. (1969): *Am. J. Clin. Nutr.* 22, 1142.
Lecocq, F.R. & McPhaul, J.J. (1964): *Metabolism* 14, 186.
Leelarthaepin, B., Woodhill, J.M., Palmer, A.J. & Blacket, R.B. (1974): *Lancet* 2, 1217.
Liebermeister, H. (1971): *Klin. Wschr.* 49, 125.
Liebermeister, H., Daweke, H., Gries, F.A., Schilling, W.H., Grüneklee, D., Probst, G. & Jahnke, K. (1968): *Diabetologia* 4, 123.
MacCuish, A.C., Munro, J.F. & Duncan, L.J.S. (1968): *Brit. Med. J.* 1, 91.
Macadam, R.F. & Jackson, A.M. (1969): *Lancet* 1, 1050.
Miettienen, T. (1971): *Circulation* 44, 842.
Moore, N.S., Young, C.M. & Maynard, L.A. (1954): *Amer. J. Med.* 17, 348.
Moore, N.S., Fryer, J.H., Young, C.M. & Maynard, L.A. (1955): *Amer. J. Clin. Nutr.* 3, 397.
Norbury, F.B. (1964): *J. Am. Med. Ass.* 188, 88.
Olefsky, J., Reaven, G.M. & Farquhar, J.W. (1974): *J. Clin. Invest.* 53, 64.
Owen, O.W., Felig, P., Morgan, A.P., Wahren, J. & Cahill, G.F. (1969): *J. Clin. Invest.* 48, 574.
Piondexter, C.A. & Bruger, M. (1935): *Arch. Intern. Med.* 56, 884.
Pozefsky, Th., Tancredi, R.G., Moxley, R.T., Dupre, J. & Tobin, J.D. (1976): *J. Clin. Invest.* 57, 444.
Preiss, H. (1970): Erfahrungen mit der diätetischen Langzeit-Therapie bei essentiellen Hyperlipämien. In *klinische Ernahrungsleher,* ed N. Zollner & K. Jahnke, p.125. Darmstadt: D. Steinkopff.
Rabast, U., Kaspar, H. & Schönborn, J. (1976): *Verh. Dtsch. Ges. Inn. Med.* 82, 1372.
V. Rekowsky, F. (1976): Zum Erfolg einer ambulanten Adipositas-Behandlung mit einer 1000 Kalorien-Mischkost. Inaugral Diss., Düsseldorf.
Ross, S.K., Thomson, W.S., Dale, R.E. & Ireland, J.T. (1971): *Postgrad. Med. J.* 47, Suppl. 447.
Runcie, J. & Thomson, T.J. (1970): *Brit. Med. J.* 3, 432.
Sandhofer, F., Dienstl, F., Bolzano, K. & Schwingshackl, H. (1973): *Brit. Med. J.* 1, 462.
Schalch, D.S. (1966): *Diabetes* 15, 527.
Schless, G.L. & Duncan, G.G. (1966): *Metabolism* 15, 98.
Schönborn, J., Eysselein, V., Rabast, U. & Kaspar, H. (1976): *Verh. Dtsch. Ger. Inn. Med.* 82, 1364.
Seltzer, C.C. (1966): *New Engl. J. Med.* 274, 254.
Society of Actuaries (1959): Build and blood pressure study, Chicago.
Sohar, E. & Sneh, E. (1973): *Am. J. Clin. Nutr.* 26, 845.
Spark, H.R.F., Arky, R.A., Boulter, P.R., Sandek, Ch. D. & O'Brian, J.T. (1975): *New Engl. J. Med.* 292, 1335.
Spencer, J.O.B. (1968): *Lancet* 1, 1288.
Stunkard, A. & Mclaren-Hume, M. (1959): *Arch. Int. Med.* 103, 79.
Swanson, D.W. & Dinello, F.A. (1970): *Psychosom. Med.* 32, 209.

Voight, K.D. & Apostolakis, M. (1969): *Klin. Wschr.* **47**, 157.
Wessells, M., Gries, F.A., Irmscher, K., Liebermeister, H., Buchenau, H. & Viehweger, I. (1970): *Dtsch. Wschr.* **95**, 382.
Yalow, R.S., Glick, S.M., Roth, J. & Berson, S.A. (1965): *Am. N.Y. Head Sci.* **131**, 357.
Yang, M-U. & Van Itallie, T.B. (1976): *J. Clin. Invest.* **58**, 722.
Zürcher, H.K., Meier, H.R., Huber, M., Lämmli, J., Wick, A. & Binswanger, U. (1977): *Schweiz. Med. Wschr.* **107**, 1025.

37
Supplemented fasting in the treatment of obesity

S.M. GENUTH, V. VERTES and I. HAZELTON
The Mt. Sinai Hospital of Cleveland, University Circle, Cleveland, Ohio 44106, USA.

The deleterious effects and lethal potential of massive obesity are well-known and amply justify medical attempts at least to palliate and, hopefully, ultimately to cure this disease. With rare exceptions, its etiology is unknown and may well be heterogeneous. Lacking a therapy based on complete understanding of the pathogenesis of obesity, the physician's recourse is to induce a negative caloric balance in the patient, largely by decreasing intake and to a lesser extent by increasing energy expenditure. Total starvation creates a maximum energy deficit which forces dissipation of the greatest amount of stored fat. It has been successfully employed in clinical medicine (Drenick *et al.*, 1964; Thompson, Runcie & Miller, 1966; Gilliland, 1968), but on a long-term basis it requires hospitalization for safety and for prevention of access to food. It is, therefore, an impractical technique for reducing any large population of obese subjects to near-ideal weight. Recent studies have shown, however, that the prominent chemical features of total starvation, ie reduction in serum glucose, elevation of serum ketoacids and elevation of serum uric acid, as well as the accompanying negative nitrogen balance, can be greatly ameliorated by the provision of very small quantities of protein and carbohydrate (Genuth, 1973; Baird, Parsons & Howard, 1974). In various reports, nitrogen balance has been maintained with 60 grams of egg albumin (Bolinger *et al.*, 1966) 55 grams of casein (Apfelbaum *et al.*, 1970), 1.2 to 1.4 grams protein/kg body weight (Bistrian *et al.*, 1976), or 30 grams protein and 20 grams carbohydrate (Baird *et al.*, 1974) per day. Furthermore, the undesirable clinical effects of starvation are lessened while its anorexigenic effect is not. Thus, it represented only a further logical step to apply these observations to the design of out-patient programs for treatment of obesity in which a total fasting regimen would be modified by the addition of a suitable protein or protein-carbohydrate supplement. A number of groups have now reported a successful experience with the use of supplemented or protein-sparing fasts over extended periods in the treatment of massive obesity (Apfelbaum, 1968; Genuth, Castro & Vertes, 1974; Blackburn, Bistrian & Flatt, 1975; Howard & Baird, 1977). This report will review the experience at Mt. Sinai Hospital in Cleveland, Ohio, USA, with approximately 1200 patients over a 5-year period. In so doing, it is hoped that the benefits, the side effects, the limitations, and the uncertainties of this approach to morbid obesity will be clearly delineated.

Some clinical characteristics of the obese population as seen by the Nutrition Service Program at Mt. Sinai Hospital is indicated in Table 1. Notable features include the great predominance of females, equal numbers of young and middle-aged individuals, and the considerable prevalence of frank diabetes mellitus or abnormal glucose tolerance, hypertension, and electrocardiographic evidence of cardiac disease. Additional complicating illnesses have included arthritis, pulmonary disease, inflammatory bowel disease, and gynecologic or orthopedic conditions requiring elective surgery. Although patients only seeking relief from the cosmetic and social-psychological liabilities of obesity are accepted, a preponderence of the patients exhibit medical problems which might be expected to benefit from significant weight reduction. Pregnancy, significant renal disease or hepatic failure,

Table 1. Characteristics of a population with morbid obesity

Age		**Hypertension**	42%
< 40	49%		
> 40	51%	**Electrocardiograms**	
		Normal	62%
Sex		Non specific ST-T	17%
Female	78%	Minor abnormalities	10%
Male	22%	Ischemia	5%
		Myocardial infarct	2%
Diabetes mellitus		Rhythm disturbance	3%
Fasting hyperglycemia	16%		
Abnormal glucose tolerance	20%		

cerebral vascular disease, recent myocardial infarction or unstable angina and severe depression with suicidal expression, currently contraindicate acceptance to this program.

Protocol

The protocol employed in most subjects calls for an initial 7-day hospitalization to institute the supplemented fast. The daily ration of supplement supplies 45 grams of protein (90 per cent egg albumin), 30 grams sucrose, 600 mg phosphorus, 40 mEq sodium, 20 mEq potassium, 2 grams essential fatty acids, 100 per cent recommended dietary allowances (RDA) of iron, magnesium, copper and zinc, 4 mg of manganese, and 100 per cent RDA of all vitamins except E. This total is provided as five equal portions from 8.00 a.m. to 11.00 p.m. An additional 20 mEq of potassium is provided daily as the chloride. During this week of hospitalization, antihypertensive medications, diuretics, oral hypoglycemic agents, and insulin are withdrawn. Other medications are generally continued. Group sessions are held for the purpose of nutritional education, exercise training, and family orientation. Following discharge, the patients remain on the same regimen. The vast majority continue to carry out their usual occupational, social and family activities throughout the entire fasting period; many begin regular forms of exercise to tolerance. They are seen weekly as outpatients in the Nutrition Service Clinic where weight and blood pressure measurement and screening for problems in adherence or side effects are carried out by paramedical personnel after which the patient sees a clinic physician. Routine blood chemistries with particular emphasis on serum potassium, uric acid, BUN, and glucose are obtained every 2 weeks and a hematocrit every 4 weeks. Fasting is terminated by physician/patient agreement at or often just above ideal body weight. Every effort is then made to transfer patients to a maintenance program where various combinations of dietary regimes augmented by individual and group therapy and intermittent supplemented fasting are used for weight maintenance. A percentage of otherwise successful patients self-terminate after losing more than 18 kg (40 lb).

Benefits

The average starting weights for our patients are 106 kg (235 lb) for women and 136 kg (300 lb) for men. Figure 1 shows a plot of weight loss versus initial weight. A linear correlation is evident and is similar for men and women. Seventy-five to 80 per cent of all patients lost at least 18 kg (40 lb) before transferring to a maintenance program or self-terminating. The weight loss averages 25 to 30 per cent of body weight, but in patients with extreme obesity, as much as 50 per cent or more of body weight has been shed. In successful patients (greater than 18 kg (40 lb) loss), the average total weight loss is 38 kg (85 lb), while the average rate of loss is 1.4 kg (3 lb) per week for women and 2.0 kg (4.5 lb) per week for

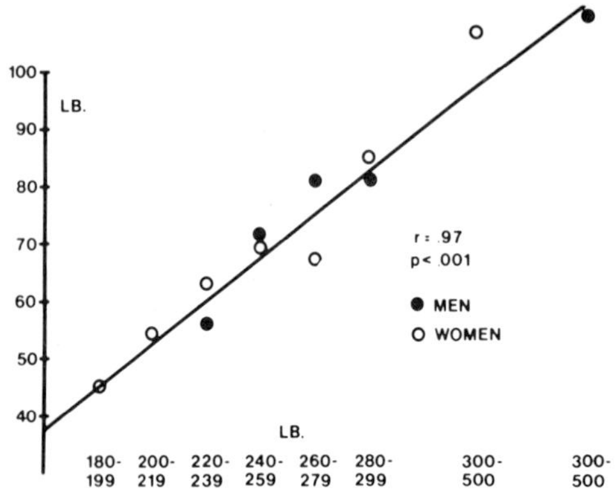

Fig. 1. Mean weight loss with supplemented fasting (ordinate) correlated with initial weight (abscissa). n=21 to 51 for groups of women and n=9 to 26 for groups of men in the various initial weight brackets

men. Although an initial one-week hospitalization was originally deemed necessary for all patients, recently approximately 200 patients with minimal medical problems and weighing less than 113 kg (250 lb) have been started on an ambulatory basis. Only slightly lower rates of adherence and slightly lesser amounts of weight loss have been noted in each starting weight category.

Palliation of obesity to the extent noted above yields definite medical benefits. Improvement in diabetes mellitus, carbohydrate tolerance and hyperinsulinism accompanying obesity is well-known to follow weight reduction (Newburgh & Conn, 1939; Hinsworth, 1949; Drenick, Brickman & Gold, 1972; Kalkhoff *et al.*, 1971; Olefsky, Reaven & Farquhar

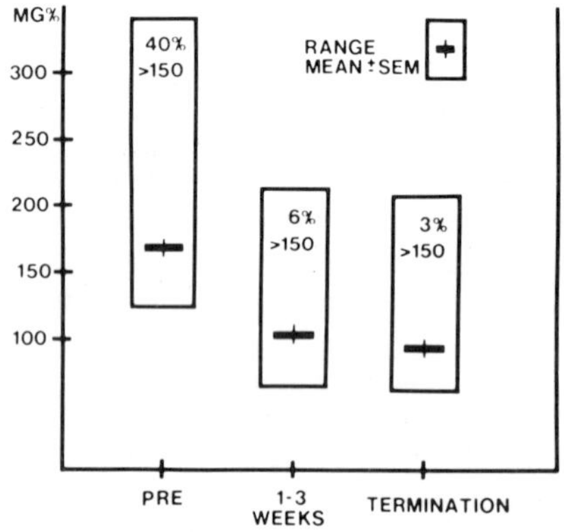

Fig. 2. Mean s.e.m. and range of plasma glucose prior to, at 1 to 3 weeks, and at termination (1 to 22 months) of supplemented fasting in 58 obese diabetics with initial fasting glucose>120 mg per cent

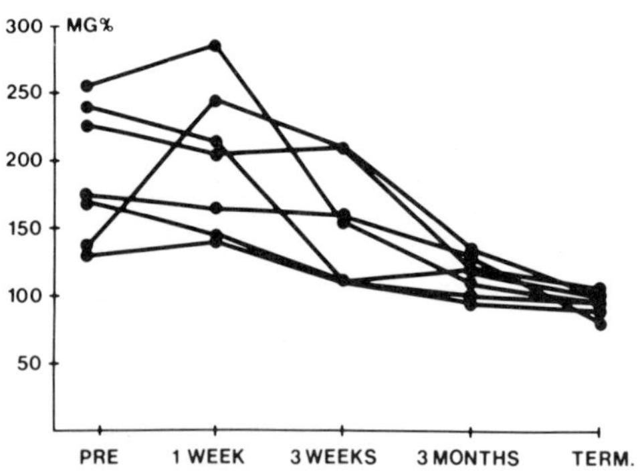

Fig. 3. Individual plasma glucose response during supplemented fasting in 7 obese diabetics taking oral sulfonylurea drugs at the outset but not thereafter. Termination at 4 to 14 months

1974). Figures 2 to 5 summarize our results with supplemented fasting in several groups of patients with clinical diabetes mellitus (fasting plasma glucose (FPG) greater than 120 mg per cent). Previously untreated patients (mean FPG 170 mg per cent) almost uniformly achieved normal plasma glucose after one week and with rare exception maintained this state throughout the period of fasting (Fig 2). A slower fall in plasma glucose is seen in patients who were on prior treatment with sulfonylurea drugs, presumably because of withdrawal of the hypoglycemic effect of these drugs (Fig. 3). Patients on previous insulin treatment respond to withdrawal of insulin and initiation of supplemented fasting in a manner related to their dose. Patients taking less than 48 units (Fig. 4) had a more rapid decline in hyperglycemia than those taking more than 48 units of insulin daily (Fig. 5). The latter tend to have a very slow fall in plasma glucose and some remained hyperglycemic for many weeks despite the intake of only 300 calories a day. This could not readily be attributed to poorer adherence to the fast because rates of weight loss were satisfactory and glycosuria was minimal or absent. Plasma beta-hydroxybutyrate levels were significantly higher after one week of supplemented fasting in the higher insulin dosage group (1.20 vs 0.58 mmol/l, $P<0.025$). As noted in Fig. 5, two patients developed significant acidosis manifested by a fall in serum bicarbonate to 10 and 12 mEq/l after 4 days of supplemented fasting and required restoration of insulin and food. Thus, this form of treatment cannot

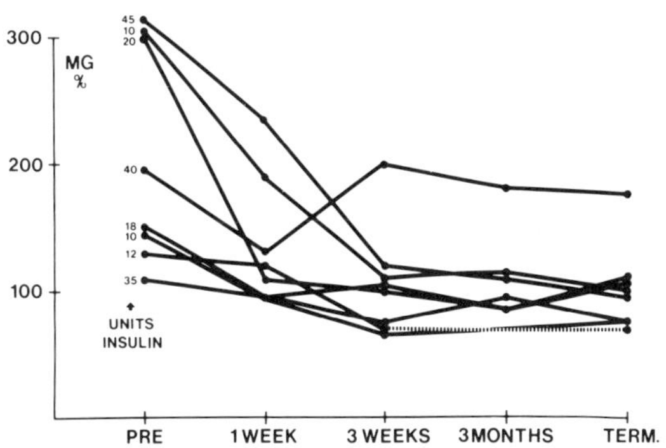

Fig.4. Individual plasma glucose response during supplemented fasting in 8 obese diabetics taking 10 to 45 units insulin at the outset but not thereafter. Termination at 1.5 to 11 months, except for individual shown by dotted line at 3 weeks

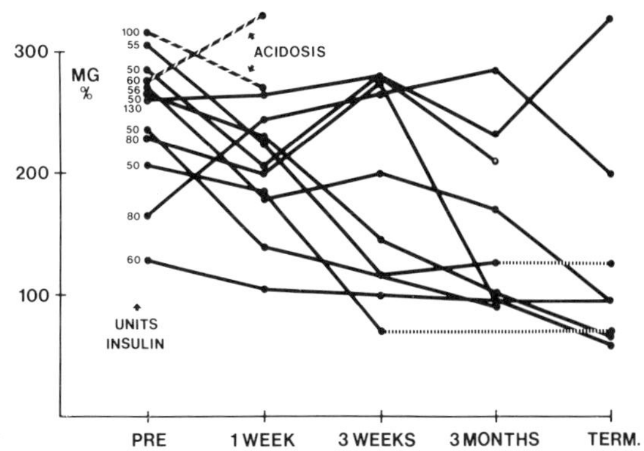

Fig.5. Individual plasma glucose response during supplemented fasting in 12 obese diabetics taking 50 to 130 units insulin at the outset but not thereafter. Termination at 4 to 16 months except for individuals shown by dotted lines at 3 weeks and 3 months, respectively, and 2 individuals still ongoing

be started with impunity outside of a hospital setting in diabetics on insulin. Studies of oral glucose tolerance in diabetics never treated previously with insulin show marked improvement after successful weight reduction. Fasting insulin levels are uniformly lowered while insulin responses to glucose are virtually unchanged. After glucose challenge, the ratios of plasma insulin levels at 30 minutes and at 60 minutes to the fasting insulin level is significantly increased following weight reduction, indicating improved sensitivity of the beta cells to glucose. However, failure to maintain the loss of weight ultimately leads to a return of carbohydrate intolerance, though a lag period may be seen before frank diabetes recurs. Ketoacidosis, reported as a possible complication of rapid weight regain (Drenick & Johnson, 1975), has thus far not been observed in this series of patients, but a renewed need for insulin has.

Hypertension, as defined by a diastolic blood pressure of 90 mm Hg is common in a morbidly obese population (Table 1). Distribution of admission blood pressures in 99 untreated obese hypertensives showed a preponderance of mild hypertension with 46 per cent of patients having diastolic blood pressures of 90 to 99 mm Hg, 32 per cent of 100 to 109 mm Hg, and 21 per cent greater than 110 mm Hg. Systolic blood pressures greater than 180 mm Hg were observed in only 16 per cent of these patients on admission. Left ventricular hypertrophy on electrocardiogram and cardiac enlargement on x-ray were very uncommon. Following one week of supplemented fasting, the distribution of blood pressures in the hypertensive population was altered radically. In 67 per cent of the hypertensive patients, diastolic blood pressure had fallen to less than 90 mm Hg, while values of only 22 per cent at 90 to 99 mm Hg and 10 per cent at greater than 100 mm Hg, respectively, were noted. Even in those patients remaining hypertensive, some blood pressure decrement was usually observed. This initial improvement in hypertension accompanied average weight losses of 15 lb in males and 10 lb in females during the first week and presumably reflected the therapeutic benefit of a sodium diuresis combined with hospitalization and the accompanying bed rest. This interpretation is supported by the fact that in a smaller number of hypertensive subjects who began supplemented fasting on an ambulatory basis, the initial improvement in blood pressure and initial fall in body weight were both less marked. At termination of supplemented fasting, a distribution of diastolic blood pressures was observed similar to that seen after one week. However, some patients who were normotensive at one week had again become mildly hypertensive at termination, while other patients who were still hypertensive at one week had become normotensive by termination, although usually within the first 4 weeks of treatment. Patients who were normotensive at termination of supplemented fasting, regardless of their status at one week, did lose a greater percentage of their excess body weight than did those patients whose blood pressures were elevated at termination. Thus, these data suggest that weight reduction by supplemented fasting is of most immediate benefit to hypertensive obese patients through its initiation of a sodium diuresis. In 13 per cent of patients, however, normotension was not achieved until body bulk had in fact been reduced significantly. Long-term follow-up results are not yet available to verify whether maintenance of this lower body weight will ensure continued freedom from hypertension. In patients whose blood pressure never became normal on supplemented fasting despite significant weight reduction (11 per cent), other factors, such as renin-angiotensin, are presumably operating to sustain their hypertension. It should also be pointed out that patients entering a supplemented fasting program already taking antihypertensive medication will, in general, tolerate withdrawal of their drugs. In only a minority has antihypertensive medication had to be resumed even though weight loss was occurring at the expected rate.

Certain medical benefits from weight reduction by supplemented fasting are difficult to quantify but are highly important to individual patients. For example, at least three patients have become pregnant following long periods of infertility. Of particular note are those rare patients with the Pickwickian Syndrome or chronic obstructive pulmonary disease further compromised by a restrictive element from obesity who have impressive relief of dyspnea and edema. Another group of cases in which results may be especially gratifying are those individuals requiring surgery of a semi-elective nature. Included in our experience have been patients requiring colectomy for ulcerative colitis, grafting for abdominal aneurysm, total hip replacement, and hysterectomy for menometrorrhagia or endometrial carcinoma following radium treatment. Though weight reduction does not invariably improve angina pectoris, it does make possible more accurate coronary angiography and safe coronary bypass surgery for those patients otherwise deemed good candidates.

Finally, the cosmetic and social benefits of weight reduction, though less tangible medically, are more easily perceived and are most appreciated by the patients. In addition to the personal sense of achievement expressed by patients, secondary gains such as occupational advancement or improved marital and familial cohesiveness have accrued. During a highly successful weight reduction phase, the approbation of others often improves the individual's self-image.

Side effects and limitations

Common side effects encountered during supplemented fasting include transient initial diarrhea, fatigue, orthostatic dizziness (rarely to the point of syncope), cold intolerance, skin dryness, hair loss, muscle cramps, amenorrhea, decrease in libido, and euphoria. These symptoms have almost never caused premature termination of supplemented fasting. Several unusual occurrences have been observed. A single case of lithium intoxication occurred with rapid transition from mild symptoms of intoxication to coma despite acceptable therapeutic blood levels of lithium. Although the patient recovered completely, great caution should be exercised in using this form of treatment in patients taking lithium carbonate and extra sodium should be provided. Several instances of cholecystitis and pancreatitis have occurred during the period immediately after cessation of supplemented fasting with uneventful recovery. Five patients have developed unilateral peroneal nerve palsy at the conclusion of weight reduction. Four recovered promptly without specific therapy; one with prior sensory complaints in this nerve distribution required a brace for nearly one year. Four patients with exceptionally large weight losses have expressed a sense of confusion or disorientation with regard to their self-identity and body image, and one required hospitalization for psychiatric treatment. Another patient with previously diagnosed schizophrenia, in remission for 5 years, decompensated 3 weeks after initiating supplemented fasting for uncontrolled diabetes mellitus. She was restored to her previous stable psychiatric state with food and electroconvulsive therapy. No identifiable instances of major renal, hepatic or cardiac failure have thus far been seen. Four sudden deaths have occurred in approximately 1200 patients in 4 years. One was in a normal individual who suffered accidental death after obstructing her airway with chewing gum; autopsy was unremarkable. Three individuals, found dead at home, had all exhibited prior clinical and/or electrocardiographic evidence of heart disease, consisting of angina, ischemic T-wave changes, remote myocardial infarction, or multifocal premature ventricular contractions.

Biochemical follow-up

With rare exceptions, serum glucose, potassium, sodium, chloride, bicarbonate, creatinine and BUN have remained normal for up to 18 months of supplemented fasting. Serum uric acid generally stabilizes in the range of 6 to 9 mg per cent. In the few patients whose uric acid persistently exceeds 10 mg per cent, Allopurinol or Benemid has been promptly effective. As a measure of ketosis, plasma beta-hydroxybutyrate usually averages 1.0 mmol/l (range 0.5 to 3.0), while semi-quantitative tests for urinary acetone are small to moderate with Acetest Tablets. An example of the stability of repeated analyses in one subject on supplemented fasting for 12 months is shown in Fig. 6. A transient rise in liver enzymes, such as SGOT and SGPT, has been noted in approximately 10 per cent of patients during the first 2 weeks with a subsequent decline thereafter. In several patients, liver enzymes were elevated on admission, probably due to fatty infiltration of the liver. In these, supplemented fasting was nonetheless undertaken for medical indications such as diabetes, and liver enzymes returned to normal during weight reduction. In two instances of Gilbert's Disease, serum bilirubin rose, and in one with a level of 7.8 mg per cent, supplemented fasting was discontinued.

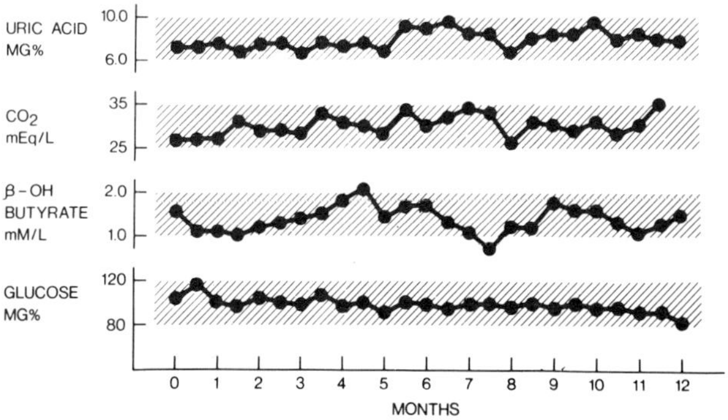

Fig.6. Weekly blood glucose, beta-hydroxybutyrate, bicarbonate and uric acid during 12 months of supplemented fasting in a man who lost 140 kg (305 lb). Shaded areas indicate the range of observations

As a standardized protocol was deemed desirable for management of large numbers of patients, all have received a supplement uniform in composition and amount, containing 45 grams of protein and 30 grams of carbohydrate. Studies of urinary nitrogen excretion were carried out on six subjects after an average weight loss of 35 kg (78 lb) in up to 6 months of supplemented fasting. The results shown in Fig. 7 indicate a wide individual variation but a mean negative urinary nitrogen balance of 2 grams was noted. Urinary excretion of phosphorus correlated well with that of nitrogen (r=0.87, P<0.025), but potassium did not. Assuming additional losses of up to 1 gram nitrogen per day via infrequent bowel movements and skin desquamation, a total negative nitrogen balance of approximately 3 grams can be estimated. This is in agreement with previously published results with slightly greater protein intake (Bistrian *et al.*, 1976). The carbohydrate component of the supplement is not likely to be accelerating nitrogen loss (Yang & Van Itallie, 1976). Hair loss, brittle nails, a tendency to low-grade anemia (Hct > 33 in women and > 38 in men), and occasionally a decrease in visible musculature or complaint of muscle weakness have been the only clinical manifestations of loss of body protein. Serum albumin and transferrin levels have remained normal.

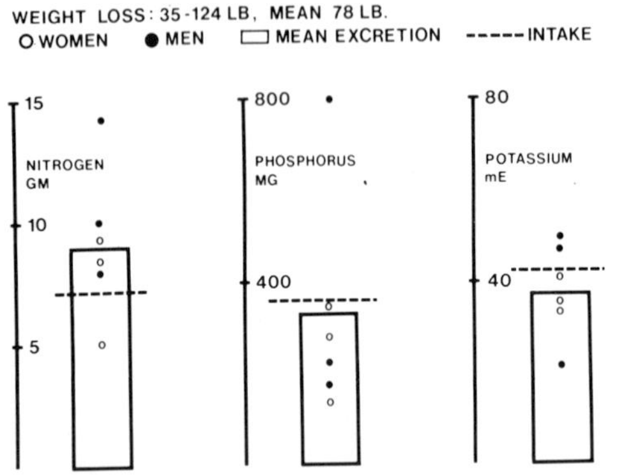

Fig.7. Urinary excretion of nitrogen, phosphorus and potassium on samples collected in hospital after 2 to 6 months of supplemented fasting. Each individual patient result is the mean of three daily collections with acceptably constant creatinine content

Weight maintenance

While highly successful weight reduction can be achieved in a majority of patients treated by supplemented fasting, maintenance of normal or near-normal body weight remains a persistent and difficult therapeutic challenge. In our original pilot study of supplemented fasting reported in 1974 (Genuth *et al.*, 1974), 47 patients had experienced successful weight reduction. These patients were recontacted without intervening systematic follow-up at an average time of 22 months later. Forty-four per cent of the patients had regained less than half of the weight originally lost, with 9 per cent of the patients having regained less than 10 per cent of the original weight lost. Fifty-six per cent of the patients had regained more than half the original weight loss. This appeared to establish that supplemented fasting, though carried on outside the hospital and in the normal environment of the patient, did not, of itself, alter subsequent eating behavior for more than a few months. Similar results have been reported following total fasting in the hospital (Johnson & Drenick, 1977). When interviewed, virtually all the subjects who had regained significant weight voluntarily expressed the desire to undergo a second course of weight reduction. The chief reasons seemed to be the tremendous gratification the patients had received from their thinned state and an unrealistic conviction that they had 'learned their lesson' and would henceforth maintain any weight loss. This experience strongly suggested that implicit in a successful weight reduction program was the obligation to provide a long-term formal maintenance program. It has become apparent that rapid weight regain should be avoided if at all possible, since a second attempt at weight reduction with supplemented fasting bears a much smaller chance of success. In 63 patients who had regained more than half of their original weight loss in the subsequent 5 to 40 months, a repeat course of supplemented fasting resulted in complete loss of the regained weight in only 15 patients (24 per cent). This compares to a success rate of 80 per cent on a first course. We have since attempted to employ supplemented fasting for weight maintenance on an intermittent basis in two fashions. In one group of patients, conventional dietary instruction and frequent follow-up visits were augmented by one week of supplemented fasting at regular intervals of 4 to 8 weeks by the calendar and irrespective of the patient's weight. It was hoped, in this fashion, to establish a cycle of modest weight gain relieved by abrupt short-term supplemented fasting. In the second group of patients, the total estimated caloric needs of the patient were divided into a 'fixed' portion of highly regimented meal plans (70 per cent) and a 'free' portion which could be ingested in any manner desired by the patient (30 per cent). The 'fixed' calories were interpreted to the patient as similar to a supplement, and hopefully divorced from the attractiveness of food. In addition, one-week intervals of supplemented fasting were employed on an *ad lib.* basis whenever the patient's body weight exceeded a pre-set upper limit. Preliminary results, covering a period of up to 15 months of follow-up, are mixed. A trend toward failure of weight maintenance is noted in each of the two groups (Fig. 8 and 9). Individual patients, however, have done strikingly well, including some with very large original weight losses. The per cent weight regain was somewhat more in the patients who attended clinic irregularly. This points up one of the major problems encountered in a weight maintenance program. Many patients exhibit resistance to continued contact with the nutritionist and physician. In some, this appears due to the unrealistic self-appraisal that they can now manage their weight alone. In others, it appears due to the embarrassment and guilt which follows weight gain. Despite much positive reinforcement, to date only approximately 30 per cent of our patients have continued to work with our maintenance programs. We have, therefore, now begun to introduce behavior modification and life-style techniques on both a group and an individual basis in hopes of sustaining greater adherence to caloric control.

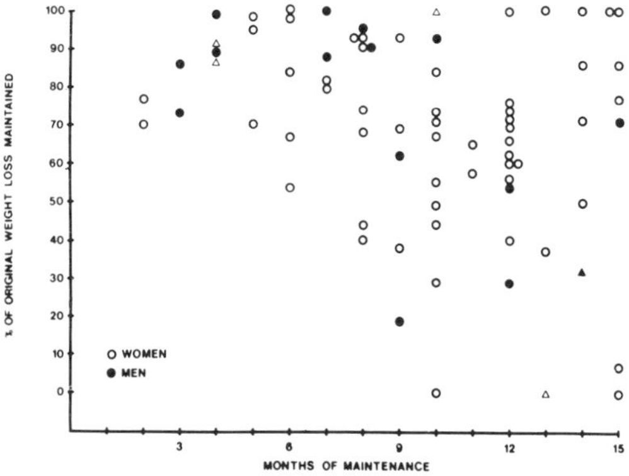

Fig. 8. Weight maintenance in individual patients plotted as a percentage of the weight originally lost during supplemented fasting. Thus, 0 per cent represents total regain of weight; 100 per cent represents no weight regain. Triangle represents patients who failed to attend maintenance clinic and in whom only telephone information was available. All patients were on a program of regularly scheduled intermittent supplemented fasting for one week

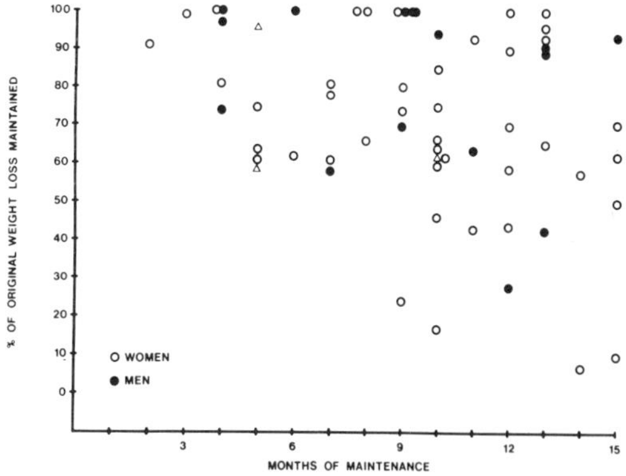

Fig. 9. Weight maintenance in individual patients, plotted as a percentage of the weight originally lost during supplemented fasting. Thus, 0 per cent represents total regain of weight and 100 per cent represents no weight regain. Triangle represents patients who failed to attend maintenance clinic and in whom only telephone information was available. All patients were on a program of 'fixed' and 'free' calories described in the text and occasional supplemented fasting for one week per physician direction

Summary

Out-patient supplemented fasting is a valuable technique for palliation of morbid obesity which subtracts little from the maximum energy deficit created by total fasting, but retains the anorectic effect of total withdrawal from food. Provision of 300 calories per day as 45 g egg albumin and 30 g of carbohydrate with appropriate mineral and vitamin additions moderates ketosis and hyperuricemia and sustains blood glucose. A small negative nitrogen balance persists. Weight loss is proportional to starting weight, averages 85 lb or 25 to 30 per cent of initial weight, exceeds 40 lb in 80 per cent of patients, and proceeds at average weekly rates of 3 lb in women and 4.5 lb in men. Untreated diabetics and those on oral sulfonylureas or less than 48 units of insulin daily, generally acieve normoglycemia within 3 weeks to 3 months. Diabetics receiving more than 48 units of insulin daily improve less rapidly and completely. Hypertensives normalize blood pressure in 67 per cent and reduce diastolic pressure to less than 100 mm Hg in 90 per cent. Side effects are generally not serious and are well-tolerated. Maintenance of weight loss may also be facilitated in some by intermittent short-term supplemented fasting, but preliminary results suggest that behavior modification or other techniques will be needed to improve long-term maintenance. Supplemented fasting is nonetheless a reliable and effective method of initial weight reduction in large numbers of out-patients which provides rapid relief of obesity and accompanying medical complications. In so doing, it provides a base from which subsequent efforts at maintenance of a normal weight can be vigorously undertaken. When a large enough group has been followed for a sufficient period of time, the long-term medical benefits of palliation of obesity by supplemented fasting can be properly assessed.

Acknowledgement – We gratefully acknowledge the contributions of the Mt. Sinai Hospital of Cleveland Nutrition Service staff to patient care, the assistance of Carol Leon and Myra Gary in data collection, and of Shirley Ehren in manuscript preparation.

References

Apfelbaum, M. (1968): *Semaine Therapeutique* **44**, 174.
Apfelbaum, M., Boudon, P., Lacatis, D. & Nillus, P. (1970): *La Presse Medicale* **78**, 1917.
Baird, I.M., Parsons, R.L. & Howard, A.N. (1974): *Metabolism* **23**, 645.
Bistrian, B.R., Blackburn, G.L., Flatt, J-P., Sizer, J., Scrimshaw, N.S. & Sherman, M. (1976): *Diabetes* **25**, 494.
Blackburn, L., Bistrian, R., Flatt, J.P. (1975): *Recent advances in obesity research: I,* ed A. Howard, p. 279. London: Newman.
Bolinger, R.E., Lukert, B.P., Brown, R.W., Guevara, L. & Steinberg, R. (1966): *Archs Intern. Med.* **118**, 3.
Drenick, E.J., Swendseid, M.E., Blahd, W.H. & Tuttle, S.G. (1964): *J. Am. Med. Ass.* **187**, 100.
Drenick, E.J., Brickman, A.S. & Gold, E.M. (1972): *Am. J. Clin. Nutr.* **25**, 746.
Drenick, E.J. & Johnson, D. (1975): *Am. J. Clin. Nutr.* **28**, 264.
Genuth, S.M. (1973): *Metabolism* **22**, 927.
Genuth, S.M., Castro, J.H. & Vertes, V. (1974): *J. Am. Med. Ass.* **230**, 987.
Gilliland, I.C. (1968): *Postgrad. Med. J.* **44**, 58.
Hinsworth, H.P. (1949): *Lancet* **1**, 465.
Howard, A.N. & Baird, M.I. (1977): *Int. J. Obesity* **1**, 63.
Johnson, D. & Drenick, E.J. (1977): *Archs Intern. Med.* **137**, 1381.
Kalkhoff, R.K., Kim, H.J., Cerletty, J. & Ferrou, C.A. (1971): *Diabetes* **20**, 83.
Newburgh, L.H. & Conn, J.W. (1939): *J. Am. Med. Ass.* **112**, 7.
Olefsky, J., Reaven, G.M. & Farquhar, J.W. (1974): *J. Clin. Invest.* **53**, 64.
Thompson, T.J., Runcie, J. & Miller, V. (1966): *Lancet* **2**, 992.
Yang, M-U. & Van Itallie, T.B. (1976): *J. Clin. Invest.* **58**, 722.

38
Nitrogen balance during weight reduction: effect of body stores of protein and fat

T.B. VAN ITALLIE and M-U. YANG
Department of Medicine and Institute of Human Nutrition, College of Physicians and Surgeons, Columbia University, and St. Luke's Hospital Center, New York 10025, USA.

When the early reports of the 'nitrogen-sparing' effects of protein-supplemented fasts were published (Apfelbaum *et al.*, 1967; Baird, Parsons & Howard, 1974; Blackburn *et al.*, 1973), they were received with scepticism by many nutritionists because the results seemed to be at odds with traditional concepts about calorie-protein interrelationships. Such concepts were based on a number of earlier observations (Allison, 1958; Munro, 1951; Swanson, 1951) indicating that, when carbohydrate and fat are completely withdrawn from the diet of previously well-nourished animals and human subjects, the protein moiety that remains can no longer support nitrogen equilibrium. These findings were generally interpreted to mean that, at very low levels of calorie intake, the energy needs of the body take precedence over the need for protein, with dietary protein being used for energy rather than anabolism.

The traditional view of calorie-nitrogen relationships as they affect nitrogen balance was well summarized in a review published a quarter of a century ago by Calloway & Spector (1954). The data they compiled indicated that when a healthy young man is deprived of all food, the nitrogen deficit in early starvation is about 12 g per day. When the daily energy intake is raised from 0 to 2.9 MJ (700 kcal) from non-protein sources, it is possible to reduce that deficit to about 7 g per day. A subsequent increase of energy intake up to levels of 11.7 MJ (2800 kcal) per day seems to be without further advantage in the sparing of body protein. When not more than 1.7 to 2.5 MJ (400 to 600 kcal) are supplied from non-protein sources, there seems to be no advantage in administering protein. If the level of non-protein calories is raised to 3.8 MJ (900 kcal) per day, any excess over 3 g of nitrogen per day in the diet (that is about 20 g protein) is virtually of no further advantage as regards nitrogen retention.

What was not given sufficient recognition by the nutritional scientists of that period is the effect of protein depletion on dietary energy-nitrogen relationships as they affect nitrogen balance. Although it was well known that as total caloric starvation (or total protein restriction) progresses, nitrogen losses gradually diminish to as low as 3 g per day (depending in part on the size of the starving individual), it was not always appreciated that nitrogen retention is more likely to occur on a very low calorie intake as protein stores are depleted. In one study reported by Allison, Anderson & Seeley (1946), it was shown that in dogs which had been fed a protein-free diet for 28 days there was a higher rate of retention of dietary nitrogen than in normal animals.

Thus, the results reported by investigators concerning the nitrogen-sparing properties of protein-supplemented fasts became more compatible with traditional nutritional thinking when it was realized that nitrogen equilibrium during supplemented fasting begins to occur only after there has been some depletion of body protein. However, it is appropriate to ask whether it is indeed the degree of protein depletion that, at any given level of energy intake, is the principal determinant of the amount of dietary protein required for nitrogen equilibrium, or whether other factors are of greater importance.

It will be recalled that in 1974, Flatt & Blackburn explained the rationale for protein-supplemented fasting in terms of a concept which came to be known to some observers as 'beneficial ketosis'. In brief, we understand the implications of this concept to be as follows: (1) Nutritional ketosis is beneficial in the sense that, during total caloric starvation, ketones can displace much of the glucose used as fuel by the brain, thereby obviating the need for wasteful gluconeogenesis from muscle protein, (2) If sufficient carbohydrate (50 g/day or more) is given to a starving individual, some nitrogen-sparing occurs; but, by eliminating or greatly reducing the ketosis, the glucose also eliminates a non-protein source of fuel for the brain, thereby creating a less-than-optimal protein-sparing effect. Also by stimulating insulin secretion, the dietary glucose reduces the rate of free fatty acid (FFA) release from adipose tissue thereby increasing the dependence of many metabolically active cells on glucose derived from gluconeogenesis, and (3) If an appropriate quantity of dietary protein is given to a starving individual, ketosis is not eliminated and ketones can continue to spare endogenous protein that might otherwise be used for gluconeogenesis. Free fatty acids continue to be mobilized because plasma insulin levels remain low, while plasma growth hormone and glucagon concentrations remain relatively high. Under these conditions, the non-neural tissues can continue to utilize FFA for energy. Finally, dietary protein of high biological value (or a suitable mixture of intravenously given amino acids, as the case may be) can be used to repair 'wear and tear' protein losses and may also be used to replenish depleted protein stores.

The concept that nutritional ketosis might be the mechanism responsible for permitting the utilization of dietary nitrogen during protein-supplemented fasting was plausible; however, this hypothesis neglected the implications of early studies like those of Allison *et al.* (1946) which called attention to the importance of the state of the body's protein stores in determining how avidly dietary nitrogen is retained for anabolic use. Recently, we (Yang & Van Itallie, 1976) published observations in obese patients showing that a 3.4 MJ (800 kcal) ketogenic diet was not more effective in sparing dietary protein than was an equicaloric mixed or non-ketogenic diet. Although the ketogenic diet induced a more rapid weight loss than did the non-ketogenic diet, the increment in rate of weight reduction was due entirely to an increase in the rate of water loss.

Concerning the effect of water balance on weight loss, it may be of interest to consider the markedly irregular rates of gross weight loss (Fig. 1A) exhibited by seven obese subjects who were studied for about 9 months on 'balanced' low calorie diets (Passmore, Strong & Ritchie, 1958). The values shown in the figure are average weight losses per day per 4.2 MJ (1000 kcal) deficit based on 5 to 7-day periods. Fig. 1B shows the mean dry weight loss of these same subjects. Taken together, these two graphs illustrate in striking fashion the confusing role played by shifts in body water content in people who are losing weight on reducing diets.

Subsequent studies by Marliss, Murray & Nakhooda (1976) have provided further evidence indicating that the attainment of nitrogen equilibrium during the ingestion of a low calorie protein diet does not always correlate well with the concurrent concentrations in the plasma of insulin and substrates derived from fat. The data of Marliss and co-workers support the notion that the level of protein intake and the antecedent degree of protein depletion play a major role in determining nitrogen balance. There is good evidence to indicate that within these constraints the body has sufficient wisdom to meet most of its energy needs from its fat stores, whether or not some carbohydrate is being ingested and regardless of the plasma level of insulin at the time.

However, there are important differences in the way in which obese and non-obese organisms tolerate caloric privation, and these differences are important to keep in mind when weight-reducing diets are prescribed.

In 1915, Benedict reported metabolic studies of his now-famous fasting man and showed

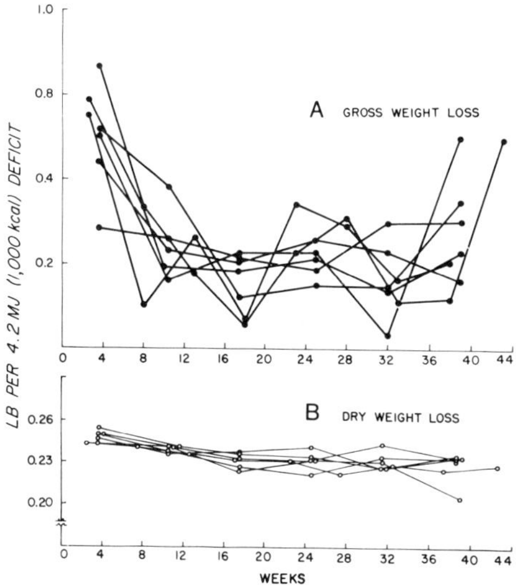

Fig. 1. Mean daily rates of weight loss exhibited by obese subjects consuming low calorie diets. Values are shown in terms of both gross weight loss (A) and 'dry' weight loss (B). All values have been normalized to lb per 4.2 MJ (1000 kcal) deficit. 'Dry' weight loss figures were derived by eliminating the contribution of water to weight loss

that after a month of starvation his subject was still excreting nitrogen at a rate of about 8.5 g per 24 hours. This represents a lean tissue loss of about 250 g per day. The early workers do not appear to have carried out comparable studies of starvation in obese humans; however, some of the data compiled by Voit (1901) concerning the responses of different animal species to starvation suggested that fat animals, notably the pig, can conserve body protein more efficiently than non-obese man, at least in relation to body surface area (Table 1).

Table 1. Nitrogen metabolism of different animals in starvation

Animal	Weight in kg	Nitrogen elimination			Percentage of calories from protein
		Total	Per kg	Per m^2 surface	
Pig	115.0	6.8	0.06	3.2	7.3
Man	63.7	12.6	0.20	6.4	15.6
Dog	28.6	5.1	0.18	5.2	13.2
Rabbit	2.7	1.2	0.46	4.8	16.5
Guinea-pig	0.6	0.4	0.65	4.2	10.8

When studies of nitrogen excretion in fasting obese men and women finally began to be carried out (Drenick, 1973;Gilder *et al.*, 1967), it became evident that the size of the fat depot was exerting a significant influence on the metabolic response to starvation. Fig. 2 shows the nitrogen excretion in g/day of Benedict's lean subject and that of an obese subject fasted for 7 weeks (Gilder *et al.*, 1967). The differences do not look very impressive until one calculates nitrogen excretion rates per hundred grams of weight loss (Fig. 3A) or per 4.2 MJ (1000 kcal) deficit (Fig. 3B) The results of these experiments, admittedly few in number, are consistent with E. Voit's observation (cited by Lusk, 1906) that, at any given time during starvation one can estimate the 'protein metabolism', that is the rate of nitrogen loss, if the ratio of total body nitrogen to total body fat is known.

If one examines the studies that provide sufficient data to permit one to estimate with reasonable confidence the composition of weight loss during starvation, it becomes plain that during a comparable period of starvation, the fuel mixture oxidized by obese persons is substantially higher in fat and lower in protein-derived substrate than that used by lean individuals. In Fig. 4, the composition of weight lost by obese persons during starvation (Runcie & Hilditch, 1974) is compared with the composition of the weight lost by Benedict's

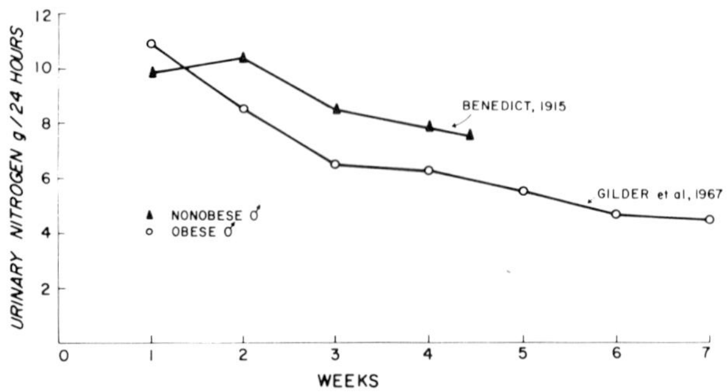

Fig.2 Mean daily nitrogen excretion rates (based on 7-day intervals)in a lean and an obese man during prolonged starvation

fasting man (Benedict, 1915) at different stages of deprivation. Not only do the obese subjects conserve nitrogen much more efficiently after 30 days of starvation but, if one compares the composition of the weight lost by obese individuals after 30 days fasting with the composition of weight lost by another series of obese subjects who remained on a 1.7 MJ (400 kcal) mixed diet for 45 days (Passmore *et al.*, 1958), no difference between the two groups can be discerned. In the figures, all values are shown as pounds of weight loss per 4.2 MJ (1000 kcal) deficit. Also, as can be seen from the same figure, obese subjects on a diet providing only 1.7 MJ (400 kcal) per day for 6 weeks lose far less nitrogen than non-obese individuals do when kept on a 6.6 MJ (1570 kcal) diet for 6 months (Keys *et al.*, 1950). Thus, non-obese individuals never adapt adequately to a low calorie diet even though they may possess normal fat stores at the outset of semi-starvation.

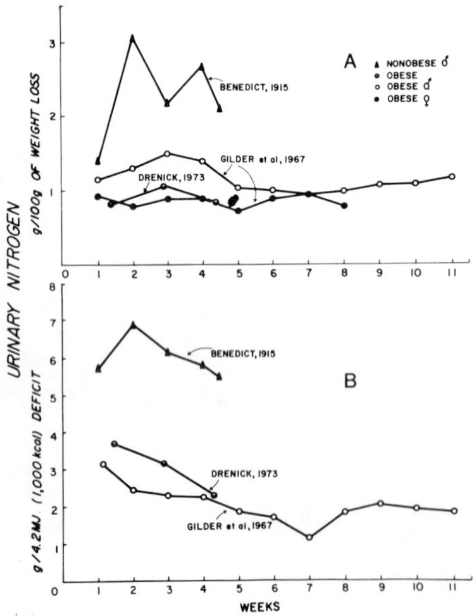

Fig.3 Mean daily nitrogen excretion rates in one lean man and several obese subjects during prolonged starvation. Values have been normalized to g/100 g of weight loss (A) or g/4.2 MJ (1000 kcal) deficit (B)

These results have implications for protein-supplemented fasting.* First, it is evident that, because obese individuals conserve protein rather well during starvation, they might, after some degree of protein depletion, retain much of the dietary protein in low calorie diets.

**In this context, protein-supplemented fasting refers only to regimens that provide proteins of high biological value together with vitamins and minerals in amounts thought to be adequate to prevent nutrient deficiency. Use of the so-called 'liquid protein diet' (collagen hydrolysate) for supplemented fasting can be extremely hazardous, especially when continued for prolonged periods, and is not recommended*

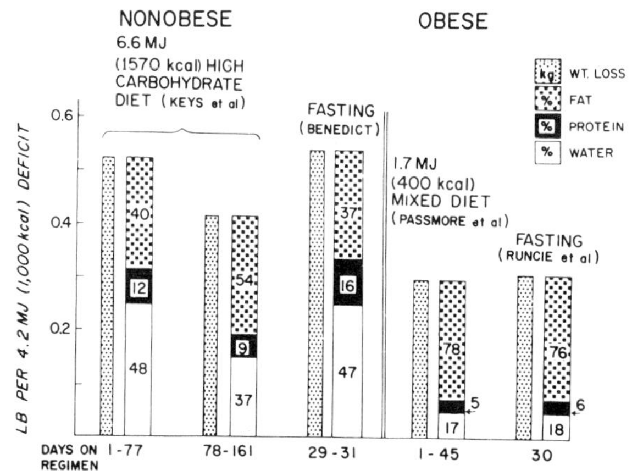

Fig.4. Composition of weight lost by obese and non-obese subjects during starvation (fasting) or calorie restriction. All values have been normalized to pounds per 4.2 MJ (1000 kcal) deficit

However, because substantial ketosis is not needed for protein-sparing under these circumstances, it would seem prudent to avoid some of the hazards known to be associated with ketogenic diets (Council on Foods and Nutrition, 1973) by providing the patient with a mixture of carbohydrate and protein rather than protein alone. Of course, if enough protein is given, sufficient glucogenic amino acids may become available to reduce or prevent ketosis.

Second, as shown by studies of composition of weight loss, non-obese individuals cannot conserve body protein well on calorie-reduced diets. It would appear to follow that mildly obese individuals also might well lose more nitrogen than is clinically desirable were they to embark on a very low calorie diet relatively high in protein content. Thus, protein-supplemented fasting and some of the variants of this regimen would seem to be indicated only for patients with severe obesity or patients with moderate obesity who are refractory to less drastic treatments.

Finally, it cannot be assumed that protein-supplemented fasting is benign just because nitrogen equilibrium may be achieved after some loss of body protein has occurred. As Nettleton & Hegsted (1975) have pointed out, the body's depletion of dietary or tissue protein is a highly complex process. 'Tissues gain or lose nitrogen at different rates and some tissues may actually gain nitrogen during a net loss of body weight or nitrogen from other tissues. Thus, dietary modifications which are incompatible with survival over the long run may temporarily result in a net increase in tissue nitrogen. Also, the results obtained are entirely dependent upon the time period over which the observations are made. Nearly all the studies upon protein requirements and the utilization of dietary protein in man are of short duration and based on overall nitrogen balance. These kinds of studies provide no information as to the distribution of nitrogen within the body tissues. Thus, moderate, but important, changes within specific tissues may be offset by compensatory changes in other tissues, and overall changes in nitrogen balance may be insufficiently sensitive to detect important changes in specific tissues.'

To answer the cogent questions raised by these workers, we need better methods than are currently available to assess the effect of varying degrees of protein depletion on body tissues and their functions.

Acknowledgement – The work in this paper was supported in part by a grant from the National Institutes of Health (Obesity Research Center AM-17624).

References

Allison, J.B., Anderson, J.A. & Seeley, R.D. (1946): *Ann. N.Y. Acad. Sci.* 47, 245.
Allison, J.B. (1958): *Ann. N.Y. Acad. Sci.* **69**, 1009.
Apfelbaum, M., Bostsarron, J., Brigant, L. & Dupin, H. (1967): *Gastroenterologia* **108**, 121.
Baird, I.M., Parsons, R.L. & Howard, A.N. (1974): *Metabolism* 23, 645.
Benedict, F.G. (1915): *A study of prolonged fasting.* Washington DC: Carnegie Institute, Publication No. 203.
Blackburn, G.L., Flatt, J.P., Clowes, G.H.A., O'Donnell, T.F. & Hensle, T.E. (1973): *Ann. Surg.* 177, 588.
Calloway, D.H. & Spector, H. (1954): *Am. J. Clin. Nutr.* 2, 405.
Council on Foods and Nutrition (1973): *J. Am. Med. Ass.* **224**, 1415.
Drenick, E.J. (1975): Weight reduction by prolonged fasting. In *Obesity in perspective,* ed G.A. Bray. p. 341. Washington DC: US Govt. Ptg. Office.
Flatt, J.P. & Blackburn, G.L. (1974): *Am. J. Clin. Nutr.* 27, 175.
Gilder, H., Cornell, G.N., Grafe, W.R., Macfarlane, J.R., Asaph, J.W., Stubenbord, W.T., Watkins, G.M., Rees, J.R. & Thorbjarnarson, B. (1967): *J. Appl. Physiol.* 23, 304.
Keys, A., Brozek, J., Henschel, A., Michelson, O. & Taylor, H. (1950): *The biology of human starvation,* Vol. 1. Minneapolis: University of Minnesota Press.
Lusk, G.L. (1906): *The elements of the science of nutrition.* Philadelphia: W.B. Saunders Company.
Marliss, E.B., Murray, F.T. & Nakhooda, A.F. (1976): *Clin. Res.* 24, 681A.
Munro, H.N. (1951): *Physiol. Rev.* 31, 449.
Nettleton, J.A. & Hegsted, D.M. (1975): *Nutr. Metabol.* **18**, 31.
Passmore, R., Strong, J.A. & Ritchie, F.J. (1958): *Br. J. Nutr.* **12**, 113.
Runcie, J. & Hilditch, T.E. (1974): *Br. Med. J.* 2, 352.
Swanson, P. (1951): *Fed. Proc.* **10**, 660.
Voit, E. (1901): *Zeitschrift für Biologie,* Bd. xli, p. 188.
Yang, M.U. & Van Itallie, T.B. (1976): *J. Clin. Invest.* 58, 722.

39
Intestinal bypass for severe obesity, a randomized trial. A report from the Danish Obesity Group

F. QUAADE and members of the Danish Obesity Group*
Department of Endocrinology, Hvidovre Hospital, University of Copenhagen, Denmark.

So much has been reported, over the years, about serious side-effects after jejuno-ileostomy, and so little is known about the prognosis of severe obesity, that grave doubt has existed as to whether the intervention is at all justified.

For these reasons, a number of departments from 11 hospitals all over Denmark agreed, in 1973, to join forces in a prospective, controlled clinical trial, in which very obese patients were allocated, on a random basis, to either conventional dietary treatment (1/3) or to jejunoileal end-to-side anastomosis with either long jejunal segment (1/3) or long ileal segment (1/3).

It is the intention of this communication to give a preliminary survey of some of our main findings.

Method

The protocol has been described in a preliminary report (Jan. 1977). The main points are recapitulated in Fig. 1 and 2.

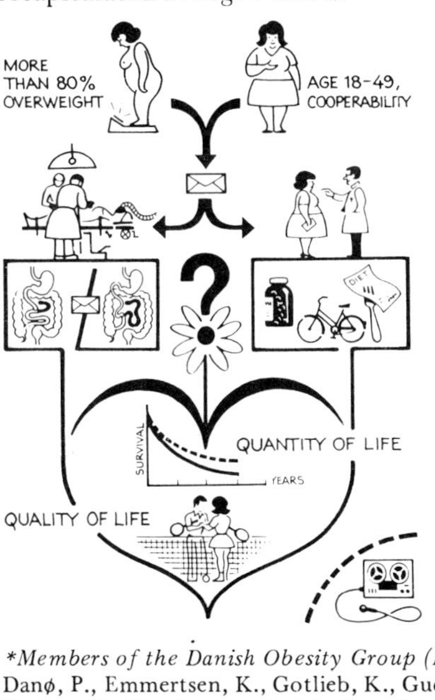

Fig. 1. The Danish Obesity Project. General principles of entry, allocation to various treatments, and evaluation of results

Members of the Danish Obesity Group (D.O.P.) are: Anderson, B., Anderson, D., Baden, H., Backer, O.G., Danø, P., Emmertsen, K., Gotlieb, K., Gudmand-Høyer, E., Halver, B., Iversen, O., Juhl, E., Madsen C.M., Madsen, S., Marckmann, A., Martiny, P.J., Mogensen, E.F., Mosekilde, L., Noring, O., Petersen, K.E., Starup, U., Stokholm, K.H., Storgard, L., Sørensen, N.S., Vagn-Nielsen, O.

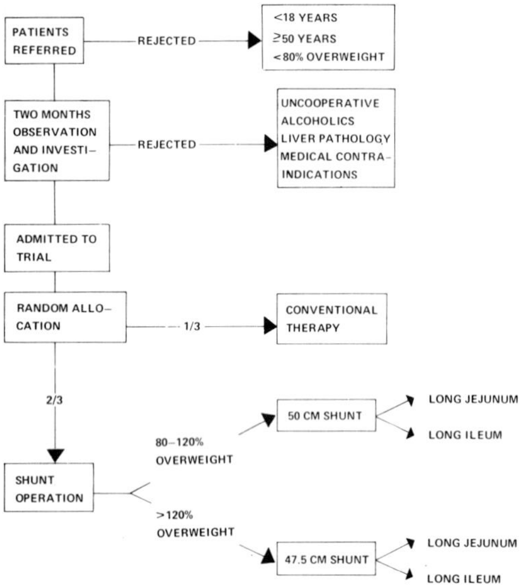

Fig. 2. The Danish Obesity Project. Flow chart for randomized controlled trial of intestinal bypass

Patients are eligible for preliminary entry if their obesity is so severe that it constitutes a physical handicap; not just a psychological one. We have felt that the patients should be legally of age, fully developed physically, and not past middle age. Ability to cooperate and a reasonable degree of mental stability are obviously important. A preallocation liver biopsy should show no cirrhosis, and if a fatty liver is found, there should be no history of alcoholism. After 2 months, the patients who meet these demands are randomly allocated to either non-surgical treatment, ie diet, exercise, possibly anorectic drugs (1/3), or to one of the following four types of bypass operation (2/3):

Long jejunal segment, total 50 cm (37.5 cm jejunum)
Long jejunal segment, total 47.5 cm (35 cm jejunum)
Long ileal segment, total 50 cm (37.5 cm ileum)
Long ileal segment, total 47.5 cm (35 cm ileum)

The 'short' shuntings are used for the most obese patients, those more than 120 per cent overweight. The relative lengths of the jejunal and ileal segments are decided by randomization.

Results

After 3 years of allocation (Sept. 1973 – Sept. 1976), the operated group consisted of 133 patients, and the control groups of 69 patients. Six patients, three from each group, were lost to follow-up immediately after allocation, which leaves 130 operated and 66 unoperated. The groups proved comparable with regard to age, sex, height, and weight.

We have been able to keep most of the control patients although 14 were lost to follow-up after 1 to 18 months (median 7 months). The remaining 52 have an observation time of 3 to 36 months (median 22 months).

In the operated group, the bypass was taken down in two patients, and two others dropped out during the second postoperative year. The observation time ranges from 6 to 45 months with a median of 24 months.

Mortality. No operated patient has died. In the control group, one patient died of complications after a liver biopsy. Autopsy showed that he had developed a cirrhosis of the liver after allocation.

Weight alterations. The curves for body weight and weight loss in the two groups are shown in Fig. 3 and Fig. 4. At 6, 12, and 24 months both groups had lost weight significantly, compared with time zero. Not surprisingly, the operated group lost significantly more than the controls. We have not yet analysed the weight data in detail, but it is evident that there are many instances of postoperative stabilization at a high level, and also of secondary weight gain.

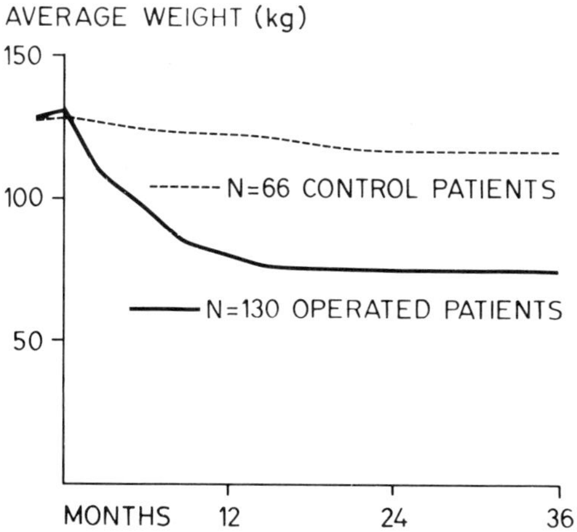

Fig. 3. Average weight curves in operated and unoperated patients

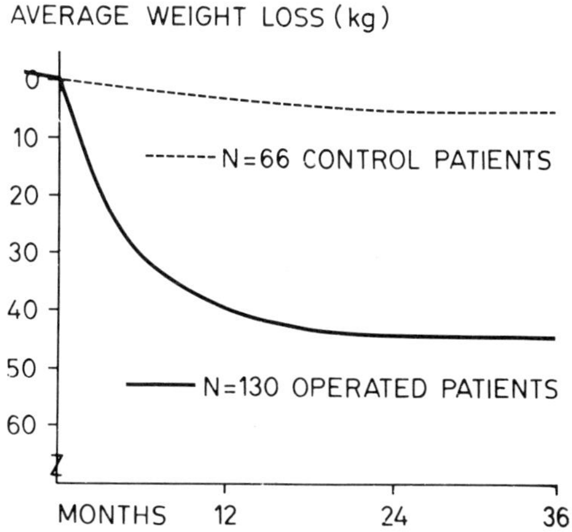

Fig. 4. Average weight loss in operated and unoperated patients

In addition to the 130 operated patients in the controlled trial, 84 have been randomized to either long or short ileal segment in other departments with whom we collaborate. Thus, a total of 214 patients are eligible for an evaluation of complications and for a comparison between the two different jejunal-ileal ratios.

Early postoperative complications. Some are listed in Table 1. They were not deterring, and furthermore there has been a statistically significant decrease in their overall frequency, from 28.9 per cent in 1973-75 to 16.1 per cent in 1975-77. Similarly, a sample of 80 patients operated in one of the participating hospitals showed a significant decrease in the duration of their postoperative stay, from 14.7 days in the first period to 7.8 days in the second.

Table 1. Early postoperative complications after jejuno-ileostomy performed for severe obesity in 214 patients

	No	%
Leakage of anastomosis	0	0.0
Wound complications	38	17.8
Lung complications	7	3.3

Late postoperative complications. The most important are shown in Table 2. Severe liver disease occurred in four cases, but three could be treated with parenteral alimentation. In the second postoperative year, cirrhosis of the liver was diagnosed by biopsy in one patient. Urinary calculi have not presented great problems, maybe because we use large doses of calcium to minimize diarrhoea.

Six women became pregnant after the operation. Two normal children were born, one

Table 2. Late postoperative complications after jejuno-ileostomy performed for severe obesity in 214 patients

	No	%
Serious electrolyte derangement (Ca, Mg, K)	16	7.5
Severe liver damage, bypass conserved	3	1.4
Severe liver damage, bypass taken down	1	0.5
Peptic ulcer, bypass taken down	1	0.5
Urolithiasis *de novo*	5	2.3
Arthritis	2	0.9

was premature, but alive and well after one year. There has been one abortion.

It has been necessary to *reoperate* quite frequently and for a variety of reasons (Table 3). It is worth noting that the patients have tolerated this secondary surgery very well.

The two groups with different jejunal-ileal ratios were entirely comparable with regard to sex, age, height, weight, drop-out frequency, and observation time. There were no significant differences between them concerning postoperative complications - with the possible exception that the patients with long ileal segment seem to be more prone to postoperative development of gall-stones. The weight curves of the two groups are seen in Fig. 5. There was no statistically significant difference.

Table 3. Reoperations after jejuno-ileostomy performed for severe obesity in 214 patients

	No	%
Bypass shortened	16	7.5
Bypass taken down	2	0.9
Gall-stones	4	1.9
Plastic surgery	26	12.2
Ventral hernia	9	4.2

'Quality of life'. Originally, we had planned to assess this by means of an elaborate prospective programme of repeated interviews, interpreted by 'blinded' collaborators. Regrettably, this part of the study proved too complex to set in motion. Instead all patients have been given an extensive and detailed questionnaire. We obtained usable answers for 94 per cent. In the operated group, we have only included answers from patients with stabilized weight and a postoperative observation time of at least 12 months. About 30 patients were excluded for these reasons from this cross-sectional study.

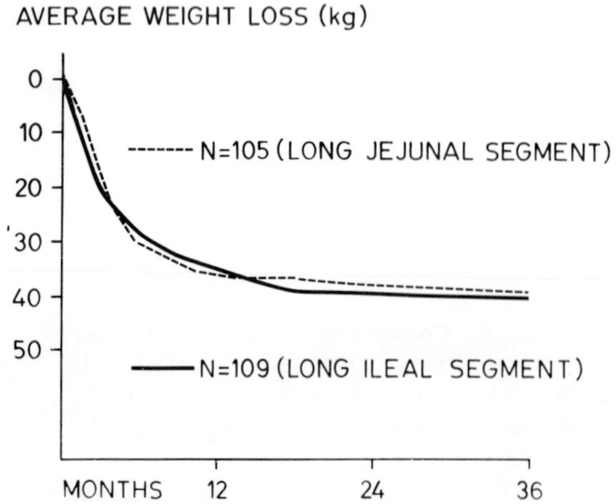

Fig. 5. Average weight loss after two types of end-to-side jejuno-ileostomy

Tables 4-7 give a comparison between operated and unoperated patients with regard to some characteristic complaints of a somatic nature. When not otherwise indicated, the differences are statistically significant. As might be expected, gastrointestinal discomfort (Table 4) dominated in the operated group, but we are reminded that it is also frequent in obesity. Shortness of breath and discomfort in the chest (Table 5) were more pronounced among the unoperated patients, as were various musculoskeletal complaints (Table 6). Table 7 shows a characteristic difference between the two groups in their adaptability to heat and cold.

The patients' rating of their psychological adaption to the operated or unoperated state (Table 8) also point to an improvement after bypass. The same is true of a list of such miscellaneous items as may indicate quality of everyday life (Table 9).

It may be added here that the number of social contacts outside the family, expressed as the monthly number of visits from or to friends, was twice as high in the operated as in the unoperated group.

Table 4. Gastrointestinal complaints in a cross-sectional questionnaire study of bypass operated and unoperated obese patients. The differences are statistically significant

	Operated %	Unoperated %
Abdominal pain	35	14
Heartburn	14	38
Bloating	65	50
Flatulence	90	49
Unpleasant odour	95	47
Abdominal rumbling	84	27

Table 5. Cardiorespiratory complaints in a cross-sectional questionnaire study of bypass-operated and unoperated obese patients. The differences are statistically significant

		Operated %	Unoperated %
Dyspnea at rest		6	26
Exertional dyspnea	1. floor	12	47
	2. –	27	84
	3. –	41	92
Heart pains		7	21

Table 6. Musculoskeletal complaints in a cross-sectional questionnaire study of bypass-operated and unoperated obese patients. The differences are statistically significant

	Operated %	Unoperated %
Pain in back	39	63
Pain in hips	15	34
Pain in knees	22	57
Pain in feet	14	49
Leg edema	41	73

Table 7. Heat regulatory complaints in a cross-sectional questionnaire study of bypass-operated and unoperated obese patients. The differences are statistically significant

	Operated %	Unoperated %
Heat intolerance	22	80
Perspiration	20	76
Cold intolerance	39	13

Table 8. Psychological complaints in a cross-sectional questionnaire study of bypass-operated and unoperated obese patients. The differences are statistically significant when not otherwise indicated

	Operated %	Unoperated %
Teased	11	66
Irritable	41	71
In good spirits	15	17 n.s.
In bad spirits	14	22 n.s.
Often depressed	36	62
Insecure	38	73
Lonely	13	38

Table 9. Various features of everyday life as rated in a questionnaire study of bypass-operated and unoperated obese patients. The differences are statistically significant

	Operated %	Unoperated %
Eat more than others	26	42
Daily exercise	54	38
Organized sport	23	12
'Normal' sex life	78	53
Sexually content	82	48
Ready-made clothes	97	51
Uninterrupted sleep	36	55
Skin folds	39	58

Discussion

The question of operative mortality, and mortality in the first years after bypass, has of course been a fundamental issue in the study. In this respect, and with regard to early post-operative complications, our data are such that they do not constitute grounds for abandoning this way of treating severe obesity. So far, our long-term side-effects, though occasionally grave, have in most cases responded well to either conservative treatment or to reestablishment of normal bowel passage, and we consider it justified to go on. Still, we feel the need for several more years of observation before a really reassuring answer can be given. Indeed the ideal, but hardly attainable, basis for our judgement would be a follow-up of both groups of patients for the rest of their lives.

Though most operated patients lost much weight, many did not lose enough. The problem of how to make the individual patient lose the right amount of weight is still unsolved and will require more of our attention in the future. We should face the possibility, among others, that bypass surgery for obesity must in many cases be a two-step procedure.

In view of the fact that mortality and somatic postoperative side-effects promise to be more favorable than we expected, increasing emphasis must, in future, be placed upon the best possible comparison between all aspects of quality of life in operated patients and in patients with conservatively treated severe obesity.

We realize that there are several weak points in our quality of life investigation. One of them is that the study is cross-sectional, and not prospective. Another is the fact that we have, in this presentation, excluded the patients whose weight had not stabilized after the operation. There are reasons to believe that these patients are less content than the others, so that our findings may be too optimistic. This may have to be revised when we have had time to process in detail the vast amount of data from our questionnaires.

The members of the Danish Obesity Project have decided to go on working together, randomizing new patients to treatment and keeping the old control patients unoperated as long as possible. However, for the future, a new and, we hope, improved protocol will have to be drawn up. In this way we hope to redeem what we have hitherto neglected, especially with regard to informed consent, individual weight loss, and prospective evaluation of psychosocial adjustment.

40
Surgical problems with intestinal bypass for obesity

D. HALLBERG
Department of Surgery, Serafimerlasarettet, S-112 83 Stockholm, Sweden.

Treatment of obesity is still a difficult medical problem. A high percentage of failures are reported with conservative methods and many obese subjects still have their problems some time after treatment. This impossible situation invited some surgeons to apply methods commonly used in other fields of surgery.

After more than 20 years of surgical practice we know that some of the available methods are effective in curing obesity and, therefore, justified when practiced under certain indications by trained surgeons. The complications and drawbacks are reasonable in relation to the magnitude of the problems at high body weight and the gain in 'quality of life' after weight reduction.

It is perhaps time to scrutinize the surgical approach and the methods in relation to some results. The common surgical methods are assumed to be known, or the reader is referred to a review (eg, Hallberg, Backman & Espmark, 1975).

The surgical approach

The surgeon's analysis of this field can be summarized as follows: (1) He can reduce undesirable adipose tissue by surgical lipectomy, (2) He can reduce the intake of food by: (a) reducing the size of the stomach by gastric bypass or gastroplasty, or (b) jaw wiring, (3) He can reduce the resorption of food from the intestine by intestinal bypass, (4) He can reduce digestion of food in the intestine by bypassing of gastro-bilio-pancreatic juices, and (5) He can reduce appetite by neurosurgical stereotactic manipulations.

Surgical problems

Each of these approaches resulted in several methodological modifications. Not only has new information about obesity, the human body and behavior been forthcoming, but also new questions have been raised. Some of the questions will be pinpointed and discussed below.

Are the deviations from control values observed in obese subjects a cause or a consequence of the obese state? If surgical methods can normalize the bodyweight, will the observed deviations disappear or increase or not be influenced? It is impossible to give a uniform answer to these two fundamental questions because they will depend both on the observed parameter and the methods used to obtain weight reduction.

The approaches outlined above present drastic procedures from a physiological viewpoint. It is, therefore, pertinent to relate these methods to other information we have.

Lipectomy removes a certain amount of subcutaneous adipose tissue. This procedure is interesting because the total number of fat cells is reduced. The metabolic consequences of this reduction for the energy homeostasis have been studied very little. What is the metabolic turnover rate of various lipids in blood and adipose tissues before and after the lipectomy? Are the changes related to the amount of tissue removed? Is there a limit for the metabolic rate in the remaining adipose tissue? The first steps to solve these questions have been taken by Kral & co-workers (Kral, 1976). Are the effects on the energy homeostasis similar to shrinking the size of the storage capacity in a warehouse? Will there be a shortage of fatty acids at high energy demand? Surgical lipectomy has turned out to be of only limited value in treatment of extreme obesity. Is this because too few fat cells are removed or are new fat cells formed all the time to store the available surplus of energy?

We have had no experience with gastric bypass. What is the mechanism for the decreased appetite and smaller meals after this procedure? Does the remaining part of the antrum influence caloric homeostasis? It seems probable that the small size of the gastric pouch is the only responsible factor. After a total gastrectomy many patients can still eat and maintain bodyweight. The studies by Bray and others (1976) of food preferences and intakes before and after intestinal shunts pointed towards an 'intestinal factor' for appetite regulation. These studies really need to be reproduced before and after gastric bypass. If there is a difference between these two surgical methods a new regulator of appetite has been demonstrated.

The intestinal bypass procedures are surgically simple and, therefore, used all over the world. Our own experiences are concerned with these methods, and some aspects of this procedure and its problems are discussed below.

The philosophy of decreasing the digestion of food in obese subjects by means of shunting away the digestive juices has not yet been studied very well. The method of cholecysto-jejunostomy described below is a combination of the creation of malresorption and maldigestion. Another experimental procedure derived from this approach is described by Scopinario and co-workers (1976). They perform a gastrojejunostomy (Billroth II) and anastomose the duodenum and upper jejunum to a distal intestinal loop. In this way the bile and pancreatic fluid, if not reabsorbed before, will not mix with food until in the distal small intestine. The principle needs much more experimental work, even if we already have a lot of information from patients treated for diseases of the upper digestive tract. Massive obesity is a new and not yet tested indication.

The neurosurgical approach of decreasing the appetite by destroying nuclei in the hypothalamus by stereotactic means has many problems. It is only mentioned as an example of ways to cope with obesity. However, in the present state of our knowledge, it is to be discouraged.

In the following text I shall assume that the methods of intestinal bypass are known to the reader: jejuno-ileostomy end-to-side (Payne *et al.*, 1973) and end-to-end (Scott *et al.*, 1971). The results after these procedures are often reliable. An early and late mortality (~2 + 3 per cent) and morbidity (~10 per cent) are still present. The advantages of a successful procedure are so great that the disadvantages are faced with a submissive mind. Some early and late problems associated with intestinal bypass procedures are given in Table 1. It is only the late complications which are of interest in this discussion. It is possible to categorize them into the areas of interest depicted in Table 2.

Intestinal length

Several authors have suggested that the results depend on a careful measurement of the intestinal length. They state than an error of 3 to 10 cm in intestinal length may be responsible for too much or too little weight loss. In our hands we have found a methodological error in measuring intestinal length of about 10 per cent (Hallberg & Backman, 1974). The total small intestinal length in obese subjects furthermore has been found to vary between 4.5 and 11 metres. One recommended measurement for a functioning shunt is 35 cm jejunum plus 15 cm ileum. This shunt length represents 11 per cent of the total intestinal length in the subject with a short intestine and only 4.5 per cent in the subject with a long intestine.

We need more information about how to handle such big inter-individual differences.

Table 1. Early and late complications after intestinal bypass for obesity

Early complications (unspecific)	**Late complications** (specific)
Wound dehiscence	Diarrhoea
infection	Flatulence
Thrombo-embolism	Too little weight loss
Anastomotic leakage	Too much weight loss
Ileus	Malnutrition
	electrolyte disturbances (K, Mg, Ca, Fe, I)
	avitaminosis
	signs of liver failure
	Hyperoxaluria (lithiasis)
	Immunological reactions (eg, erythema nodosum)
	Psychological-psychiatric disturbances
	psycho-social imbalance
	crisis reactions
	depressions
	suicide

Table 2. Problem areas associated with intestinal bypass for obesity

Methods for measurement of intestinal length
Intestinal reflux
Diarrhoea and flatulence
Nutritional and metabolic problems
Adaptation of the intestinal mucosa
How to perform reoperations: too little weight loss
too much weight loss
Insight into psychodynamic mechanisms

Otherwise we will have difficulties in performing the procedure with high precision (see preface in Atkins, 1969).

The subject with a very long intestine probably needs a longer shunt. It is difficult to explain that one obese subject has excess of small intestine when another has not. One possible explanation is that the gut length or resorptive surface area has adapted to metabolic circumstances before surgery. We have adjusted the shunt length according to information obtained from each patient. We use a fixed length of jejunum (35 to 40 cm) and a piece of ileum which is not less than 2 per cent of the total intestinal length (measured from the ligament of Treitz to the valvula of Bauhini). If the ileum is shorter than 2 per cent, the rate of weight loss was too fast and malnutrition became obvious (Hallberg *et al.*, 1975).

The measurement of intestinal length has the same errors as measuring a rubber band. Each surgeon must therefore test and calculate his own error by repeated measurements.

Reflux

X-ray of the intestine demonstrates that after most bypass procedures there is reflux of contrast medium into the blind intestinal loop (after the end-to-end and end-to-side procedures). The barium may be seen several metres up into the blind loop during several hours. This probably also occurs with food. Some patients lose weight fairly slowly after the intestinal shunt. We, therefore, consider reflux as an important source of error in determining the size of the postoperative resorptive surface area. The phenomenon makes it difficult to explain weight loss purely by a decreased resorptive area because these areas are larger than expected. Some cases with too little weight loss may be explained this way. Therefore, methods have been developed to prevent reflux and increase the precision of surgery (Hallberg *et al.*, 1975). The best method to prevent intestinal blind loop reflux has not yet been described.

In spite of a considerable reflux most subjects lose weight anyhow. This fact gives us a difficult question to answer. Does the reflux of food into the blind loop decrease our appetite, which could explain the weight loss (Bray *et al.*, 1976)?

Is the adaptation of the intestinal mucosa less marked in cases where reflux into the blind loop? Is the final resorptive surface area (the sum of the shunt area and the resorptive area in the blind loop) constant?

We cannot yet answer these questions. It is important for our future work to increase the precision in our methods so we can avoid reflux and then allow us to draw our conclusions.

Diarrhoea and flatulence

The most constant finding after intestinal shunts is diarrhoea. This phenomenon seems to be a predictable necessity given the philosophy which initiated the procedure. Increased amounts of semidigested food mixed with unresorbed bile acids enter the colon. The bacterial flora will both increase and change. These factors have been considered to contribute to diarrhoea and flatulence. Patients chosen for intestinal bypass are, therefore, informed about these 'complications'.

Are there any means of minimizing the drawbacks by decreasing the amount of bile acids in the colon? Recently we have tested a surgical method in which the end-to-side jejuno-ileal shunt is performed, but is modified by anastomosing the top of the blind jejunal loop to the functioning gall-bladder (Fig. 1). This new anastomosis drains most of the bile from the gall-bladder into the blind loop, where it is absorbed without coming into contact with food and colon. The enterohepatic circulation of bile acids is thus preserved. During digestion the sphincter of Oddi will relax and some bile will reach the duodenum and mix with food. During the fasting state the sphincter is closed and the bile will enter the gall-bladder and continue into the blind loop and be recycled.

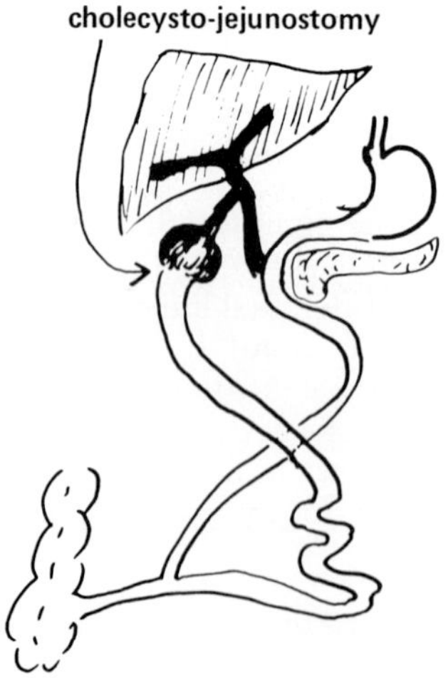

Fig. 1. Schematic illustration of a modified intestinal bypass procedure (jejuno-ileostomy end-to-side plus cholecysto-jejunostomy) aimed to preserve the entero-hepatic bile acid circulation

Our experience with this method is limited to six cases and a one-year observation time (Hallberg & Holmgren, in press). The results, up to now, may be designated as excellent. The rate of weight loss is similar to the usual Payne procedure. The frequency of diarrhoea and flatulence is much lower.

The procedure is a combination of decreasing the resorptive surface area and decreasing the fat digestive ability in the intestine. The method has interesting aspects and advantages in preservation of the enterohepatic circulation. It is, however, still too early to recommend.

Nutritional and metabolic problems

The intestinal bypass forces the patient into a negative energy balance. This continues for a variable time depending on several factors. During this time interval imbalances in a number of parameters may occur (Table 1). The most common are losses of minerals (K, Mg, Ca, Fe, I) vitamins and proteins.

As time passes the remaining part of the small intestine has adapted and the resorptive surface has grown to such an extent that a new balance is reached.

During the time of weight loss it is, therefore, important to follow these patients carefully. If the weight loss is too fast it may be necessary to supplement with nutrients given by the intravenous route (supplemental parenteral feeding) until the bodyweight has stabilized. Most of our current views on these problems have been published elsewhere (Hallberg *et al.,* 1975).

Intestinal adaptation

The resorptive surface area of the small intestine is a function of several parameters: the small intestinal length, the circumference and the number and height of the villi and folds in the intestinal mucosa. All these parameters are subjected to changes. The causes inducing these changes are only partly known (see review by Fenyő, 1976). The best known stimulus to induce changes is to shorten the small intestinal length. The remaining part of the intestine starts adaptation in order to restore the resorptive surface area eg, both by elongation and increasing the diameter of the intestine as such and also the size and number of the villi and folds in the mucosa. These phenomena are an almost consistent finding, after intestinal bypass for obesity and work against our aim to reduce the resorptive area. The ability to adapt is probably one explanation for why it is possible to perform extensive intestinal exclusions (see Table 3). The figures in Table 3 are chosen as examples of the effect of adaptation on the surface area. The figure 1.8 for the Kerckrings folds needs to be explained. The number of these folds per unit length is not counted but probably the number has not decreased. The height of the folds has increased as the diameter of the gut has increased. This has been verified by inspection at reoperations. The length of the folds is dependent on the circumference ($2\pi r$) of the gut. As this has increased by a factor of 2, the length of these folds has also increased. In order not to exaggerate the calculations, the low figure 1.8 has been chosen because then the surface area is restored to the initial figure (1.8 x 56 = 100 per cent). The importance of adaptation of the Kerckrings folds is probably larger than this figure shows. The calculations demonstrate that the mucosa has considerable ability to adapt.

Table 3. Adaptation factors and importance for the resorptive surface area after intestinal bypass

	Example		Adaptation factor	% of preoperative surface area	
Factor	Before adaptation	After adaptation		Before adaptation	After adaptation
Intestinal length/cm	60	84	1.4	10	1.4x10=14
diameter/cm	4	8	2		2 x14=28
Villus no/cm^2	?	?	1		1 x28=28
height μ	500	>1000	2		2 x28=56
Kerckrings folds					
length ($2\pi r$) cm	—	—	2 } ~1.8*		
no/cm	?	?	? } ~1.8*		
height/cm	?	>1	>1 } ~1.8*		1.8x56=100

*See text

Another facet of obesity may be linked to the atrophy of the intestinal mucosa seen in the disease celiaca. The mucosal atrophy and poor absorption in this disorder depends on the oral intake of gluten. If we could, by some pharmacological means reduce the surface area of the intestinal mucosa in obese subjects, then it would be possible to reduce the absorption of food without surgery.

In this context it may be of interest to mention one obese woman treated by intestinal shunt. She lost weight from 170 to 70 kg. She had nutritional difficulties for almost three years. Parenteral nutrition now and then was necessary in order to keep her free from symptoms. She was at last reoperated and the intestinal shunt was then observed to have the same measurement as at the initial surgery (40 cm + 15 cm). Biopsy of the mucosa showed that the villi were unchanged in height. There were few signs of reflux into the blind loop. One possible explanation of her difficulties is that this woman had no intestinal adaptation. This is in contrast to most other subjects with intestinal shunts reoperated because of other indications. I think that future observations of such patients will be of particular value towards our understanding of intestinal adaptation.

How to handle too little weight loss

About 5 to 10 per cent of shunted subjects consider that their weight loss is too little and ask for another operation. Our attitude in these cases is conservative. We ask them to wait as least one year and restrict their food intake. This year of expectancy usually takes away several kilograms of bodyweight. Only a few come to surgery. What is done for them? We perform a laparotomy and measure the intestinal length and compare it with the measurement at the first operation. The length of the intestine in the shunt is usually longer than expected or there are obvious signs of reflux into the blind loop. The cause of these observations are in several cases either measurement errors at the first operation or an unusual ability for elongation or adaptation. We resect the anastomosis and parts of the intestine leaving an intestinal length in the shunt which is 35 to 40 cm. We have tried taking away only jejunum in some cases and leaving only 10 cm of ileum in other cases. The results up to now are such that no definite recommendations can be given. After the jejunum resection the bodyweight decreased further but in a few cases not enough, according both to the patients' opinions and our bodyweight determinations.

In a few cases with a loss of bodyweight which may satisfy the surgeon (~ 50 kg) but not the patient, we have given a small dose of thyroxin by mouth. The response is usually very good. The background for this medication may be that iodine and thyroxin are normally excreated in the bile and then reabsorbed from the intestine. The postoperative course with a short intestine, diarrhoea and loss of bile constituents, may produce a biological shortage of thyroxin.

How to handle loss of too much bodyweight

In our hands this situation has appeared only three times in 178 patients. One patient developed signs of liver injury and anorexia in the postoperative course and vomited. After intense psychotherapy her problems were partly solved and the nutritional problems and signs of liver failure disappeared.

In two other patients with rapid and considerable weight loss, in spite of supporting parenteral nutrition, we have elongated the shunt by adding 35 cm of the jejunum from the blind loop back into the shunt. Both patients had signs of protein malnutrition. One of the patients is very well after the reoperation. The other patient has been mentioned because there were no signs of mucosal adaptation. She has improved after the last operation, but still has not stabilized.

Psychodynamic aspects

Understanding and insight into the psychodynamic aspects of obesity and weight loss is important for all surgeons performing any kind of weight losing operations.

The obese individual has very often unconsciously adjusted her personality to obesity. After surgery, when the weight decreases, the patient begins sooner or later, to meet new situations. The new situation may give rise to difficulties, where we can help by understanding.

Postoperative behaviour varies according to preoperative personality and the degree of conscious insight into adjustments. Some subjects are very happy all the time, when other subjects may show various degrees of crisis reaction or even suicide. For the pre- and postoperative assessments it is important to have an understanding attitude.

The aspects given above are examples of problems and thoughts related to our intestinal bypass surgery. The surgical approach in this field is unphysiological, but as long as the obese subjects have their problems unsolved, it is one way out of their dilemma. In the meantime we hope to learn more about these subjects.

Summary

The surgical approach in treatment of obesity has been categorized. The importance of methodological errors and precision in measuring the intestinal length are mentioned as important steps in intestinal bypass surgery. The degree of reflux in the blind loop is mentioned as one erroneous factor for determination of the resorptive surface area. The postoperative intestinal adaptation is considerable and thus counteracts the surgical aim to reduce the resorptive surface area. A modified intestinal bypass procedure is described which preserves the enterohepatic bile acid circulation. The occurrence of diarrhoea is less frequent with this method. A number of questionmarks pertaining to this kind of surgery are mentioned.

References

Atkins, H. (1969): *Measurement and precision in surgery*. Oxford: Blackwell.

Bray, G.A., Barry, R., Benfield, J., Castelnuovo-Tedesco, P. & Rodin, J. (1976): *Am. J. Clin. Nutr.* 29, 779.

Fenyö, G. (1976): *Acta Chir. Scand.* Suppl. 469.

Fenyö, G., Backman, L. & Hallberg, D. (1976): *Acta Chir. Scand.* **142**, 154.

Hallberg, D. & Backman, L. (1974): *Acta Chir. Scand.* **140**, 57.

Hallberg, D., Backman, L. & Espmark, S. (1975): *Progress in surgery* **14**, 46.

Hallberg, D. & Holmgren, U. (in press): *Acta Chir. Scand.*

Kral, J.G. (1976): Surgical reduction of adipose tissue. Effects of adipectomy and intestinal bypass on adipose tissue cellularity. Thesis. Gothenburg.

Payne, J.H., De Wincl, L., Schwab, C.E. & Kern, W.H. (1973): *Archs Surg.* **106**, 432.

Scopinaro, N., Gianetta, E., Pandolfo, N., Anfossi, A., Berretti, B. & Bachi, V. (1976): *Min. Chir.* **31**, 560.

Scott, H.W., Sandstead, H.H., Brill, A.B., Burk, H. & Younger, R.K. (1971): *Ann. Surg.* **174**, 560.

41
Medical aspects of jejunoileal bypass for morbid obesity

D. H. LOCKWOOD
Endocrine-Metabolism Unit, Department of Medicine, University of Rochester, School of Medicine and Dentistry, Rochester, New York 14642, USA.

When an individual's weight reaches 100 per cent above ideal the diagnosis of morbid obesity is customarily made. This terminology serves to emphasize the impression that serious health hazards are present and life will be significantly shortened. The exact morbidity and mortality in this group of patients are unknown since life insurance companies, the primary provider of these statistics, are reluctant to provide coverage. However, in a group of 47 patients whose mean ideal weight was 196 per cent, Genuth, Castro & Vertes (1974) reported a high incidence of diabetes (74 per cent), hypertension (30 per cent), gall-bladder disease (28 per cent), gout (13 per cent) and coronary artery disease (11 per cent). In a larger study of the prevalence of cardiovascular risk factors in obesity, Berchtold & co-workers (1977) concluded that patients with gross obesity are at high risk with respect to coronary artery disease. Thus, despite the absence of precise information concerning the risks of morbid obesity, vigorous attempts directed towards weight reduction appear warranted. Unfortunately, this task is not easily achieved.

Since the review by Stunkard & McLaren-Hume in 1959 indicating that less than 5 per cent of patients who needed to lose 40 or more pounds were successful, several newer therapeutic modalities have been introduced and assessed. Prolonged fasting insures weight loss but is accompanied by a substantial loss of body protein along with the desired fat loss. Moreover, a generalized failure to maintain weight loss coupled with large costs and inconvenience of hospitalization diminish significantly the benefits of this therapeutic approach (Drenick, 1975). When morbidly obese outpatients are placed on a fast, modified by the intake of small amounts of protein, significant weight loss usually occurs and lean body mass is preserved (Genuth *et al.*, 1974; Bistrian *et al.*, 1976). However, the long-term benefits of these protein-sparing modified fasts are currently unknown although several deaths have now been reported. The use of behavior modification as an approach to the treatment of obesity shows considerable promise (Stuart, 1975; Stunkard & Mahoney, 1976) but its effectiveness in the morbidly obese has not been rigorously evaluated.

With the knowledge that the results of medical management of the morbidly obese are dismal, it is not surprising that our surgical colleagues became intrigued with the possibility of introducing successful operative procedures. Payne, DeWind & Commons (1963) were able to demonstrate that jejunocolic shunts produced enough intestinal malabsorption to cause significant weight reduction. Unfortunately, the complications of this initial surgical approach were numerous (Payne *et al.*, 1963; Salmon, 1971) and one was left with the impression that the 'cure' was worse than the disease. Particularly discouraging was the progressive, unrelenting weight loss which frequently necessitated revision and an ultimate return to the morbidly obese state. It is my view that the poor results of the jejunocolic shunt, although recognized early, have undeservedly continued to contribute to the controversy surrounding small bowel bypass surgery. In contrast to the jejunocolic shunt, the results of jejunoileostomy first introduced by Payne & DeWind (1969) and later modified by Scott & co-workers (1971) have been found to be generally satisfactory.

Between 1970 and 1976, over 100 morbidly obese patients at the Johns Hopkins Hospital were treated with the small bowel bypass. Most of these patients were evaluated preoperatively and on a continuing basis postoperatively by a team of physicians which included experienced surgeons, internists knowledgeable in acute and chronic postoperative complications, and a concerned psychiatrist. The criteria for acceptance for surgery were similar to those of other centers (Payne & DeWind, 1969; Sandstead, 1975). They include: an age between 15 and 50 years; a weight greater than 100 per cent above ideal; proven failure on medical regimens; evidence by psychiatric evaluation that the patient can emotionally tolerate surgery, weight loss and potential complications; absence of a history of significant alcohol ingestion; absence of any related or unrelated significant disease which might increase operative risk; and assurances of the patient's cooperation in preoperative and prolonged postoperative follow-up evaluation. All acceptable patients were submitted to a jejunoileal bypass in which 36 to 38 cm of proximal jejunum was anastomosed end-to-end with 10 to 13 cm of terminal ileum. The remaining segment of small intestine was closed proximally and anastomosed distally end-to-side with the transverse colon. Although the large series at Hopkins is primarily a result of multiple investigational interests, we have been able to gain considerable clinical experience regarding many aspects of the bypass procedure.

Table 1. Presumed beneficial effects of jejunoileal bypass

Benefit	Reference
Significant weight loss	Scott *et al.*, 1973; Campbell *et al.*, 1977
Relief of hypertension	Campbell *et al.*, 1977
Improvement in pulmonary function	Soterakis *et al.*, 1976
Reduction in serum triglycerides and cholesterol	Scott *et al.*, 1973
Improvement in carbohydrate tolerance	Rehfeld, Juhl & Quaade, 1970; Campbell *et al.*, 1977
Improvement of varicosities and leg stasis	Iber & Cooper, 1977
Relief of low back pain	Weismann, 1973
Rehabilitation to job	Iber & Cooper, 1977
Improvement in psychosocial function	Solow, 1977

The results of our series and most others indicate that following end-to-end jejunoileostomy two important objectives concerning weight loss are achieved. First significant weight loss amounting to 30 to 40 per cent of initial weight usually occurs within the first 1 to 2 years following surgery (Campbell *et al.*, 1977; Dean *et al.*, 1977). After this weight losing phase, the patient's weight usually stabilizes or increases only slightly. Table 1 shows that there are other presumed benefits secondary to jejunoileal bypass and subsequent weight loss. The reduction in blood pressure is most striking in patients with preoperative hypertension. Campbell & co-workers (1977) found that the incidence of hypertension preoperatively was 74 per cent and decreased to 30 per cent after surgery. Following substantial weight loss there is considerable improvement in pulmonary function, as measured by forced 1 s expiratory volume, minute ventilation and responsiveness to elevated PCO_2. The decrease in serum cholesterol is observed in virtually all patients. The serum concentration postoperatively is usually less than 150 mg/100 ml. The low cholesterol reflects at least in part increased cholesterol turnover induced by surgical interruption of the enterohepatic circulation and consequent fecal loss of bile acids (Moore, Frantz & Buchwald, 1969). It has been suggested that the low cholesterol may also be due to a decrease rate of cholesterol synthesis in the bypassed intestine (Faloon *et al.*, 1977). The fall in serum triglycerides is variable. The improvement in carbohydrate tolerance following bypass has been gratifying. In the series from the University of California (Campbell *et al.*, 1977) 22 patients preoperatively had an elevated fasting plasma glucose and all reverted to normal postoperatively. Associated with the improved glucose tolerance there is a reduction of the hyperinsulinemia characteristic of obesity and an improvement in insulin sensitivity. We and others (Iber & Cooper, 1977) have been impressed with a significant improvement in socioeconomic status following successful surgery but the results of others have not been encouraging (Campbell *et al.*, 1977). Previously Solow (1977) has provided convincing evidence that the psychological and social status of bypassed patients is improved. This will be discussed more fully in a subsequent manuscript (Solow *et al.*, this volume).

Table 2. Intestinal malabsorption following jejunoileal bypass

Fats	Scott *et al.*, 1971; Faloon *et al.*, 1977
Amino acids	Moxley *et al.*, 1974; Lockwood *et al.*, 1977
Glucose	Barry *et al.*, 1977; Dowling & Booth, 1966
Water and fat soluble vitamins	Scott *et al.*, 1973; Teitelbaum *et al.*, 1977
Electrolytes - potassium, calcium and magnesium	Sandstead, 1975; Teitelbaum *et al.*, 1977

Although the presumed benefits of bypass appear considerable, many adverse complications may be expected following massive reduction of the small bowel surface area, interruption of enterohepatic circulation and production of a 'blind loop'. Table 2 indicates that the aim of jejunoileal bypass, namely intestinal malabsorption, is achieved at least during the weight losing phase. Excessive fecal fat loss is seen in virtually all patients postoperatively but surprisingly the amount of weight loss is not related to the degree of steatorrhea (Faloon *et al.*, 1977). This lack of correlation probably serves to emphasize that reduced caloric intake following surgery is a major determinant of postoperative weight loss (Bray *et al.*, 1976). Our laboratory has provided evidence that protein malnutrition is a consequence of bypass surgery (Moxley, Pozefsky & Lockwood, 1974). Postabsorptive amino levels determined 4 months after surgery were characteristic of protein malnutrition. Oral amino acid tolerance tests performed at the same time indicate that the reduced plasma amino acid levels are in part attributable to decreased intestinal absorption. Employing intraluminal techniques, S.A. Adibi (personal communication) has substantiated our finding that free amino acid absorption is significantly reduced after surgery. We have been unable to prevent protein malnutriton by vigorous oral supplementation with essential amino acids (Lockwood *et al.*, 1977). One study (Barry *et al.*, 1977) of intestinal segmental glucose absorption indicates an impairment during the weight losing phase while another shows an increased rate of uptake (Dowling & Booth, 1966). In any case, carbohydrate deficiency does not appear to be extreme in view of observations that postoperatively patients are non-ketotic and maintain normal plasma glucose concentrations and liver glycogen content. Furthermore, it is our belief that the hepatic steatosis characteristically seen during the early months following bypass is a reflection of protein malnutrition coupled with adequate carbohydrate stores (Moxley *et al.*, 1974). These metabolic findings are similar to those seen in kwashiorkor, where fatty liver is common. Further support of this concept comes from the demonstration that intravenous infusion of amino acids can reverse the fatty hepatic infiltration in bypassed patients (Heimburger *et al.*, 1975).

Scott & co-workers (1973) have not found any evidence for vitamin B_{12} deficiency following bypass but Barry *et al.* (1977) have. We routinely give our patients 100 μg of vitamin B_{12} intramuscularly every 3 to 6 months. Scott & co-workers (1973) found a low incidence of hypovitaminosis C and a moderate incidence of low serum folate levels. Of the fat soluble vitamins there is little evidence clinically that vitamin K deficiency occurs. Vitamin E and A levels fall after surgery but the clinical significance is unknown. The effect of bypass on vitamin D has been carefully assessed (Teitelbaum *et al.*, 1977). Sixty-one per cent of 44 patients who had undergone jejunoileal bypass had low circulating levels of 25-OH vitamin D. In two patients studied intestinal absorption of 25-OH vitamin D was impaired. It is of interest that 25-OH vitamin D, the predominant form of vitamin D in plasma appears to be recycled through the enterohepatic circulation and thus bypass surgery could contribute to a deficiency state by interruption of recycling (Arnaud *et al.*,

1975). Although the hypovitaminosis D tends to normalize with postoperative duration, the possibility that bypass surgery promotes clinically significant skeletal abnormalities remains unanswered. Bone densitometry studies and bone biopsies have suggested that some patients may develop problems (Teitelbaum *et al.*, 1977).

An increase in stool excretion of magnesium, calcium and potassium is a consequence of the procedure. In addition, about one-half of the patients develop abnormally low serum magnesium levels and one-quarter low calcium levels (Teitelbaum *et al.*, 1977). In our experience hypocalcemia is usually associated with hypomagnesemia. In general, clinical problems of malabsorption are most prevalent during the weight losing phase following bypass and are unlikely to appear as a late complication. Whether the decrease in these complications results from improved intestinal function (Moxley *et al.*, 1974) and/or increased dietary intake (Bray *et al.*, 1976) and/or other factors remains unclear. The effect of bypass surgery on other aspects of intestinal function clearly needs evaluation. Investigations should consider the influence of bypass on drug absorption and on intestinal immunologic and endocrine function. We have recently accumulated data suggesting that postoperatively there is a loss of an enteric insulinotrophic factor(s) normally released by the intestine in response to ingested protein (Moxley *et al.*, 1977).

Table 3. 'Minor' medical complications of jejunoileal bypass which are usually transient and/or treatable

Complication	Treatment
Diarrhea	Low fat diet; diphenoxylate or deodorized tincture of opium
Transient bloating and flatulence	Simethicone
Perianal irritation	Topical treatment with lidocaine, steroids or cholestyramine paste
Electrolyte abnormalities	Oral supplementation
Vitamin deficiencies	Oral supplementation
Anemia	Usually iron; folate and parenteral vitamin B_{12} if indicated
Menstrual abnormalities	
Hair loss	

As a result of the bypass-induced malabsorption, every patient experiences a marked increase in stool frequency. A shortened intestinal transit time, steatorrhea, an intraluminal accumulation of fluids in response to unabsorbed sugars and bile salts, and a change in bacterial flora are all known factors contributing to the diarrhea. Somewhat surprising is the observation that stool frequency decreases significantly with increasing postoperative duration. It is not unusual for patients to pass eight to 20 stools per day during the initial 3 months after bypass, but this rate progressively declines to three or four stools per day by the time of weight stabilization. When indicated the diarrhea can be adequately controlled by lowering the fat content of the diet and administering drugs which decrease intestinal motility (Table 3). It should be noted that two of our patients developed problems of addiction while on deodorized tincture of opium. The massive diarrhea is sometimes accompanied by gas pangs, mild bloating, excessive flatulence and eructation. This symptom complex presents in a much milder form than the more serious 'bacterial overgrowth' syndrome which will be discussed subsequently by Drenick. The use of antiflatulents like simethicone frequently provides symptomatic relief. In our experience, perianal burning pain is the gastrointestinal complication which is most troublesome for the patient. The symptoms are frequently exacerbated by prolonged diarrhea and examination of the rectum reveals anal cryptitis and/or inflamed hemorrhoids. The goals of therapy should include reduction of stool frequency and symptomatic relief. The latter is usually accomplished with a local anesthetic (5 per cent xylocaine ointment) and topical glucocorticoids. In some cases, application of a cholestyramine 'paste' is beneficial, suggesting that at least part of the irritation is due to bile acids in the feces. In some patients the recurrence rate is so high that hemorrhoidectomy is required.

Hypokalemia, hypocalcemia and hypomagnesemia as well as the vitamin deficiencies are usually associated with marked diarrhea and thus are an early complication. With the exception of vitamin B_{12} deficiency, these deficits are usually satisfactorily managed by appropriate oral supplementation. Anemia with hematocrit readings in the range of 28 to 34 per cent has been found in 10 to 20 per cent of bypass patients (Starkloff *et al.*, 1975; O'Leary, 1976). The anemia tends to occur in the first year after surgery and is most commonly due to iron deficiency. Although overt gastrointestinal bleeding may be responsible for the loss of iron stores in some patients, we have been unable to detect evidence of blood loss in the majority.

The effect of jejunoileal bypass on menstruation and fertility is confusing since morbid obesity itself is associated with a high incidence of menstrual irregularity and amenorrhea (Rogers & Mitchell, 1952). With weight loss following surgery some patients experience a correction of these abnormalities and become pregnant for the first time while others develop amenorrhea. In a review of the literature, O'Leary (1976) found 20 pregnancies occuring after bypass. It is our impression that menstrual problems are most prominent during the weight losing phase suggesting that malnutrition is a causal factor. Transient hair loss is an infrequent but disturbing complication for the patient. The cause of this complication is unknown.

Table 4. Moderate to severe medical complications of jejunoileal bypass

Hepatic failure
Cholelithiasis
Bacterial overgrowth
- 'bypass enteritis'
- colonic pseudo-obstruction
- polyarthritis

Urinary calculi

As shown in Table 4, there are additional medical complications of bypass surgery which are associated with a greater degree of morbidity and mortality than those problems in Table 3. These more severe complications tend to differ from those related to malabsorption in other ways. With the exception of progressive liver failure which characteristically appears during the weight losing phase, the major complications can occur at any time after surgery. Thus, data concerning the prevalence of these complications are less precise but are of more importance as we continue to evaluate the pros and cons of this procedure. Long-term follow-up studies to date indicate that with the exception of urinary calculi the incidence of these major complications is less than 10 per cent.

Hepatic and biliary disease, along with problems associated with intestinal bacterial overgrowth, are topics to be discussed subsequently by Drenick. However, a few general comments based on our experience at Johns Hopkins are warranted. We have been most concerned with postoperative liver disease since hepatic failure has been the cause of two of the four deaths in a hundred patients studied. This incidence of deaths is identical to that found by Holzbach (1971) in a review of the literature. Our deaths have occurred despite comprehensive preoperative and postoperative evaluation of liver function and assessment of liver tissue obtained at the time of surgery and serially thereafter until weight stabilization occurs. Although we are impressed with the association between protein malnutrition and hepatic steatosis (Moxley *et al.*, 1974), we are not convinced that this is the primary cause of the infrequent hepatic fibrosis and cirrhosis. With the knowledge that altered hepatic morphology is common in morbid obesity (Juhl *et al.*, 1971; Manes, Taylor & Starkloff, 1973), we have embarked on a long-term study searching for preoperative risk factors. Very preliminary results suggest that preoperative hepatic changes (fat and/or fibrosis) may be useful in identifying patients at high risk for severe hepatic disease following bypass (Hamilton *et al.*, 1976). No predictors of hepatic steatosis observed during the weight losing phase have been found.

The hazards of gall-stones postoperatively is another condition which may not be solely related to the bypass procedure. In a careful study by Faloon & co-workers (1977), 19 of 44 patients had evidence of biliary tract disease or gall-stones before surgery. Of the remaining 25 patients with normal preoperative cholecystograms, four developed gall-stones within the first year after surgery. However, chemical analysis of the bile several months postoperatively did not demonstrate changes in the bile saturation ratio or lithogenic index, which are measures of the propensity for stone formation. However, the lithogenic index is increased in the first few weeks which may enhance gall-stone formation (Barry *et al.*, 1977).

In our experience, the problems presumed to be related to bacterial overgrowth in the bypassed intestine are becoming more alarming because they are appearing in patients 3 to 5 years following successful surgery. To date 3 per cent of our patients have developed polyarthritis which is considerably less than the incidence of 23 per cent observed by Shagrin, Frame & Duncan (1971). Oral administration of tetracycline has provided an excellent response in all three cases adding further support to the work of Wands & others (1976) who first suggested that bacterial overgrowth was involved in the pathogenesis of this complication.

Dickstein & Frame (1973) were the first to focus on the high incidence of renal calculi after small bowel bypass. In a 6-year experience with 34 patients, 11 (32 per cent) were found to have renal calculi. The clinical appearance of stone formation occurred as early as 24 days and as late as 6 years following bypass surgery. Of the stones analyzed all contained calcium oxalate. In other studies the incidence of renal stones appears to be somewhat less (O'Leary, Thomas & Woodward, 1974; Starkloff *et al.*, 1975). In evaluating their 475 patients, Starkloff & co-workers (1975) found a 6 per cent incidence of urinary calculi but also reported that of 80 postoperative patients studied, 60 per cent had elevated 24-hour urinary oxalate excretion in the range of 80 to 120 mg/day (Gregory *et al.*, 1975). O'Leary (1976) reported that over 75 per cent of his patients developed hyperoxaluria. The observations that most stones are composed of calcium oxalate and that hyperoxaluria is the rule following surgery strongly suggest that alterations in oxalate metabolism are important in the pathophysiology of stone formation.

Identification of these alterations has largely been a result of studies in patients with inflammatory bowel disease or ileal resection where there is an enhanced risk of renal stone formation (Gelzayd, Brener & Kirsner, 1968). Initially it was felt that the hyperoxaluria seen in patients with ileal resection was a consequence of interruption of the enterohepatic circulation (Smith, Fromm & Hofmann, 1972). They proposed that bile salts escaping into the colon underwent bacterial deconjugation releasing glycine which was further metabolized to glyoxalate. The glyoxalate was then absorbed, converted to oxalate by the liver and excreted in the urine. However, further studies following the fate of orally administered 1-^{14}C cholyl glycine demonstrated that bile salt glycine was not the precursor of urinary oxalate.

The more recent demonstration that the administration of cholestyramine, a non-absorbable anion exchange resin, could reverse hyperoxaluria in patients with ileal resection suggested that the source of urinary oxalate was the intestinal lumen (Stauffer, Humphreys & Weir, 1973). Additional studies provided convincing evidence that in these patients hyperoxaluria is the result of hyperabsorption of dietary oxalate which can be reversed by treatment with diets low in oxalate (Stauffer *et al.*, 1973; Chadwick, Modha & Dowling, 1973; Earnest *et al.*, 1974). Recent studies of urinary excretion of ^{14}C-oxalate following oral or caecal administration indicate that the colon is the site for enhanced oxalate absorption following jejunoileal bypass (Earnest, 1977). In ileal resected patients, Earnest & colleagues (1974) were able to correlate hyperoxaluria with the degree of steatorrhea. The absence of hyperoxaluria in some patients following jejunoileal bypass can be explained by severe maldigestion of oxalate-containing foods (Earnest, Williams & Admirand, 1975*a*).

Enhanced absorption of oxalate in the presence of steatorrhea suggests an altered intraluminal solubility of oxalate. It is likely that high levels of malabsorbed free fatty acids combine with intraluminal calcium, and thereby foster formation of other more soluble oxalate salts, which are available for absorption by passive diffusion in the colon. Earnest, Williams & Admirand (1975*b*) have shown that increasing calcium concentrations within a range normally found in the intestinal lumen enhances formation of insoluble and unabsorbable calcium oxalate. In the presence of increasing amounts of sodium oleate, calcium becomes progressively less effective in precipitating oxalate. The demonstration by Stauffer (1977) that high calcium diets (3000 mg/day) lower urinary oxalate excretion in bypass patients confirms the importance of oxalate solubility as a determinant for hyperabsorption. Dobbins & Binder (1976) in studies using everted rodent gut sacs have demonstrated that exposure of colonic mucosa to high levels of bile salts or fatty acids increases absorption of oxalate. Since fecal fat and bile acids are increased following bypass it is intriguing to consider altered colonic permeability as another cause for hyperabsorption of oxalate. However, studies in man including those with jejunoileal bypass do not support this hypothesis (Earnest & Graham, 1976; Earnest, 1977).

Table 5. Management of hyperoxaluria in patients with jejunoileal bypass

Low oxalate diet
Low saturated fat diet
Calcium supplementation
Cholestyramine
Medium-chain triglycerides

With a clearer understanding of the pathogenesis of renal calculi following bypass, we should, by proper medical management, significantly reduce this complication in the future (Table 5). We place all our postoperative patients on a low-oxalate diet (<50 mg/day). Compliance has not been a problem since most of the foods high in oxalate are leafy green vegetables (Stauffer, 1977). However, Earnest (1977) has noted that our knowledge of oxalate content in many foods is incomplete. Similarly, patients do not mind decreasing the fat content of their diet since it also decreases stool frequency. In addition, substituting medium-chain triglycerides for long-chain fats can further lower oxalate excretion in patients with jejunoileal bypass (Earnest, Williams & Admirand, 1975*c*). If necessary calcium and/or cholestyramine are included as adjunctive therapy for the purpose of lowering intraluminal oxalate solubility and absorption. Aluminum antacids are also effective in causing oxalate precipitation (Earnest, 1977). It should be noted that an occasional patient continues to have hyperoxaluria and recurrent stone formation while on maximal therapy (Stauffer, 1977; O'Leary, 1976). The reason for this phenomenon remains unknown.

At present, it appears that the benefits of jejunoileal bypass surgery outweigh the risks of excessive adiposity and the hazards of the procedure only for the morbidly obese individual. I have not discussed the surgical complications of jejunoileal bypass which have been responsible for two of the four deaths at Johns Hopkins. This aspect was discussed earlier by Hallberg. Prevailing evidence would indicate that the morbidity and mortality associated with this drastic procedure are at their lowest in programs which adhere to strict criteria for acceptance into surgery and provide close follow-up from a multidisciplinary approach, ie surgeons, knowledgeable internists and psychiatrists. Iber & Cooper (1977) substantiated this point very clearly by showing that the mortality rate in the two 'bypass centers' in Baltimore, Maryland is 4 per cent while it remains an unsatisfactory 13 per cent at community hospitals in the same area. In my view, we will probably detect new complications of bypass surgery in the future. The final answer concerning the justifiability of surgery for obesity must rely on comparative prospective studies such as the Scandinavian Obesity

Project (Quaade, 1977 and this volume) and a continuing high level of patient surveillance and investigation.

Summary

The health hazards associated with morbid obesity appear to be considerable although the exact morbidity and mortality are unknown. Since medical management of the massively obese has traditionally been unsuccessful, considerable attention has been focused on surgical approaches developed over the past 15 years.

The results of end-to-end jejunoileostomy indicate that patients lose 30 to 40 per cent of initial weight and maintain significant weight loss thereafter. Other presumed beneficial effects of the weight loss include relief of hypertension, improvement in pulmonary function, reduction in serum triglycerides and cholesterol, improvement in carbohydrate tolerance and improvement in socioeconomic and psychosocial status. However, these benefits are only achieved by surgically creating intestinal malabsorption of fat, protein and perhaps carbohydrate. In addition, there is malabsorption of some fat soluble vitamins as well as potassium, calcium and magnesium. Intestinal malabsorption appears to be most severe during the weight losing phase and is associated with a number of correctable medical complications including fatty liver, diarrhea, perianal irritation, electrolyte abnormalities, vitamin deficiencies and anemia.

A number of more severe medical complications are associated with bypass surgery. These include hepatic failure, gall-stones, renal calculi and problems associated with bacterial over-growth in the bypassed bowel. Patients with jejunoileal bypass are at an increased risk of forming calcium oxalate renal calculi because of increased colonic absorption of dietary oxalate. An increase in intraluminal solubility of oxalate as a result of sequestration of calcium by malabsorbed fats is the most likely cause for hyperabsorption of this anion. Medical management with low oxalate, low fat diets and if necessary calcium supplementation and/or cholestyramine has proved to be beneficial.

Despite these multiple complications, jejunoileal bypass surgery appears to be an acceptable mode of therapy for the morbidly obese patient who is refractory to more traditional, safer forms of management. The morbidity and mortality associated with this procedure seem to be at their lowest in a program which includes an experienced surgeon, a physician knowledgeable in acute and chronic postoperative complications and a concerned psychiatrist.

References

Arnaud, S.B., Goldsmith, R.S., Lambert, P.W. & Go, V.L.W. (1975): *Proc. Soc. Exp. Biol. Med.* **149**, 570.

Barry, R.E., Barish, J., Bray, G.A., Sperling, M.A., Morin, R.J. & Benfield, J. (1977): *Am. J. Clin. Nutr.* **30**, 32.

Berchtold, P., Berger, M., Greiser, E., Dohse, M., Irmscher, K., Gries, F.A. & Zimmerman, H. (1977): *Int. J. Obesity* **1**, 219.

Bistrian, B.R., Blackburn, G.L., Flatt, J., Sizer, J., Scrimshaw, N.S. & Sherman, M. (1976): *Diabetes* **25**, 494.

Bray, G.A., Barry, R.E., Benfield, J.R., Castel-Nuovotedesco, P. & Rodin, J. (1976): *Am. J. Clin. Nutr.* **29**, 779.

Campbell, J.M., Hunt, T.K., Karam, J.H. & Forsham, P.H. (1977): *Archs Intern. Med.* **137**, 602.

Chadwick, V.S., Modha, K. & Dowling, R.H. (1973): *New Engl. J. Med.* **289**, 172.

Dean, R.H., Scott, H.W., Jr., Shull, H.J. & Gluck, F.W. (1977): *Am. J. Clin. Nutr.* **30**, 90.

Dickstein, S.S. & Frame, B. (1973): *Surg. Gynecol. Obstet.* **136**, 257.

Dobbins, J.W. & Binder, H.J. (1976): *Gastroenterology* **70**, 1096.

Dowling, R.H. & Booth, C.C. (1966): *Lancet* **2**, 146.

Drenick, E.J. (1975): In *Obesity in perspective*, ed G.A. Bray. Washington DC: US Govt. Ptg. Office.

Earnest, D.L., Johnson, G., Williams, H.E. & Admirand, W.H. (1974): *Gastroenterology* **66**, 1114.

Earnest, D.L., Williams, H.E. & Admirand, W.H. (1975*a*): *Gastroenterology* **68**, 1072.

Earnest, D.L., Williams, H.E. & Admirand, W.H. (1975*b*): *Trans. Ass. Am. Physicians* **88**, 224.

Earnest, D.L., Williams, H.E. & Admirand, W.H. (1975*c*): *Clin. Res.* 23, 130.
Earnest, D.L. & Graham, D.Y. (1976): *Gastroenterology* 70, 881.
Earnest, D.L. (1977): *Am. J. Clin. Nutr.* 30, 72.
Faloon, W.W., Rubulis, A., Knipp, J., Sherman, C.D. & Flood, M.S. (1977): *Am. J. Clin. Nutr.* 30, 21.
Gelzayd, E.A., Breuer, R.I. & Kirsner, J.B. (1968): *Am. J. Digest. Diseases* 13, 1027.
Genuth, S.M., Castro, J.H. & Vertes, V. (1974): *J. Am. Med. Ass.* 230, 987.
Gregory, J.G., Starkloff, E.B., Miyai, K. & Schoenberg, H.W. (1975): *J. Urol.* 113, 521.
Hamilton, S.R., Boitnott, J.K., Lockwood, D.H. & Bedine, M.S. (1976): *Lab. Invest.* 34, 317.
Heimburger, S.L., Steiger, E., LoGerfo, P., Biehl, A.G. & Williams, M.J. (1975): *Am. J. Surg.* 129, 229.
Holzbach, R.T. (1977): *Am. J. Clin. Nutr.* 30, 43.
Iber, F.L. & Cooper, M. (1977): *Am. J. Clin. Nutr.* 30, 4.
Juhl, E., Christoffersen, P., Baden, H. & Quaade, F. (1971): *New Engl. J. Med.* 285, 543.
Lockwood, D.H., Amatruda, J.M., Moxley, R.T., Pozefsky, T. & Boitnott, J.K. (1977): *Am. J. Clin. Nutr.* 30, 58.
Manes, J.L., Taylor, H.B. & Starkloff, G.B. (1973): *J. Clin. Path.* 26, 776.
Moore, R.B., Frantz, I.D., Jr. & Buchwald, H. (1969): *Surgery* 65, 98.
Moxley, R.T. III, Pozefsky, T & Lockwood, D.H. (1974): *New Engl. J. Med.* 290, 921.
Moxley, R.T. III, Lockwood, D.H., Amatruda, J.M., Tobin, J.D. & Pozefsky, T. (1977): *Diabetes* (in press).
O'Leary, J.P., Thomas, W.C. & Woodward, E.R. (1974): *Am. J. Surg.* 127, 142.
O'Leary, J.P. (1976): *Clins Endoc. Metab.* 5, 481.
Payne, J.H., DeWind, L.T. & Commons, R.R. (1963): *Am. J. Surg.* 106, 273.
Payne, J.H. & DeWind, L.T. (1969): *Am. J. Surg.* 118, 141.
Quaade, F. (1977): *Am. J. Clin. Nutr.* 30, 16.
Rehfeld, J.F., Juhl, E. & Quaade, F. (1970): *Metabolism* 19, 529.
Rogers, J. & Mitchell, G.W. (1952): *New Engl. J. Med.* 247, 53.
Salmon, P.A. (1971): *Surg. Gynec. Obstet.* 132, 965.
Sandstead, H.H. (1975): In *Obesity in perspective,* ed G.A. Bray. Washington DC: US Govt. Ptg. Office.
Scott, H.W. Jr., Sandstead, H.H., Brill, A.B., Burko, H. & Younger, R.K. (1971): *Ann. Surg.* 174, 560.
Scott, H.W., Jr., Dean, R., Shull, H.J., Abram, H.S., Webb, W., Youngerm R.K. & Brill, A.B. (1973): *Ann. Surg.* 177, 723.
Shagrin, J.W., Frame, B. & Duncan, H. (1971): *Ann. Int. Med.* 75, 377.
Smith, L.H., Fromm, H. & Hoffman, A.F. (1972): *New Engl. J. Med.* 286, 1371.
Solow, C. (1977): *Am. J. Clin. Nutr.* 30, 103.
Soterakis, J., Glennon, J.A., Ishimara, A.M., Tyler, J.M. & Iber, F.L. (1976): *Am. J. Digest. Diseases* 21, 533.
Starkloff, G.B., Donovan, J.F., Ramach, K.R. & Wolfe, B.M. (1975): *Archs Surg.* 110, 652.
Stauffer, J.Q., Humphreys, M.H. & Weir, G.J. (1973): *Ann. Int. Med.* 79, 383.
Stauffer, J.Q. (1977): *Am. J. Clin. Nutr.* 30, 64.
Stuart, R.B. (1975): In *Obesity in perspective,* ed G.A. Bray. Washington DC: US Govt. Ptg. Office.
Stunkard, A.J. & McLaren-Hume, M. (1959): *Archs Intern. Med.* 103, 79.
Stunkard, A.J. & Mahoney, M.J. (1976): In *Handbook of behavior modification and behavior therapy,* ed H. Leitenberg. Englewood Cliffs, NJ: Prentice-Hall.
Teitelbaum, S.L., Halverson, J.D., Bates, M., Wise, L. & Haddad, J.G. (1977): *Ann. Int. Med.* 86, 289.
Wands, J.R., LaMont, J.T., Mann, E. & Isselbacher, K.J. (1976): *New Engl. J. Med.* 294, 121.
Weismann, R. (1973): *Am. J. Surg.* 125, 437.

42
Bacterial complications of intestinal bypass

E.J. DRENICK, S.M. FINEGOLD, T.M. STANLEY and W.A. BORDER
Veterans Hospital, Wadsworth Hospital Center, Wilshire and Sawtelle Boulevards, Los Angeles, California 90073, USA.

Several distinct mechanisms lead to the various complications of intestinal bypass operations. This discussion will focus on the consequences of bacterial overgrowth in the bypassed bowel segment which can cause an enteropathy (Barry *et al.*, 1975; Drenick *et al.*, 1976; Passaro, Drenick & Wilson, 1976) with its systemic manifestations and secondarily, disorders involving distant organs. Appropriate therapeutic measures to treat this complex of disorders have been effective in many cases when aimed at the suppression of the anaerobic flora. Unrelated to bacterial overgrowth there appeared to develop in some patients a decrease in resistance to new infections or to the reactivation of old inactive bacterial infection (Pickleman *et al.*, 1975).

As originally devised, intestinal bypass operations were to produce a state of 'controlled' malabsorption. The diarrhea which almost invariably commenced shortly after the operation was expected as the sequel of the shortened bowel, and aggravated by bile salts irritating the colonic mucosa. However, it was soon noted that the severity of the diarrhea, the pattern of exacerbations and partial remissions, continuing for years in some patients, differed markedly from the diarrhea of the typical short bowel syndrome that follows extensive resection. In this latter situation, after an initial adaptation period, the diarrhea tended to decrease to a stable pattern of several semi-solid stools. In most bypass patients, stool frequency decreased to three to six per day over a period of about 6 months. However, in a sizeable proportion of patients this pattern was interrupted by severe exacerbations occurring at irregular intervals without apparent cause and without prior dietary indiscretions. These episodes were associated with an increase in digestive discomfort, nausea, bloating, flatus and occasionally with fever, weakness and accelerated weight loss.

Upright abdominal x-rays during these periods revealed distended segments of small and large bowel and the presence of gas/fluid levels of variable size (Fig. 1). Extreme distention, noted on occasion, permitted luminal gas to penetrate through the intestinal wall. Subserous, gas filled blebs developed, giving rise to a condition termed pneumatosis cystoides intestinalis (Fig. 2). Rupture of these cysts resulted in subphrenic accumulation of free gas. This finding was readily misinterpreted as a sign of a ruptured abdominal viscus, but the characteristic x-ray features of pneumatosis should serve to avoid unnecessary laparotomies.

When the bowel in several instances was entered and drained, the organisms generally had the characteristics, both in species and numbers, of fecal flora (Table 1). Since the small bowel, generally, is free of significant numbers of anaerobic organisms the colonization with this 'foreign' flora was associated with mucosal damage, demonstrable by changes in size and shape of villi and disarray of the cell nuclei, mononuclear infiltrates and submucosal edema (Fig. 3). The gross appearance of the serosa reflected the transmural inflammatory process with intense injection and reddening. After remission, extensive adhesions tended to form along the entire bypassed segment.

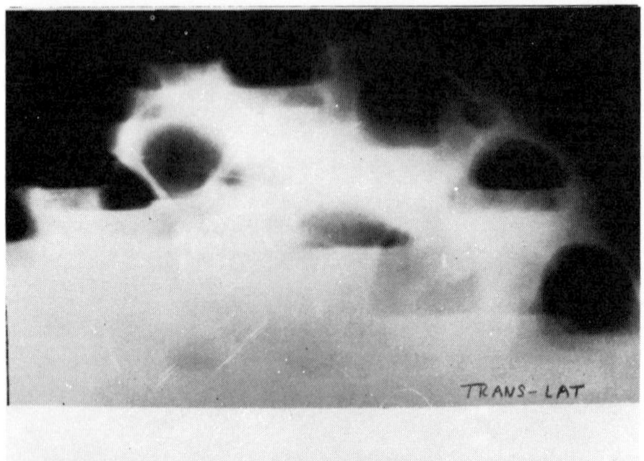

Fig. 1. Gas fluid levels in distended, excluded small bowel and in colon due to enteropathy

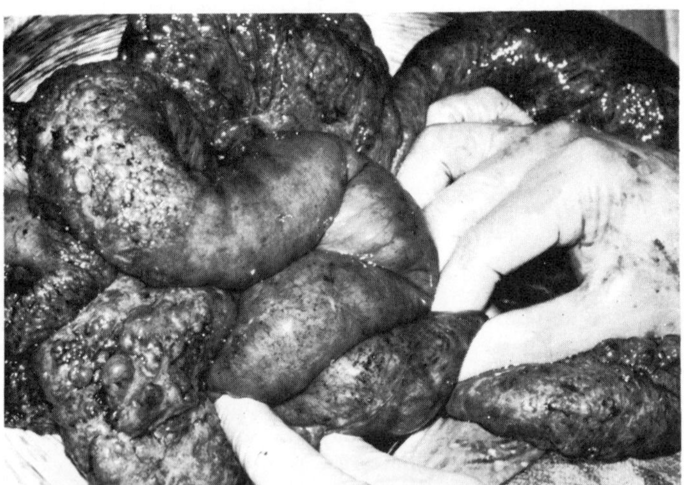

Fig. 2. Enteritis and pneumatosis intestinalis of bypassed small bowel

Table 1. Number of aerobic and anaerobic organisms in the excluded segment and functioning small bowel of patients with evident bypass enteropathy

Subjects without antibiotics	Interval after bypass (months)	Flora in excluded jejunum		Flora in functioning small bowel	
		aerobic	anaerobic	aerobic	anaerobic
1	14	6×10^7	2×10^7	4×10^7	1×10^5
2	8	5×10^8	2.7×10^9	1×10^5	1.3×10^5
3	48	3×10^6 (E. coli)	0		
Subjects with antibiotics					
1	36	1.8×10^4	0	0	0
2	21	0	7.2×10^6	4×10^6	3.8×10^6

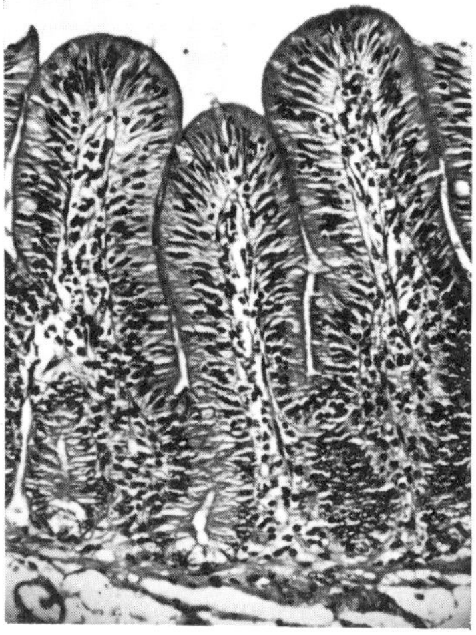

Fig. 3. Shortened villi in bypassed ileum in a patient with enteropathy, 4 years after the operation

The incidence, severity and course of this enteropathy varied greatly. Mild degrees were probably present, off and on, in the majority of bypass patients and may have passed unnoticed. Symptomatic forms probably occurred in one-half the patients and severe cases were seen in no more than 10 per cent. The frequency of recurrent episodes tended to decrease in all but a few cases. In some, there seemed to be little relief for as long as 10 years after the operation, and eventually the bypass had to be dismantled to terminate the distressing symptoms as well as the recurrent episodes of electrolyte and nutrient depletion. It was of interest that in several of the more severe cases exudative protein loss could be documented by the use of ^{51}Cr-labelled albumen which, after i.v. injection, appeared in the feces in excessive amounts.

The abnormalities of the enteropathy induced by bacterial overgrowth was not limited to the small bowel, but in some cases involved colon as well (Barry *et al.*, 1975). Whether this was an extension of the small bowel disorder or a secondary phenomenon remained unclear. Massive distention by gas and fluid occurred soon after the operation in some instances, or after an interval of more than 2 years in others. Some patients with this complication actually complained of constipation, because a functional colonic ileus caused infrequent evacuation despite the presence of liquid bowel contents. Grotesque degrees of distention were erroneously thought to reflect persistent obesity. Terms applied to this phenomenon have been colonic pseudo-obstruction or toxic megacolon. The possible mechanisms producing this manifestation include: impairment of motility resulting from exposure to the irritant effects of degraded bile acids and hydroxylated fatty acids leading to spasm of anorectal musculature and the use of opiates or related synthetics for relief of diarrhea. Bacteria convert the abundant bile acids which have escaped reabsorption to secondary bile acids, which are thought to be more irritating than the primary forms. The question arose why postbypass patients appeared to have more serious difficulties than patients with steatorrhea from other causes or patients with short bowel syndromes. There is at present no conclusive explanation, but a reasonable hypothesis would suggest that nutrients, refluxing into the excluded loop, were subject to stagnation and prolonged exposure to the fecal flora prevailing in this area. Therefore, greater quantities and concentrations of irritants may have been generated.

Procto-cryptitis

Aside from diarrhea one of the most common complaints was anorectal distress and this had generally, but probably erroneously, been ascribed to diarrhea. However, other mechanisms may also be responsible, as some patients developed this disorder in the absense of significant diarrhea. On the other hand, this disorder is quite uncommon in patients with pancreatic insufficiency who have frequent bowel movements. The incidence of anorectal disorders during the postoperative course has been 50 per cent in our series of patients. The symptoms tended to become distressing within the first few months after the operation and receded subsequently in most but not all cases. Anorectal burning, soreness and pain, occasionally with radiation into the retropubic area, was either constant or intermittent and was exacerbated when the patients experienced descent of fecal material toward the anus. Generally, the distress increased when 'acid' food, pepper or larger quantities of fatty foods were consumed. The pain was so severe in one patient as to precipitate a suicide attempt.

Examination of the anorectal area revealed increased sphincter tone. Inspection of the mucosa, in general, failed to reveal any overt abnormalities. Yet, biopsies in five of six subjects so examined demonstrated attenuation of the surface epithelium, variable degrees of inflammatory infiltrates of the lamina propria and mild edema. Late secondary sequelae were fissures, rectal abscess and hemorrhoids.

No immunoglobulin deposits or complement components were found. Fibrinogen was present in a non-specific pattern. No pathogens were discovered in the submucosal tissues. Bacterial cultures of biopsied tissue revealed only the usual fecal flora. To assess the effect of various irritants, cholic acid and chenodeoxycholic acid were instilled into the rectal ampulla, but these proved inert while dilute acetic acid and rhizinoleic acid (castor oil) reproduced the typical distress.

Of 17 patients with severe distress, refractory to routine measures, fourteen were treated with metronidazole and experienced dramatic improvement in 1 to 3 days. Small maintenance doses averted recurrent distress. In a single instance a second rectal biopsy after metronidazole treatment revealed disappearance of the inflammatory changes.

Although not strictly a direct manifestation of the enteropathy, in one patient a secondary complication of this disorder had arisen in the form of obstruction of one ureter. Periureteritis had resulted from the inflammatory bowel disease contiguous to the ureter with ensuing hydroureter and hydronephrosis. This condition was promptly relieved with antibiotic treatment and alleviation of the enteropathy.

Extra-enteric manifestations

To causally connect distant organ involvement to the bacterial overgrowth in the excluded loop requires that active episodes of enteropathy be associated with active pathological processes in the various involved organs. Conversely, if relief of the enteropathy by medications was followed by regression in distant organ disease, then the presumption of cause and effect was favoured. Such temporal associations have in fact been observed for most of the complications cited below.

Hepatic damage

Among the extra-intestinal complications of bypass operation, liver disease has been the most common and also the most ominous, since it caused some of the late postoperative deaths. Preoperatively, variable degrees of steatosis have been frequently seen in gross obesity, but hepatic function was generally unimpaired. A weight loss by dietary restriction nearly always normalized hepatic morphology. After the operation most if not all patients developed hepatic steatosis, and among these, about 3 to 5 per cent progressed to cirrhosis. The etiology of liver damage has remained unclear and responses to various treatment measures have been used to infer pathogenetic mechanisms. Several reports ascribed hepatic damage to protein-calorie malnutrition. With restoration of good nutrition via oral or parenteral alimentation, improvement of hepatic morphology and function was observed in some cases (Moxley, Pozefsky & Lockwood, 1974; Heimberger *et al.*, 1975; Ames *et al.*, 1976). However, there have been instances of progressive hepatic deterioration, despite adequate nutritional support (Brown, O'Leary & Woodward, 1974) suggesting alternative explanations.

Among a group of 18 patients, followed with liver bipsies at regular intervals, increasing steatosis developed in all but two. It was noted as early as 7 weeks after the operation in one patient who died in hepatic failure, but was generally maximal 6 to 12 months later and receded subsequently in all but three cases. Fatty deposits decreased moderately in one and remained unaltered in another 6 months before diminishing. Two years after the operation only one patient continued to show greater than baseline fat content.

In order to assess the anaerobic enteropathy as a possible underlying cause, patients were treated with metronidazole either immediately after the operation or during the period 3 to 6 months after the operation when maximal changes obtained in most patients. In several patients, 3-month treatment periods were alternated with drug-free periods and liver biopsies were performed at 3-month intervals to elucidate more clearly a possible drug effect. No attempts were made to regulate nutritional support. During 11 periods of metronidazole administration, in the course of the first 12 postoperative months, there was a dramatic decrease in steatosis in 11 out of 12 treatment courses involving 12 subjects. There was a slight to moderate increase in hepatic fat deposition in one patient.

On the other hand, in seven of the same patients during ten drug-free periods of the same 12-month postoperative interval, there was a marked increase in steatosis in nine out of ten instances. In one patient fat content remained unchanged. It is particularly significant that in five out of six patients treated with metronidazole during the initial 6-month period, the degree of steatosis diminished, while it almost uniformily increased in all the untreated subjects during the same interval. Since alleviation of the enteropathy occurred with the institution of metronidazole administration, it appeared reasonable to postulate that suppression of the anaerobic flora in the bypassed intestinal segment had been a critical factor in the prevention or reversal of hepatic steatosis. An example of the alternating deterioration and improvement of liver morphology is shown in Fig. 4. It should be noted that these changes occurred irrespective of alterations in rates of weight loss and without any consistent directional changes of serum protein levels. However, it may be reasonable to invoke protein malnutrition as an additional factor in the causation of liver

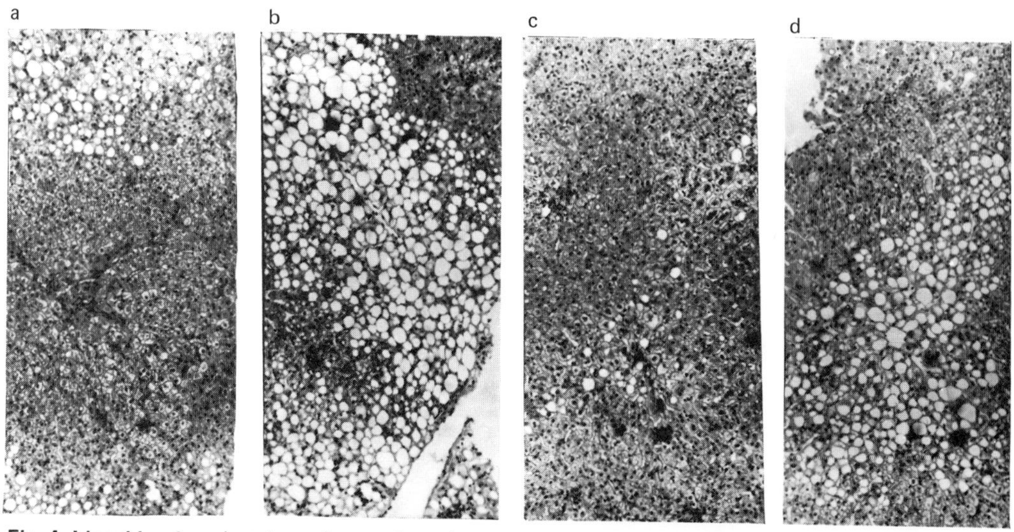

Fig. 4. Liver biopsies: a) at time of operation, b) 3 months postop., no drugs, c) 6 months postop. with metronidazole for preceding 3 months, d) 9 months postop., no drugs for the preceding 3 months demonstrating the effect of metronidazole upon hepatic fat content. Serum albumen always >4.2 g/dl. Weight loss rate identical during first and second 3-month period and lower during third period

damage in some patients, since toxic insults to the liver are known to be graver during states of protein depletion. The improvement in liver morphology with nutritional support may be explainable on the same basis.

At present it is not known whether the control of enteropathy can prevent the development of fibrosis or cirrhosis and of progressive hepatic failure.

In two subjects a distinct granulomatous hepatitis was recognized. The granulomata were non-caseating. No organisms were found on stain or culture biopsy tissue. Lesions of this type have been considered suggestive of a non-specific reaction to chronic inflammatory bowel diseases. In one of the patients, mesenteric lymph nodes were found to be involved as well.

Several reports have dealt with the occurrence of active tuberculosis in postbypass patients (Pickleman *et al.*, 1975). Both the pulmonary form and tuberculous cervical adenitis have been reported. Two patients in our series developed active tuberculous adenitis. One, a female, had had scrofula in childhood. Within 4 months after the operation and after a minimal weight loss she suffered a recurrence. The other patient developed tuberculous adenitis *de novo* after a 2-year postoperative interval. The mechanisms leading to the development of infection or reinfection are unknown, but malnutrition does not appear to be a necessary concomitant.

Arthritis

A 23 per cent incidence of polyarthritis in bypass patients was first reported by Shagrin, Frame & Duncan (1971). Several other reports have confirmed their observations (Buchanan & Willkens, 1972; Mir-Madjlessi, MacKenzie & Winkelman, 1974; Wands *et al.*, 1976; Hess, 1975). Wands examined several such patients and proposed that absorbed intestinal bacteria antigens led to the formation of circulating immune complexes, activating complement pathways and producing joint disease. Elevated serum antibody titers against *E. coli* and *B. fragilis* during active illness regressed when symptoms subsided. This syndrome appeared to resemble the joint manifestations known to be associated with several types of intestinal inflammatory diseases, such as regional enteritis or ulcerative colitis.

Among 79 patients operated upon in this center, eight developed arthritic symptoms. In addition, 13 others with this syndrome were seen among a group of 26 who had been operated on elsewhere and referred for evaluation. Evidence of enteropathy was present during the phases of active joint disease in all cases. Joint symptoms tended to arise and subside in phase with the enteropathy. Hepatic steatosis was present in all but two of these patients while joint symptoms were acute. The postoperative interval to the onset of symptoms varied from 1 month to 2 years. Minimal migratory arthralgia, lasting only hours and recurring irregularly, occurred in two patients. Stiffness and pain, lasting days to months, affected various joints at different times and were, generally, of moderate severity in 12 patients. In the remaining nine the distress was severe and disabling. Visible swelling of joints varied from mild to marked but redness was absent. Effusions were present at times in six patients of this group but large joint effusions were rare. Aspiration of fluid was successful in only one patient. Overt synovitis with redness and swelling was noted over the wrists in three instances. Extension of pain and tenderness into juxta-articular tissue was common. Tests for rheumatoid disease were negative in all but one patient who had developed typical seropositive rheumatoid arthritis. One patient had a positive ANA test.

Cryoglobulins were not found in the serum of three patients so tested. Circulating immune complexes were searched for in several of these patients but not in a systematic manner. Some sera had been obtained during periods when the patients were asymptomatic or had been treated with antibiotics, leading to remission of the bypass enteropathy. Elevated Clq levels were detected in three out of six patients.

In the single patient with a massive joint effusion, fluid was obtained. Bacterial cultures were negative. The protein content was 2.05 g/dl and synovial tissue revealed the presence of chronic inflammatory cells. There was mucoid degeneration of collagen, proliferation of synovial cells and thickening of the walls of blood vessels. The x-rays of involved joints were negative in all but one subject who manifested juxta-articular demineralization involving the hands. A second patient had typical and extensive changes of rheumatoid arthritis in multiple joints.

Anti-inflammatory medicines such as salicylates and Indocin were employed routinely as a first therapeutic measure and found effective in four out of 15 cases. In some of the non-responders who had disabling symptoms, adrenal steroids were employed and in one out of four, partial benefit was obtained. In five patients, relief of arthritic complaints followed dismantling of the bypass which had become necessary for alleviation of other serious complications.

Antibiotic therapy was instituted in 11 patients. Metronidazole was effective in eight out of 11 subjects. Relief was noted in some patients within 24 hours and recurrence could almost always be averted with a minimum maintenance dose of one to three 250 mg tablets per day. Exacerbations were common when metronidazole was discontinued but improvement was prompt with reinstitution. In three patients this drug was ineffective. In one of the three, tetracycline caused transient improvement and ampicillin brought relief in another. It was assumed that an aerobic organism was related to the arthritic process in these subjects.

The correlation of enteropathy with the joint disease and the response of both syndromes to antibiotics were strongly suggestive for a bacterial origin of this syndrome. The response to metronidazole in the majority of patients implicated anaerobic organisms as the more common etiologic agents.

Renal damage

Seven to 108 months after the bypass operation, kidney biopsies were performed in 18 patients. Twelve of these had developed overt bypass enteropathy. All biopsy specimens revealed evidence of a focal interstitial nephritis with tubular atrophy, fibrosis and secondary glomerular hyalinization. The extent of injury varied from mild to extensive, but because of the focal distribution renal function had remained normal in all but four patients. In ten of the subjects, no renal oxalate deposits were discovered. In the other eight, oxalate crystals were present, but numerous areas of nephrotic involvement were found distant from any crystal deposits.

Immune complex deposits, containg IgM and C3 in glomerular capillary walls and in mesangium were noted in five out of 15 patients. Circulating immune complex-like material was detected in six out of 16 patients tested with a Clq binding assay.

The renal complications appear to be due to the combined effect of oxalate and immune complex induced injury. The latter factor most likely had its origin with bacterial byproducts in the excluded bowel segment. Another mechanism may be the release of proteins from damaged intestinal epithelium into the circulation which then acts as an antigen, stimulating antibody production and formation of immune complexes on cell membranes of similar protein structure.

Skin lesions

Skin lesions of different forms were observed in the aftermath of the bypass operation in 12 instances, and, with one exception, always in association with active enteropathy. Of 59 patients actually operated on and followed at this center, six developed skin lesions. Among 61 other bypass patients, referred for consultation, four such cases were found. The character of the lesions varied from tender erythematous nodules to macular, vesicular or pustular lesions. No overt ulcerative lesions were observed. One patient developed scaly psoriatic lesions over back, chest and abdomen. Erythema nodosum-like lesions in five patients were noted on lower legs, forearm and hands. Lesions persisted for variable periods, from a few days to several months, and in all but one the presence coincided with active enteropathy. The histological description in one lesion, grossly diagnosed as erythema nodosum, revealed a predominantly lymphocytic perivascular infiltrate throughout the dermis and subcutaneous tissue with endothelial swelling of vessels, leading to the diagnosis of vasculitis. In another patient with a similar lesion on the forearm the diagnosis of nodular vasculitis with venous thrombus formation was made. The lesion with vesicle formation was interpreted as showing leucocytoclastic angiitis. Patients with macular lesions exhibited non-specific dermal and subcutaneous inflammatory changes with giant cells.

In one case, in whom the biopsy tissue was examined by immunofluorescent staining, deposition of IgG and C3 and fibrinogen at the dermal-epidermal junction and in capillary walls was revealed. The pattern appeared more indicative of thrombosis of the microvasculature and not of immune complex disease.

The lesions disappeared following institution of metronidazole in five patients and after dismantling of the bypass in two. In three others, improvement was spontaneous and in one patient the psoriatic lesions persisted.

Similar lesions have been reported in several types of inflammatory bowel disease and it appears reasonable to assume that bacterial overgrowth in bypassed bowel loops indirectly induced the skin lesions observed in bypass patients.

The metronidazole-induced improvement in the extra-enteric manifestations generally paralleled the alleviation of the enteropathy. This drug was effective in reducing diarrhea, digestive discomfort and bloating while the offensive odor of stools and flatus was eliminated. Once megacolon had fully developed, only partial improvement could be obtained with this drug. Whether immune complex mediated renal damage can be averted by the use of antibiotic therapy is doubtful since focal nephritis was found in patients who had been on almost continuous treatment with metronidazole.

Summary

Many manifestations following jejunoileal bypass are due to chronic inflammation of the excluded bowel rather than short bowel malabsorption. Diarrhea, abdominal distention and gas-fluid levels were common diagnostic features of 'bypass enteropathy'. Exploration showed the bypassed bowel to be dilated, with serosal inflammation and pneumatosis cystoides intestinalis. The bypassed loops contained a fecal flora and the mucosa demonstrated non-specific chronic inflammatory changes. Exudative protein losses were noted.

Systemic complications of bypass enteropathy were similar to other inflammatory diseases of the bowel. Improvement following treatment with metronidazole or after dismantling of the bypass suggested that bacterial byproducts originating in the excluded bowel were causally related.

References

Ames, F.C., Copeland, E.M., Leeb, D.C., Moore, D.L. & Dudrick, S.J. (1976): *J. Am. Med. Ass.* 235, 1249.

Barry, R.E., Benfield, J.R., Nicell, P. & Bray, G.A. (1975): *Gut* 16, 903.

Brown, R.G., O'Leary, J.P. & Woodward, E.R. (1974): *Am. J. Surg.* 127, 53.

Buchanan, R.F. & Willkens, R.F. (1972): *Arthritis Rheum.* 15, 644.

Drenick, E.J., Ament, M.E., Finegold, S.M., Corrodi, P. & Passaro, E. (1976): *J. Am. Med. Ass.* 236, 269.

Heimburger, S.L., Steiger, E., LoGerfo, P., Biehl, A.G. & Williams, M.J. (1975): *Am. J. Surg.* 129, 229.

Hess, R.J. (1975): *Oklahoma State Med. J.* p. 283.

Mir-Madjlessi, S.H., MacKenzie, A.H. & Winkelman, E.I. (1974): *Cleveland Clinic Quarterly* 41, 119.

Moxley, R.T., Pozefsky, T. & Lockwood, D.H. (1974): *New Engl. J. Med.* 290, 921.

Passaro, E., Drenick, E. & Wilson, S.E. (1976): *Am. J. Surg.* 131, 169.

Pickleman, J.R., Evans, L.S., Kane, J.M. & Freeark, R.J. (1975): *J. Am. Med. Ass.* 234, 744.

Shagrin, J.W., Frame, B. & Duncan, H. (1971): *Ann. Int. Med.* 75, 377.

Wands, J.R., LaMont, J.T., Mann, E. & Isselbacher, B.S. and K.J. (1976): *New Engl. J. Med.* 294, 121.

43
Psychological and behavioral consequences of intestinal bypass

C. SOLOW, P.M. SILBERFARB and K. SWIFT
Department of Psychiatry, Dartmouth Medical School, Hanover, New Hampshire 03755, USA.

Most publications concerning intestinal bypass surgery for massive and intractable obesity have emphasized the experimental nature of this therapeutic approach. This may still be a valid label, but much is now known about assessing the odds in the therapeutic gamble for enhanced quality of life; furthermore, much has been learned, from this surgical experiment, about obesity itself. Such progress can be seen in the psychological-behavioral area as well as in the surgical management-metabolic area.

In a prospective study of 29 consecutive, massively and intractably obese patients treated with jejunoileal bypass we found that the response to weight loss, at an average of 34 months (range, 26 to 46) after surgery, included improvement in activity levels, mood, self-esteem, body image, self-consciousness, interpersonal and vocational effectiveness, and a trend towards more normal satiety mechanisms and eating behavior (Solow, Silberfarb & Swift, 1974). Other notable changes included decreased use of denial as a coping style, and replacement of a self-reinforcing sense of entrapment, resignation, and ineffectiveness by hope and awareness of increased opportunity. The sailing was by no means entirely smooth. Unhappiness over somatic symptoms and (usually) short-term irritability, fatigue and depression were common, especially in the first postoperative year, during the phase of rapid weight loss. Increased self-assertiveness and enhanced feelings of independence and autonomy constituted a mixed blessing for some patients, requiring painful interpersonal realignments: six experienced marital conflicts or break-up. At some point in the follow-up period six patients suffered from frank psychiatric illness. In every instance but one, this illness represented either a continuation of a preexisting pattern of care-requiring psychiatric disturbance, or a response to unusually stressful events (for example, depression following hysterectomy). In one instance psychiatric hospitalization was occasioned by emotional turmoil related to marital break-up, which in turn was related to weight loss. In each instance of psychiatric illness, the patient eventually emerged with apparently more flexible and adaptive modes of coping than evident before weight loss. We concluded that many of the components of the psychological syndrome associated with obesity (low self-esteem, passive-dependency, vulnerability to depression, marked self-consciousness, and a sense of helplessness and ineffectiveness) were reversible to a surprising degree by jejunoileal bypass surgery. It was inferred that this psychological constellation may be as much a result of obesity as a cause of it in this particular population.

In a review of 14 other reports concerning psychosocial consequences of intestinal bypass (Solow, 1977), there was found to be substantial agreement with this impression of rather surprisingly favorable effects upon mood, self-esteem and confidence, attitudinal body image, and vocational effectiveness – and of general patient satisfaction. There was support of the specific findings relating to decreased recourse to denial in coping with problems and painful emotions, to increased self-assertiveness and independence with the not uncommon consequence of difficult family adjustments, and to the phenomenon of an apparent improvement in satiety mechanisms and eating behavior. Most observers were impressed with the importance of somatic dysfunction and distress during the first postoperative year for most patients, and longer for some. Psychosocial clues to increased risk of postoperative difficulties were cited in two reports: Kalucy & Crisp (1974) found that two older female patients with long histories of severely deficient interpersonal attachments and social phobias became more depressed after surgery, no longer able to blame the emptiness of their lives upon obesity; they were clearly dissatisfied with the results of surgery. Starkloff & co-workers (1975) suggested that patients with a history of somatization of emotional difficulties were vulnerable to developing psychogenic vomiting postoperatively, and were thus at increased risk for liver failure. Several other reports gave a much more pessimistic view of the psychiatric hazards of this operation, but these accounts suffered from the failure to view the psychosocial problems encountered in the context of the patients' past experience and performance, and their current somatic status. Furthermore, the conclusions to be drawn from all these studies were limited by a relatively short average follow-up period, in all cases under 2 years except for the report of Solow & co-workers (1974). It was suggested (Solow, 1977) that a valid assessment of psychosocial results requires a minimum of 3 years: the first year is burdened with major somatic stresses; the second year, with the challenge of adjustment to new intrapsychic and interpersonal conditions; it is only during the third year that many patients begin to experience the full benefits of surgically induced weight loss.

Follow-up study

It was from a sense of the need for a longer longitudinal view of the patient's course after bypass that the authors undertook to reassess their status at an average of 78 months (range 61 to 100) following surgery.

All patients were given a semi-structured psychiatric interview by one of the authors following the format used for the original study of the same group (Solow *et al.*, 1974). In two instances this had to be done by telephone as the patient had moved a considerable distance away. Two patients could not be located, leaving a total of 27 patients studied. One 60-year-old woman died while spending the winter in Florida, 93 months postoperatively, reportedly of liver failure associated with sepsis. Her husband was interviewed several months later. She was dissatisfied and bitter at the time of the first follow-up (45 months post surgery), suffering from continued disabling diarrhea and having lost only 13 kg. Following a shunt revision at 48 months after initial surgery, she lost an additional 19 kg and functioned somewhat more comfortably and happily. She failed to return for follow-up care at this center, and apparently contributed to her demise by resisting her husband's entreaties to seek medical attention, even though ill for several months, until she was preterminal. Preoperatively she had been assessed as being one of the better emotionally adjusted individuals in the series.

At the time of the first follow-up study there had been a mean weight loss of 55 kg. By the second follow-up, 17 patients had gained an average of 8.6 kg (range 1.8 to 21) over the lowest weight achieved postoperatively; nine patients had lost a further 8.6 kg (range 0.5 to 28). The net change in the group was a total gain of 68 kg. Clearly, weight loss had been maintained. Two patients had revision of their shunts to achieve greater weight loss, and went on to further reductions of 37 and 31 kg, respectively. One man was found to have Hodgkin's disease at age 27 and, because of this, was reanastamosed at 45 months. Predictions notwithstanding, he regained only 21 kg following this, still 44 kg below his prebypass weight, and has remained at that level for 2 years. A woman who achieved only a 7 kg weight loss after her bypass was reanastamosed at age 49, 37 months after original surgery, because of weakness, nausea, persistent diarrhea, and cirrhosis on liver biopsy. In the subsequent 4 years she dieted to a level 27 kg below that at reanastamosis, and has essentially remained there.

Other than the one death, there have been no major late somatic complications. The patients, as a group, have come to accept and live with and around the remaining alteration of bowel function. Of 25 patients still having shunts, ten reported diarrhea as no problem, ten as a mild problem, and four as a moderate problem; six had mild difficulties with foul smelling stools or flatus, and four were moderately inconvenienced by this. Four individuals were mildly bothered by abdominal bloating, while two were moderately so. Most patients continued to enjoy an improvement in energy and stamina.

While food intake had increased somewhat (compared to the end of the original follow-up period), as a group the patients continued to report a definite normalization of eating behavior (total intake reduced, satisfied with smaller portions, less snacking, diminished preoccupation with food, finding it easier to resist temptation). Twenty report maintenance of this change, four report no change, and two allege increased food intake compared with preoperative levels.

Improvement in various psychosocial parameters (self-esteem, self-assertiveness and autonomy, activity levels, attitudinal body image, sexual satisfaction, and vocational effectiveness) has persisted, and many continue to manifest a reduction in use of denial.

There has been only one additional instance of psychiatric illness: a woman who had had repeated hospitalizations for psychosis since age 16, and had experienced another psychotic decompensation shortly after bypass (but before weight loss) at age 29, was hospitalized briefly 5 years after in reaction to exceptional situational stress. Her overall psychiatric status is remarkably improved since she lost weight. A schizophrenic patient treated in preparation for bypass has required no further treatment and has done well. Three patients who received psychiatric outpatient treatment following bypass have subsequently fared well and needed no further psychiatric assistance. One patient continues to see her psychiatrist occasionally at times of stress, as she did before surgery. A man who required hospitalization almost a year after bypass because of marital break-up precipitated by his weight loss has continued in monthly psychotherapy. He views this treatment as having been of great and lasting benefit to him, above and beyond helping him through his postoperative temporary life crisis.

The pattern of marital disruption and realignment noted at 34 months after surgery has become more prominent. Seven patients have been divorced (in six instances at the patient's instigation; in one it was the spouse's choice). Three have married new partners; four have remained single but socially active or are living in a stable non-marital relationship. In all cases of divorce it is apparent that the original marriage choice had been largely determined by the patient's low self-esteem, the marriages had been unsatisfying, and the patients were happy to be free of them. One woman left her husband for some months, but ultimately, rather unhappily returned. One husband is having some continued dissatisfaction with the patient's newfound assertiveness. On the other hand, two single patients have married since bypass one of them giving birth to two healthy children. Most marriages remained improved or have continued satisfying and stable.

Global assessment by patients of the results of surgery has remained very favorable. Twenty-three are very satisfied (although two would have preferred to have lost more weight). One patient, when asked if again faced with the decision, she would choose to have surgery, replied, 'Oh, yeah! Even if it means dying early, at least the years I'm living are *living*.' Two patients remained dissatisfied: one who required reanastamosis because of persistent somatic problems in the face of inadequate weight loss, and one who remains in a virtual social morass of deprivation and frustration which antedated the surgery.

Discussion

While the long-term psychological/behavioral effects of this operation emerge as basically salutory in our small study population, recent literature in this area leaves the matter somewhat problematic. Crisp & colleagues (1977), reporting on the completion of a prospective investigation of 25 subjects, confirmed the findings of their retrospective pilot study (Kalucy & Crisp, 1974) and of our work: for most patients, surgically induced weight loss results in considerable psychological gains; for many, reduction in use of denial and increased assertiveness involves difficult interpersonal adjustment. In addition to severely isolated, socially phobic older women, they suspect that young, unstable sociopathic males and older males who do not devalue their obese bodies represent types of cadidates at risk for less than satisfactory results.

Contrary to our impressions, the concept of obesity as a needed defense for a good many candidates for bypass continues to hold strong appeal. Thus Faloon (1977) states, 'For some people obesity appears to be an escape from certain kinds of social responsibility - as it were, a way of hiding from the world beneath a blanket of fat. When the fat is removed, they are unable to cope with the new expectations produced in the people around them'. Further reports of considerable psychiatric morbidity following bypass would seem to lend credence to this concern. DeWind & Payne (1976) commenting on the course of 330 patients observe: 'Major emotional upsets were encountered in 20 patients; these patients either required psychiatric care or their behavior became socially unacceptable or irresponsible, in the presence of quite normal preoperative personality'. Telmos (1977) cites only two patients out of 169 who presented psychiatric problems as 'long-term morbidity' of this operation, while Prian & co-workers (1976) mention that one of their 129 patients required reanastamosis for 'emotional instability'. More significantly, Wise (1976) discusses five adverse psychologic reactions to bypass in a series of 33 patients in which he places heavy emphasis on the defensive need for obesity and the morbidity to be expected from loss of this prop. His interpretations do not seem convincingly supported by his data, and he attacks a straw man when he erroneously claims that, 'Recent investigations have uniformly demonstrated the innocuous psychologic effects on these individuals' of bypass. He concedes that, 'surgery, even in the cases cited above, has been a useful attempt to try to help these individuals with a life-threatening medical condition'. He concludes quite justifiably that, 'continued psychiatric follow-up is as important a part of the ileal bypass procedure as are the frequent medical check-ups of hepatic, renal, and metabolic functioning'. Hallberg, Backman & Espmark (1975) report a very high incidence of psychiatric morbidity. Forty-nine of their 66 patients experienced anxiety or depressive reactions (during the first 2 years postoperative) of sufficient severity to require psychotherapy, and four of the patients made serious suicide attempts. Interestingly, a few instances of psychogenic vomiting were noted. Hallberg & colleagues (1975) cite these problems without concluding that the ultimate effect of bypass surgery was unfavorable. Sixty-three of 66 patients were satisfied with their results, and 'the great majority of the patients have experienced a radical and positive change in their life situation'. Comparison of Rorschach tests before and 1 to 2 years after surgery showed a positive change in the variable for 'mental health'. This change was most notable in those individuals who scored most negatively before operation.

It would seem that the implication for the clinician of this rather variable data concerning psychosocial morbidity following bypass is, as previously noted (Solow, 1977), a need to consider actual and potential emotional disturbances in the context of the patient's past adjustment, current somatic status, and future potential. Psychiatric difficulties following surgery must not be viewed as an isolated event, automatically signalling an unfavorable response to surgery. 'It is unfair to expect that surgically-induced weight loss will "cure" or prevent all psychiatric illness', especially in a massively obese population that is preoperatively at high risk for emotional disturbance (Castelnuovo-Tedesco & Schiebel, 1975; Webb *et al.*, 1976), is subjected to severe somatic stresses postoperatively, and has to meet the challenge of increased opportunity after years of disability. A justifiable and widely accepted conclusion is that the surgeon must have ready, if not routine, access to psychiatric consultation if intestinal bypass surgery is to be undertaken.

Others have drawn more specific conclusions from the available evidence and have evolved fairly formal programs of psychological evaluation preoperatively in order to screen out patients at risk for postoperative psychosocial problems (Harrington, 1976; Starkloff *et al.*, 1975; Wehlage & Bechtold, 1976; Lundgren *et al.*, 1977). These programs have the attraction of plausibility. However, they are all based upon *a priori* reasoning without any convincing validation of underlying hypotheses. Reduction in incidence of complications is cited as confirmation of the success of such screening, but this reduction has occurred at a time of increasing sophistication in understanding and preventing the somatic complications of bypass. Carried to an extreme, one might follow MacLean's (1976) advice to select 'only mature, intelligent patients who have an appropriate emotional demeanor, (and) have a good chance to succeed vocationally...' (and thus do no surgery at all!) Our experience with our study series and numerous other patients leads us to wonder about the justification for leaving the patients, screened out by plausible but untested programs, to their miserable fates. A much more appealing program for preoperative psychological assessment is outlined by Wright & Wright (1975) in relation to candidates for cosmetic nasal surgery. This program stresses the goal for detecting and *controlling* the effects of personality disorders, rather than the rejection of questionable candidates.

Several recent reports are of theoretical interest in furthering understanding of the effects of bypass surgery, and indeed the understanding of obesity itself. The view has been expressed (Castelnuovo-Tedesco & Schiebel, 1976; Solow, 1977) that somatic difficulties are highly significant determinants of postoperative psychological distress. The findings of Spanier *et al.* cited by MacLean (1976) of two patterns of weight loss following surgery, one involving loss of fat and one involving loss of body cell mass, might help to explain why some patients have much more difficulty with weakness and lassitude than others. Crisp and his colleagues (1977) discuss the likelihood of a critical weight threshold, approximately 25 per cent above mean matched population weight, below which the psychological mechanism of denial becomes much less available. Garner & co-workers (1976), using Rotter's Locus of Control Scale in studying body image abnormalities in the obese, found a correlation between the obese individual's sense of external control ('ineffectiveness') and his/her body image distortion. This lends support to our view that a sense of ineffectiveness is a basic variable in the psychological constellation affected by this operation.

Kalucy (1976) discusses intestinal bypass in the context of a comprehensive review of current psychobiological understanding of the syndromes of obesity. Finally, Mills & Stunkard (1976) have retrospectively examined eating behavior following operation and have admirably evaluated postoperative status in the context of the patients' past experience. Confirming ours and others' observations (Bray *et al.*, 1976; Crisp *et al.*, 1977; Solow, 1977), they noted: 'postoperative voluntary restriction of food intake, "normalization" of eating patterns, resistance to eating during intense emotion, and far less dysphoria during post-surgical weight loss than during previous weight loss efforts'. The reasons for these changes are unknown; reconditioning of satiety mechanisms may be involved (Stunkard, 1975; Booth, 1977). It would seem that the challenge for the future is to discover what enables patients to lose weight *relatively* free of emotional discomfort after intestinal bypass, and to attempt to provide this without the anatomical and metabolic disruption involved in intestinal shunt surgery.

References

Booth, D.A. (1977): *Psychosom. Med.* 39, 76.

Bray, G.A., Barry, R.E., Benfield, J.R., Castelnuovo-Tedesco, P. & Rodin, J. (1976): *Am. J. Clin. Nutr.* 29, 779.

Castelnuovo-Tedesco, P. & Schiebel, D. (1975): *Int. J. Psychiat. Med.* 6, 465.
Castelnuovo-Tedesco, P. & Schiebel, D. (1976): *Am. J. Psychiat.* 133, 26.
Crisp, A.H., Kalucy, R.S., Pilkington, T.R.E. & Gazet, J-C. (1977): *Am. J. Clin. Nutr.* 30, 109.
DeWind, L.T. & Payne, H.J. (1976): *J. Am. Med. Ass,* 236, 2298.
Faloon, W.W. (1977): *Hospital practice* (1), 73.
Garner, D.M., Garfinkel, P.E., Stancer, H.C. & Moldovsky, H. (1976): *Psychosom. Med.* 38, 327.
Hallberg, D., Backman, L. & Espmark, S. (1975): *Prog. Surg.* 14, 46.
Harrington, M. (1976): *Bypass Byword* 3, (4), 1.
Kalucy, R.A. (1976): Obesity! an attempt to find a common ground among some of the biological, psychological, and sociological phenomena of the obesity/overeating syndromes. In *Modern trends in psychosomatic medicine,* Vol. 3, p. 404. London: Butterworth.
Kalucy, R.S. & Crisp, A.H. (1974): *J. Psychosom. Res.* 18, 465.
Lundgren, K.D., Scott, G. & Grabski, D.A. (1977): *Am. J. Surg.* 133, 569.
MacLean, L.L. (1976): *Can. J. Surg.* 19, 387.
Mills, M.J. & Stunkard, A.J. (1976): *Am. J. Psychiat.* 133, 527.
Prian, G.W., Buerk, C.A., Norton, L., Sawyer, R.B. & Sawyer, K.C. (1966): *Am. J. Surg.* 132, 691.
Solow, C., Silberfarb, P.M. & Swift, K. (1974): *New Engl. J. Med.* 290, 300.
Solow, C. (1977): *Am. J. Clin. Nutr.* 30, 103.
Starkloff, G.B., Donovan, J.F., Ramach, K.R. & Wolfe, B.M. (1975): *Archs Surg.* 110, 652.
Stunkard, A. (1975): *Psychosom. Med.* 37, 383.
Telmos, A.J. (1977): *Am. Surg.* 43, 389.
Webb, W.W., Phares, R., Abram, H.S., Muxel, S.A., Scott, H.W. & Gerdes, J.T. (1976): *J. Clin. Psychol.* 32, 82.
Wehlage, D.F. & Bechtold, D.L. (1976): *J. Indiana State Med. Ass.* 69, 833.
Wise, T.N. (1976): *Sth Med. J.* 69, 1533.
Wright, M.R. & Wright, W.K. (1975): *Archs Otolaryngol.* 101, 145.

44
DRUGS, APPETITE, AND OBESITY IN MAN

T. SILVERSTONE
Academic Unit of Human Psychopharmacology, Medical Colleges of St. Bartholomew's and the London Hospitals, German Hospital, Ritson Road, London, E8 IDF, England.

The effects which drugs can have on appetite are of obvious relevance to all who are involved in the study and management of patients with disorders of body weight such as obesity.

The clinical practice of using drugs to suppress appetite in the treatment of obesity originated from the unexpected clinical observation that patients with narcolepsy who were being treated with amphetamine frequently lost weight. Among the first of such reports was that by Prinzmetal & Bloomberg (1935) who noted that one of their narcoleptic patients who had previously gained 30 lb (13.5 kg) as a result of an 'insatiable appetite', was greatly benefited, in terms of his weight, by amphetamine 20 mg daily. Shortly afterwards Davidoff & Reifenstein (1937) remarked that weight loss occurred in the majority of their subjects who had been given amphetamine; and, on the basis of this finding, suggested that amphetamine 'may be of use in reducing weight'. Lesses & Myerson (1938) were quick to act on this suggestion, and they were impressed with the results: '...... on the one hand it (amphetamine) decreases the appetite, and on the other it so increases the sense of well-being and of energy that physical activity is increased'. Seven out of their eight overweight patients lost weight without feeling hungry.

That was 40 years ago. What is the position today regarding the use of drugs affecting appetite in the management of obesity?

Clinical psychopharmacology of anorectic drugs

The anorectic drugs in current clinical use include amphetamine itself (although to a rapidly diminishing degree), diethylpropion (Tenuate, Tepanil, Apisate), fenfluramine (Ponderax, Ponderal, Pondimin), mazindol (Teronac, Sanorex), phenmetrazine (Preludin), and phentermine (Fastin, Duromine, Ionamin). All but mazindol are chemical derivatives of phenylethylamine (Fig. 1).

Anorectic action

Before we can talk of a drug having an anorectic action we must be in a position to measure its effect on hunger and on food intake. In the case of hunger, as with other purely subjective states, we cannot make direct, quantitative measurements. We are limited to quantifying changes in the experience and awareness of hunger which may occur in a given subject over a period of time. For this purpose visual analogue scales (Fig. 2) have been repeatedly shown to be useful, particularly when assessing the effect of drugs on appetite (Silverstone & Fincham, 1977).

For example: when we examined the anorectic effect of dextroamphetamine sulphate in normal volunteers using visual analogue scales we found that the drug reduced hunger ratings in a dose related manner, suggesting a true pharmacological effect (Silverstone &

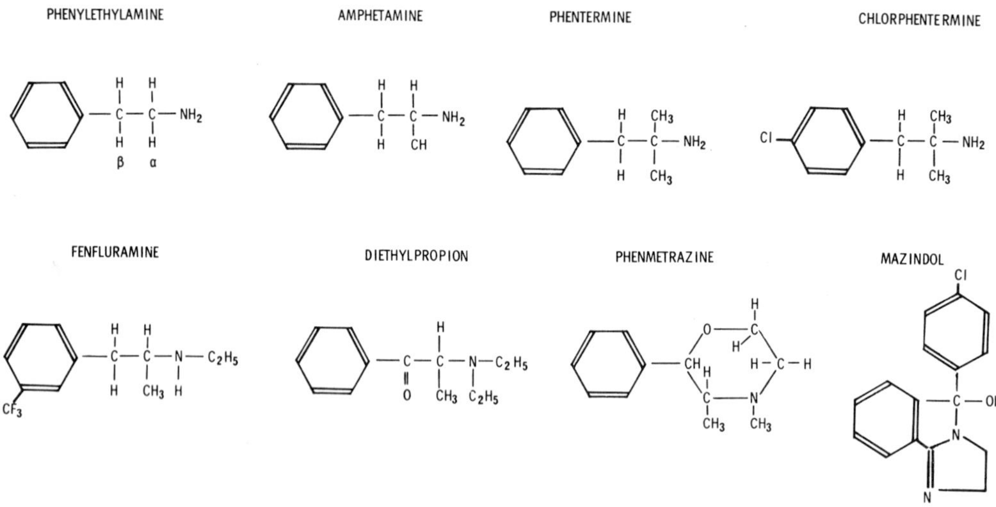

Fig.1. Formulae of anorectic drugs

Stunkard, 1968). Subsequent investigations have indicated that the anorectic effect of dextroamphetamine sulphate is maximal some 2 hours after oral administration (see Fig. 5).

Other drugs which have been evaluated in a similar fashion and which have been shown to have definite anorectic properties include phentermine, diethylpropion, fenfluramine and mazindol (Silverstone, 1975). The anorectic effects of both fenfluramine (Silverstone, 1974) and mazindol (unpublished observations) tends to be more prolonged with a pronounced anorectic effect being present some 8 hours after oral adminsitration of 80 mg fenfluramine or 2 mg mazindol.

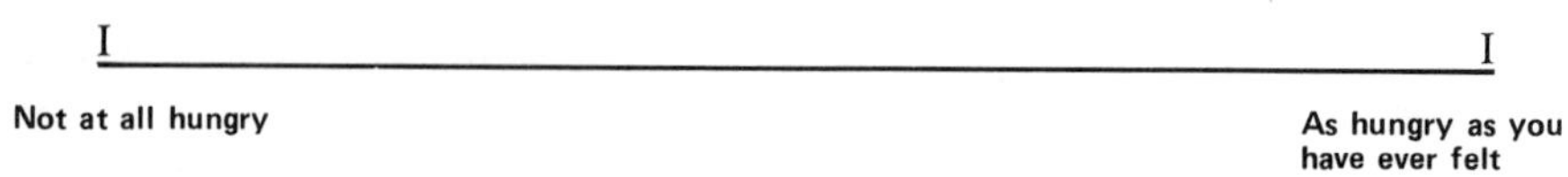

Fig. 2. Visual analogue scale for hunger. The subject is instructed to mark the line at a point which he considers most closely reflects his subjective hunger sensations at that time

In order to evaluate, in man, the effect of drugs on solid food intake over an extended period we have recently developed an automated food dispenser (Silverstone & Fincham, 1977) (Fig. 3). Using this dispenser to examine the effect of a new anorectic compound, tiflorex, on food intake, we were able to show a close correspondence between the effect of the drug on subjective hunger ratings, as determined by hunger visual analogue scales on one occasion and its effect on food intake, as measured by the food dispenser on another occasion (Fincham & Silverstone, 1977). Such close concordance between drug-induced changes in subjective hunger ratings and directly measured food intake strongly supports the view that anorectic drugs do have a primary effect on appetite, and that reliable and valid assessment of their anorectic action is possible.

Arousal

Amphetamine often produces central stimulation as had been originally noted by Prinzmetal & Bloomberg (1935). This may cause symptoms of restlessness and insomnia. Using an

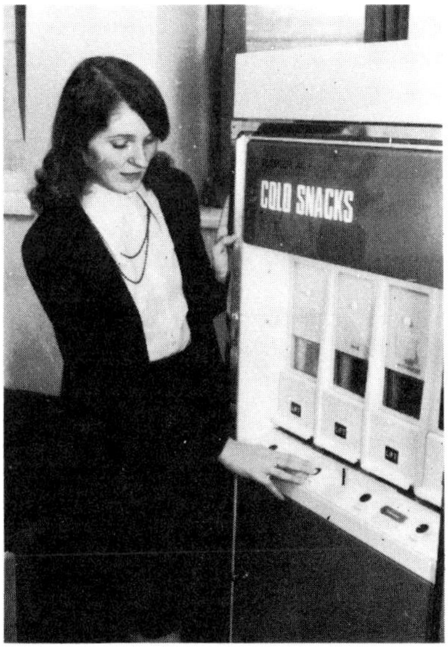

Fig.3. The automated food dispenser in use

appropriate visual analogue scale to rate the subjective 'arousal' induced by dextroamphetamine, we found it to be dose related; furthermore, objective measurements of arousal, such as critical flicker frequency are consistent with the subjective ratings (Turner, 1971). Of the other anorectic drugs studied in this way phenmetrazine and diethylpropion were found to increase critical flicker frequency, whereas fenfluramine and tiflorex did not. If anything fenfluramine countered the stimulant effect of amphetamine (Kramer & Turner, 1971). Such differences in laboratory findings between fenfluramine and some of the other anorectic compounds are in keeping with the differences in side effects reported during clinical trials; with fenfluramine causing sedation, and diethylpropion, phentermine and amphetamine being more frequently associated with increased arousal (Bray, 1976).

Mood changes

Amphetamine can elevate mood (Lasagna, von Felsinger & Beecher, 1955), and does so in a dose related manner, according to changes in visual analogue scale. Similar findings have been obtained using other rating scales (Smith & Davis, 1977). It is this euphoriant property of amphetamine which is largely responsible for the widespread abuse of the drug (Martin *et al.*, 1971).

In a comparison of the subjective effects of amphetamine, mazindol and fenfluramine in former amphetamine addicts, mazindol bore a slight resemblance to amphetamine in the opinion of these subjects, whereas fenfluramine had no such effect (Götestam & Gunne, 1972).

Mechanism of action

The centrally acting anorectic drugs are presumed to act on neurotransmitter systems within the brain. It is though, largely on the basis of animal studies, that amphetamine, phenmetrazine, diethylpropion, phentermine and mazindol act on catecholaminergic pathways, although there is uncertainty as to whether the noradrenergic or the dopaminergic pathway is the more important in this respect (Garattini & Samanin, 1976). In contrast to the other compounds, fenfluramine is generally believed to act via serotonergic pathways.

As far as amphetamine is concerned it is also not known whether its anorectic effect is mediated via the same pathways as its stimulant and euphoriant actions. Prior administration of alpha-methylparatyrosine, a compound which blocks the synthesis of both noradrenaline and dopamine, virtually abolished the euphoriant and stimulant effect of large intravenous doses of amphetamine given to previous amphetamine abusers (Jonssen, Anggard & Gunne, 1971). Similar inhibition of amphetamine-induced euphoria and arousal was obtained with the specific dopamine receptor blocking drug pimozide (Jonssen, 1972). This latter finding would indicate that euphoriant and stimulant actions of amphetamine are mediated via dopaminergic pathways. Our own findings are in keeping with this view. Pimozide 2 mg administered 2 hours before an oral dose of 10 mg dextroamphetamine attenuated the stimulant activity of amphetamine. In contrast, this small dose of pimozide had no effect on amphetamine-induced anorexia. If confirmed, this latter finding would suggest that the anorectic action of amphetamine may not be mediated via dopaminergic pathways (Silverstone & Fincham - to be published) (Fig. 4 & 5).

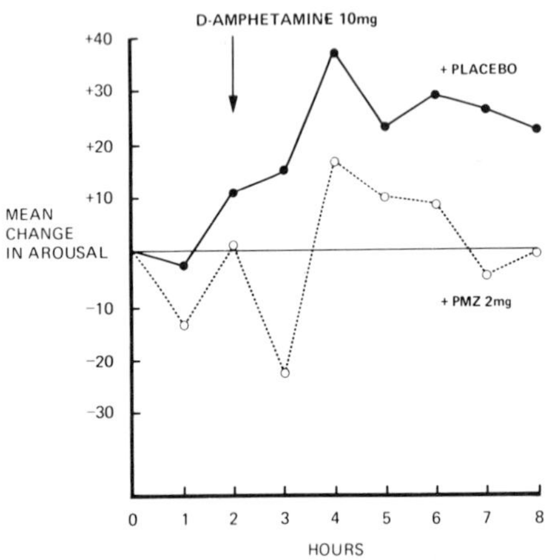

Fig.4. The attenuating effect of a single oral 2 mg dose of pimozide (a dopamine receptor blocking compound) on the stimulant activity of a single oral 10 mg dose of d-amphetamine, given 2 hours later

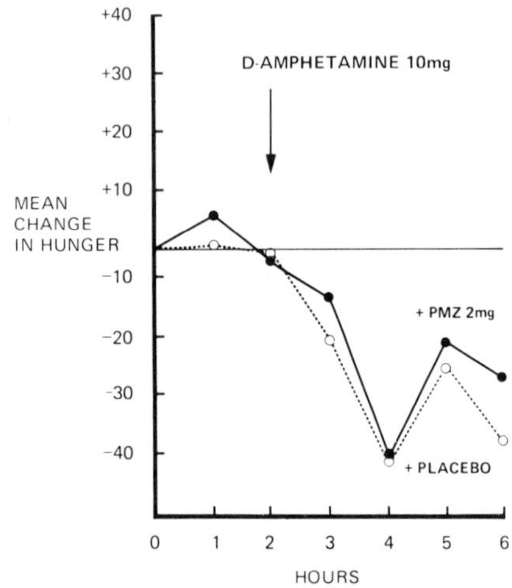

Fig.5. The lack of effect of a single 2 mg dose of pimozide on the anorectic action of a single oral 10 mg dose of d-amphetamine, given 2 hours later

If it is true that anorectic drugs such as diethylpropion act via a catecholaminergic mechanism, and fenfluramine acts via a serotonergic one, then the two types of drug could conceivably act synergistically in terms of appetite suppression, whereas fenfluramine might, at the same time, antagonise the central stimulant effect of the others. We examined this proposition in normal volunteer subjects using combinations of fenfluramine and diethylpropion (Silverstone, Salkind & Fincham, in preparation). Unfortunately for this hypothesis, neither 20 mg nor 40 mg fenfluramine added at all to the anorectic effect produced by 25 or 50 mg diethylpropion; in fact the combination of 40 mg fenfluramine with 50 mg diethylpropion was significantly less anorectic than diethylpropion alone. We can therefore only conclude that, far from enhancing the anorectic effect of diethylpropion, fenfluramine would appear to antagonise it; and there would be little potential clinical advantage in combining the two drugs. Furthermore, there was no significant attenuation by fenfluramine of the slight stimulant effect seen after diethylpropion.

Drugs causing weight gain

Another pharmacological approach to appetite regulation in man is through the study of drugs which appear to increase, rather than decrease hunger. One such compound is cyproheptadine which, in addition to its antihistamine properties, is thought to act by inhibiting serotonergic pathways in the CNS. It is in keeping with the view that serotonergic mechanisms are involved in the regulation of food intake that cyproheptadine was found to cause increased hunger, and consequently increased food intake and weight gain, in normal volunteers (Silverstone & Schuyler, 1975). Another serotonin antagonist, methysergide, has also been reported to cause weight gain in patients prescribed the drug for migraine (Blundell, 1977).

Other compounds causing weight gain secondary to an increase in food intake include chlorpromazine, given as a long-term treatment of chronic schizophrenic patients (Robinson, McHugh & Folstein, 1975), and amitriptyline, used in the long-term prevention of relapse from depressive illness (Paykel, Mueller & de la Vergne, 1973). Chlorpromazine has a number of neurochemical actions in the brain among which are blocking of dopaminergic and noradrenergic pathways. It is, therefore, of interest that anorectic drugs such as amphetamine, which are also thought to act on catecholaminergic pathways, are not effective in the treatment of chlorpromazine-induced obesity, presumably because the pathways by which they act are already blocked by the chlorpromazine. Fenfluramine, on the other hand, which probably acts on serotonergic pathways, does help overweight schizophrenics on chlorpromazine to lose weight (Jensen & Kirk, 1972).

The more specific dopamine receptor blocking compounds such as pimozide do not seem as prone as chlorpromazine to cause weight gain (Silverstone, 1976); this might be another pointer towards implicating noradrenergic as opposed to dopaminergic pathways in appetite control in man.

Amitriptyline prevents the neuronal reuptake of both noradrenaline and of serotonin, thereby increasing their availability at the receptor site; it is not known which of the two neurotransmitters is involved in its hunger-stimulating effect.

The use of appetite suppressant drugs in obesity

However striking may be the effects of single doses of anorectic drugs on hunger ratings in normal volunteers under laboratory conditions, and however intriguing the pharmacological interactions observed, such observations do not answer the crucial clinical question: 'Are appetite suppressant drugs of any real value in the management of obesity?' Furthermore, this question needs to be answered not only in terms of efficacy; if these drugs are to be useful clinically they must also be shown to be safe and to be free from long-term undesirable effects such as the tendency to produce drug dependency. It is particularly with regard to the possibility of dependence that anorectic compounds have become suspect, and their overall value questioned. Furthermore, as a result of widespread abuse of amphetamine, and to a lesser extent of phenmetrazine, both these drugs have ceased to be recommended for the treatment of obesity. This is in spite of the fact that the abuse of compounds was not a significant problem among obese patients prescribed these drugs by doctors; it was largely confined to teenagers using illicitly obtained drugs (Lasagna, 1973; Willis, 1978).

Excluding amphetamine and phenmetrazine for the reasons stated, there are four centrally acting appetite suppressant drugs in general clinical use: three with some central stimulant activity - diethylpropion, phentermine, mazindol; and one, fenfluramine, with a sedative action. Certain other preparations such as thyroid derivatives, diguanide compounds, human chorionic gonadotrophin and bulk fillers have all at some time been recommended in the treatment of obesity. However, as none of these latter groups of compounds have proved generally clinically effective (Garrow, 1973; Munro, 1973; Samuel & Burland, 1974; Silverstone, 1975; Bray, 1976) they need not be considered further.

Efficacy of anorectic drugs in obesity

The usual way to determine whether a given drug is an effective treatment in a particular condition is to compare it to a placebo or control treatment under the conditions of a double blind clinical trial. Many such trials have been undertaken with anorectic drugs, and most show a clear superiority of the active drug under test over placebo, at least in the short term (Samuel & Burland, 1974; Garrow, 1974; Silverstone, 1975; Bray, 1976; Craddock, 1976). Analysis of the results of 206 placebo controlled trials, involving over 7500 patients for which the US Food and Drug Administration had the individual case records on file, revealed that 'administration of an active anorectic drug will result in a weight loss of approximately 0.5 pounds more each week than if he or she were taking placebo' (Scoville, 1975) (Fig. 6). It is a reflection of the controversy within the medical profession which surrounds the use of anorectic drugs in obesity, that the drug-placebo differences presented in this analysis were dismissed by some as 'clinically trivial' (International Herald Tribune, 1972), while others hailed the findings as 'significant and desirable' (Lasagna, 1973).

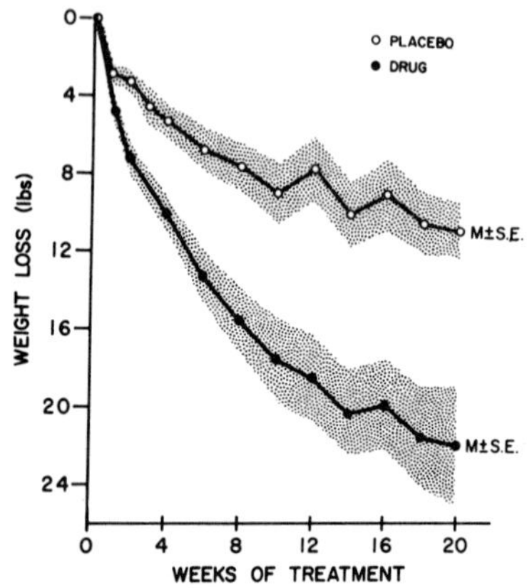

Fig.6. Representative clinical trial result comparing the efficacy of an anorectic drug to placebo over 20 weeks. (From Bray, 1976)

Diethylpropion

This compound, particularly in its long-acting form is currently the anorectic drug most frequently prescribed by general practitioners in the United States (Lasagna, 1973) and in the United Kingdom (Craddock, 1973). A number of trials have consistently demonstrated the short-term superiority of diethylpropion to placebo in helping obese patients lose weight (Silverstone, 1975) and one trial, that by McKay (1973), showed that the advantage of the active drug over placebo can persist for at least 25 weeks (Fig. 7).

Le Riche & Csima (1967) demonstrated that intermittent administration of diethylpropion (as Tenuate Dospan) 75 mg daily was as effective as continuous administration over a 24-week period. Unfortunately the drop-out rate was high in both groups with only 18 per cent of the initial 200 patients remaining at the end of the trial. Nevertheless, this study has obvious relevance to the clinician concerned with minimising the risks of dependence which might be greater with continuous than with intermittent medication.

In terms of drug tolerance, it is of interest to note that continuous medication was as good as intermittent; if significant pharmacological tolerance were occurring then one might expect less anorectic effect after a period of continuous administration than after intermittent administration. At the end of the sixth month of the trial the 14 patients who had been on diethylpropion continuously had attained 34.5 per cent of the desired weight loss, compared to the 24.7 per cent achieved by those 22 patients who had been on the drug intermittently. Furthermore, in the final month, the group with continuous treatment showed a significant advantage over the group with intermittent treatment and who were on placebo that month; in other words the active drug still appeared to be exerting a clinically significant anorectic effect even after 6 months. Such a finding argues against pharmacological tolerance. Nevertheless, it is a common clinical experience that patients lose ever-decreasing amounts of weight the longer they are in treatment. Such a diminution in efficacy has often been attributed to pharmacological tolerance, and the development of tolerance has been used as an argument against the usefulness of anorectic drugs in general (Lasagna, 1973). In my view the phenomenon is more likely to be due, at least

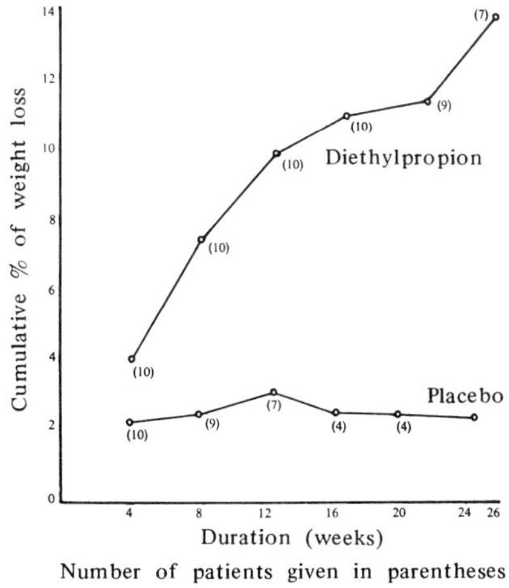

Fig.7. The continuing efficacy of diethylpropion over 26 weeks. (From McKay, 1973)

partly, if not largely, to a general non-specific lessening of enthusiasm on the part of the patient than to true pharmacological tolerance. As evidence, I would quote some data from a study of my own, in which I compared two different regimens of intermittent diethylpropion to continuous medication over a period of 16 weeks (Silverstone, 1974) (Fig. 8). One of the intermittent groups started on active drugs, the other on placebo. If tolerance were taking place then the weight loss in the second month should have been less in those patients who were continuing on diethylpropion, having already had it for a month, than in those patients who were starting it for the first time; in fact there was virtually no difference between the two groups.

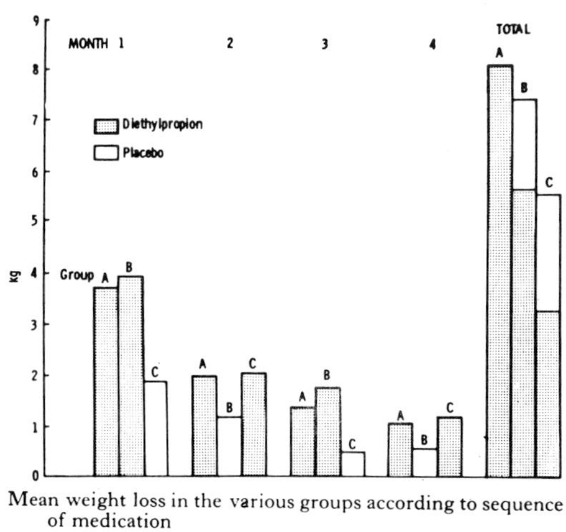

Fig. 8. The pattern of weight loss following three different therapeutic regimens using diethylpropion 75 mg daily: Group A received diethylpropion 75 mg daily continuously for 4 months; Group B received diethylpropion during months 1 and 3, and placebo in months 2 and 4; Group C received placebo in months 1 and 3, and diethylpropion in months 2 and 4. (From Silverstone, 1974)

Phentermine

Convincing evidence that both continuous and intermittent administration of phentermine is superior to placebo has been provided by Munro *et al.* (1968) in a 36-week controlled trial involving over 100 obese female patients. Phentermine 30 mg daily was significantly more effective than placebo and the drug was still exerting a useful effect during the ninth month (Fig. 9).

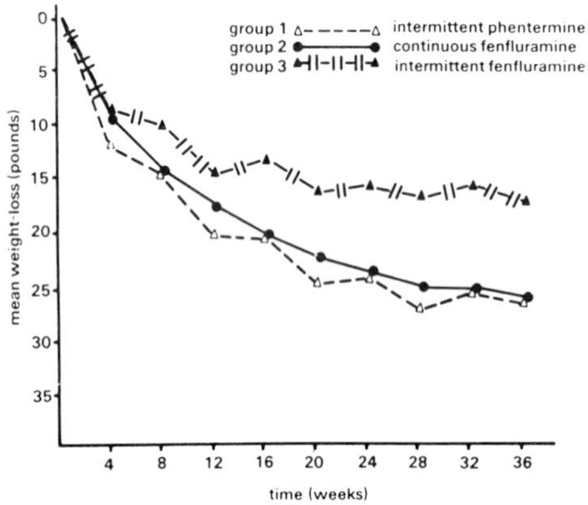

Fig.9. A comparison of continuous and intermittent fenfluramine medication with intermittent phentermine over a 36-week period in obese patients. (From Munro, 1973)

Mazindol

Unlike the other compounds we are considering, mazindol, the newest of the generally available anorectic drugs, is not a phenylethylamine derivative. It is, however, thought to act on catecholaminergic systems in the brain in a similar fashion to phentermine and diethylpropion. Smith, Innes & Munro (1975) showed that mazindol 2 mg daily, when given to what they term 'refractory' obese patients, was better than placebo for some 6 weeks, but after this its relative superiority waned sharply. However, a report from general practice has indicated a continuing efficacy of mazindol 2 mg daily over a period of 12 weeks (Murphy *et al.*, 1975).

Fenfluramine

Fenfluramine has been the most widely studied of the anorectic drugs apart from amphetamine (Burland, 1975; Pinder *et al.*, 1975). This compound is of particular interest as it was the first effective appetite suppressant which did not have any central stimulant action. In a trial involving patients with refractory obesity given fenfluramine 80 mg daily there was a clear superiority of the active drug over placebo which persisted throughout the 12 weeks of the trial (Munro, Seaton & Duncan, 1966). This persistent efficacy of fenfluramine was confirmed in a subsequent comparative study lasting 36 weeks (Steel, Munro & Duncan, 1973) (Fig. 9). The weight loss accompanying fenfluramine administration is closely related to plasma levels, with the best results occurring when these exceed 200 ng/ml (Innes *et al.* - unpublished observations).

Which drug to use?

Having established that all four of the drugs reviewed are clinically useful, the next question is, 'Which one to use?' Is any one of the four clearly superior to the others? In terms of weight loss the answer is, probably not. A number of comparative trials have been undertaken, most of which show little difference between one drug and the other. For example, Steel *et al.* (1973) found continuous fenfluramine to be as effective as intermittent phentermine, and Goldrick, Nestel & Havenstein (1974) found no significant difference in weight loss in patients treated with mazindol and fenfluramine. Similarly, we observed no statistically significant advantage of diethylpropion over fenfluramine, in terms of weight loss (Silverstone, Cooper & Begg, 1970); and, although Murphy *et al.* (1975) in their study did find mazindol to be better than diethylpropion, a comprehensive review of

145 double blind comparative studies by the Food and Drug Administration of the US Government failed to reveal any real differences in efficacy between the anorectic drugs (Bray, 1976).

Where these drugs do differ is in the side effects they cause. Diethylpropion, phentermine and mazindol have all been reported to cause central stimulant effects such as irritability and insomnia, although diethylpropion appears less likely to do so than the other two (Silverstone & Cleary, 1967; Bray, 1976). In contrast, fenfluramine is prone to cause drowsiness, and may be associated with depression, particularly on withdrawal (Steel & Briggs, 1972). Due to this tendency fenfluramine unlike the other drugs, should not be given intermittently, and, in fact, intermittent fenfluramine treatment was found to be not so effective as continuous (Steel *et al.*, 1973). Another side effect which occurs more commonly with fenfluramine than with the other drugs is diarrhoea; the proportion of patients reporting this symptom occurred in 18 per cent of our patients (Silverstone *et al.*, 1970), and 14 per cent of those of Steel *et al.* (1973). It is possibly because of the nature of the side effects associated with fenfluramine that it appears to be a somewhat less popular drug among patients than the others (Ashwell, 1973) (Fig. 10)

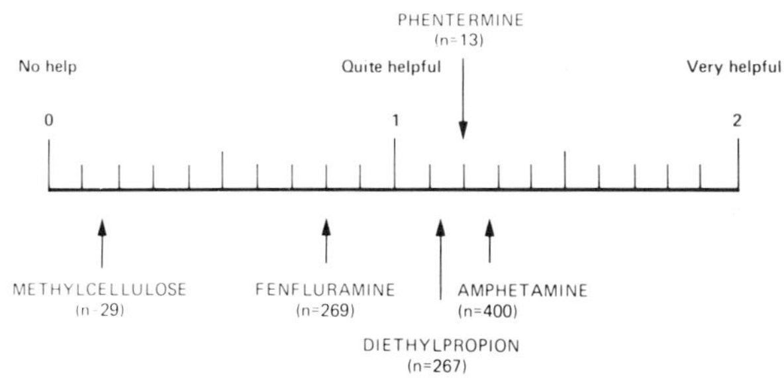

Fig.10. The attitudes of patients towards particular anorectic drugs.
(Based on data presented by Ashwell, 1973)

For the obese patient, who is somewhat lethargic or depressed, intermittent treatment with diethylpropion 75 mg daily, phentermine 30 mg daily or mazindol 2 mg daily should prove helpful, provided that it is fully appreciated by both the patients and the prescribing doctor that the drug can only be regarded as an adjunct to dietary measures. By reducing hunger these drugs may make dieting easier, they can never replace it. In fact, when dietary treatment is stringent (Baird & Howard, 1977) or when there is close and frequent personal support given by the therapist (Atkinson *et al.*, 1977) anorectic drugs have little to add. For the tense, anxious obese patient continuous administration of fenfluramine is best; the dosage being adjusted upwards from 40 mg daily according to effectiveness and side effects, with some patients requiring 120 mg a day in divided doses.

Attitudes to anorectic drugs

Even if anorectic drugs do suppress hunger and thereby help obese patients lose weight, should they have any place in clinical practice? According to some members of the medical profession the answer is clearly 'no'. Such physicians roundly denounce the practice of giving anorectic drugs to obese patients partly on the grounds that anorectic drugs do not work in the long term, and partly because they believe that anorectic drugs are very likely to lead to psychological dependence, and to widespread abuse. For instance Bruch (1974) speaks of prescribing anorectic drugs as 'perpetuating some form of quackery', while the quasi-official British National Formulary (1976) declaims '...... there is no substitute for willpower'. In contrast to such puritanical views come firm statements in support of drug treatment, such as that of Mayer (1968): 'It is fortunate for many people who hope to reduce weight that anorexigenic agents do exist'. Lasagna (1973) adopts a similar stance.

More common than either of these what might be termed 'polar' views concerning anorectic drugs is a half-hearted acceptance of their possible short-term value. For example: 'amphetamine and some related drugs are quite powerful anorectics but after a time their reducing effect is lost and the danger of addiction to them is great' (Garrow, 1973), or, 'anorectic drugs therefore make it easier for the patients to keep to a low energy diet for a while, but there is no published evidence that the majority of obese patients do regain normal weight' (James, 1976).

Most doctors have a similarly somewhat ambivalent attitude to anorectic drugs. Yudkin (1968) analysed questionnaires completed by over 1500 doctors, mainly general practitioners, in the United Kingdom (Table 1). It appeared that UK doctors were much more prepared to give anorectic drugs to their overweight women patients (70 per cent doctors) than to their male patients (56 per cent) even though they believed the results of drug treatment were better in men than in women. When it came to treating their own obesity, of the 832 who admitted trying to lose weight only 7 per cent had taken anorectic drugs. In his random survey of doctors in the United States, Lasagna (1973) also found that a minority (31 per cent) considered drugs to be of any real value, yet some 78 per cent of general practitioners used them in practice (Table 1).

Table 1. Doctors' attitudes towards anorectic drugs

	Total number surveyed	Number using anorectic drugs	Results (% doctors)		
			Good or fairly good	Equivocal	Poor
Yudkin UK	1562 (Treating others)	1095 (70%) (Female patients)	20%	26%	54%
		882 (56%) (Male patients)	42%	22%	36%
	832 (Treating themselves)	55 (7%) (On themselves)			
			Excellent or Good	Fair	Poor
Lasagna USA	450	117 G.P.s (78%)			
		75 Internists (50%)	31%	42%	27%
		86 Obst. and Gyn. (57%)			

While it is true that anorectic drugs do not afford a permanent cure for obesity, I would agree with Scoville (1975) when he says this is 'no reason to reject them out of hand; partial success is clearly better than failure'. It is also clear, as Bray (1976) remarks, that what is needed is a long-term trial of these drugs in the severely obese, before we can reach a final conclusion about their value.

The oft-repeated criticism directed against anorectic drugs, ie that they cause dependence, is only partly, if at all, a criticism of the drugs themselves. First of all I believe that we confuse the problems of abuse with those of dependence. Abuse is the use of a drug for non-therapeutic purposes. This is not, as we have already seen, a particular problem among patients prescribed anorectic drugs for slimming. Because a drug can be abused by a section of the population who are not patients is no reason to limit its legitimate use. Dependence, like abuse, is also a word with emotive overtones. Patients can be dependent on drugs for their physical health; diabetics requiring insulin affords an example. Patients can also be dependent on drugs to the extent that they feel better and accomplish more when taking their drug, osteoarthritics on analgesics are such. Just because many obese patients lose weight only while they are taking anorectic drugs should not be a reason for not giving the drugs in the first place. I suspect that many doctors believe, in spite of no real supporting evidence (Garrow, 1974), that most cases of obesity are due to gluttony, one of the seven deadly sins; as such it is a moral rather than a medical problem, and penance rather than pills is what is required.

It is my opinion that drug treatment of obesity should be limited to those who are at least 30 per cent overweight (and whose eating behavior is not pathological) and who consequently run a significant risk of developing cardiovascular complications (Bray, 1976), and to those who although not 30 per cent overweight have serious symptoms directly related to their obesity, symptoms such as hypertension, diabetes, or arthritis. I would suggest that the rest, who probably form the majority of patients seeking treatment where the weight is of cosmetic rather than clinical significance, should be referred to specialised slimming groups whose record of success is generally much better than that of doctors (Garrow, 1975).

Within the limited group of patients who are significantly obese, I believe that we should use anorectic drugs more vigorously and for longer periods than we have been accustomed to doing in the recent past. Surely the risk of central nervous stimulation is preferable to the morbidity (not to mention the risk of mortality) accompanying such drastic alternative measures as intestinal bypass surgery. Let us by all means be circumspect in our application of anorectic drugs, but when we do use them let us use them to their full potential and for as long as necessary.

References

Ashwell, M.A. (1973): *Practitioner* 211, 653.

Atkinson, R.L., Greenway, F.L., Bray, G.A., Dahms, W.T., Molitch, M.E., Hamilton, K. & Rodin, J. (1977): *Int. J. Obesity* 1, 113.

Baird, I.M. & Howard, A.N. (1977): *Int. J. Obesity* 1, 271.

Blundell, J.E. (1977): *Int. J. Obesity* 1, 15.

Bray, G.A. (1976): *The obese patient*. Philadelphia: W.B. Saunders.

British Medical Association and The Pharmaceutical Society of Great Britain (1976): British National Formulary.

Bruch, H. (1974): *Obesity, anorexia nervosa and the person within.* London: Routledge and Kegan Paul.

Burland, W.L. (1975): A review of experience with fenfluramine. In *Obesity in perspective,* ed G.A. Bray, p. 429. Washington DC: US Govt. Ptg. Office.

Craddock, D. (1973): *Obesity and its management.* Edinburgh: Churchill Livingstone.

Craddock, D. (1976): *Drugs* 11, 378.

Davidoff, E. & Reifenstein, E.C. (1937): *J. Am. Med. Ass.* 108, 1770.

Fincham, J. & Silverstone, T. (1977): Abstr. Second International Congress on Obesity 1977. *Int. J. Obesity* 2, (in press).

Garattini, S. & Samanin, R. (1976): Anorectic drugs and brain neurotransmitters. In *Appetite and food intake,* Dahlem Konferenzen, ed T. Silverstone. Berlin: Abakon.

Garrow, J.S. (1973): *Prescribers Journal* 13, 50.

Garrow, J.S. (1974): *Energy Balance and obesity in man.* Amsterdam: North Holland Publishing Co.

Garrow, J.S. (1975): A survey of three slimming and weight control organisations in the UK. In *Recent advances in obesity research:* I, ed A. Howard, p. 301. London: Newman.

Goldrick, R.B., Nestel, P.J. & Havenstein, N. (1974): *Med. J. Aust.* 1, 882.

Göstestam, K.G. & Gunne, L-M. (1972): *Brit. J. Addict.* 67, 39.

International Herald Tribune (1972): Experts call most dietary pills useless. Wed. Oct. 11.

James, W.P.T. (1976): *Research on obesity.* London: HMSO.

Jensen, P.S. & Kirk, L. (1972): Fenfluramine (Ponderal) in the treatment of adipositas caused by neuroleptics. Paper presented at the Annual Meeting of the Scandinavian Society of Psychopharmacology, Copenhagen.

Jonssen, L-E., Anggard, E. & Gunne, L-M. (1971): *Clin. Pharm. Therap.* 12, 889.

Jonssen, L-E. (1972): *Eur. J. Clin. Pharm.* 4, 206.

Kramer, R.L. & Turner, P. (1971): *J. de Pharmacol.* 48.

Lasagna, L. (1973): *J. Am. Med. Ass.* 225, 44.

Lasagna, L., von Felsinger, J.M. & Beecher, K.H. (1955): *J. Am. Med. Ass.* 157, 1006.

Le Riche, W.H. & Csima, A. (1967): *Canad. Med. Ass. J.* 97, 1106.

Lesses, M.F. & Myerson, A. (1938): *New Engl. J. Med.* 218, 119.

McKay, R.H.G. (1973): *Curr. Med. Res.* 1, 489.

Martin, W.R., Sloan, J.W., Sapira, J.D. & Jasinski, D.R. (1971): *Clin. Pharm. Therap.* 12, 245.
Mayer, J. (1968): *Overweight.* Englewood Cliffs, New Jersey: Prentice Hall.
Munro, J. (1973): *Brit. J. Hosp. Med.* 10, 8.
Munro, J.F., MacCuish, A.C., Wilson, E.M. & Duncan, L.J.P. (1968): *Brit. Med. J.* 1, 352.
Munro, J.F., Seaton, D.A. & Duncan, L.J.P. (1966): *Brit. Med. J.* 2, 624.
Murphy, J.E., Donald, J.F., Molla, A.L. & Crowder, D. (1975): *J. Int. Med. Res.* 3, 202.
Paykel, E-S., Mueller, P.S. & de la Vergne, P.M. (1973): *Brit. J. Psychiat.* 123, 501.
Pinder, R.M., Brogden, R.N., Sawyer, P.R., Speight, T.M. & Avery, G.S. (1975): *Drugs* 10, 241.
Prinzmetal, M. & Bloomberg, W. (1935): *J. Am. Med, Ass.* 105, 2051.
Robinson, R.G., McHugh, P.R. & Folstein, M.F. (1975): *J. Psychiat. Res.* 12, 59.
Samuel, P. & Burland, W. (1974): Medicinal treatment of obesity. In *Obesity.* ed P. Samuel, W. Burland & J. Yudkin. Edinburgh: Churchill Livingstone.
Scoville, B.A. (1975): Review of amphetamine-like drugs by the food and drug administration. In *Obesity in perspective,* ed G.A. Bray, Washington DC: US Govt. Ptg. Office.
Silverstone, J.T. (1974): *Practitioner* 212, 245.
Silverstone, T. (1975): Anorectic drugs. In *Obesity: pathogenesis and management,* ed T. Silverstone, Lancaster: M.T.P.
Silverstone, T. (1976): Appetite and psychiatry: a psychopharmacological approach. In *Appetite and food intake,* Dahlem Konferenzen, ed T. Silverstone. Berlin: Abakon.
Silverstone, J.T. & Cleary, T. (1967): *Clin. Trials J.* 4, 837.
Silverstone, J.T., Cooper, R.M. & Begg, R.R. (1970): *Brit. J. Clin. Pract.* 24, 423.
Silverstone, T. & Fincham, J. (1977): Experimental techniques for the measurement of hunger and food intake in man for use in the evaluation of anorectic drugs. In *Central mechanisms of anorectic drugs,* ed S. Garattini & R. Samanin. New York: Raven Press.
Silverstone, T. & Fincham, J. (1977): Experimental techniques for measuring hunger and food intake in man. Paper presented as 6th International Conference on Physiology of Food and Fluid Intake, Paris.
Silverstone, T. & Schuyler, D. (1975): *Psychopharmacologia* 40, 335.
Silverstone, T. & Stunkard, A.J. (1968): *Brit. J. Pharmacol. Chemother.* 33, 513.
Smith, R.C. & Davis, J.M. (1977): *Psychopharmacology* 53, 1.
Smith, R.G., Innes, J.A. & Munro, J.F. (1975): *Brit. Med. J.* 3, 284.
Steel, J.M. & Briggs, M. (1972): *Brit. Med. J.* 3, 26.
Steel, J.M., Munro, J.F. & Duncan, L.J.P. (1973): *Practitioner* 211, 232.
Turner, P. (1971): *Seminars in Drug Treatment* 1, 335.
Willis, J. (1978): In Central mechanisms of anorectic drugs, ed S. Garattini & R. Samanin. New York: Raven Press.
Yudkin, J. (1968): *Practitioner* 201, 330.

45
Importance of serotonin for explaining the action of some anorectic agents

S. GARATTINI
Istituto di Ricerche Farmacologiche 'Mario Negri', Via Eritrea, 62–20157 Milan, Italy.

Previous work by this laboratory has demonstrated that it is possible to dissociate various pharmacological effects of d-amphetamine such as hyperthermia, anorexia, locomotor stimulation and stereotyped behavior, suggesting that they may be mediated by different mechanisms.

For instance, C_3H mice respond to the anorectic effect of d-amphetamine but they are insensitive to the hyperthermic effect (Jori & Garattini, 1973; Garattini, Jori & Samanin, 1976*b*). In rats, a selective degeneration of central noradrenergic neurons markedly reduces the anorectic effect of d-amphetamine without affecting the increase of locomotor activity and stereotyped behaviour (Garattini *et al.*, 1976*b*; Quattrone *et al.*, 1978). Furthermore, amineptine, a new type of stimulant, at doses causing marked stimulation of locomotor activity and stereotyped behaviour in the rat produces no significant reduction of food intake (Samanin *et al.*, 1977*c*). Conversely, drugs such as fenfluramine induce marked anorexia in the rat without behavioural signs of central stimulation (Bizzi *et al.*, 1970; Garattini *et al.*, 1978; Le Douarec, Schmitt & Laubie, 1966). These findings suggest that mechanisms regulating food intake can be dissociated from those involved in the stimulatory effects. Research into the interaction between anorectic agents and monoaminergic systems in the brain appears to be the most promising way of obtaining knowledge of the mechanisms specifically involved in anorectic activity.

This report summarizes the main criteria used and experimental results in support of the hypothesis that some monoaminergic mechanisms are specifically involved in anorectic activity. Emphasis is laid on the serotoninergic system, since its role in anorexia appears to be further supported by new data obtained in our laboratory.

Criteria applied for evaluating the mechanism of action of anorectic agents on monoaminergic systems

Two main approaches have been used to investigate the possibility that the anorectic activity of various compounds may be mediated by one or more monoaminergic systems in the brain.

The first consists of evaluating the effects of different doses of anorectics on several amine parameters by *in vivo* and *in vitro* tests in order to identify which biochemical effects correlate best with pharmacological activity. These tests include: (a) determination of steady-state levels of serotonin (5HT), noradrenaline (NA), dopamine (DA) and some of their metabolites -5-hydroxyindoleactic acid (5HIAA), 3-methoxy-4-hydroxyphenylethylglycole sulphate (MOPEG–SO_4) and homovanillic acid (HVA). HVA was measured in the striatum, an area particularly rich in dopaminergic terminals but all the other substances were determined in the whole brain; (b) uptake of labelled monoamines in brain synaptosomal preparations; (c) indirect *in vivo* methods to measure uptake inhibition. The event where anorectics interfere with catecholamine uptake is assessed by studying their effects on the depletion of brain NA and DA induced by an intraventricular injection of 6-hydroxydopamine (6OHDA) (Garattini *et al.*, 1978); blockers of CA uptake specifically counteract the effect of 6OHDA (Samanin, Bernasconi & Garattini, 1975*b*). Inhibition of the depletion of brain 5HT induced by fenfluramine has been taken to indicate interferences with the uptake mechanism in 5HT neurons. This effect is shown specifically by 5HT uptake blockers such as chlorimipramine, fluoxetine (Ghezzi *et al.*, 1973; Garattini *et al.*, 1975*a*).

In some cases, the effects of anorectic agents on the uptake and release of 5HT in rat blood platelets (Garattini *et al.*, 1975*a*) were studied.

The second approach consists of establishing whether manipulations of monoaminergic systems can affect the decrease of food intake induced by anorectics. The rationale of this approach is that if brain monoamines do play a role in the activity of anorectics, a disruption of these systems in the brain sould modify the effect of these drugs.

Table 1 lists the procedures used to manipulate monoaminergic systems in the brain. It is necessary to use procedures which are supposed to act pre or postsynaptically in order to clarify whether the reduction of food intake is mediated by the anorectics acting on presynaptic nerve endings and/or directly on postsynaptic receptors.

Table 1. Procedures used to block monoaminergic transmission at various levels

Experimental condition	Monoamine involved	Site of action
Electrolytic lesions of raphe nuclei (MR)	5HT	presynaptic
Electrolytic lesions of NA neurons, (ventral bundle, VNB)	NA	presynaptic
Pargyline plus intraventricular 6OHDA	NA, DA	presynaptic
Desipramine plus intrastriatal 6OHDA	DA	presynaptic
α-Methylparatyrosine	NA, DA	presynaptic
Parachlorophenylalanine	5HT	presynaptic
Methergoline	5HT	postsynaptic
Penfluridol	DA	postsynaptic
Phenoxybenzamine	NA (α-receptors)	postsynaptic
Propranolol	NA (β-receptors)	postsynaptic

Although the use of procedures such as those listed in Table 1, particularly when combined with biochemical studies, have helped differentiate the role of monoamines in the activity of various anorectics, it should be borne in mind that various factors, such as the relative specificity of the means used to alter monoaminergic systems, metabolic interactions when two drugs are used and others, can make it particularly difficult to assess the specificity of effects on a single brain monoamine. There is also the possibility that an effect on one monoamine may cause changes in other systems as a consequence of interaction between the relative neurotransmitters in the brain (Blondaux *et al.*, 1973; Kostowski *et al.*, 1974; Samanin & Garattini, 1976; Consolo *et al.*, 1975). These changes can be overlooked when work is done on the whole brain. Knowledge of these problems is important is results are to be interpreted properly.

This general approach has generated a large amount of data during the last few years (Garattini *et al.*, 1978; Garattini & Samanin, 1976; Garattini *et al.*, 1974; Garattini *et al.*, 1975*b*) and we shall, therefore, only summarise the findings here.

Differences and similarities between anorectic drugs

d-Amphetamine at anorectic doses (2.5 mg/kg i.p.) slightly increases brain NA and striatum DA while it decreases striatum HVA (Garattini *et al.*, 1978). At higher doses it decreases brain NA (Garattini *et al.*, 1975*a*) and increases HVA (Garattini *et al.*, 1975*a*). No effects were observed on 5HT, 5HIAA (Garattini *et al.*, 1978; Garattini *et al.*, 1975*a*) and MOPEG-SO_4 (Calderini, Morselli & Garattini, 1975). The uptake of NA is inhibited more than that of DA both *in vitro* and *in vivo*, while no effect on 5HT uptake was observed *in vivo* (Garattini *et al.*, 1978).

The anorectic activity of d-amphetamine was inhibited by manipulation of the catecholaminergic system but not of the serotoninergic system (Garattini *et al.*, 1978; Samanin *et al.*, 1975*a;* Samanin *et al.*, 1972; Samanin *et al.*, 1977*a*). Overall evaluation of the results suggests that the anorectic effect of d-amphetamine could be mediated by noradrenaline, either alone or in combination with dopamine, depending on the dose employed.

dl-Fenfluramine at anorectic doses (5 mg/kg i.p.) considerably reduces brain 5HT (Duhault & Verdavainne, 1967; Ghezzi *et al.*, 1973) while it increases striatum HVA (Garattini *et al.*, 1978). At higher doses there is a reduction of 5HIAA (Garattini *et al.*, 1975*a*), a decrease of NA (Garattini *et al.*, 1975*a*) and a slight increase of MOPEG-SO_4 (Calderini *et al.*, 1975). 5HT uptake *in vitro* is inhibited by concentrations of fenfluramine smaller than those required to inhibit the uptake of NA and DA (Garattini *et al.*, 1978). *In vivo* fenfluramine does not affect brain uptake of NA or DA, as shown by the 6OHDA test (Garattini *et al.*, 1978).

The anorectic activity of fenfluramine is selectively inhibited by lesions of the serotoninergic system (Samanin *et al.*, 1972) and by 5HT antagonists (Garattini *et al.*, 1974). 5HT uptake inhibitors such as chloroimipramine have the same effect presumably by preventing fenfluramine entering the serotoninergic system (Ghezzi *et al.*, 1973). Manipulation of the noradrenergic and/or dopaminergic systems has no effect on anorexia induced by fenfluramine (Garattini *et al.*, 1978; Samanin *et al.*, 1975*a;* Samanin *et al.*, 1972). These findings suggest that the anorectic effect of fenfluramine requires an intact serotoninergic system.

Mazindol, phentermine and *diethylpropion* are other anorectic agents which appear to resemble d-amphetamine more than fenfluramine in their mechanism of action (Garattini *et al.*, 1978; Garattini *et al.*, 1975*a;* Samanin *et al.*, 1975*a*). DA seems to play a more important role in the anorectic effect of mazindol than in that of d-amphetamine (Garattini *et al.*, 1978; Samanin *et al.*, 1977*a*).

Table 2 summarizes the findings obtained for d-amphetamine, mazindol and fenfluramine.

Table 2. Effect of procedures affecting central monoaminergic mechanisms on the anorectic activity of amphetamine, mazindol and fenfluramine in the rat. See Garattini *et al.* (1978; 1975*a*); Garattini & Samanin (1976); Garattini *et al.* (1974; 1975*b*); Samanin *et al.* (1975*a*; 1972; 1977*a*) for details

Experimental condition	Effect on			Anorexia by		
	5HT	NA	DA	Amphetamine	Mazindol	Fenfluramine
5HT antagonists	↘	—	—	unchanged	unchanged	reduced
MR lesion	↘	—	—	unchanged	unchanged	reduced
pargyline + 6OHDA	—	↘	↘	reduced	reduced	unchanged
VNB lesion	—	↘	—	reduced	reduced	unchanged
striatial 6OHDA	—	—	↘	unchanged	reduced	unchanged
DA antagonists	—	—	↘	reduced or unchanged	reduced	unchanged

All these compounds, particularly at doses higher than those required to cause anorexia, increase striatal HVA (Jori & Dolfini, 1974). However, animals made resistant to the effect of d-amphetamine show cross resistance to other anorectic agents, with the exception of fenfluramine (Jori & Bernardi, 1972; Jori, Caccia & Dolfini, 1974). It is, therefore, suggested that fenfluramine acts on the striatal dopaminergic system by a different mechanism from that of d-amphetamine. Some experimental findings support the hypothesis that fenfluramine increases striatal HVA by blocking dopaminergic receptors (Jori *et al.*, 1974). While it is also possible that this drug's effect on HVA may be mediated, at least partially, by the serotoninergic system (Samanin, unpublished results).

The bulk of data suggests that food intake can be decreased in rats at least by two different mechanisms, one involving the catecholaminergic system (d-amphetamine, diethylpropion, phentermine and mazindol), the other by the serotoninergic system (fenfluramine). The second type of anorexia seems to occur without the stimulation and stereotyped behaviour induced by the amphetamine and the other compounds which preferentially act on brain catecholamines.

Further evidence that the serotoninergic system may be important for anorectic effect of drugs

The two optimal isomers of fenfluramine show different biochemical and pharmacological effects. The d-isomer is more effective than the l-form as an inhibitor of 5HT uptake *in vitro* (Garattini *et al.*, 1978) while the l-isomer increases striatal HVA more than the d-form (Jori *et al.*, 1973). These biochemical differences can hardly be explained by different availability of the two isomers in the brain (Caccia, unpublished results). Table 3 summarizes these findings. It is interesting to note that d-fenfluramine is more effective than the l-isomer in decreasing food intake (Le Douarec *et al.*, 1966), supporting the hypothesis of serotoninergic involvement in this effect.

Table 3. Differential effects of d- and l-isomers of fenfluramine (F) on various parameters

Parameters	Dose mg/kg i.p.	d-fenfluramine	l-fenfluramine	References
Striatal HVA (% of control)	15	151	306	Jori *et al.*, 1973
Striatal levels (μg/g)	7.5	11 ± 0.7	9 ± 0.8	Caccia *et al.*, unpublished
Food intake (% of control)	5	15	75	Samanin *et al.*, unpublished
in vitro 5HT uptake (IC_{50})	–	5.2×10^{-7}	8.9×10^{-6}	Garattini *et al.*, unpublished

A corollary of this conclusion is that if 5HT is important for the anorectic action of drugs, all drugs that act specifically on 5HT receptors, either directly at the postsynaptic sites or indirectly by releasing and/or making available more 5HT, should have anorectic activity.

Table 4 shows that in fact a number of agents such as quipazine, a 5HT agonist (Hong *et al.*, 1969) Organon 6582 (dl-8-chloro-11-anti-amino-benzo-(b)-bicyclo-[3.3.1]-nona-3, 6a-(10_a)-diene hydrochloride) and *m*-chlorophenylpiperazine, both powerful inhibitors of 5HT uptake (Sugrue, Goodlet & Mireylees, 1976; Garattini *et al.*, 1976*a*) reduce food intake in rats without being stimulants or inducing overt behavioral abnormalities, unless higher doses are used.

Table 4. Decrease of food intake induced in rats by quipazine, Organon 6582 and *m*-chlorophenylpiperazine (*m*CPP). The animals were trained for 10 days to take their daily food during 4 hours (from 10 a.m. to 2 p.m.). *$P<0.01$ compared with control (Duncan's test)

Treatment	Dose mg/kg i.p.	Food intake (g/rat/1h ± s.e.)
Control	–	9.8 ± 0.4
Organon 6582	10.0	5.7 ± 0.5*
Quipazine	2.5	4.6 ± 0.45*
*m*CPP	1.25	5.6 ± 0.9*

Although these findings appear to bear out the importance of 5HT in mediating anorexia, more specific studies are necessary to confirm or contradict this hypothesis. Such studies have been partially performed for quipazine and *m*-chlorophenylpiperazine.

Quizapine (Q), as shown in Table 5, produces a dose dependent decrease of food intake with no apparent gross changes in behaviour (Samanin *et al.*, 1977*b*). On synaptosome preparations, *in vitro* Q inhibits 5HT more than NA uptake, while it inhibits DA uptake only at much higher concentrations (Samanin *et al.*, 1978*a*) (Table 6). *In vivo* small doses (2.5 mg/kg) reduce brain 5HIAA without affecting striatal HVA (Samanin *et al.*, 1978*b*).

Table 5. Dose dependent decrease of food intake induced by quipazine in rats. *$P<0.01$ compared with saline (Tukey's test). See Samanin *et al.* (1977*b*) for experimental details

Treatment	Dose mg/kg. i.p.	Food intake (g/rat/2h ± s.e.)
Saline	–	8.3 ± 0.4
Quipazine	2.5	5.9 ± 0.7
Quipazine	5.0	3.3 ± 0.4*
Quipazine	10.0	2.0 ± 0.5*

Table 6. Effect of quipazine on *in vitro* uptake of C^{14}-monoamines by rat brain synaptosomes. Synaptosomes were obtained from pooled striata (for DA) or whole brain (for 5HT and DA) according to Gray & Whittaker (1962) and suspended in Krebs-Henseleit buffer to obtain a final protein concentration of 0.5 to 1.0 mg/ml (Samanin *et al.*, 1977*a*). Samples of 0.6 ml were incubated at 30°C with C^{14}-monoamines, 1 x 10^{-7}, for 5 min. Quipazine was added during a preincubation of 5 min. Data are mean values + s.e. of 4 replications

Concentration mmol/l	% inhibition		
	C^{14}-5HT	C^{14}-NA	C^{14}-DA
10^{-7}	28 ± 2	12 ± 9	0
10^{-6}	68 ± 1	49 ± 4	0
10^{-5}	87 ± 1	64 ± 4	38 ± 5
10^{-4}	89 ± 2	88 ± 12	69 ± 1

Only at a dose of 10 mg/kg does Q reduce the concentrations of HVA while brain 5HT and NA levels were not affected (Samanin *et al.*, 1978*b*). (Table 7). As indicated in Table 8, *in vivo* Q inhibits brain 5HT uptake while it has no effect on the uptake of NA and DA (Samanin *et al.*, 1978*b*). Table 9 summarizes a number of studies aimed at elucidating the mechanisms involved in the anorectic effect of Q.

Table 7. Effect of quipazine on 5-hydroxyindolacetic acid (5HIAA) and homovanillic acid (HVA) in the rat brain. The animals were killed 1 h after treatment. *$P<0.01$ compared with saline, **$P<0.05$ compared with saline. 5HIAA and HVA were determined by the method of Giacalone & Valzelli (1969) and Korf, Van Praag & Sebens (1971) respectively

Treatment	Dose mg/kg i.p.	brain 5HIAA	striatal HVA
		μg/g ± s.e.	
Saline	–	0.31 ± 0.03	0.63 ± 0.03
Quipazine	2.5	0.22 ± 0.01*	–
Quipazine	5.0	0.21 ± 0.01*	0.69 ± 0.02
Quipazine	10.0	0.17 ± 0.02*	0.53 ± 0.02**

Table 8. Effect of quipazine on the depletion of brain serotonin (5HT) and catecholamines induced by fenfluramine and 6-hydroxydopamine (6OHDA) respectively. Quipazine was administered 30 minutes before dl-fenfluramine (15 mg/kg i.p.) or 6OHDA (300 μg/rat intraventricularly) and the animals were killed 2 h or 7 days after fenfluramine and 6OHDA respectively. *$P<0.01$ compared with saline + fenfluramine treated rats (Duncan's test)

Pretreatment mg/kg i.p.	6OHDA or fenfluramine	Effect on 6OHDA		fenfluramine
		NA	DA	5HT
Saline	–	0.38 ± 0.01	1.28 ± 0.05	0.40 ±0.02
Quipazine 10	–	0.40 ± 0.03	1.34 ± 0.04	0.46 ±0 03
Saline	+	0.06 ± 0.01	0.50 ± 0.08	0.20 ±0.01
Quipazine 2.5	+	–	–	0.30 ± 0.01*
Quipazine 5.0	+	0.06 ± 0.01	0.47 ± 0.07	0.40 ± 0.01*
Quipazine 10	+	0.06 ± 0.01	0.44 ± 0.01	0.46 ± 0.02*

The decrease of food intake induced by Q is inhibited by a 5HT antagonist such as methergoline (Samanin *et al.*, 1977*b*; 1978*a*) but is not affected by lesions causing degeneration of the catecholaminergic system, by a specific dopaminergic antagonist such as penfluridol or by α or β noradrenergic antagonists such as phentolamine and propanolol (Samanin *et al.*, 1978*b*). It is interesting that lesion of the median raphe antagonizes the anorectic effect of 5 but not that of 10 mg/kg of Q (Samanin *et al.*, 1977*b*; 1978*a*) on postsynaptic 5HT receptors or through a different mechanism.

Table 9. Effect of quipazine on food intake of rats injected intraventricularly with 6-hydroxydopamine (6OHDA) or treated with penfluridol, methergoline, phentolamine or propranolol. Quipazine was administered intraperitoneally at a dose of 5 mg/kg. * $P<0.01$ compared with saline, ** $P<0.01$ compared with control (Duncan's test). See Samanin *et al.* (1978*b*) for experimental conditions

Treatment	**Food intake (g/rat/2h ± s.e.)**	
	Saline	**Quipazine**
Vehicle	8.5 ± 0.7	4.2 ± 0.3*
6OHDA	8.0 ± 0.6	4.5 ± 0.5*
Control	8.7 ± 0.8	4.3 ± 0.7*
Phentolamine	9.5 ± 0.6	2.3 ± 0.5*
Propranolol	7.7 ± 0.5	3.6 ± 0.7*
Control	7.2 ± 0.5	4.3 ± 0.4*
Penfluridol	7.8 ± 0.5	3.6 ± 0.5*
Methergoline	6.5 ± 0.8	6.6 ± 0.7**

m-Chlorophenylpiperazine (*m*CPP) is a possible metabolite of trazodone but it is a much stronger inhibitor of 5HT uptake in platelets (Garattini *et al.*, 1976*a*). At doses of 1.25 and 2.5 mg/kg, *m*CPP decreases food intake in proportion to the dose employed, while causing no signs of excitation or any other behavioural abnormalities (Table 10). At doses of 5 to 10 mg/kg, it elicits a complex motor syndrome consisting mainly of arching of the back and abduction of the hindlimbs. These effects also appear to depend on 5HT stimulation since they are completely prevented by pretreatment with methergoline (Samanin, unpublished results).

Table 10. Dose dependent decrease of food intake induced by *m*-chlorophenylpiperazine (*m*CCP) in the rat. *$P<0.01$ compared with saline (Tukey's test)

Treatment	**Dose mg/kg i.p.**	**Food intake (g/rat/1 h + s.e.)**
Saline	–	9.8 ± 0.5
*m*CPP	1.25	5.6 ± 0.9
*m*CPP	2.5	2.6 ± 0.7
*m*CPP	5.0	1.0 ± 0.3

Studies *in vitro* revealed that this agent inhibits 5HT and to a lesser extent NA uptake while DA uptake is affected at much higher concentrations. Also, *in vivo* data suggest that this compound, at a dose of 5 mg/kg, can preferentially act on brain serotonin, as indicated by the fact that it counteracts the effect of fenfluramine on 5HT but not that of 6OHDA on CA (Table 11). Findings after manipulation of the monoaminergic systems are also in progress in our laboratory to establish whether the effect on 5HT is responsible for the decrease of food intake induced by *m*CPP in the rat.

Interactions of the serotoninergic system with other monoamines

It is becoming apparent that an effect on any one monoaminergic system may induce changes in other monoaminergic systems, particularly when discrete brain areas are considered rather than the whole brain (Kostowski *et al.*, 1974; Samanin & Garattini, 1976; Consolo *et al.*, 1975; Stadler *et al.*, 1973; Agid *et al.*, 1975). Thus, today it is accepted that

Table 11. Effect of *m*-chlorophenylpiperazine (*m*CCP) on the depletion of brain serotonin (5HT) and catecholamines induced by fenfluramine and 6-hydroxydopamine (6OHDA) respectively. *m*CPP was administered 30 minutes before dl-fenfluramine (15 mg/kg i.p.) or 6OHDA (300 μg/rat intraventricularly) and the animals were killed 2 h or 7 days after fenfluramine and 6OHDA respectively. *$P<0.01$ compared with saline + fenfluramine treated animals (Duncan's test)

Pretreatment mg/kg i.p.	6OHDA or fenfluramine	Effect on		
		6OHDA		5HT
		NA	DA	fenfluramine
saline	−	0.35 ± 0.02	1.11 ± 0.03	0.45 ± 0.02
*m*CPP 5	−	0.36 ± 0.01	1.20 ± 0.02	0.49 ± 0.02
saline	+	0.09 ± 0.02	0.52 ± 0.07	0.21 ± 0.02
*m*CPP 5	+	0.07 ± 0.01	0.49 ± 0.02	0.31 ± 0.02*

there is a link between the dopaminergic and cholinergic systems in the striatum (Consolo *et al.*, 1975; Ladinsky *et al.*, 1978*a*) and an interaction between noradrenergic and serotoninergic neurons originating in the locus coeruleus and raphe nuclei respectively (Kostowski *et al.*, 1974; Samanin & Garattini, 1976; Blondeaux *et al.*, 1973).

It seems interesting, therefore, to study whether agents acting on the serotoninergic system indirectly affect other monoaminergic systems.

The two isomers of fenfluramine have been found to have a differential effect on striatal acetylcholine (ACh); the d-isomer significantly increases ACh levels (Samanin *et al.*, 1978*c*; Ladinsky *et al.*, 1978*b*), while the l-isomer (and the racemate) either has no effect or it causes a small decrease (Garattini *et al.*, 1974; 1975*a*).

Table 12 shows that d-fenfluramine and Q (7.5 mg/kg i.p.) both increase the levels of ACh in the striatum and to a lesser extent in the hippocampus and n.accumbens septituberculum olfactorium, while they have no effect on the brainstem ACh (Samanin *et al.*, 1978*c*). ACh in the telencephalon is significantly increased by d-fenfluramine but not by Q.

Table 12. Effect of quipazine and d-fenfluramine on ACh in rat brain areas. *$P<0.01$ Student's *t*-test. Quipazine was dissolved in distilled water and administered at a dose of 10 mg/kg i.p. d-Fenfluramine was dissolved in distilled water and administered at a dose of 7.5 mg/kg i.p. The animals were killed 60 min after quipazine and 30 min after d-fenfluramine. ACh was determined by the radiochemical method of Saelens, Allen & Simke (1970). The number of animals for each experiment is indicated in brackets

Brain area	ACh (nmol/g wet wt ± s.e.)		
	Control	Quipazine	d-fenfluramine
Striatum	31.5 ± 0.7 (11)	45.1 ± 1.8* (10)	53.6 ± 2.5*(11)
Hippocampus	15.5 ± 0.6 (9)	20.2 ± 0.6* (9)	23.9 ± 0.7*(8)
n-Accumbens septituberculum olfactorium	34.1 ± 1.3 (14)	41.2 ± 1.5* (6)	40.8 ± 1.5*(14)
Telencephalon	15.2 ± 0.6 (14)	13.3 ± 0.3 (4)	18.9 ± 0.4*(14)
Brainstem	22.3 ± 0.5 (14)	21.4 ± 0.7 (4)	23.8 ± 0.5 (13)

The increase of striatal ACh caused by either d-fenfluramine or Q is inhibited by previous treatments which antagonize 5HT such as methergoline or by treatments which block 5HT synthesis such as *p*-Cl-phenylalanine (Samanin *et al.*, 1978*c*; Ladinsky *et al.*, 1978*b*). In addition, the effect of d-fenfluramine was completely antagonized by degeneration of the serotoninergic system induced by lesion of both nuclei medianus and dorsalis raphe (Ladinsky *et al.*, 1978*b*) or by agents such as fluoxetine (Ladinsky *et al.*, 1978*b*) which prevent the release of 5HT by fenfluramine. Conversely degeneration of the dopaminergic nigro-striatal neurons induced by local injection of 6OHDA, inhibition of catecholamine synthesis by alpha-methyl-*p*-tyrosine or administration of specific dopaminergic antagonists such as penfluridol and pimozide did not affect the increase of striatal ACh obtained after treatment with d-fenfluramine or Q (Samanin *et al.*, 1978*c*; Ladinsky *et al.*, 1978*b*).

Table 13 summarizes some of these results, strongly suggesting that agents which increase the serotoninergic activity either directly or indirectly, also increase the levels of ACh in relation to their serotoninergic activity. The role played by this 'serotoninergic-cholinergic link' in the decrease of food intake induced by 'serotoninergic anorectics' remains to be established.

Table 13. Procedures affecting monoaminergic mechanisms on the quipazine and d-fenfluramine-induced increase of striatal acetylcholine. See Ladinsky *et al.* (1978*b*) and Samanin *et al.* (1978*c*) for details

Experimental condition	Striatal ACh increase induced by	
	Quipazine	d-fenfluramine
MR lesions	unchanged	antagonized
methergoline	antagonized	antagonized
parachlorophenylalanine	antagonized	antagonized
α-methylparatyrosine	unchanged	unchanged
pimozide	unchanged	unchanged
6-hydroxydopamine	unchanged	unchanged

Conclusions

The present results support the view that amphetamine and fenfluramine reduce food intake in rats through different mechanisms. Drugs such as amphetamine, mazindol, diethylpropion and phentermine may act by stimulating the noradrenergic and/or dopaminergic system, while drugs such as fenfluramine, quipazine and *m*-chlorophenylpiperazine may act by stimulating the serotoninergic system. These conclusions are reached by both biochemical and pharmacological approaches.

In addition, stimulation of the serotoninergic system results in increased ACh levels in the striatum, hippocampus and n.accumbens septi-tuberculum olfactorium. Whether this effect is important for the anorectic action remains to be elucidated.

References

Agid, Y., Guyenet, P., Glowinski, J., Beaujouan, J.C. & Javoy, F. (1975): *Brain Res.* **86**, 488.

Bizzi, A., Bonaccorsi, A., Jesperson, S., Jori, A. & Garattini, S. (1970): In *Amphetamines and related compounds*, ed E. Costa & S. Garattini, p. 577. New York: Raven Press.

Blondaux, C., Juge, A., Sordet, F., Chouvet, G., Jouvet, M. & Pujol, J-F. (1973): *Brain Res.* 50, 101.

Calderini, G., Morselli, P.L. & Garattini, S. (1975): *Eur. J. Pharmac.* 34, 345.

Consolo, S., Fanelli, R., Garattini, S., Ghezzi, D., Jori, A., Ladinsky, H., Marc, V. & Samanin, R. (1975): *Adv. Neurol.* 9, 257.

Duhault, J & Verdavainne, C. (1967): *Archs Int. Pharmacodyn. Ther.* 170, 276.

Garattini, S., Bizzi, A., de Gaetano, G., Jori, A. & Samanin, R. (1975*a*): In *Recent advances in obesity research:* I, ed A. Howard, p. 354. London: Newman.

Garattini, S., Bonaccorsi, A., Jori, A. & Samanin, R. (1974): In *Obesity: causes, consequences and treatment*, ed L. Lasagna, p. 70. New York: Medcom Press.

Garattini, S., Borroni, E., Mennini, T. & Samanin, R. (1978): In international symposium on *Central mechanisms of anorectic drugs.* New York: Raven Press (in press).

Garattini, S., Buczko, W., Jori, A. & Samanin, R. (1975*b*): *Postgrad. Med. J.* 51, (Suppl. 1), 27.

Garattini, S., de Gaetano, G., Samanin, R., Bernasconi, S. & Roncagliono, M.C. (1976*a*): *Biochem. Pharmac.* 25, 13.

Garattini, S., Jori, A. & Samanin, R. (1976*b*): *Ann. N.Y. Acad. Sci.* 281, 409.

Garattini, S. & Samanin, R. (1976): In *Dahlem workshop on appetite and food intake*, ed T. Silverstone, p. 83. Berlin: Abakon.

Ghezzi, D., Samanin, R., Bernasconi, S., Tognoni, G., Gerna, M. & Garattini, S. (1973): *Eur. J. Pharmac.* 24, 205.

Giacalone, E. & Valzelli, L. (1969): *Pharmacology* 2, 171.

Gray, E.G. & Whittaker, V.P. (1962): *J. Anat.* 96, 79.

Hong, E., Sancilio, L.F., Vargas, R. & Pardo, E.G. (1969): *Eur. J. Pharmac.* 6, 274.

Jori, A. & Bernardi, D. (1972): *Eur. J. Pharmac.* **19**, 276.
Jori, A., Caccia, S. & Dolfini, E. (1978): In international symposium on *Central mechanisms of anorectic drugs.* New York: Raven Press (in press).
Jori, A.,Cecchetti, G., Ghezzi, D, & Samanin, R. (1974): *Eur. J. Pharmac.* **26**, 179.
Jori, A. & Dolfini, E. (1974): *Pharmacol. Res. Commun.* **6**, 175.
Jori, A., Dolfini, E., Tognoni, G. & Garattini, S. (1973): *J. Pharm. Pharmac.* **25**, 315.
Jori, A. & Garattini, S. (1973): In *Frontiers in catecholamine research,* ed E. Usdin & S.H. Snyder, p. 939. New York: Pergamon Press.
Korf, J., Van Praag, H.M. & Sebens, J.B. (1971): *Biochem. Pharmac.* **20**, 659.
Kostowski, W., Samanin, R., Bareggi, S.R., Marc, V., Garattini, S. & Valzelli, L. (1974): *Brain Res.* **82**, 178.
Ladinsky, H., Consolo, S., Bianchi, S., Ghezzi, D. & Samanin, R. (1978*a*): In international symposium on *Interactions among putative neurotransmitters in the brain,* Milan, October 26-28, 1976. New York: Raven Press (in press).
Ladinsky, H., Consolo, S., Peri, G., Crunelli, V. & Samanin, R. (1978*b*): In international symposium on *Cholinergic mechanisms and psychopharmacology,* La Jolla, California, March 28-31, 1977. New York: Raven Press (in press).
Le Douarec, J.C., Schmitt, H. & Laubie, M. (1966): *Archs Int. Pharmacodyn. Ther.* **161**, 206.
Quattrone, A., Bendotti, C., Recchia, M. & Samanin, R. (1978): *Commun. Psychopharmac.* (in press).
Saelens, J.K., Allen, M.P. & Simke, J.P. (1970): *Archs Int. Pharmacodyn. Ther.* **186**, 279.
Samanin, R., Bendotti, C., Bernasconi, S., Borroni, E. & Garattini, S. (1977*a*): *Eur. J. Pharmac.* **43**, 117.
Samanin, R., Bendotti, C., Bernasconi, S. & Pataccini, R. (1978*a*): In international symposium on *Central mechanisms of anorectic drugs.* New York: Raven Press (in press).
Samanin, R., Bendotti, C., Candelaresi, G. & Garattini, S. (1978*b*): *Life Sci.* (in press).
Samanin, R., Bendotti, C., Miranda, F. & Garattini, S. (1977*b*): *J. Pharm. Pharmac.* **29**, 53.
Samanin, R., Bernasconi, S. & Garattini, S. (1975*a*): *Eur. J. Pharmac.* **34**, 373.
Samanin, R., Bernasconi, S. & Garattini, S. (1975*b*): *Eur. J. Pharmac.* **34**, 377.
Samanin, R. & Garattini, S. (1976): *Life Sci.* **17**, 1201.
Samanin, R., Ghezzi, D., Valzelli, L. & Garattini, S. (1972): *Eur. J. Pharmac.* **19**, 318.
Samanin, R., Jori, A., Bernasconi, S., Morpurgo, E. & Garattini, S., (1977*c*): *J. Pharm. Pharmac.* **29**, 555.
Samanin, R., Quattrone, A., Consolo, S., Ladinsky, H. & Algeri, S. (1978*c*): In international symposium on *Interactions among putative neurotransmitters in the brain,* Milan, October 26-28, 1976. New York: Raven Press (in press).
Stadler, H., Lloyd, K.G., Gadea-Circia, M. & Bartholini, G. (1973): *Brain Res.* **55**, 476.
Sugrue, M.F., Goodlet, I. & Mireylees, S.E. (1976): *Eur. J. Pharmac.* **40**, 121.

46
Novel pharmacological approaches to the treatment of obesity

A.C. SULLIVAN and J. TRISCARI
Department of Biochemical Nutrition, Roche Research Center, Hoffman-La Roche Inc., Nutley, New Jersey 071100, USA.

Obesity results when an imbalance occurs between intake and expenditure, which is manifested by excessive expansion of the adipose tissue mass. Current pharmacological therapy for the obese patient focuses primarily on one side of this equation, the reduction of energy intake. However, there are many levels within this equation relating intake and expenditure, where modification may be achieved theoretically with resultant effects on energy balance. A careful assessment of the metabolic, morphologic, and endocrine differences between obese and lean individuals suggests new approaches to the development of antiobesity agents. The following discussion outlines potential mechanisms of action for antiobesity drugs, indicating where pharmacological modifications have been assessed, and where future explorations should be directed. These approaches include the following: (1) suppression of food intake, (2) reduction of the availability of nutrients by modulating intestinal absorption, (3) modification of lipid metabolism, (4) alteration in the efficiency of lipid and/or carbohydrate oxidation, and (5) normalization of hormone levels.

Suppression of food intake

In the overall management of the obese patient, anorectic agents* continue to be used as short-term adjuncts to a nutritionally and/or behaviorally designed weight reduction program. Several reviews described the therapeutic efficacy and safety of these agents in reducing appetite and promoting weight loss (Bray, 1976; Craddock, 1976; Silverstone, 1975; Sullivan, Cheng & Hamilton, 1976; Sullivan & Cheng, in press; Sullivan & Comai, in press). Most of the anorectics utilized currently in the treatment of obesity produce their effects by interacting with central systems involved in appetite regulation. Current views on appetite regulation support the involvement of both central and peripheral components, which are integrated by metabolic processes. Brain neurotransmitters constitute an important element in the transcription of metabolically and peripherally generated information regarding the energy status of the organism, which is then translated into the behavioral activity defined as appetite. The anorectics employed today in antiobesity therapy produce their effects on food intake by modifying the release, concentration or uptake of biogenic amines involved in appetite regulation. Catecholamines appear to play an important role in the suppression of food intake induced by amphetamine, phentermine, diethylpropion and mazindol, whereas fenfluramine produces its anorectic effect by interacting with brain serotonin (Garattini & Samanin, 1976). Furthermore, procedures which affect brain monoamines alter the anorectic activity of these drugs (Garattini *et al.*, 1975; Garattini & Samanin, 1976; Hoebel, 1977).

*Anorectic agents currently employed for the treatment of obesity in the US include d, l-amphetamine, methamphetamine, phenmetrazine, phendimetrazine, benzphetamine, chlorphentermine, clortermine, mazindol, fenfluramine, diethylpropion, and phentermine.

Various new anorectics are currently undergoing evaluation in clinical and animal studies (for chemical structures and experimental details see Sullivan *et al.*, 1976; Sullivan & Cheng, in press; Sullivan & Comai, in press). Although the mechanism of action of these drugs has not been established clearly, these novel anorectics resemble those described above in terms of modifying central systems involved in appetite regulation. Several phenethylamine-like drugs such as the fenfluramine analogs, 780 SE (Miller *et al.*, 1975) and flutiorex (Giudicelli, Richer & Berdeaux, 1976) reduce food intake in man. Flucetorex (Bourillet & Buzas, 1975) and, particularly a number of fenfluramine glycinates (Duhault *et al.*, 1975) produce anorexia in animals.

Of the novel non-phenethylamine anorectics which have been reported, 11698 JL suppressed appetite in man (Dorf, Louis & Benedetti, 1975). DITA (Abdallah & White, 1976), APMO (Abdallah, 1973) and PR-F-36-CL (Oliver, 1974), although less potent than amphetamine in suppressing appetite in animals, possessed less central nervous system or cardiovascular side effects. UP 507-04 also suppressed food intake and decreased weight in experimentally-induced obesity in rats and mice (Dumeur *et al.*, 1976). Quipazine produced anorexia in rats, apparently by directly stimulating brain serotonin receptors (Samanin *et al.*, 1977).

Although some anorectics, particularly fenfluramine and mazindol, also produce effects on peripheral energy metabolism (for review see Sullivan *et al.*, 1976), it is unclear whether these metabolic effects are involved in the production of anorexia. However, the modulation of peripheral rather than central mechanisms regulating appetite appeared to explain the anorexia produced by (±)-trans-epoxyaconitic acid and (-)-hydroxycitrate. These compounds probably do not enter the brain, and thus produce neither tolerance nor CNS side effects such as stimulation or sedation, characteristic of other anorectic agents. Although, both (±)-trans-epoxyaconitic acid and (-)-hydroxycitrate reduced food intake and weight gain, the mechanisms underlying these activities differed. Anorexia and inhibition of hepatic lipogenesis *in vivo* in rats was observed by the oral administration of both (±)-trans-epoxyaconitic acid and (-)-hydroxycitrate. However, only (-)-hydroxycitrate was effective in reducing appetite and lipogenesis after intraperitoneal administration; (±)-trans-epoxyaconitate was inactive under these conditions (Sullivan *et al.*, 1973). The anorectic effect of (±)-trans-epoxyaconitic acid appeared to be related to a selective reduction in the rate of stomach emptying. (-)-Hydroxycitrate produced little or no inhibition of gastric emptying. When (±)-trans-epoxyaconitic acid was given orally to rats 30 min before a load of [^{14}C] glucose the rate at which the [^{14}C] disappeared from the stomach and entered the serum and liver was inhibited significantly (Fig. 1A). At 30, 60, and 90 minutes after the oral administration of [^{14}C] glucose, significantly more radioactivity was retained in the stomachs of the (±)-trans-epoxyaconitic acid treated rats; this was reflected in significant decreases in the radioactivity appearing in the blood and liver. Rats given (±)-trans-epoxyaconitic acid as a dietary admixture for 38 days gained weight at a significantly reduced rate compared to *ad lib.* fed controls, but at the same rate as rats pair-fed to the (±)-trans-epoxyaconitic acid animals (Fig. 1B). These weight reductions were reflected in body fat losses.

(-)-Hydroxycitrate also significantly reduced food consumption, but in contrast to (±)-trans-epoxyaconitic acid, it additionally altered the metabolic flux of dietary nutrients by diverting carbohydrate and its metabolites from lipid biosynthesis in liver, even under pair-feeding conditions (Fig. 2A). Some of this carbon was diverted apparently into hepatic glycogen. Significant increases in both the rate of glycogen synthesis (Fig. 2B) and glycogen content (Fig. 2C) were observed. These changes in carbohydrate metabolism may be involved in the anorexia produced by (-)-hydroxycitrate (Sullivan & Triscari, 1976). It was postulated that information regarding hepatic glycogen and/or glucose levels may be transmitted to the vagus by the brain, where it is translated into feeding behavior (Russek & Stevenson, 1972). This hepatic glucoreceptor hypothesis has been reviewed recently (Wolff *et al.*, 1976).

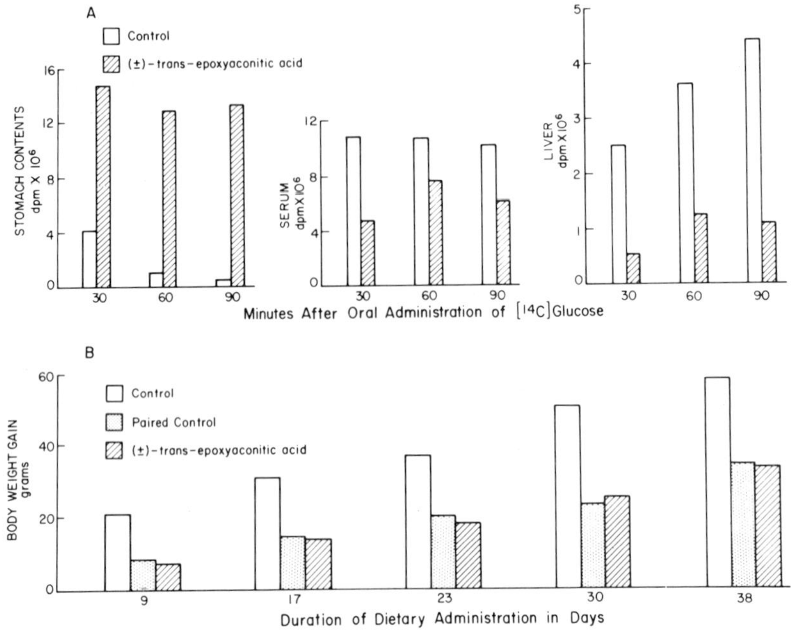

Fig. 1. Effect of (±) -trans-epoxyaconitic acid on rates of stomach emptying (A) and body weight gain (B). Rats (five per group in panel A and ten in panel B) were prefasted 48 hr, then meal-fed (8 to 11 a.m.) a 70 per cent glucose diet for 1 week prior to each experiment. In the stomach emptying experiment (A) rats were given either saline or (±)-trans-epoxyaconitic acid (by gastric intubation) 21 hr after their last meal, and ½ hr prior to a gastric load of 500 mg glucose (12.5μCi [u-^{14}C] glucose). Rats were killed 30, 60 or 90 min following the glucose load. (±)-trans-Epoxyaconitic acid increased the retention of glucose in the stomach, decreased serum radioactivity at 30 and 90 min, and decreased liver radioactivity at all points ($P<0.05$). In the feeding experiment (B) rats were meal fed for 38 days either a 70 per cent glucose diet (control and pair-fed) or 70 per cent glucose containing (±)-trans-Epoxyaconitic acid (26.3 mmol/kg diet). Paired control rats were fed an amount of food equivalent to that eaten by (±)-trans-epoxyaconitic acid fed rats. (±)-trans-Epoxyaconitic acid reduced food intake significantly compared to control at each time point ($P<0.05$)

The chronic administration of a non-toxic dose of (-)-hydroxycitrate as a dietary admixture significantly reduced body weight (due to a selective reduction in body fat) and food intake in several obese models including mature fat rats, genetically obese Zucker rats, and rats and mice made obese by hypothalamic lesions (Sullivan *et al.;* 1974*b*; Sullivan & Triscari, 1977). Analyses of body composition of the (-)-hydroxycitrate treated mature rats demonstrated a significant depression of body lipid levels and an unaltered protein content (Fig. 3A). Citrate administered as a control produced no significant effect on weight gain, food intake or body lipid (Sullivan & Triscari, 1977). The (-)-hydroxycitrate-induced decrease in appetite was not mediated by the ventromedial hypothalamus (VMH), a locus in the brain involved in satiety, because anorexia and reduced weight gain were observed in the presence or absense of an intact VMH nucleus (Fig. 3B). Recent conditioned aversion studies suggest that the food intake suppression produced by (-)-hydroxycitrate was not a consequence of any aversive effects of the drug (Panksepp *et al.*, 1977).

In summary, the mechanism by which (-)-hydroxycitrate reduced body weight gain appears to have two components: (1) suppression of appetite, and (2) inhibition of lipid synthesis (see 'Modification of lipid metabolism' for further discussion of (-)-hydroxycitrate). (±)-trans-Epoxyaconitic acid reduced body weight gain primarily by decreasing food consumption.

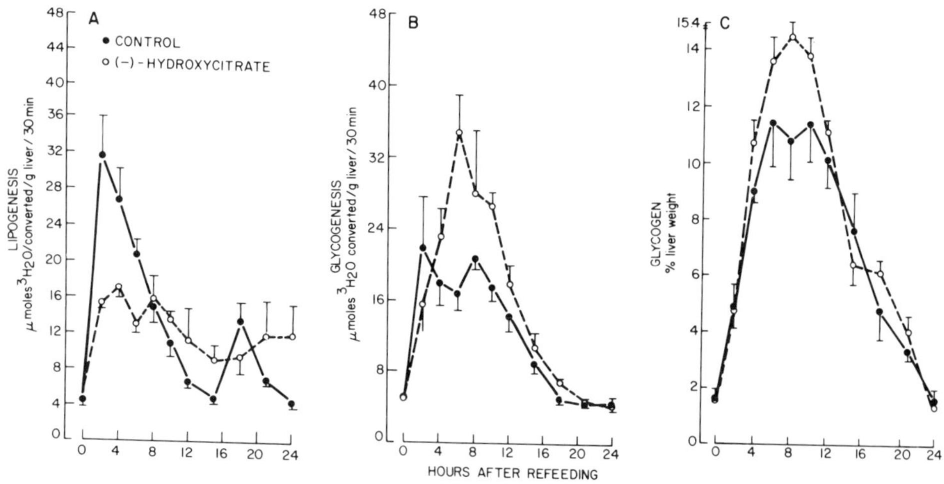

Fig. 2. Effect of hydroxycitrate on hepatic rates of lipogenesis (A), glycogenesis (B), and glycogen levels (C) determined over a 24-hr period. Rats (ten per group) were prefasted 48 hr, then meal-fed (8 to 11 a.m.) a 70 per cent glucose diet for 6 days. On day 7, rats were given either saline or (−)-hydroxycitrate (2.63 mmol/kg) by gastric intubation immediately before receiving 8.7 g of food. ^3H_2O was administered intravenously at the indicated times and animals killed 30 min later. (−)-Hydroxycitrate: (1) reduced significantly lipogenesis at 2, 4, and 6 hr after the initiation of the meal, (2) increased significantly glycogenesis 6 and 8 hr after refeeding, and (3) increased significantly glycogen levels at 6 to 10 hr after refeeding ($P < 0.05$)

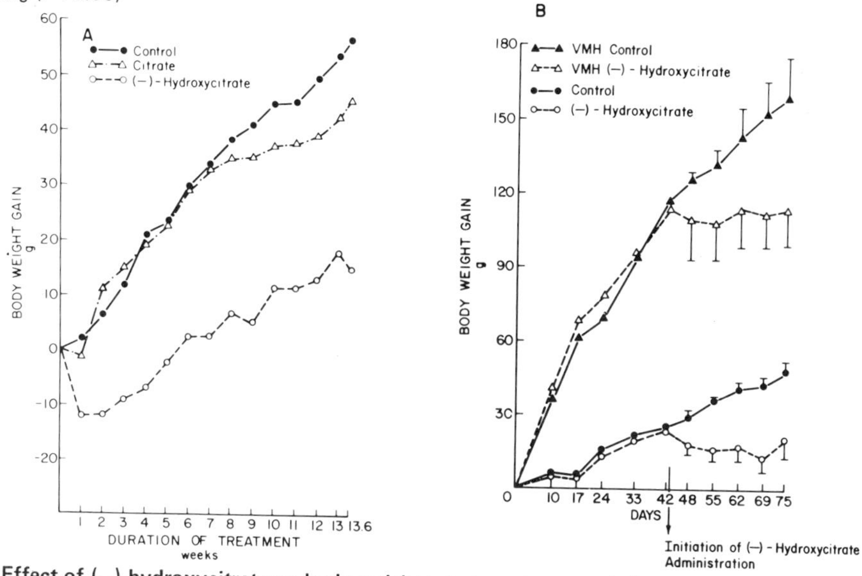

Fig. 3. Effect of (−)-hydroxycitrate on body weight gain in mature rats (A) and in VMH-lesioned rats (B). In the mature rat study, three groups of 12 to 29 rats per group (mean age 10 months) were fed *ad lib.* 70 per cent glucose diet (control), 70 per cent glucose containing citrate (52.6 mmol/kg diet) or 70 per cent glucose containing (−)-hydroxycitrate (52.6 mmol/kg diet) for 13.6 weeks. Cumulative body weight gain of the (−)-hydroxycitrate treated group was reduced significantly compared to control or citrate groups ($P < 0.05$). There were no significant differences in the weight gained by the citrate treatment compared to controls. In the VMH study, ten VMH rats (VMH region was destroyed bilaterally by electrocauterization) and 15 non-lesioned rats were fed *ad lib.* the G-70 diet for 42 days. On day 43, one-half of each group was given (−)-hydroxycitrate (52.6 mmol/kg diet) as a dietary admixture for 33 days. (−)-Hydroxycitrate reduced significantly body weight gain in both groups ($P < 0.05$). Adapted from Sullivan & Triscari, 1977

Other agents also decrease appetite by mechanism(s) which may originate in the periphery with subsequent translation by the central nervous system. Glucagon administration decreased hunger contractions (Stunkard, Van Itallie & Reis, 1955), and body weight and food intake (Schulman *et al.*, 1957) in man. Cholecystokinin (CCK) a polypeptide gut hormone, was postulated to function as a short-term satiety signal (Smith & Gibbs, 1976). Although CCK inhibited gastric emptying, its satiety effect was not mediated by gastric distension, because CCK inhibited feeding in a rat gastric fistula preparation in which food could not accumulate in the stomach, thus preventing any gastric distension. Injections of CCK decreased food intake but not water consumption, and elicited the complete behavioral sequence of satiety in rats and monkeys under sham feeding conditions (Antin *et al.*, 1975; Gibbs, Falasco & McHugh, 1976). A preliminary report suggested that CCK may not function in producing satiety in man (Goetz & Sturdevant, 1975). Elevation of body glycerol levels by multiple daily injections of glycerol produced hypophagia and body weight loss in rats (Wirtshafter & Davis, in press). These studies suggest that blood glycerol levels may be a signal by which the brain monitors body lipid content, and may play a role in the control of body weight.

Prostaglandins have been implicated in appetite regulation. Injections of prostaglandin E_1 into selected areas of the hypothalamus caused a significant decrease of food intake in rats with no apparent effect on behavior or water intake (Baile *et al.*, 1973). These data suggested that endogenous prostaglandin levels may represent a satiety signal, since prostaglandins are found in the brain and released in response to nervous stimuli. Additionally, circulating prostaglandin levels may vary with the degree of adiposity (prostaglandins are produced in adipose tissue) and thereby modulate hypothalamic activity by functioning as a component of a feedback signal for the regulation of energy balance. Recent studies suggested that the inhibitory activity of prostaglandin $F_{2\alpha}$ on food intake occurred at both peripheral and central sites (Doggett & Jawaharal, 1977*a*). A significant decrease in feeding was noted in rats following the subcutaneous injection of prostaglandin E_2 (Scaramuzzi, Baile & Mayer, 1971). Furthermore, intraperitoneal and intragastric administration of prostaglandin precursors, arachidonic, linolenic and linoleic acids to fasted rats reduced food intake (Doggett & Jawaharal, 1977*b*). Prior treatment with the prostaglandin synthesis inhibitors, indomethacin and paracetamol, specifically reversed the anorexia and biochemical satiety induced by these three fatty acids, while not affecting prostaglandin $F_{2\alpha}$-induced suppression of food intake. These findings suggest that both physiological and pharmacological modification of appetite could be produced by modulating prostaglandin generating systems.

Reduction of the availability of nutrients by modulating intestinal absorption
The search for oral agents which might produce a chemically-induced, reversible form of altered intestinal absorption has been encouraged by the success of intestinal bypass operations for the treatment of obesity. Compounds have been reported which reduce selectively either lipid absorption or carbohydrate absorption, or decrease non-selectively the absorption of all nutrients.

Significant lipid malabsorption (equivalent to 20 to 50 per cent of the dietary fat consumed) was demonstrated in a short-term study of obese subjects using neomycin (Faloon *et al.*, 1966). This compound produced steatorrhea by apparently antagonizing micelle formation in the intestinal lumen, due to interaction between the polybasic neomycin molecule and ionized fatty acids and bile acids in the lumen of the small intestine; pancreatic lipase was unaffected (Thompson *et al.*, 1971). The use of neomycin to produce fat loss in the chronic treatment of obesity is limited by the marked morphological alteration in the intestinal mucosa produced by this drug (Dobbins, Herrero & Mansbach, 1968). Cholestyramine, a non-absorbable anion exchange resin which binds intraluminal bile acids, thus preventing their availability for micellar solubilization has also been investigated. Although cholestyramine produced steatorrhea in man, the degree of fecal fat excretion was too small to produce a significant weight loss (Bray, 1976; Campbell, Jukl & Quaade, 1970). Other drugs inducing lipid malabsorption in man have been reviewed (Rahman & Cain, 1973). Fenfluramine inhibited the intestinal absorption of dietary triglycerides in rats (Bizzi, Veneroni & Garattini, 1973), but failed to alter fat excretion in man at the recommended therapeutic doses (Evans *et al.*, 1975).

An alternate approach to producing lipid malabsorption of digestible fats is the replacement of conventional dietary fats with a non-caloric, unabsorbable synthetic fat. An example of this is sucrose polyester (SPE), a preparation of sucrose with six, seven or eight of its hydroxyl groups esterified with long-chain fatty acids which possesses physical properties similar to dietary triglyceride. The negligible metabolism and absorption of SPE has been confirmed in rats (Mattson & Nolen, 1972; Mattson, Jandacek & Webb, 1976) and man (Fallat *et al.*, 1976). Since SPE is neither digested nor absorbed, there is the continued presence of an oil phase of SPE in the intestinal lumen. Exogenous and endogenous cholesterol will distribute into this oil phase and be excreted in the feces. The graded replacement of each 1 per cent dietary triglyceride with SPE resulted in a 1.2 per cent decrease in cholesterol absorption (Mattson *et al.*, 1976). In normal subjects, SPE (50 g/day for 10 days) induced a significant reduction in total plasma cholesterol and LDL cholesterol; no changes were observed in hypercholesterolemic subjects (Fallat *et al.*, 1976). The use of SPE as a weight controlling agent is suggested by the numerous varieties of food in which conventional fats could be theoretically replaced by SPE.

Recent studies suggest that the inhibition of carbohydrate digestion in the intestinal tract by inhibitors of pancreatic α-amylase may provide a possible approach to the treatment of obesity and diabetes mellitus. The rationale for this approach is as follows. Amylase plays a key role in carbohydrate digestion by hydrolyzing starch to maltose, which is further degraded to glucose. Since neither starch nor maltose can be absorbed by the intestinal mucosa, inhibition of amylase prevents the metabolic utilization of starch. Bay d 7791, an amylase inhibitor from wheat, consisting of thermostable proteins (Frerichs *et al.*, 1974) and Bay e 4609, an inhibitor from microorganisms comprised of complex oligosaccharides (Keup & Puls, 1975*a*) have been described. These inhibitors diminished the intestinal digestion of starch (Puls & Keup, 1973; Puls & Keup, 1975) and attenuated the hyperglycemic and serum insulin responses to starch ingestion in healthy volunteers and diabetic subjects (Frerichs *et al.*, 1974; Keup & Puls, 1975*a*). The reduced bioavailability of carbohydrate was further demonstrated by the depressed conversion of starch into lipids of adipose and aortic tissues in rats receiving Bay e 4609 orally (Keup & Puls, 1975*b*).

Other pharmacological approaches to a carbohydrate malabsorption are possible. Mazindol may interfere with intestinal glucose absorption since acute administration produced significant improvement in oral glucose tolerance and a concomitant reduction of insulin secretion, without an effect on intravenous glucose tolerance in human subjects (Harrison, 1975; Harrison, King-Roach & Sandy, 1975).

The non-selective prevention of food absorption from the gastrointestinal tract has been reported recently. Perfluoroctyl bromide (PFB), a chemically and biologically inert, non-absorbable, high molecular weight fluorocarbon used as a radiopaque contrast medium (Long & Liu, 1972; Clark, Becattini & Kaplan, 1972) was employed to coat the stomach and intestines of rats and thus reduce nutrient absorption (Hussain *et al.*, 1977). When administered prior to and during a 3-hr meal in rats, PFB prevented weight gain throughout the 13-day study.

The effects on energy balance of substituting non-absorbable carbohydrate or lipid for well absorbed nutrients in the diet stressed the importance of evaluating potential antiobesity agents or approaches in both lean and obese model systems. Lean and obese Zucker rats were fed diets in which either non-absorbed carbohydrate (fiber) was substituted for glucose, or poorly absorbed lipid (hydrogenated soybean oil) was substituted for

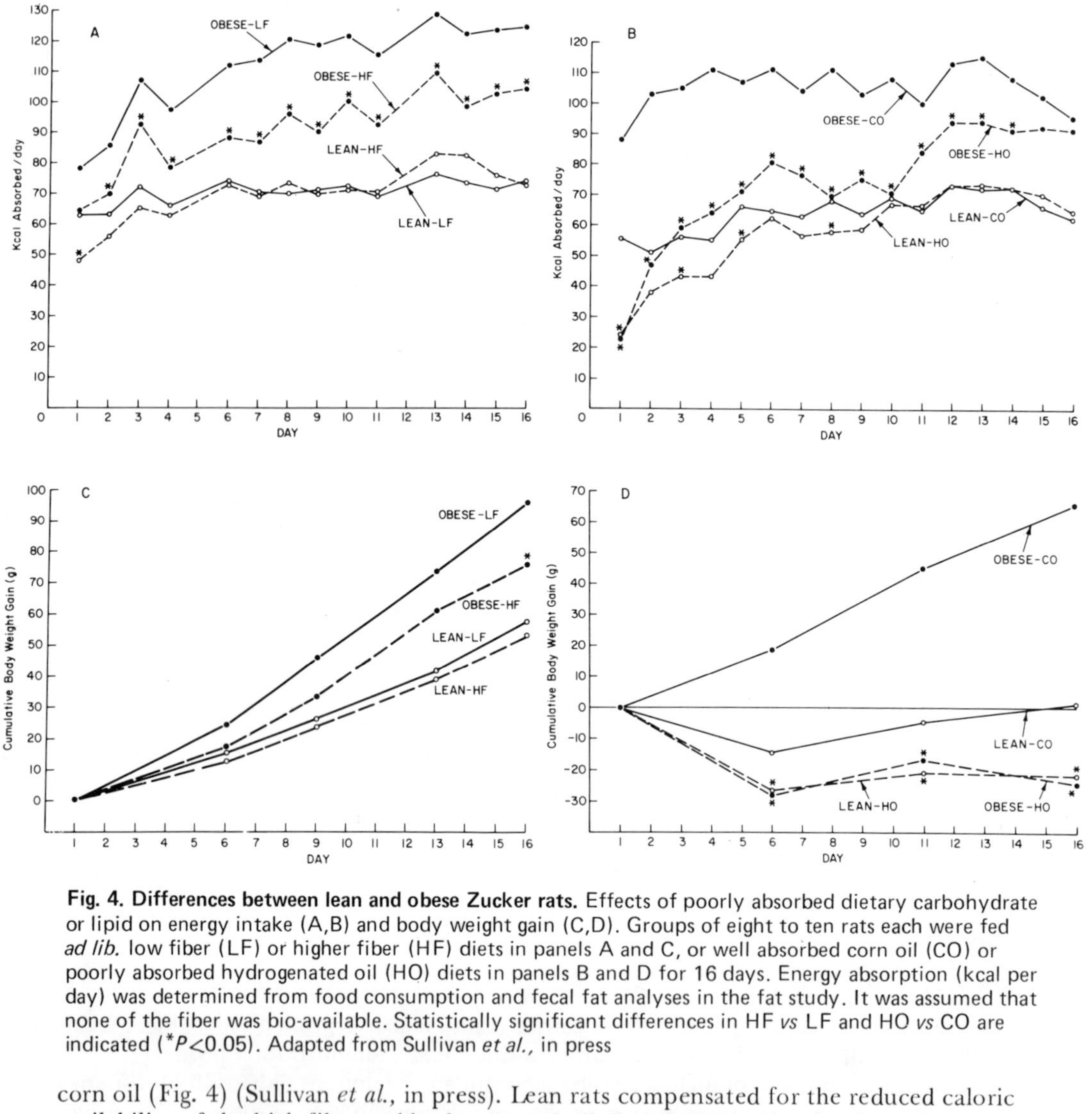

Fig. 4. Differences between lean and obese Zucker rats. Effects of poorly absorbed dietary carbohydrate or lipid on energy intake (A,B) and body weight gain (C,D). Groups of eight to ten rats each were fed *ad lib.* low fiber (LF) or higher fiber (HF) diets in panels A and C, or well absorbed corn oil (CO) or poorly absorbed hydrogenated oil (HO) diets in panels B and D for 16 days. Energy absorption (kcal per day) was determined from food consumption and fecal fat analyses in the fat study. It was assumed that none of the fiber was bio-available. Statistically significant differences in HF *vs* LF and HO *vs* CO are indicated (*$P<0.05$). Adapted from Sullivan *et al.,* in press

corn oil (Fig. 4) (Sullivan *et al.*, in press). Lean rats compensated for the reduced caloric availability of the high fiber and hydrogenated oil diets by increasing food consumption, so that equivalent kilocalories were absorbed per day (Fig. 4A,B). In contrast, obese rats did not respond to these dietary alterations by significant hyperphagia, and thus consistently absorbed fewer calories. There were no differences in the amount of weight gained by lean rats fed either the high or low fiber diets, due to compensatory hyperphagia in the high fiber group (Fig. 4C). Lean rats fed the hydrogenated oil diets gained less weight than corn oil fed controls, even in the presence of compensatory hyperphagia, due to the increased fecal elimination of water and lipid caused by the poorly absorbed fat diet (Fig 4D). Due to a delayed and incomplete response to reduced caloric availability, obese rats fed the high fiber and hydrogenated oil diets gained significantly less weight than obese rats fed low fiber and corn oil diets (Fig. 4C,D).

Modification of lipid metabolism

Agents which inhibit lipid biosynthesis or enhance lipid metabolism may prevent the development and/or maintenance of obesity. (-)-Hydroxycitrate, a natural product from the fruit rinds of the Indian plant *Garcinia cambogia,* is a potent competitive inhibitor of citrate cleavage enzyme, a key enzyme involved in the production of acetyl CoA for lipid biosynthesis (Watson, Fang & Lowenstein, 1969). As expected from this activity, studies in rats demonstrated that fatty acid and cholesterol synthesis in liver were inhibited significantly after the oral administration of (-)-hydroxycitrate (Lowenstein, 1971; Sullivan *et al.*, 1972; Sullivan *et al.,* 1974*a*; Sullivan, 1975). The utility of (-)-hydroxycitrate as a hypolipidemic agent was suggested by studies in which normal and hyperlipidemic rats given (-)-hydroxycitrate demonstrated significant reductions in the synthesis and circulating levels of triglycerides and cholesterol (Sullivan *et al.,* 1977*a,b*). A non-toxic dose of (-)-hydroxycitrate significantly reduced appetite and weight gain which was reflected in decreased levels of total body lipid in rats (Sullivan *et al.,* 1974*b*). The antiobesity activity of (-)-hydroxycitrate was discussed above under 'Suppression of food intake'.

Dehydroepiandrosterone (DHEA) is an inhibitor of mammalian glucose-6-phosphate dehydrogenase, one of the enzymes required for the generation of reducing equivalents for lipid biosynthesis. This compound prevented the development of obesity in $A^{vy}a$ mice, a strain characterized by a mature onset type of obesity (Yen *et al.,* 1977). Hepatic lipogenesis and body fat, but not food intake, were reduced significantly by DHEA administration. Fenfluramine reduced glyceride synthesis *in vitro* $K_i \sim 1$ mmol) in human adipose tissue (Ashwell, 1974) and rat liver, apparently by inhibiting phosphatidate phosphohydrolase (Brindley & Bowley, 1975). However, the dose required to produce these effects was approximately hundredfold greater than the serum concentrations of fenfluramine reported following therapeutic doses in man (Campbell, 1970).

The concept of developing agents to enhance lipid mobilization has not been pursued vigorously, but represents a useful area for future exploration. Prostaglandins may antagonize lipolysis (Gorman, Hamberg & Samuelsson, 1976) and several unpublished studies employing agents to modify this prostaglandin activity were cited (Curtis-Prior, 1975). Adipose tissue from obese Zucker rats which was 'insensitive' to the lipolytic action of norepinephrine and ACTH *in vitro* readily released glycerol in the presence of polyphloretin phosphate, a prostaglandin antagonist (unpublished). Indomethacin, a prostaglandin synthetase inhibitor, reduced the body weight of lean and obese Zucker rats (unpublished). An explanation of the paradoxical activities of prostaglandins on energy balance, ie anorexia (see Suppression of food intake) and inhibition of lipolysis awaits further study.

Alternation in the efficiency of lipid and/or carbohydrate oxidation

Compounds which either enhance oxygen consumption with a concomitant increase in the ratio of heat to energy production or increase futile cycles have potential value in antiobesity therapy. Thyroid hormones potentiate weight loss in obese subjects by increasing the basal metabolic rate (oxygen consumption). Dinitrophenol, an uncoupler of oxidative phosphorylation, markedly reduced body weight when administered to obese subjects (Tainter, Stockton & Cutting, 1935). Increased metabolic rate and heat production characterized by sweating, flushed skin and warmth were experienced by all subjects. However, this compound's toxicity precludes its use as an antiobesity agent (Simons, 1953).

Salicylate uncouples oxygen utilization from the production of adenosine triphosphate resulting in increased oxygen consumption, depletion of liver glycogen, and increased production of heat (for review see Smith & Dawkins, 1971). Oxygen uptake was increased at a dose of aspirin which also produced tinnitus in obese and lean subjects (Bray, 1976). However, the multiple actions of this drug (Collier, 1969) limit its use in the treatment of obesity.

Normalization of hormone levels

Obesity is characterized by several endocrine abnormalities. The most prominent is hyperinsulinemia, which is manifested by enhanced pancreatic insulin secretion, elevated plasma insulin levels and increased peripheral insulin resistance. Inhibition of insulin release may constitute a potential treatment of obesity (Sullivan *et al.*, 1976). Somatostatin suppresses the secretion of various pituitary, pancreatic and gastrointestinal hormones (Vale, Rivier & Brown, 1977). A somatostatin analog which selectively inhibits insulin secretion, but produces no effect on glucagon or growth hormone, could prove useful as an antiobesity agent. Several somatostatin analogs have been prepared which appear to possess this type of selectivity in animals (Brown, Vale & Rivier, 1977; Efendic, Luft & Sievertsson, 1975). In man, both the linear (reduced) and cyclic (oxidized) form of somatostatin appeared to be more potent in suppressing insulin release as compared to glucagon release, with no discernible change in growth hormone levels (Leblanc & Yen, 1975). Weight loss in rats treated for 2 weeks with a protamine-zinc preparation of cyclic somatostatin was reported recently (Micossi *et al.*, 1976).

Growth hormone levels and secretory responsiveness are reduced in obese subjects. The evaluation of L-Dopa as an antiobesity agent seems reasonable, since it is known to stimulate growth hormone release in normal subjects, and Parkinsonian patients demonstrated weight loss when treated with this drug (Vardi *et al.*, 1976). L-Dopa was ineffective in eliciting growth hormone release in obese patients; lean subjects showed a marked increase in growth hormone (Pinter, Tolis & Friesen, 1975). The administration of L-Dopa to obese patients in a double blind study up to a maximum dose of 4.8 g/day for 6 months failed to alter body weight compared to placebo (Quaade, Pakkenberg & Juhl, 1974).

Summary

The critical need for more effective pharmacological agents for the treatment of obesity is obvious. Multiple pharmacological approaches to the problem of energy balance in obesity need to be assessed. With the increasing evidence that human obesity rather than being a single disease is a heterogenous group of disorders, selective pharmacological treatments for these specific types of obesities may be useful. The preclinical evaluation of novel antiobesity agents should include: (1) analysis in both lean and obese model systems as differential responses such as those demonstrated in our non-absorbable carbohydrate and lipid study may be expressed, and (2) investigations into the possible compensatory responses to such agents, which may become evident with chronic administration or after cessation of treatment. The development and evaluation of novel antiobesity agents in these ways could at the minimum assist us in defining the hierarchy of importance of the metabolic aberrations in obesity and identifying redundancies in the systems involved in the regulation of energy balance and perhaps could at a maximum constitute useful and effective treatments.

Acknowledgement – The authors wish to thank Ms Sandra Zvolensky for her excellent assistance in the preparation of this manuscript.

References

Abdallah, A.H. (1973): *Toxicol. Appl. Pharmacol.* 25, 344.

Abdallah, A.H. & White, H.D. (1976): *Fed. Proc.* 33, 564.

Antin, J., Gibbs, J., Holt, J., Young, R.C. & Smith, G.P. (1975): *J. Comp. Physiol. Psychol.* 89, 784.

Ashwell, M. (1974): *Brit. J. Clin. Pharmacol.* 1, 413.

Baile, C.A., Simpson, C.W., Bean, S.M., McLaughlin, C.L. & Jacobs, H.L. (1973): *Physiol. Behav.* 10, 1077.

Bizzi, A., Veneroni, E. & Garattini, S. (1973): *Eur. J. Pharmacol.* 23, 131.

Bourillet, F. & Buzas, A. (1975): Abstracts of the Intl. Congress of Pharmacol., 6th Helsinki, p. 357.

Bray, G.A. (1976): Drug therapy for the obese patient In *The Obese patient*, p. 353. Philadelphia: W.B. Saunders.

Brindley, D.N. & Bowley, M. (1975): The effects of fenfluramine and related compounds on the synthesis of phospholipids and glycerides by rat liver. In *Recent advances in obesity research:* I, ed A. Howard. p. 374. London: Newman.

Brown, M., Vale, W. & Rivier, J. (1977): *Diabetes* 26, (Suppl. 1), 360.

Campbell, D.B. (1970): *Chromatogr.* 49, 442.
Campbell, V.D., Julk, E. & Quaade, F. (1970): *Nord. Med.* **84**, 1628.
Clark, L.C. Jr., Becattini, F. & Kaplan, S. (1972): *Triangle* **11**, 115.
Collier, H.O.J. (1969): *Adv. Pharmacol. Chem. Ther.* 7, 333.
Craddock, D. (1976): *Drugs* **11**, 378.
Curtis-Prior, P.B. (1975): *Lancet* **1**, 897.
Dobbins, W.O., Herrero, B.A. & Mansbach, C.M. (1968): *Am. J. Med. Sci.* **255**, 63.
Doggett, N.S. & Jawaharal, K. (1977*a*): *Br. J. Pharmac.* **60**, 409.
Doggett, N.S. & Jawaharal, K. (1977*b*): *Br. J. Pharmac.* **60**, 417.
Dorf, G., Louis, A. & Benedetti, M.S. (1975): Clinical and pharmacokinetic studies of a new anorectic drug. In *Recent advances in obesity research:* I, ed A. Howard, p. 404. London: Newman.
Duhault, J., Beregi, L., Boulanger, M. & Hugon, P. (1975): New glycinates with high anorectic activity. In *Recent advances in obesity research:* I, ed A. Howard. p. 409. London: Newman.
Dumeur, G., Hui, B., Lwoff, J.M., Mouries, M.A. & Tremblay, D. (1976): *Br. J. Pharmacol.* **58**, 437P.
Efendic, S., Luft, R. & Sievertsson, H. (1975): *FEBS Letters* **58**, 302.
Evans, E., Miller, D.S., Samuel, P.D. & Burland, W.L. (1975): *Postgrad. Med. J.* **51**, (Suppl. 1), 115.
Fallat, R.W., Glueck, C.J., Lutmer, R. & Mattson, F.H. (1976): *Am. J. Clin. Nutr.* **29**, 1204.
Faloon, W.W., Paes, I.C., Woolfolk, D., Nankin, H., Wallace, K. & Haro, E.N. (1966): *Ann. N.Y. Acad. Sci.* **132**, 879.
Frerichs, F., Daweke, H., Gries, F. Gruneklee, D., Hessing, J., Janke, K., Keup, U., Miss, Otto, H., Puls, W., Schmidt, D. & Zumfelde, C. (1974): *Diabetologia* **9**, 68.
Garattini, S., Bizzi, A., de Gaztano, G., Jori, A. & Samanin, R. (1975): Recent advances in the pharmacology of anorectic agents. In *Recent advances in obesity research:* I ed. A. Howard, p. 345, London: Newman.
Garattini, S. & Samanin, R. (1976): Anorectic drugs and brain neurotransmitters. In *Appetite and food intake,* Dahlem Konferenzen, ed T. Silverstone, p. 83. Berlin: Abakon.
Gibbs, J., Falasco, J.P. & McHugh, P.R. (1976): *Am. J. Physiol.* **230**, 15.
Giudicelli, J.F., Richer, C. & Berdeaux, A. (1976): *Br. J. Clin. Pharmac.* **3**, 113.
Goetz, H. & Sturdevant, R. (1975): *Clin. Res.* **23**, 98A.
Gorman, R.R., Hamberg, M. & Samuelsson, B. (1976): *Adv. Prostaglandin Thromboxane Res.* **1**, 325.
Harrison, L.C. (1975): Effect of mazindol on carbohydrate-lipid metabolism *in vivo* and *in vitro*, In *Recent advances in obesity research:* I, ed A. Howard, p. 401. London: Newman.
Harrison, L.C., King-Roach, A.P. & Sandy, K.C. (1975): *Metabolism* **24**, 1353.
Hoebel, B.G. (1977): Pharmacologic control of feeding. In *Ann. Rev. Pharmacol. Toxicol. 1977,* p. 605. New York: Annual Reviews Inc.
Hussain, M., Niazi, S., Arambulo, A. & Long, D.M. (1977): *J. Pharm. Sci.* **66**, 907.
Keup, U. & Puls, W. (1975*a*): *Archs Pharmacol.* **287**, (Suppl.), R85.
Keup, U. & Puls, W. (1975*b*): Influence of an amylase inhibitor, Bay e 4609, on the conversion of orally applicated starch into total lipids of rat adipose tissue. In *Recent advances in obesity research:* I, ed A. Howard, p. 412. London: Newman.
Leblanc, H. & Yen, S.S.C. (1975): *J. Clin. Endoc. Metab.* **40**, 906.
Long, D.M. & Liu, M.S. (1972): *Radiology* **105**, 323.
Lowenstein, J.M. (1971): *J. Biol. Chem.* **246**, 629.
Mattson, F.H. & Nolen, G.A. (1972): *J. Nutr.* **102**, 1171.
Mattson, F.H., Jandacek, R.J. & Webb, M.R. (1976): *J. Nutr.* **106**, 747.
Micossi, P., Dunbar, J.C., Pontiroli, A.E., Baker, B.A., Lengel, F., Walsh, M.F. & Foa, P.P. (1976): *Diabetologia* **12**, 410.
Miller, D.S., Evans, E., Samuel, P. & Burland, W.L. (1975): *Postgrad. Med. J.* **51**, 117.
Oliver, J.T. (1974): *Archs Int. Pharmacodyn. Ther.* **211**, 253.
Panksepp, J., Pollack, A., Meeker, R.B. & Sullivan, A.C. (1977): *Pharmacol. Biochem. Behav.* **6**, 683.
Pinter, E.J., Tolis, G, & Friesen, H.G. (1975): *Int. J. Clin. Pharmacol. Biopharm.* **12**, 277.
Puls, W. & Keup, U. (1973): *Diabetologia* **9**, 97.
Puls, W. & Keup, U. (1975): Metabolic studies with an amylase inhibitor in acute starch loading tests in rats and men and its influence on the amylase content of the pancreas. In *Recent advances in obesity research:* I, ed A. Howard, p. 391, London: Newman.
Quaade, F., Pakkenberg, H. & Juhl, E. (1974): *Acta Med. Scand.* **195**, 129.
Rahman, F. & Cain, G.D. (1973): *Southern Med. J.* **66**, 724.
Russek, M. & Stevenson, J.A.F. (1972): *Physiol. Behav.* **8**, 245.
Samanin, R., Bendotti, C., Miranda, F. & Garattini, S. (1977): *J. Pharm. Pharmacol.* **29**, 53.
Scaramuzzi, O.E., Baile, C.A. & Mayer, J. (1971): *Experientia* **27**, 256.
Schulman, J.L., Carleton, J.L., Whitney, G. & Whitehorn, J.C. (1957): *J. Appl. Physiol.* **11**, 419.
Silverstone, T. (1975): Anorectic drugs. In *Obesity: its pathogenesis and management,* ed T. Silverstone, p. 193. Massachusetts: Publishing Sciences Group, Inc.

Simons, E.W. (1953): *Biol. Rev.* 28, 453.
Smith, G.P. & Gibbs, J. (1976): Cholecystokinin and satiety: Theoretic and therapeutic implications. In *Hunger: basic mechanisms and clinical implications,* ed D. Novin, W. Wyrwicka & G.A. Bray, p. 349. New York: Raven Press.
Smith, M.J.H. & Dawkins, P.D. (1971): *J. Pharm. Pharmacol.* 23, 729.
Stunkard, A.J., Van Itallie, T.B. & Reis, B.B. (1955): *Proc. Soc. Exp. Biol. Med.* 89, 258.
Sullivan, A.C., Hamilton, J.G., Miller, O.N. & Wheatley, V.R. (1972): *Archs Biochem. Biophys.* 150, 183.
Sullivan, A.C., Triscari, J., Hamilton, J.G. & Miller, O.N. (1973): *Fed. Proc.* 32, 887.
Sullivan A.C., Triscari, J., Hamilton, J.G., Miller, O.N. & Wheatley, V.R. (1974*a*): *Lipids* 9, 121.
Sullivan, A.C., Triscari, J., Hamilton, J.G. & Miller, O.N. (1974*b*): *Lipids* 9, 129.
Sullivan, A.C. (1975): Effect of (-)-hydroxycitrate on lipid metabolism. In *Modification of lipid metabolism,* ed E.G. Perkins & L.A. Witting, p. 143. New York: Academic Press.
Sullivan, A.C. & Triscari, J. (1976): Possible interrelationship between metabolite flux and appetite. In *Hunger: basic mechanisms and clinical implications,* ed D. Novin, W. Wyrwicka & G. Bray, p. 115. New York: Raven Press.
Sullivan, A.C., Cheng, L.C. & Hamilton, J.G. (1976): Agents for the treatment of obesity. In *Annual reports in medicinal chemistry, Vol. 11,* p. 200. New York: Academic Press.
Sullivan, A.C. & Triscari, J. (1977): *Am. J. Clin. Nutr.* 30, 767.
Sullivan, A.C., Triscari, J. & Spiegel, H.E. (1977*a*) *Am. J. Clin. Nutr.* 30, 777.
Sullivan, A.C., Triscari, J., Hamilton, J.G. & Ontko, J.A. (1977*b*): *Lipids* 12, 1.
Sullivan, A.C. & Cheng, L.: Appetite regulation and its modulation by drugs. In *Nutrition and drug interrelations,* ed J. Hathcock & W. Coons. New York: Academic Press (in press).
Sullivan, A.C., Triscari, Joseph, & Comai, Karen: *Am. J. Clin. Nutr.* (in press).
Sullivan, A.C. & Comai, K. (in press): *Int. J. Obesity* 2, 167.
Tainter, M.L.; Stockton, A.B. & Cutting, W. (1935): *J. Am. Med. Ass.* 105, 332.
Thompson, G.R., Barrowman, J., Gutierrez, L. & Dowling, R.H. (1971): *J. Clin. Invest.* 50, 319.
Vale, W., Rivier, C. & Brown, M. (1977): *Ann. Rev. Physiol.* 39, 473.
Vardi, J., Oberman, Z., Rabey, I., Streifler, M., Ayalon, D. & Herzberg, M. (1976): *J. Neurol. Sci.* 30, 33.
Watson, J.A., Fang, M. & Lowenstein, J.M. (1969): *Archs Biochem. Biophys.* 135, 209.
Wirtshafter, D. & Davis, J.D. (in press): Body weight *Science.*
Wolff, F.W. *et al.* (committee report) (1976): Peripheral and hormonal mechanisms, Group Report. In *Appetite and food intake,* Dahlem Konferenzen, ed T. Silverstone, p. 219. Berlin: Abakon.
Yen, T.T., Allan, J.A., Pearson, D.V., Acton, J.M. & Greenberg, M.M. (1977): *Lipids* 12, 409.

47
Cholecystokinin and satiety

G.P. SMITH
Department of Psychiatry, Cornell University Medical College and Edward Bourne Behavioral Research Laboratory, The New York Hospital-Cornell Medical Center, Westchester Division, 21 Bloomingdale Road, White Plains, New York 10605, USA.

Duodenal infusions of food inhibit food intake. This could occur when food stimulates the numerous mucosal receptors that activate the neural and endocrine mechanisms of the gut. For the past 5 years, our laboratory has investigated the possibility that such stimuli inhibit food intake by releasing one or more gut hormones. To test this hypothesis we studied the effects of gut hormones on sham feeding in rats with chronic gastric fistulas.

After an overnight food deprivation, rats with chronic gastric cannulas will sham feed a liquid food continuously for several hours (Young *et al.*, 1974). They do not display the fixed behavioral sequence of satiety, ending in rest and apparent sleep, which characterizes satiety in the rat (Antin *et al.*, 1975).

As the sham-feeding rat with a gastric fistula does not satiate spontaneously under these conditions, this preparation provides a reliable bioassay system for testing the effectiveness of gut hormones to produce satiety.

Method

Adult male rats were implanted with stainless steel gastric cannulas located in the rumen of the stomach. After recovery from surgery, they were adapted to a 17-hour schedule of overnight food deprivation. Gastric cannulas were opened and cleared 15 minutes before presentation of a diluted, balanced liquid diet. Sham feeding was immediate and vigorous. Each rat received a 1 ml intraperitoneal injection of one or more gut hormones, or 0.15 mmol/l sodium chloride as a control, 17 minutes after sham feeding began. Sham intake was measured and behaviors of individual animals were recorded during the succeeding 1-hour period.

Hormones and sources were as follows: 20 per cent pure cholecystokinin and pure natural secretin, purchased from GIH Research Unit, Karolinska Institutet; synthetic C-terminal octapeptide of cholecystokinin, the gift of Dr Miguel Ondetti, Squibb Institute for Medical Research; gastrin I and II, purchased from Sigma; pure gastrin II, the gift of Dr M.I. Grossman; gastric inhibitory polypeptide, purchased from Dr J.C. Brown.

Results

Of the six preparations of gut hormones tested, only cholecystokinin (CCK) and the synthetic C-terminal octapeptide of CCK (OCT) produced significant inhibition of sham feeding and elicited the behavioral sequence characteristic of satiety (Table 1). Gastrin, secretin and gastric inhibitory polypeptide (GIP) not only had no effect when given alone, they also failed to increase or decrease the satiety effect of OCT significantly when given in combination with the OCT (Lorenz, Gibbs & Smith, in press).

The satiety effect of CCK and OCT is also dose-related in intact rats and monkeys (Smith & Gibbs, 1976). The effect is specific for food: CCK has no effect on water intake

Table 1. Effects of gut hormones on sham feeding. All hormones were injected intraperitioneally in a minimum of six rats 17 minutes after sham feeding began

Hormone	Dose	Effect on sham feeding
Cholecystokinin (20 per cent pure)	5-160 Ivy dog units/kg	inhibition
Octapeptide of CCK	20-640 Ivy dog units/kg	inhibition
Gastrin II	0.1-100 μg/kg	none
Gastrin I and II	100-1000 μg/kg	none
Secretin	0.1-100 clinical units/kg	none
Gastric Inhibitory Polypeptide	0.1-100 μg/kg	none

in rats. The effect does not appear to be due to sickness. Rats begin to eat eagerly after CCK; they just stop eating sooner.

Although we have not been able to demonstrate a significant interaction between other gut hormones and CCK, we have recently observed a potent interaction between the food contingent stimuli of sham feeding and the satiating potency of CCK.

By varying the relation between the time of adminstration of CCK (40 u/kg, i.p.) and the time of the beginning of sham feeding Antin, Gibbs & Smith (in press) observed profound differences in the satiating potency of CCK (Table 2). Note the trivial effect of CCK administered 12 minutes before sham feeding began (-12) compared to the large inhibition produced by CCK administered 12 minutes after sham feeding began (+12). Furthermore, the inhibition produced by CCK administered 12 minutes after sham feeding began was significantly larger than the inhibition produced by CCK administered 6 minutes after sham feeding began. These results demonstrate that the inhibitory effect on sham feeding observed after administration of CCK is the result of a synergistic interaction between the food contingent stimuli of sham feeding and CCK.

Table 2. Sham feeding by 11 rats after injections with CCK (40 u/kg) or saline which preceded, coincided with, or followed presentation of liquid food at time 0)

Time of injection min	Intake after 0.15 mmol/l NaCl injection (ml, $\bar{x} \pm$ s.e.m.)	Intake after CCK injection 40 u/kg (ml, $\bar{x} \pm$ s.e.m.)	Mean per cent suppression
−12	56 ± 3	50 ± 3 ^{a,d}	11
− 6	55 ± 3	35 ± 7 ^{a,c,d}	36
0	52 ± 2	24 ± 5 ^{b,c,d}	54
+ 6	50 ± 3	24 ± 7 ^{b,c,d}	52
+12	47 ± 3	11 ± 4 ^{b,c}	77

1. Sham intakes were measured during the 30 min interval that began 12 min after an injection of saline or CCK. This delay permitted comparison of sham intake during the same interval relative to the time of an injection. It was the minimal delay allowed by the temporal constraint of the −12 min injection.
2. Suppression is defined as a sham intake during any 6 min interval after CCK below the range of sham intakes in any 6 min interval for the same rat after saline on an adjacent day.
3. Statistical differences from saline control: $^{a}P<0.05$, $^{b}P<0.0005$, matched pairs *t*-test, one-tailed.
4. Statistical differences from −12 CCK injection: $^{c}P<0.025$, matched pairs *t*-test, one-tailed.
5. Statistical differences from +12 CCK injection: $^{d}P<0.05$, matched pairs *t*-test, one-tailed.
6. The results after injections of CCK at −6, 0, +6 min are not statistically different in any category.
7. Intakes after saline injections were not different (1 way ANOVA, $F(4, 50) = 1.39$).

Discussion

We did these experiments to test the idea that the release of gut hormones mediates the satiety effect of food in the intestine (intestinal satiety). A comparison of the effects of duodenal infusions of liquid diet and intraperitoneal injections of CCK (40 u/kg) shows that: (1) both inhibit sham feeding in a dose-related manner (2) both elicit the behavioral sequence of satiety, and (3) both have a synergistic interaction with the pregastric stimuli of sham feeding. The striking similarity of the effect is consistent with the hypothesis that CCK mediates intestinal satiety, but similar effects do not prove much about mechanism. Crucial evidence for the hypothesis will come from an experiment in which the inhibitory effect of a duodenal infusion into a *denervated* small intestine can be abolished by the selective block of CCK release or by specific antagonism of its effect at the receptor site(s) for satiety. Such an experiment has not yet been reported. At the current time it cannot be attempted because neither a selective blocker of CCK release nor a specific antagonist is available and the receptor site(s) for its effect on satiety is not known.

It remains to be seen if CCK or OCT will be useful in the treatment of obesity. In normal weight volunteers Sturdevant & Goetz (1976) reported a small, significant inhibition of food intake after an intravenous injection of CCK and a slight increase of food intake during a slow, intravenous infusion of CCK. A therapeutic trial in obese patients has not yet been reported. The consistent and clear results in rats and rhesus monkeys suggests that a trial is worth doing. Such a trial should be designed to take advantage of the synergistic interaction of pregastric food stimuli and CCK.

Acknowledgement – Supported by N.I.H. research grants (AM 17240, MH 70874) and a Career Development Award (MH 00149).

References

Antin, J., Gibbs, J., Holt, J., Young, R.C. & Smith, G.P. (1975): *J. Comp. Physiol. Psychol.* 89, 784.
Antin, J., Gibbs, J. & Smith, G.P. (in press): *Physiol. Behav.*
Lorenz, D., Gibbs, J. & Smith, G.P. (in press): *Proc. Int. Congr. Gastroint. Endocrinol.*
Smith, G.P. & Gibbs, J. (1976): Cholecystokinin and satiety: theoretic and therapeutic implications. In *Hunger: basic mechanisms and clinical implications,* ed D. Novin, W. Wyrwicka & G. Bray, p. 349. New York: Raven Press.
Sturdevant, R.A. & Goetz, H. (1976): *Nature* 261, 713.
Young, R.C., Gibbs, J., Antin, J., Holt, J. & Smith, G.P. (1974): *J. Comp. Physiol. Psychol.* 87, 795.

48
Clinical use of anorectic drugs and other pharmacologic agents in treating obesity

P.J. COLLIPP
Nassau County Medical Center, East Meadow, New York 11554, USA.

With respect to medications, we stand in the treatment of obesity where we stood in the treatment of pneumonia before penicillin was discovered. The significance of obesity as a health problem affecting 10 to 20 per cent of the population of western civilization is virtually unquestioned. Increased risk for atherosclerosis, hypertension, coronary artery disease, breast, bowel and uterine (Alcantara & Speckmann, 1976) cancer, debilitating bone and joint disease, as well as psychological and social pathology have been documented. If ever there was a health problem in need of an effective remedy it is obesity. Tanner has reported that the skin fold thickness norms for children in the British Isles have increased approximately one standard deviation in the last 25 years (Tanner & Whitehouse, 1975).

Impediments to developing an effective therapy have included a lack of agreement regarding the seriousness of the problem among health professionals, significant constraints imposed on the pharmaceutical industry in the development of new medications, and a cultural and at times social public impression that 'all this attention we are paying to obesity is the cause of psychological problems of the obese'. In effect, the attitude is that until a better remedy comes along, we would do better to forget about the problem and stop making obese people feel bad. There have also been those who have emphasized the documented lack of physical activity among the obese, or the improper eating habits, or the behavioral and cultural aspects, and thereby indirectly discouraged others working on metabolic or pharmacologic therapy. None of the available non-pharmacologic methods has a success rate of greater than 40 to 50 per cent, and we do need a good drug therapy for obesity.

Obesity is inherited as a polygenic characteristic, and this suggests that multiple metabolic and enzymatic steps are involved and potentially modifiable with suitable medications. Other polygenic characteristics include height and intelligence. Some short children are treated successfully with human growth hormone, others with thyroid or anabolic steroid hormones, and some with vitamin D or better diets, and some with a better emotional environment at home. Some potentially retarded children are treated with specific diets, some with vitamins, and others with anticonvulsants or thyroid hormone.

As we become more sophisticated and more successful in the pharmacologic treatment of obesity we can imagine two general areas of attack on the problem; first in prevention, and second, in treatment of the established process. The currently available agents are discussed next.

Anorectic drugs

Amphetamines

The available amphetamine drugs are listed in Table 1. They include dextroamphetamine, benzphetamine, amphetamine, and methamphetamine. These medications have a high potential for abuse, and tolerance, drug dependence, and severe social disability have occurred. Abrupt cessation after prolonged high doses results in extreme fatigue and depression. They should not be taken during pregnancy, and have no role in the treatment of childhood obesity.

Adult patients who are refractory to alternative therapy and are entering upon a comprehensive weight control program receive some benefit during the first 4 to 12 weeks, and then the medication should be discontinued.

They are contraindicated in patients with advanced arteriosclerosis, symptomatic cardiovascular disease, moderate to severe hypertension, hyperthyroidism, glaucoma and known hypersensitivity to sympathomimetic amines.

Table 1. Pharmaceutical preparations containing amphetamines

Drug	Company	Usual daily adult dose
Benzedrine	Smith Kline & French	15-30 mg
Biphetamine	Pennwalt	7.5-20 mg
Delcobese	Delco	5-30 mg
Desoxyn	Abbott	5-15 mg
Dexamyl	Smith Kline & French	10-15 mg
Dexedrine	Smith Kline & French	10-30 mg
Didrex	Upjohn	25-150 mg
Eskatrol	Smith Kline & French	15 mg
Fetamin	Mission	10-20 mg
Obetrol	Obetrol	5-30 mg
Obotan	Mallinckrodt	15-30 mg

Non-amphetamines

Table 2 lists the available non-amphetamine anorexics. Phentermine, chlorphentermine and clortermine are sympathomimetic amines pharmacologically similar to the amphetamines. There is less information regarding the problems of drug dependence, tolerance, and withdrawal symptoms, but they are recommended only as short-term (4 to 12 weeks) adjuncts in a comprehensive weight control program. Phenylpropanolamine (Hoebel, 1975), phendimetrazine and diethylpropion are also sympathomimetic amines with similar properties which are recommended only as short-term adjuncts to a comprehensive weight control program.

Table 2. Appetite suppressing drugs other than amphetamines

Drug	Generic name	Company	Usual daily adult dose
Adipex-P	phentermine	Lemmon	15-30 mg
Anorexin	phenylpropanolamine plus caffeine & vitamins	SDA	25 mg
Bacarate	phendimetrazine	Tutag	70-105 mg
Bontril PDM	phendimetrazine	Carnrick	70-105 mg
Fastin	phentermine	Beecham	30 mg
Ionamin	phentermine	Pennwalt	15-30 mg
Melfiat	phendimetrazine	Reid-Provident	70-105 mg
ObeNil	phendimetrazine	TheraMedic	70-105 mg
Plegine	phendimetrazine	Ayerst	70-105 mg
Pondimin	fenfluramine	Robins	60-120 mg
Preludin	phenmetrazine	Boehringer Ingelheim	50-75 mg
Pre-Sate	chlorphentermine	Warner Chilcott	65 mg
Sanorex	mazindol	Sandoz	2-3 mg
Statobex	phendimetrazine	Lemmon	50-210 mg
Tenuate	diethylpropion	Merrell National	75 mg
Tepanil	diethylpropion	Riker	75 mg
Trimtabs	phendimetrazine	Mayrand	70-105 mg
Voranil	clortermine	USV	50 mg

Fenfluramine is a sympathomimetic amine pharmacologically different from the amphetamines. It produces sedation more often than stimulation at therapeutic dosages, and did not produce dependence in animals. While drug abuse has been reported with it in patients, the potential for abuse seems less than with the other amphetamine-like drugs. The most common side effects (2 to 10 per cent of patients) have been drowsiness, diarrhea and dry mouth. It is recommended in doses of 20 to 30 mg three times daily, and unlike the other amphetamine-like drugs the possibility of successful long-term usefulness in treating obese patients exists. Fenfluramine should not be used during pregnancy or given to children. It is contraindicated in patients with glaucoma, patients hypersensitive to it, and should not be given within 14 days following administration of monamine oxidase inhibitors since hypertensive crises may develop. It has recently been found useful in children with congenital total lipodystrophy, a rare condition associated with diminished subcutaneous fat (Seip, Trygsted & Oseid, 1977).

Mazindol is an imidazoisoindole anorectic agent chemically unrelated to amphetamines. It produces some amphetamine-like actions including CNS stimulation. It does not cause brain norepinephrine depletion in animals, as is seen with amphetamines. It is recommended in doses of 1 to 3 mg daily and can be given as a single daily dose. The possibility that it may have long-term usefulness in the treatment of obesity still exists. It is contraindicated in glaucoma, hypersensitivity to it, manic-depressive and agitated states, and within 14 days following administration of monamine oxidase inhibitors. It should not be given during pregnancy or to growing children. We have recently documented a reduction of growth rate in children receiving mazindol and have successfully used it to treat excessively tall stature in several girls (Collipp *et al.*, 1977).

The explanation for the value of amphetamines and the non-amphetamine anorexics in promoting weight loss in obese patients may not rest entirely on their anorexic properties. Fenfluramine and mazindol (Harrison & King-Roach, 1975) have both been reported to reduce intestinal glucose absorption recently. Other mechanisms have not been ruled out.

In summary, the available anorexic medications are generally useful only as a short-term adjunct to a comprehensive program. They should be limited to those patients who are refractory to the comprehensive program without a medication, and should deliberately be discontinued after the short-term use because of their potential for abuse. Two possible exceptions to this general recommendation are fenfluramine and mazindol, whose abuse potential seem to be reduced significantly, and whose role in long-term management of obesity remains to be determined.

Gastrointestinal antacids and bulk-fillers

Gastric acidity, a feeling of emptiness, and the physical act of putting things in the mouth and swallowing, contribute to the human hunger and satiety mechanisms. The use of these products permits the patient to ingest something that is 'filling' several times each day without significant calories. Patients use water and low-calorie soda in the same way. They are generally given 15 to 30 minutes before meals (Jordan, 1974). If they were more appealing to the palate, and more varied in form ar.   sistency, they would be more useful. At present they are not very helpful in a weight control program and have not been documented to be of long-term benefit. Prolonged excessive ingestion of antacids can result in potassium depletion.

Hormones

Thyroid hormone has no role in the treatment of obesity. It is indicated in patients who are thyroxine-deficient as indicated by low serum levels of T_3, and T_4 and elevated TSH. Most hypothyroid patients are not significantly obese. Patients with above average serum PBI do not lose weight better than those with below average PBI (Collipp, Schmierer & Greensher, 1971). Thyroxine dosages which will cause weight loss are associated with unacceptable side effects.

Growth hormone is, among other things, lipolytic and during the first 6 months of its administration to hypopituitary children there is a loss of subcutaneous fat and an increase in lean body mass (Collipp *et al.*, 1973). This effect levels off at a normal subcutaneous fat mass. Acromegalic patients with markedly increased growth hormones are rarely obese. Administration of growth hormone for treatment of obesity is likely to be associated with an acceptable incidence of side effects (similar to acromegaly), even if large quantities were available.

Chorionic gonadotropin has been used occasionally for the treatment of obesity and has been shown recently to be no better than placebo (Shetty & Kalkhoff, 1977).

Nicotine

Cessation of cigarette smoking is often associated with a gain in weight. The explanation for the effect is uncertain and probably not simple. The psychological advantage of putting something in the mouth which contains no calories, and of relieving anxiety with an alternative activity to consuming food, as well as the anorexic and lipolytic effects of nicotine are all plausible explanations for the effect of smoking on body weight. The potential harmful effects on health known to be associated with smoking cigarettes make this an unacceptable remedy at present.

Caffeine

Caffeine is ingested by many in our population. The principal sources are coffee and tea. Its depressant effect on appetite is recognized, and restaurants as well as custom dictate that it is served at the end of a meal. It is a CNS stimulant tending to increase physical activity, and it is an inhibitor of the phosphodiesterase that catalyzes the destruction of cyclic AMP. This probably accounts for its lipolytic effects. One of the available anorexic medications contains caffeine (Table 2). Due to its strong effect on CNS stimulation it is limited in usefulness for obesity, but can be employed in a supportive role in weight loss programs.

Other CNS medications

L-Dopa has been used primarily as a treatment for patients with Parkinson's disease, and is known as a test for hypopituitarism because of its ability to acutely stimulate growth hormone production following oral administration. Toxic symptoms and side effects include weight loss and nausea, and it has been proposed as a treatment for obesity but in one study was ineffective (Quaade, 1974).

Phenytoin was proposed as a treatment for 'compulsive eaters' who are obese, but has not been found helpful (Greenway, Dahms & Bray, 1977).

Medications causing intestinal malabsorption

Cholestyramine binds bile acids and thereby reduces lipid absorption as well as reducing serum cholesterol. It has not been found helpful in obesity so far, although additional studies using it as part of a long-term program may be worthwhile. It also reduces absorption of fat soluble vitamins and, therefore, patients receiving it need supplements of vitamins A, D, and K.

Hypothetical medications

The medication we need for obesity must be tasty, inexpensive, long-acting, safe, attractive and potent. To the extent that the available medications fit this description they are effective, but patient compliance with long-term pharmacologic therapy is a problem the available medications have not faced.

The relative lack of success of the available medications in dealing with the problem of obesity leads me to speculate a little further. One of the problems faced by obese patients is that they have slightly elevated insulin levels in their serum, which stimulates fat synthesis. Somatostatin is a new peptide which suppresses serum insulin levels, as well as other hormonal levels. It has not yet been evaluated in obesity.

Summary

Amphetamines and amphetamine-like drugs are the most widely used and most available medications for the treatment of obesity. Their use should be restricted to adults (over 18 years), and they should not be prescribed unless they are part of a comprehensive weight loss program. They should be discontinued after 4 to 12 weeks of therapy because of their abuse potential. Mazindol and fenfluramine are two recent drugs which need further evaluation in long-term (1 to 3 years) trials before their role in obesity therapy is clear.

New and better medications are needed if this serious health problem is to be cured. We are permitting surgery with its 2 to 10 per cent mortality rate for morbid obesity, and more serious effort must be directed toward developing successful medical therapy.

References

Alcantara, E.N. & Speckmann, E.W. (1976): *Amer. J. Clin. Nutr.* 29, 1035.

Collipp, P.J., Schmierer, B. & Greensher, J. (1971): *Med. Times* 99, 155.

Collipp, P.J., Gupta, K.B., Amin, S., Maddaiah, V.T. & Chen, S.Y. (1977): *Ped. Res.* 11, 424.

Collipp, P.J., Curti, V., Sharma, R.K., Thomas, J., Maddaiah, V.T. & Cohn, S. (1973): *Metabolism* 22, 589.

Greenway, F.L., Dahms, W.T. & Bray, G.A. (1977): *Current Therapeutic Research* 21, No. 3.

Harrison, L.C., Sandy, K.C. & Ling-Roach, A.P. (1975): *Metabolism* 24, 1353.

Hoebel, B.G. (1975): *J. Comp. Physiol. Psychol.* 89, No. 9.

Jordan, H.A. (1974): *Med. Com. Press* 20.

Quaade, F. (1974): In *Obesity symposium*, ed W. Burland, P. Samuel & J. Yudkin. London: Churchill Livingstone.

Seip, M., Trygsted, O. & Oseid, S. (1977): *Ped. Res.* 11, 1015.

Shetty, K.R. & Kalkhoff, R.K. (1977): *Archs Int. Med.* 137,

Tanner, J.J. & Whitehouse, R.H. (1975): *Archs Dis. Childh.* 50, 142.

49
The American food scene: food choices and affluent malnutrition

A.M. ALTSCHUL and J. GROMMET
Division of Nutrition, Georgetown University School of Medicine, Washington DC 20007, USA.

Thus far, discussions at this conference have centered principally on the problems of energy balance in the individual and on problems of correction of obesity through interaction with the patient in clinical procedures. It is not the purpose of this paper to propose or advocate specific solutions, but instead to consider the condition of the society in which the individual lives and which, surely, has an important and perhaps an overriding impact on chances of coping or not coping with problems of energy balance.

As a society moves from a condition of relative scarcity to one of sufficiency and then to abundance, obesity emerges as a problem. Here the problem differs from society to society and among different segments of the same society as, for example, different socioeconomic groups in the same society.

In societies where obesity is a problem, it is tempting to consider interventions that would reduce the prevalence of obesity at any given level of abundance or affluence. Even though the theories of intervention in matters of abundance are less well developed than in matters of scarcity and no better developed than theories of clinical intervention, intuitively, one would seek to consider societal intervention not in place of clinical intervention but as an adjunct to those procedures. The intuition is reinforced by the knowledge that for certain groups in any affluent society, for example, people in the higher socioeconomic groups, certain external elements operate on personal matters and personal resources. This leads to the question - which conditions would make it possible to broaden the population base that copes better with this problem? One might expect that society could help in two ways: (1) prevention, by creating conditions where it becomes more difficult for obesity to develop, (2) facilitating clinical management of obese patients. Where there is a socioeconomic bias in the prevalence of obesity there is also a socioeconomic bias in the effectiveness of its clinical treatment, if only because of cost.

An example of the complexities that must be reckoned with in an affluent, highly technological society, is the problem of food choices that form part of the fabric within which personal decisions are made and which could affect energy balance.

Nutrient choice

An individual has two ways of handling the intake of specific nutrients such as salt and sugar. He can either add the pure nutrient to other foods being eaten, or he can choose among sources of food that have varying contents of the nutrients in question. In both instances, there is discretion, but of a different order. In the first instance, it is a simple choice of adding salt or not, or adding sugar or not, or putting more or less fat in the foods on the table. The alternative is not quite so simple because it involves making decisions about foods to be eaten, and it assumes a knowledge of the specific nutrient composition in those foods. Classically, the control over salt and sugar intake was primarily of the first type, viz., individual control by adding or not adding sugar or salt in the kitchen or at the table. Control over fat intake was never so simple because of the major contribution of meat and dairy products to fat consumption. Nevertheless, there was room for some discretionary addition of fat as table spreads. The availability of synthetic vitamins is relatively new but has added a dimension to the exercise of discretion in obtaining these nutrient choices. Protein classically is obtained entirely from foods. Pure protein is an artifact from the food industry and has been available primarily for incorporation into processed foods. Gelatin is an outstanding exception. It is only in very recent years that pure protein has been made available to the consumer market as, for ėxample, in connection with weight reduction programs or in 'fad' diets.

Sugar

An analysis of sucrose consumption is given in Table 1. There has been a profound change in the type of discretionary use of sucrose in the diet. Whereas in 1920 the discretionary use of sucrose in the diet was over 60 per cent, this had been lowered to close to 20 per cent by the 1970s.

Table 1. Caloric sweetener consumption in the American diet. Caloric sweetener consumption data from 1920 to 1965 was obtained from Gray (1971) and classified into the categories of discretionary and less discretionary. Gray's tabulations were based on data from Jones and Thomason (1951) and the US Dept. of Agriculture (USDA, 1949-1968). Data for the 1970s are available for beet and cane sugar in terms of the subcategories shown in the table, but the data are no longer reported according to these subcategories for other sweeteners. Thus, the more recent data for the 1970s is expressed only in the broad terms of discretionary and less discretionary. Total sweetener data for 1970 and 1975 were derived from US Dept. of Agriculture, Sugar and Sweetener Report, 1976 (USDA, 1976a) and were fractionated into discretionary and less discretionary according to the suggestions of Gray (1976): cane and beet sugar, 20 per cent home use; corn sugar, 0 per cent home use; cane, sorgo, and maple syrups, 100 per cent home use; corn syrup, 5 per cent home use; refiners and edible can molasses, 20 per cent home use; and honey, 80 per cent home use. Home use was equated with discretionary consumption, and the balance was considered to be utilized by the food industry, thus becoming less discretionary consumption

Source	1920	1925	1930	1935	1940	1945	1950	1955	1960	1965	1970	1975
	lb/capita/year											
Discretionary												
Household use	66	75	69	67	59	36	41	37	36	31	23	20
% Consumption	63%	64%	60%	61%	53%	34%	37%	34%	32%	27%	18%	17%
Less discretionary												
Commercial food use	31	36	39	35	45	51	61	64	67	75	–	–
Eating & drinking places	6	6	6	6	7	7	8	8	7	7	–	–
Institutions including military	1	1	1	1	1	1	1	1	1	1	–	–
Sub-total	38	43	46	42	53	69	70	73	75	83	98	94
% Consumption	37%	36%	40%	39%	47%	66%	63%	66%	68%	73%	82%	83%
Total sweetener consumption	104	118	115	109	112	105	111	110	111	114	121	114

Similar data for Sweden in 1970 indicate considerably more simple choice in the consumption of sugar and syrup: 48 per cent discretionary consumption including lump and powdered sugar and syrup and 52 per cent less-discretionary consumption, composed primarily of chocolates and confectioneries, fruit and vegetables, bakery products, and beverages.

Fat

The official statistics of the US Department of Agriculture divide fat consumption into categories of visible and invisible fats. Visible fats are those identifiable as such. Visible fats may be consumed as table or household butter, margarine, shortening, or salad oil, or may be part of an industrial food preparation in which they are incorporated into; for example, baked foods, prepared foods for institutional feeding, french fried potatoes or potato chips. The invisible fats classically are those originally part of meat, fish, eggs, or in whole milk or milk products.

The consumption of visible fats is relatively unchanged (see Table 2). The proportion of fats calculated as involving simple discretion by the consumer was always relatively low and seems even to have become lower.

Table 2. Fat consumption in the American diet. Data on the annual per capita consumption of fats were obtained from publications of the US Department of Agriculture. Container size was the criterion for determining if the fat classified as visible was under individual control (discretionary) or was put into processed foods (less discretionary). As an example, salad oil sold in one gallon containers or smaller was considered to be for direct consumer consumption whereas that sold in container sizes larger than one gallon was considered an industrial consumption. Data on shortening, lard, and salad and cooking oils were obtained from the Institute of Shortening and Edible Oils; that on margarine from the Fats and Oils Situation; analagous container data for butter were not available, hence, all butter consumption was designated as discretionary, recognizing that this overestimates the case (USDA, 1973; USDA, 1976b; USDA, 1975; Shortening, 1947-75). As in the other instances, the data is for disappearance and not consumption; there is no accounting of wastage. Nor were there any data from which to estimate discretionary consumption of margarine and salad oils in restaurants

Discretionary fat	1947-49	1957-59	1960	1965	1970	1975
			g/day			
Discretionary fat						
Butter	13.2	10.2	9.3	8.0	6.6	5.8
Margarine	7.0	10.2	10.7	11.2	12.2	11.9
Lard and shortening	12.8	10.3	8.3	6.3	6.3	6.2
Cooking and salad oils	0.6	2.2	2.9	4.2	6.2	6.1
Sub-total	33.6	33.4	31.2	29.7	31.3	30.0
% of total	23%	23%	21%	20%	20%	19%
Less discretionary fat						
Dairy products (excluding butter) and eggs	30.5	29.3	27.4	26.1	25.0	23.8
Meat, poultry, game, fish	47.2	47.2	48.8	48.7	54.8	50.1
All fruits and vegetables	8.2	7.9	8.2	8.7	8.8	8.9
Flour and cereals	2.7	2.1	2.1	2.2	2.0	2.1
Margarine	0.0	0.7	1.0	1.1	1.5	2.0
Lard and shortening	14.6	15.4	16.8	19.2	21.0	18.9
Cooking and salad oils	8.5	11.2	11.4	13.3	16.0	19.2
Sub-totals	111.7	113.8	115.6	119.3	129.1	125.0
% of total	77%	77%	79%	80%	80%	81%
Total fat consumption	145.3	147.2	146.8	149.0	160.4	155.0

Convenience

Every year, it is easier to obtain foods away from home. This affects two aspects of consumer choice: it is easier to obtain foods of relatively high caloric density, such as snacks with high fat content or high sugar content or both; and it is easier to eat without being involved in the preparation of food. Eating in restaurants places much of the choice in the hands of the cook. In both instances there has been an increase in the amount of money spent of food items.

Table 3 gives the volume of sales of vended foods for selected years 1960-1975. When sales of cigarettes, cigars, and others are subtracted from the total, it can be seen that there was a sixfold increase in consumption of those foods.

Table 3. Total vended dollar volume, United States* (in millions)

	1960	1965	1970	1975	1976
Hot drinks	143	314	452	712	775
Cold drinks – cup	132	269	380	675	675
– canned	–	(50)	420	1300	1425
– bottled	306	454	697	945	989
Confections/snacks	305	409	671	1115	1190
Bulk vending	55	65	305	273	330
Milk	62	90	153	244	248
Ice cream	26	36	51	64	63
Pastries	–	(36)	80	205	214
Hot canned foods	22	31	74	114	111
All-purpose food	(45)	(130)	224	410	440
Cigarettes, cigars, all others	1491	1917	2718	3275	3366
Total	2587	3801	6225	9332	9826
Food items	1096	1884	3507	6057	6460

* Taken from Vending, 1977

Table 4 gives the amounts and proportion of expenditures for food eaten at home and away from home for the period 1960-1976. There is a continuing decrease in the proportion of expenditure for food at home and an increased expenditure for food away from home.

Table 4. Expenditure for food at home and away from home (United States)*

	At home		Away from home	
Year	Amount (bil. dol.)	Per cent of total	Amount (bil. dol.)	Per cent of total
1960	56.3	79.9	14.2	20.1
1965	66.8	77.9	19.0	22.1
1970	91.8	77.4	26.8	22.6
1975	141.0	76.3	43.8	23.7
1976**	149.2	75.7	47.9	24.3

* Calculated from USDA, 1976*c*.
** First three quarters

The changes and their consequences

The changes in the American diet in this century did not take place for trivial, capricious, or malevolent reasons. They have come about because of increased income. A graphic description of the qualitative changes in diet with income is given by Perisse *et al.* (1969); this curve was revised to include changes in total food energy intake. Hollingsworth (1974) showed the same distribution in the United Kingdom. There is ample evidence that this is so almost anywhere where there are differences in socioeconomic level.

A speculative description of this general change is summarized in Figure 1. Curve A depicts the effect of personal income on desire for convenience in foods for eating out of the home. Curve B suggests that good nutrition bears a complex relationship to income. In region I (underconsumption), an increase in income makes it possible to eat more total food and more of certain constituents. In region II (adequate consumption), a further improvement in income does not improve nutritional status; there is enough disposable income and, presumably, adequate education to properly meet food and nutritional needs. In region III (overconsumption), a further increase in income tends to reverse the gains reached by an increase in income up to that point. This condition could be described as affluent malnutrition. The dimensions of this problem are just beginning to appear. The poor in an affluent society are in double jeopardy; they could occupy portions of regions I and III simultaneously. There are still remnants of undernutrition among the poor; they

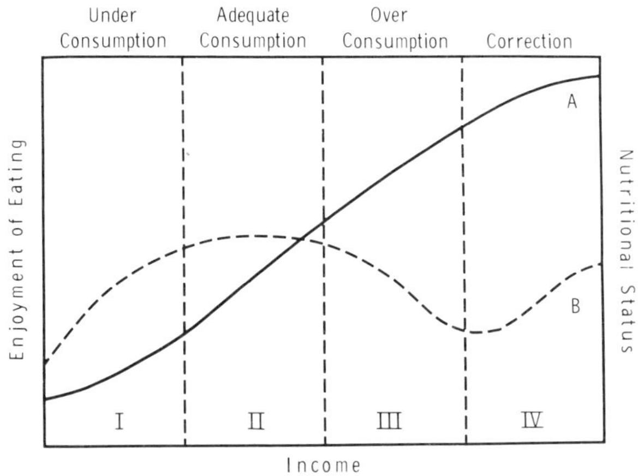

Fig. 1. A general view of the direction of changes in an affluent society, which comes under the rubric of enjoyment of eating (Curve A), and include the desire for taste, status, and convenience in foods, and the consequences as they relate to nutritional status (Curve B). Regions I, II, III, and IV describe, respectively, conditions of underconsumption, adequate consumption, overconsumption, and correction. The authors acknowledge helpful discussions on this matter with Professor Sanford A. Miller

have more risk of being low or borderline in vitamin status, in iron and other mineral consumption and, perhaps, for certain parts of the life cycle in total calorie or protein consumption. Infant mortality (in part nutrition-related) is higher among the poor than for the average of their society. At the same time, the poor are apparently more susceptible to the problems of affluent malnutrition; hence, there is a higher percentage of obesity. In region IV (correction), further increase in income tends to produce a new set of conditions. Life-style is managed in such a way that despite the higher amount of money available for consumption, corrections are made, for reasons of vanity, or health or both, that maintain energy balance and, therefore, produce a tempering effect on the diseases of affluent malnutrition.

The role of society

In the matter of undernutrition, American society has made serious contributions towards reducing the number of individuals who cannot cope, by making available abundant food supplies, by encouraging fortification of some foods with certain vitamins and minerals, by the food stamp program, and by the school lunch program.

Let us consider what society can do to help individuals who would like to reduce their risk of obesity. For the individual who is able to cope with obesity by one means of counselling or another, the personal problem is solved. However, this is usually an expensive solution. As pointed out earlier, there is more obesity among the poor than the non-poor. The reasons are complex and interrelated with other problems of the poor. It seems clear that the difficulty is at both ends: it is more difficult to avoid becoming obese and more difficult to take advantage of available tools to reverse the process. Society can, of course, help to defray the cost of treating obesity just as other personal costs for food, welfare, and medical services are defrayed. A more logical role, however, would be in prevention.

Some countries have favored educational programs to encourage change in food habits and to promote more exercise. Quasi public groups or medical societies have evolved programs. There are other opportunities: any means that favors less fat in meat or less fat in dairy products helps to reduce fat intake. Any programs that encourage less saturated fat in the diet facilitate more dietary options. Non-caloric sweeteners make it possible for the food industry to produce a greater variety of foods, which may help people to shift more easily away from food habits which favor excesses.

Care in advertising can reduce the pressures towards gluttony or a misunderstanding of nutritional needs. Labelling of caloric value and content (preferably quantitatively) of certain critical nutrients may help the consumer to exercise more choice.

The role of school education remains largely unexplored. This is particularly important since it might be easier, especially for those in low socioeconomic groups, to deal with children than to wait until the problem has fully developed and then try to deal with it in adult life.

The political problem is that an overwhelming consensus on specific risk factors does not and may never exist. This creates problems on a personal level but generates even greater problems on a political level since clear-cut decisions with widespread popular support are not possible. Since there is a lack of consensus and because clear political decision is often not possible, conflicting policies co-exist. One agency in the government supports the growing of tobacco whereas another agency in the same government condemns cigarette smoking as a major risk factor. One agency in the government furthers the consumption of meat and milk whereas another agency talks about the problems of saturated fat and cholesterol. School lunch authorities do not concern themselves with the salt content of foods while the regulatory agencies encourage lower limits on the salt content of baby foods.

The food manufacturing industry and the institutional food industry could play a major role. People can minimize the stresses of overnutrition by reducing the role of hedonism in food, in their life-style, and by returning to the more modest food habits that would characterize region II of Figure 1. This may be possible for some but these would be a minority. It would also be contrary to the trends shown in Tables 1 to 4. The majority of people would like to retain their life-styles. They need a solution characterized by region IV of Figure 1. They need attractive options for foods with lower caloric concentration. Let the marketplace decide which foods will remain. Just as the marketplace has decided that non-fat and low-fat milks are now a viable option, so it is quite likely that options of foods with lower caloric concentrations and lesser amounts of sodium may attract more public attention. Moreover, their availability will make it possible for more effective education.

Institutional feeding establishments can also provide consumers with options of smaller portions and alternative spreads and seasonings. This would reduce wastage and provide the opportunity to enjoy meals away from home without the danger of overeating.

Acknowledgement—supported, as part of a program, by the Brunner Foundation.

References

Abramson, E. (1973): In *The role of sugar in modern nutrition*, p. 39, Marabou Symposium, Marabou, Sundyberg, Sweden, Aug. 18.

Altschul, A.M. editor (1974): In *New protein foods*, Vol. 1, p. 3. New York: Academic Press.

Cantor, S.M. (1975): In *Sweeteners—issues and uncertainties.* Washington DC: National Academy of Sciences.

Gray, F.D. (1971): *Sweetener consumption, utilization, and supply patterns in the United States: past trends and relationships, and prospects for target years 1980 and 2000*, p. 335. Ph.D. Dissertation, University of Maryland.

Hollingsworth, D. (1974): *Nutr. Rev.* 32, 353.

Jones, P.E. & Thomason, F.G. (1951): *Competitive relationships between sugar and corn sweeteners*, Agr. Inf. Bull. No. 48, PMA, p. 214. US Dept. Agr., Washington DC.

Page, L. & Friend, B. (1974): In *Sugars in nutrition*, ed H.L. Sipple & K.W. McNutt. New York: Academic Press.

Perisse, J., Sizaret, F. & Francois, P. (1969): *FAO Nutrition Newsletter*, 7 (3), 1.

Shortening (1947-1975): *Analysis of domestic shipments of edible oils and fats*, 1947-49, 1957-59, 1960, 1965, 1970, 1975. Institute of Shortening and Edible Oils Inc, Washington DC.

USDA (1949-68): *Sugar reports,* ASCS, US Dept. Agr., Washington DC.
USDA (1973): *Food consumption, prices, and expenditures,* AER No. 138, Tables 12, 38, and 39, Economic Research Service, US Dept. Agr., Washington DC.
USDA (1975): *National food situation* (NFS-154), Nov., Tables 9 and 10, Economic Research Service, US Dept. Agr., Washington DC.
USDA (1976*a*): *Sugar and sweetener report,* Vol. 1, No. 8, Economic Research Service, US Dept. Agr., Washington DC.
USDA (1976*b*): *Fats and oils situation,* No. 282, April, Tables 17 and 19, Economic Research Service, US Dept. Agr., Washington DC.
USDA (1976*c*): *National food situation* (NFS-158), Nov., Table 5, Economic Research Service, US Dept. Agr., Washington DC.
Vending (1977): *Vending Times* 17 (6-A), June, 15.

50
The obese individual and society

F. R. DAVIDSON
Department of Community Medicine and International Health,
Division of Nutrition, Georgetown University School of Medicine,
Washington DC 20007, USA.

Food deprivation and hunger are a constant reality for more than two-thirds of the world's population. In the United States, the more common problem is that of overnutrition or obesity. This continual abundance of food does not necessarily result in a healthier population, ie a population using its food resources to its benefit. Many of the ills becoming more prevalent in our society are a direct or indirect result of overconsumption of foodstuffs. The correlation with diabetes mellitus, hypertension, cardiovascular disease, other chronic debilitating diseases, as well as complications following surgery and childbirth, seem crucial. The link between obesity and disease is a complex one and not a simple cause and effect condition (Mayer, 1972).

Americans are obsessed with their health and diet, and spend at least $600 000 000 a year on self-prescribed vitamin supplements. What is the allure of food fortification, or dietary supplementation - does it express ignorance, or desire for reassurance? We are, to be sure, not the first inhabitants of this earth to make the connection between what we put in our mouths and the kind of lives we are able to lead. A proverb found on an ancient Egyptian papyrus states quite simply: 'We live off a quarter of all we eat, doctors live off the other three quarters.'

A recent public health survey stated that 79 000 000 Americans were obese or 30 per cent overweight (Lowenstein, 1976). A further 12 per cent of the population are said to be overweight. Since these estimates are based on averages and reference people, it is doubtful whether this should, in fact, be our sole criteria for defining the magnitude of the problem. Weight reduction programs of all kinds, and there are indeed many variations on this theme, proliferate. They would not thrive if there were no market for them, and this is the clearest indication of public interest in body weight and its control.

The definition of obesity is variable and while it is agreed to be 20 to 30 per cent overweight, means simply that an individual possesses considerable expansion of the adipose tissue mass. However, because of body shape and bone structure, some look heavier with less weight than others with a different body structure. So, while there may be a commonly held medical definition of overweight and obesity, the ways in which we look at each other and come to subjective judgments about the way people look, are much more variable and must, like other things, be conditioned by our own background; our social and cultural ideas. Thus, we invest the words obesity or overweight with certain meanings that apply only in one context. Even the act of defining a population on the basis of its body weight is culture bound. The value judgments we make on this division reveal our own ideas and those with which we have been inculcated with regard to body size and image. Whether the medical concern for overweight people is product or inspiration for our cultural concepts is arguable.

Even within what we think of as the American culture, different groups have differing values about body weight. Thus, the higher incidence of obesity in poor black women may seem less a social liability than for a middle class professional white woman. Is the expectation mother to the incidence or the reverse? As Goldblatt, Moore & Stunkard (1965) have stated in their discussion of social factors in obesity: 'Obesity may always be unhealthy, but it is not always abnormal.'

Greater mutual understanding between the approaches of different scientists in the field of weight control would be of considerable benefit in this and other health problems. For food biochemists and plant geneticists, food is a material which they have been taught how to modify, with little consideration devoted to the motives and preferences of the human race. The biochemist tries to use scientific knowledge to alter the results of habits, the human beings, rather than the habits themselves. Parents and educators try to teach children to eat foods of greater rather than less nutritional value. And physiologists believe that if the human organism were not tainted by various pressures man could freely choose the correct nutrients. Economists insist the problem hinges on the absence or availability of the food itself. To them, the all important element is the purchasing power of the consumer and the group with the most available food should be the best nourished.

The work of psychologists, especially that relating to eating cues, their cause and effect, and the social stigma of obesity, has brought into serious consideration the interpersonal aspects of this condition. Clinical research delineating 'critical periods' and type of adipose cell development and the roles this plays in juvenile and adult onset obesity will help to identify individuals at high risk and aid in targeting resources in treatment programs. Physicians, for many years the only source of professional advice for the obese, either through lack of interest or time give support to the theory of obesity as a personal failing. Our highly individualized society holds each of us responsible for so very much in our lives. Results of preliminary research by us on health and illness beliefs of children (in which being ill was equated with misbehavior) reveals the subtle but organized ways in which individual responsibility for health and well being are transmitted.

Each of these approaches is partially valid. I suggest that the study of food habits should integrate all of them, to provide the optimum understanding of what can be done in the area of eating behavior. Thus, new scientific discoveries, changes in methods of child rearing, incidence of disease, as well as emergence of new diseases and knowledge of the relationships between these and eating, can be integrated. Social and political/economic changes and changes in the natural environment require adjustments in the food habits of populations. Eating habits in one situation may be adaptive while in another, maladaptive.

In understanding what people eat, it is important to have in hand a body of data regarding food habits. The way in which children learn to eat or reject foods, and the way in which foods are categorized as good or bad, of high or low status, needs to be comprehended. The whole complicated set of beliefs and practices that regulate the way in which each human being, born with the needs common to all mammals, becomes a socialized individual, accepting and rejecting parts of his environment as edible and non-edible, at different times, for different purposes, in different situations, are also important to evaluate.

All those things that go to make us the individuals we are, play a role in determining our body weight, the importance it has for us, and what actions we might take to alter it. These aspects include innate properties of our biological identity, ie our genetic heritage, our metabolism, our parentage and the sociocultural milieu in which we integrate all the influences to which we are subject and begin to learn in a conscious and an unconscious way all that we must do in order to take our rightful places as fully fledged members of our own society.

What we learn is - what is delicious, what less so, and how much is enough. What we think about food and, consequently, the way we deal with it, all have their bases here. Food must be eaten for us to survive, but the manner in which it is chosen, cooked, served, and eaten, is determined by a myriad of factors. The old saw that some live to eat and others eat to live, is a good illustration of what food means to us. Are our families blue ribbon members of the clean plate club, do they choose mealtime as a pleasant family social occasion, or use it as a battleground? Did our parents use food as punishment or reward, and what kinds of foods came to represent these values for us? Did eating all our food and maybe more win approval or disapproval? Where did we learn that food can be a consolation, and for what - the lack of love, companionship, success? Once learned as a child, was it reinforced through repetition of the same circumstances in our adult life? How difficult it is to break old habits, especially those associated with deeply seated feelings of self-image and importance. The vicious circle of a child eating more than needed to show a parent how the food was appreciated may well continue with an adult insisting her family eat what she considers a good portion - in reality too much, to confirm feelings of worth. Are there specific physiologies for whom this is exclusively true or are we all equally vulnerable?

What we eat is influenced by what is available, our budget, our family, friends, our attitudes, and our culture. Eating is one of the first activities we engage in. How we do it, and with whom, and what sort of experience it is from then influences greatly the way we feel about food and about eating.

In discussing the eating habits of groups of people, it is thus important to recognize that these shared beliefs about food are not simply preferences for certain foods but, rather, a whole interrelated system of food production, preservation, distribution, and consumption. As such, it is inextricably interwoven with our entire way of life. Any attempts at altering food patterns must take this into consideration. Only in this way will points of leverage for change be found and points of resistance be anticipated or understood. Margaret Mead (1945) cautioned this when discussing changed eating requirements and habits in post war societies: 'Whether food is regarded by public officials as something to sell or something to eat; whether the need for food ... is regarded as a natural inalienable right ... whether eating food (and in the appropriate quantity) is regarded as a duty to society, which is denied in a hunger strike ... - all of these attitudes, which stem from the whole cultural attitude toward food, condition the acceptance of any scientific improvement in nutrition'.

The physical environment includes crucial factors. If high density, high caloric value products were not readily available, and in quantity, they could not be consumed. In our society, some highly noxious foods are vigorously promoted by advertisers. Indeed, supermarkets place great store by impulse purchases. The grocers have carefully researched ways to influence the consumer to purchase products with higher profit margins. I have yet to see at the checkout counter a display inviting one to buy celery and carrot sticks. No, loaded with pretzels and candy, you leave the store, get into a car, where physical activity is discouraged. Our great contemporary technology includes considerable calorie saving devices. Is this really a favor to us? A sedentary life-style has required us to make great efforts to perform physical exercise ... and this has become an important feature of weight management.

Within the set of influences comprising the physical environment, let us also consider the 'new consumerism'. By this I mean, the greater public awareness and concern about institutions affecting peoples' lives eg, supermarkets, purity of food laws. It derives, I think, from a strong urge to seek an improved quality of life. A feature of the 'new consumerism' is the growth of a substantial political lobby which has arisen subjectively because of greater public awareness and objectively because of changing political norms.

The growth of consumer powers is an important force and has direct impact in health matters. People are told that some things for sale are bad and bad for them, and laws are enacted outlawing some of these.

The new consumerism is not the be all and end all of obesity or poor nutritional practices but is in itself one of many factors that impinge on nutrition related behavior we are considering here. Consumer advocacy is not a god but should be put alongside all other aspects of an individual's environmental context that we have been discussing.

The new consumerism has modified the physical environment in which we live by making us more aware of passive influences on our values and thereby altering these. Responsibility for good food choice was previously ascribed to the individual. Bad choices resulting in, for example, obesity, and bad health, revealed inadequacies in individual performance.

Food intake is intimately related to our cognitive sense, our body image, self-worth concepts, our priorities of health, and our immediate psychosocial state. Everything that happens about us, especially with those people who mean most to us or who most often come into contact with us, must be considered, ie family and peer pressures.

Most workers in the field agree that sociocultural factors play a crucial role in obesity. The midtown study in New York (Langner, 1963) found that obesity was six times more common among women of lower socioeconomic status than among those of high status, the corresponding ratio among men was only 2:1. Movement in social classes resulted in weight changes for women and men. Among women, those who moved down in social status had a higher prevalence of obesity (22 per cent), those who moved upwards a lower prevalence (12 per cent). Among men both these factors also applied but, again, to a less dramatic degree. Thus, increased social status resulted in a movement from obese to normal categories. Among the women, movement was from obese to thin categories.

This study is useful in helping us understand why it is that some groups of the population have a higher prevalence of either obese or thin individuals and may not actively seek change. This would appear to suggest that the standards for normalcy vary between groups. Once a habit develops, the younger generation will naturally accept it as part of their perceptual framework as members of this group. If change is deemed necessary, the 'normative' behavior of the group must be taken into account, and the implications of attempting to shift the norm carefully weighed.

Obesity is an elusive concept embracing a number of interrelated factors in the human environment eg, social, psychological, physical and cultural. The importance attached to each component varies between individuals and across subgrouping within the population. Aesthetic and health considerations, themselves multifaceted concepts, play an important part.

Because obesity arises from deep seated and complex problems, dramatic reform cannot be expected, particularly in the context of a complex consumer society. A useful step would be increased communication among the different disciplines concerned with food, in academic, social, clinical, and commercial fields. Mitigation of the problems of obesity is not the exclusive preserve of any one of the various disciplines involved. Indeed amelioration of this many-sided human ill can best be expected through the cross-fertilization of research, better mutual understanding, and improved cooperation among the various branches of academicians, physicians and food industrialists involved.

References

Goldblatt, P.B., Moore, M.E. & Stunkard, A.J. (1965): *J. Am. Med. Ass.* 192, 12.

Langner, T.S. & Michael, S.T. (1963): *Life stress and mental health: Midtown Manhattan study.* New York: The Free Press of Glencoe, Inc.

Lowenstein, F.W. (1976): *Am. J. Clin. Nutr.* 29, 918.

Mayer, J. (1972): *Human nutrition.* Springfield, Illinois: Charles C. Thomas.

Mead, M. (1945): National Academy of Sciences, *National Research Council Bulletin* 111.

51
The obese individual and government regulatory agencies

A.L. FORBES
United States Bureau of Foods, Food and Drug Administration, Washington DC 20204.

Most of what I have to say is a recounting of fact, but occasionally I express opinions of my own. Let me emphasize that my opinions do not necessarily reflect those of the Commissioner of Food and Drugs or of the Agency.

Three federal regulatory agencies have activities that relate in a number of different ways to the obese individual, namely The Food and Drug Administration (FDA), The Federal Trade Commission (FTC), and The Department of Agriculture (USDA). I think all of us working in these agencies understand that our activities on behalf of the obese individual are adjuncts to clinical management, and recognize that they are secondary to: basic research elucidating the fundamental etiologies; the evolution of various dietary, behavioral, surgical, and pharmacologic approaches to therapy; and the individual patient-physician relationship to achieve weight reduction and maintenance. Nevertheless, I believe our activities are useful adjuncts, since they are aimed for the most part directly at consumers. I would, therefore, like to review briefly with you the current status of regulatory approaches and a number of proposals that are in the 'works'.

Probably the most useful single activity is the FDA nutrition labelling program, which is now 5 years old and working rather well. Today, nutrition labelling is widely used by the public, particularly by the calorie-conscious individual. The labelling provides the consumer with precise information on caloric content, as well as protein, fat, and carbohydrate content in grams per serving. In addition, protein and a minimum of seven vitamins and minerals are presented as percentages of the US recommended daily allowance (US RDA) per serving. All foods for which any type of nutrition claim is made in labelling or advertising (except for fresh fruits and vegetables, and meat and poultry products regulated by USDA) must bear nutrition labelling. This is also true when any specific nutrient is added to a food. Hence, all fortified or enriched foods bear nutrition labelling. Otherwise, the program is voluntary. However, many food processors are now using nutrition labelling voluntarily, particularly many national brands of canned vegetables and fruits. Currently, we do not know what proportion of the national food supply carries nutrition labelling. Several years ago, it was estimated that approximately 10 billion dollars worth of the food supply was so labelled, but this figure is no doubt obsolete. We have a study underway now (scheduled to be completed in about 6 months), which will give us a very precise estimate of the extent of use of nutrition labelling in both economic and volumetric terms, according to specific classes of foods. It is our intent to repeat this study about every 2 years in order to track the evolution of the total program. We are working intensively with the fresh fruit and vegetable industry to develop a reasonable analytical data base for nutrients which will be commensurate with the precision required for nutrition labelling. The problem with this particular segment of the food supply is that the existing data base is old, outdated, and generally insufficient. There is now a degree of momentum which should solve the problem commodity by commodity over time. We are particularly pleased to see certain segments of the snack food industry also developing data bases to commence nutrition labelling. In addition, USDA officials have recently stated that they intend to finalize their program for nutrition labelling for the meat and poultry products regulated by USDA. Many luncheon-type and other processed meat products are already labelled according to the FDA requirements.

A voluntary addition to standard nutrition labelling is the declaration of cholesterol and/or polyunsaturated and saturated fatty acid content per serving. Although the general nutrition labelling program is developing well, we are not satisfied with the extent of cholesterol and fatty acid labelling. It simply is not very widely used. As a result, and also in response to a number of petitions submitted by industry to the Agency, we are developing a proposal to modify the regulation in such a manner as to encourage expanded use of cholesterol and fatty acid labelling.

At present, sodium content can be voluntarily added to the standard nutrition label. Again, this is not widely practiced. We are working on a regulatory proposal now that would require sodium and potassium content to be declared as part of all nutrition labels. Although perhaps not relevant to obesity *per se*, this certainly should assist consumers who either already have essential hypertension or are predisposed to development of this disease, which is so frequently associated with obesity.

The last fact about nutrition labelling is that we are launching an extensive series of studies to determine the most effective means of communicating nutrition information to consumers in labelling and also ways in which such information may be applied to advertising. In other words. we are trying to find out if there is a better way to do it than our present system. Pictographic and bar graph systems and the like will all be explored. We are more than willing to change format and detail. The one thing we will not do is decrease the accuracy of information provided to consumers.

Now, let me change the subject to that of low calorie and reduced calorie foods, regulated as particular types of foods for special dietary use. Since the 1940s and 50s, there has been a regulation which requires label declaration of calories per serving, and the percentage by weight of protein, fat, and carbohydrate, for any food, for which claims are made, of usefulness in weight reduction or weight control. This regulation remains in effect today, the only difference being that full nutrition labelling is now required for foods for which such claims are made. The problem was, and remains, that there is as yet no legal definition of the nature of such foods for which weight control claims could reasonably be made. Hence, in June 1962, FDA published for comment the first proposal to define these foods. This was followed by an enormously complex series of procedural events concerning all types of foods for special dietary use, including: the filing of numerous exceptions to the proposals; publication of new regulations in 1966; staying of these regulations pending a hearing; a 2-year-long public hearing from mid-1968 to mid-1970; and preoccupation for the next several years with aspects of special foods other than those for weight control, ultimately leading to a congressional amendment to The Food, Drug, and Cosmetic Act in 1976.

At last, 3 months ago, on July 19, 1977 (over 15 years after the original proposal), we issued a tentative final order encompassing two regulations: one for foods claiming usefulness in reducing or maintaining caloric intake or body weight, and a second pertaining to foods for use in the diet of diabetic patients. Even this is not the end of the matter, because under current procedural requirements the order had to be issued on a tentative basis, subject to comment. The comment period ended on October 18, 1977. It will be a matter of months before we issue the final regulation.

With that little bit of history, I would like to describe to you the key points of the tentative order for low calorie and reduced caloric foods which are still subject to change on the basis of final comments. All such foods must bear nutrition labelling. The original requirement alerting consumers to the role of the food in the total diet has been modified to read: 'Weight control by diet requires limiting total intake of calories'. A statement is also required on foods fabricated or altered to lower caloric intake, describing how the calorie adjustment was achieved eg, by the use of non-nutritive sweeteners, and non-nutritive fillers.

On the basis of testimony from the public hearing, the concept of caloric density has been introduced into the definition of 'low calorie' foods, which are now to be defined as providing no more than 40 calories per serving, and containing no more than 0.4 calories per gram. We think that this new definition will be quite helpful for a number of reasons, particularly because many of the lower caloric density fruits and vegetables, as well as a good many calorically dilute fabricated foods and drinks, can now be identified clearly as being low calorie foods, and because the definition goes a long way to resolving the problem of the wide variation in the number of servings of such foods that may be ingested by consumers in the course of the day.

Reduced calorie foods have also been redefined on the basis of the testimony so that there must be a caloric reduction of at least one-third (rather than the previously proposed reduction of 50 per cent); there must be a reduction of at least 25 calories per serving; the food must be nutritionally equivalent to the food it resembles, ie in terms of protein, vitamin and mineral content per serving; and there must be a statement of comparison with a serving of the food without the calorie alteration, including the caloric content of the unaltered food. There are similar provisions for foods of lower caloric content which do not exactly resemble another specific food, but which can logically replace the food in the diet. In this case, the lower calorie food must meet the same caloric reduction and nutrition equivalency requirements, and, although such a food cannot be called 'calorie-reduced', the statement 'for calorie restricted diets' can be used. An example of such a food is canned fruits packed in unsweetened water contrasted with such fruits packed in heavy syrup. The testimony supported very clearly the idea that a 50 per cent reduction in calories excluded many foods, which in fact are useful in clinical management of obesity, from being considered as 'calorie-reduced'. A typical example is skim milk, which does meet the one-third reduction requirement, but not the 50 per cent reduction.

The regulation also addresses the use of a number of special terms, which heretofore have been very loosely used in the marketplace, to the point of producing a good deal of consumer confusion. One is the word 'dietetic', and similar terms such as 'artifically sweetened', implying usefulness in weight control to consumers. Under the provision of the tentative order, the use of such terms would be limited to foods which meet the requirements for 'low calorie' or 'reduced calorie' foods, or otherwise can be labelled 'for calorie restricted diets'. The exceptions to this limitation are: when the label clearly demonstrates usefulness for some other special purpose, eg 'for low sodium diets'; in the case of a few regulations which may require their use; and lastly, for whole meals or replacements, pending issuance of a new regulation defining the nutritional characteristics of these meals.

Similarly, the use of the term 'sugarless', and similar terms such as 'sugar-free' is limited to 'low calorie' and 'reduced calorie' foods, and 'foods for calorie-restricted diets', unless it is very clearly stated that the food is not a reduced or low calorie food. It seems reasonable that clarification of the use of these dietetic and sugar-related terms will substantially reduce the degree of consumer confusion which currently exists.

I would like to take just a moment to describe the key provisions of the companion regulation concerning foods for use in the diet of diabetic patients. Currently, there are no regulations which specifically address the subject of foods for diabetic patients. Such foods are labelled in accordance with a very general regulation for foods used in the dietary management of disease. The new regulation would require three key things:

(1) a specific label statement: 'Diabetic patients: this product may be useful in your diet on the advice of a physician'.

(2) nutrition labelling.

(3) that the food's usefulness to diabetic patients shall not be solely on the basis of its being a food useful in reducing or maintaining caloric intake or body weight; in other words, the food must have a clinical value other than (or in addition to) being a low or reduced calorie food.

In my opinion, this last provision is an important one. It is obvious that many diabetic patients, but by no means all, need to lose weight. It is equally obvious that this applies to enormous numbers of people without diabetes, and with or without other chronic diseases. Although there may be some differences in the diet used for weight reduction of a diabetic patient, depending on the management problems for that particular patient, the basic principles for achieving weight control remain the same. It, therefore, is logical that a food marketed with specific reference to diabetic patients should have some particular attribute relative to the management of that particular disease. Otherwise, reference to a whole host of diseases could be made on the labels of low calorie and reduced calorie foods; a situation that would constitute the practice of medicine on food labels in an appropriate manner.

Lastly on this matter of the tentative final order, the responses we received during the initial 30-day comment period were not very revealing. An early review disclosed only three substantive comments from health professionals, and a considerable collection of requests for extension of the comment period from firms individually or collectively representing industry. We granted this extension for an additional 60 days to October 18, 1977. We have now received numerous and detailed exceptions from industry, which will take a considerable amount of time to evaluate. I frankly do not know what we are going to do about encouraging responsiveness from the professional community on these kinds of regulatory matters, but we definitely need to do something. The paucity of professional contributions does not serve the public well. At least we recognize that we have a problem, and we are certainly open to suggestions on how to improve the system.

Another area of activity at FDA concerning the obese individual, which may be of interest to you, is the matter of the so-called liquid 'predigested' protein products now being widely marketed as the principal or only source of nutrients for purposes of achieving rapid weight loss. Our major concern is the use of these products without medical supervision. Clear-cut evidence of harm to consumers has begun to accumulate* and enough circumstantial evidence of possible adverse effects has been brought to our attention to cause us concern. These adverse effects include electrolyte imbalance, dehydration, potential ill-effects in the presence of pregnancy, and renal, hepatic, or cardiac insufficiency, possibly further aggravated by the concomitant use of diuretics. As I am sure you know, these products are advocated as a means of applying the nitrogen-sparing concept to weight reduction. Most of them are partial hydrolysates of collagen or gelatin, ie they are derived from protein of very low nutritional quality. Some contain one or more added essential amino acids, and/or vitamins and minerals; others do not. None that we are aware of is nutritionally complete. Several products have recently been identified with swollen containers from bacterial outgrowth. Hence, our concerns are both nutritional and microbiological. We currently have a program underway to clearly define the safety and/or potential hazards of these products. The program includes: inspection of production plants and processing methods; label reviews of finished products at the retail level; composition analyses to identify individual amino acid and peptide content; augmented efforts to document possible adverse clinical effects; studies to determine the potential of the products to support growth of microorganisms of public health significance; and development of consumer information materials with emphasis on the need for medical supervision in the use of these products.

**This situation changed substantially and quickly as numerous deaths associated with use of these diets were reported, starting in the month of October 1977. Since that time, numerous actions have been taken by FDA. The reader is referred particularly to: (1) Federal Register Notice, Volume 42, pages 61285-61287, December 2, 1977, proposing strong warning statements on labels; (2) Morbidity and Mortality Weekly Report of November 18, 1977, Volume 26/No. 46, page 383, describing clinical findings.*

Before leaving the subject of the relationship of the FDA to the obese individual, I would like to mention one more activity that is currently underway. In the Federal Register of October 14, 1977, the Commissioner published an announcement that a public hearing will be held on December 2, 1977, at the Parklawn Building in Rockville, Maryland, 'to receive information and views from interested persons on the issue of the current patterns of medical use and abuse of amphetamines'. I commend the October 14 announcement to you because it contains a scholarly review of the history of the evolution of the anorectic drugs, both in terms of their value for short-term adjunctive therapy in obesity and in terms of their abuse for non-medical purposes. One rarely recommends the Federal Register as a scientific journal, but this case is an exception. In very abbreviated form, the Commissioner is considering the initiation of proceedings intended to accomplish the following:

(1) Remove the anorectic indication from the labelling of amphetamine products. If done, the recommended production quotas for amphetamines could be sharply reduced.
(2) retain the indication of narcolepsy for dl-amphetamine and dextro-amphetamine and retain the indication of minimal brain dysfunction for dl-amphetamine, dextro-amphetamine, and methamphetamine.
(3) require patient labelling for amphetamine products, including warnings about using these drugs in weight reduction.

Approved anorectic drug products, other than amphetamines, will remain on the market labelled for their anorectic indication. However, these approved drugs will continue to be reviewed periodically to determine whether additional controls may prove to be necessary. The basic objective is for long-term marketing of only those effective anorectic drugs which have the lowest potential for abuse.

In any discussion of the relationships of regulatory agencies to the obese individual today, it is important to include the activities of the Federal Trade Commission because the FTC regulates all food advertising, whereas FDA regulated food labelling, which includes written, printed, or graphic matter appearing on the article of food or accompanying the package. In November of 1974, FTC proposed a complex trade regulation rule governing food advertising, a very large part of which involved nutrition advertising. One of the ten sections of the proposed rule is concerned specifically with energy and calorie claims. The latter being concerned primarily with advertising of foods for weight control. The key provisions of this section are that:

(1) the food must comply with FDA regulations for foods claiming usefulness in reducing or maintaining caloric intake or body weight.
(2) the advertisment must clearly disclose calories per serving.
(3) if the product is artificially sweetened, the advertisement must disclose the caloric content of the food made with sugar or other nutritive sweeteners.
(4) terms such as 'sugarless' can only be used when the food contains no sugars of any sort, including the sugar alcohols.

Since issuance of their proposal, FTC has held numerous public hearings around the country on the various sections, including the one on energy and calorie claims. We at FDA have also conferred with them on numerous occasions and provided them with our views. Although we may not agree with every detail of their various sections, we certainly strongly support the general thrust and purposes of the trade rule. In the case of the calorie-related parts, we are in close accord. FTC is working hard on finalizing the rule, although they are not ready to predict when this will be an accomplished fact.

The current activities of the regulatory agencies as they may influence the obese individual have been considered here. It is not an idle area, and I hope the description of it has been more helpful than confusing, although I realize that the fine points of regulation are not the favored cup of tea for most clinical professionals concerned with a serious health problem such as obesity.

52
Diet and exercise: assessment of the Swedish programme. A Swedish approach to nutrition in obesity

B. ISAKSSON
Institute of Clinical Nutrition, Annedalsklinikerna, Sahlgren's Hospital,
S-413 45 Gothenburg, Sweden.

In 1963 a Swedish Governmental Committee planning for the national farming policy appointed Professors Blix and Wretlind to state the nutritional points of view which, in their opinion, should be considered in the Swedish farming policy. This was a good initiative, but when the results were studied - for instance a proposal to reduce the production of fat so that it would cover only 35 per cent of the calorie intake of the consumers - the committee panel just shook their heads, patted the professors on their shoulders and disregarded their proposal completely. The effect of this, however, was that Blix and Wretland published a more extensive report (Blix *et al.*, 1965) on the national diet in Sweden and a programme for its revision, in a journal issued by the National Institute of Public Health. The article aroused attention and interest only within a narrow sector of the medical branch, as there were no professional nutritionists in the country at that time; nutrition was not a part of the medical curricula; there was no academic training in nutrition at all; and there were no dietitians, only people with a Diploma in home economics or institutional management.

We, who found the report important and who realized that the development of the dietary habits in this country indicated a continued worsening of conditions with medical consequences, determined to try to have these recommendations endorsed within the field of medical sciences. Therefore, a Nutrition Section within the Swedish Medical Society was established in 1965. This section then published a memorandum entitled 'Medical viewpoints on the Swedish public diet' which in 1966, after having been somewhat modified, was accepted by the sections of cardiology, internal medicine and geriatrics of the Medical Society.

The next step was to contact nutritionists in other Scandinavian countries. This resulted, in 1967, in a joint memorandum entitled 'Medical aspects of the national diet in the Nordic countries'. With this memorandum at our disposal we then approached the National Board of Health and Welfare in its capacity as the supreme health authority. The board found the matter of great significance, and together with the corresponding medical boards in Finland and Norway (but not in Denmark), supported this memorandum as an 'Official collective recommendation on diet in the Scandinavian countries'. It was released on May 3 1968, probably the industrialized world's first official recommendation on changes in the dietary pattern (Keys, 1968).

The National Board of Health and Welfare soon realized, however, that a statement of this type would have no effect whatsoever if it was not followed by a number of practical measures. Considering the extremely high medical service expenses they decided to start a nation-wide campaign, the 'Diet and exercise' campaign (Fig. 1). The purpose of this campaign was 'to give the individual more opportunities to improve his health by means of different health policy measures'. The task of organizing the campaign was given to its

Kost och motion

Fig. 1. The diet and exercise campaign symbol

Committee on Health Education which, in 1969, appointed an organizing committee and a medical expert group. Thus, it was considered that the campaign had to be based on scientific material and the assignment was to investigate previous statements with respect to this question and, in the capacity of the board's own expert group, express an opinion on the matter. A new component was the desire to connect the campaign for better dietary habits with a campaign for increased exercise, because of the natural relationship between diet and exercise via energy balance. Here I will give you some background data on the development of dietary habits in Sweden, their effect on public health and the changes that were proposed. These changes are in complete agreement with the four memoranda which I mentioned before.

Changes in the Swedish dietary pattern

Considerable changes in food habits have occurred during this century in Sweden (Fig. 2).

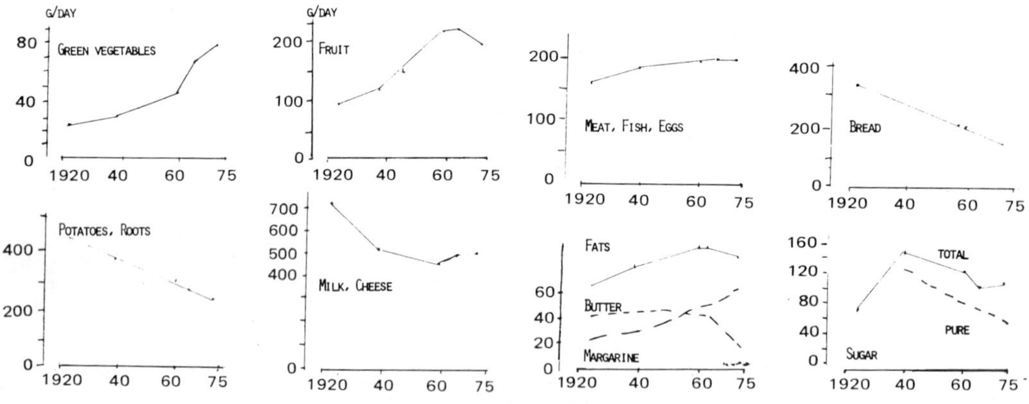

Fig. 2. Per capita consumption changes in Sweden 1920-1975

Some of these changes must be regarded as favourable for the health of the population, such as an increased consumption of green vegetables and fruit, especially as our intake was very low during the first decades of this century. In many other respects, however, the nutritional situation had changed in the wrong direction. A decreased consumption of bread and other cereals with a high caloric density eg, potatoes and roots in the 1920s, could perhaps be regarded as desirable in order to avoid a positive energy balance at a time when people increasingly could afford to buy more food. However, it could not be regarded as positive to have such a low consumption of bread as we had in Sweden - among the lowest in the world. Moreover, the expected decrease in energy intake failed to occur, as there was a simultaneous and considerable increase in the consumption of pure fat and of sugar-rich products, such as sweets, beverages and pastries.

The high level consumption of milk products, also decreased remarkably, while the fat-rich dairy products, cheese and cream, increased in consumption. Finally, for meat, the changes in quantity were small, while the changes in quality tended to turn towards more fat meat products such as pork and sausages.

These changes in food habits had resulted in a traditional diet which, on average, had a lower nutrient density, ie the amounts of the essential nutrient per unit of energy were low, and a higher caloric density, ie the amount of energy-yielding nutrients per unit of weight was higher than in the past (Fig. 3).

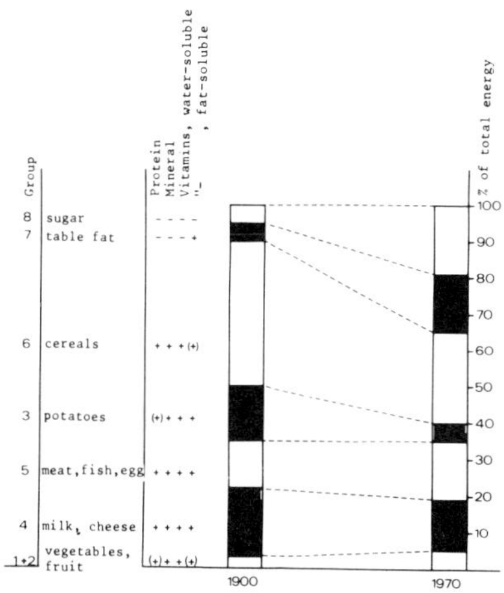

Fig. 3. Changes in energy and nutrient density of the Swedish national diet due to changed dietary pattern during this century

Moreover, data collected from a number of dietary surveys in Sweden showed that the nutrient density was remarkably constant across the whole energy scale for each nutrient studied except ascorbic acid (Blix, 1965). This meant that the content of, for example, protein, iron, thiamine per unit of energy was the same in the diets consumed by hard-working forest workers as in the diets of white collar workers or pensioners, regardless of sex and age. This undoubtedly reflected a certain monotony in the Swedish dietary habits: prinicipally, we ate the same kind of food and has the same type of meals, the basic difference being the size of the portions.

These data showed that you must consume more than 10 MJ (about 2500 kcal) per day of the average Swedish diet in order to obtain the recommended amount of the different essential nutrients. However, simultaneously with these changes in food habits, which have caused a lowering of the nutrient density, the physical activity of the average Swede has decreased due to the continued mechanisation of our society. So, today, there are few people who have a daily need of 10 MJ (about 2500 kcal) or more; perhaps only 20 per cent of the male adult Swedish population.

Medical consequences

Thus, these dietary changes have resulted in a fat and sugar-rich diet which, because of its composition, can lead to diseases of both overnutrition and undernutrition (Table 1).

The high proportion of fat and sugar results in a high caloric density and, combined with a low physical activity level, must necessarily increase the risk of a caloric over-consumption which leads to obesity and concomitant complications among which diabetes is particularly serious. The effect of the saturated fat itself on the blood cholesterol content must, in our opinion, be largely responsible for the development of atherosclerosis. The fact that the sugar-rich products are responsible for dental caries is today denied by hardly anyone, including the candy manufacturers.

The reduced nutrient density, as a consequence of the high fat and sugar content, applies particularly to iron, with a resulting iron deficiency anemia. There is also perhaps a sub-clinical iron deficiency with a generally impaired physical condition, due to the lack of other minerals and perhaps also vitamins. Modern foodstuffs, highly refined by industrial methods, lead to constipation, perhaps also to diverticulosis and may increase the risk for colon cancer.

Table 1. Diet related diseases in Sweden

Malnutrition	Cause	Effect
Overconsumption	Energy	Obesity (Diabetes, arthroses)
	Saturated fat	Atherosclerosis
	Sucrose	Caries
Underconsumption (secondary or primary)	Fe, I, Ca (?), K	Deficiency symptoms
	Trace elements	'Suboptimal health'
	Vitamins	
	Fibre	Constipation, diverticulosis, (colon cancer ?)

All these conditions were, and still are, common in Sweden, so common that during the 1960s I did not hesitate to describe the average family in the following manner: The mother is obese, the father has started to get his first symptoms of coronary heart disease, the daughter has anaemia, the boy has been given his first false teeth, all of them are generally fatigued, suffer from cold, and are constipated.

The diet and exercise campaign

This background information was published by the medical expert group (MEK) in a pamphlet in 1971, intended for the informed, but published with an edition of 150 000 copies for a population of eight million, and thus could be read by many others. A more comprehensive second edition with 102 pages and references was published in 1975 (MEK, 1975). The recommendations made by MEK are summarized in Table 2.

Table 2. Summary of the medical expert group on diet and exercise (MEK) recommendations in 1975

Fat ↓ to ⩽ 35 cal %, Saturated fat ↓, PUFA ↑
Sugar ↓ to ⩽ 10 cal %

Proposed changes in per cent of consumption 1960

Green vegetables	+100	Meat, fish and eggs	± 0 (fat ↓ lean ↑)
Fruit	+ 50	Flour, bread	+25
Potatoes	+ 25	Fats and oils	−25
Roots	+100	Others: sugar, syrups, sweets	−25
Milk	+ 25 (lean)		

Breakfast: 1/4 of daily energy need. Most food groups
Lunch: 1/3 of daily energy need. All 7 food groups
Dinner: 1/3 of daily energy need. All 7 food groups

Dental health:

Sugar-containing products ↓	Promote mastication
Regular meals	Promote secretion of saliva
Few snacks	Oral hygiene

Regular exercise

In the meantime, the campaign organization had been increased with a number of project groups (Fig. 4). It was clear that the information campaign to the public should be preceded by information to and discussions with existing key position organizations, such as large institutions, the sports movements, mass media and the schools.

A special project group called Institutions was, therefore, created and became activated in the first major campaign as soon as the MEK report was available in 1971. A basic investigation was made in 225 lunch canteens. This investigation showed that good nutrition was strived for only in exceptional cases. Therefore, several conferences were held all over the country and the project group worked out dietary recommendations for employee restaurants, institutions for care of the elderly, and nursery schools. Furthermore, they produced special information packages to be used in the training of the staffs of large catering units.

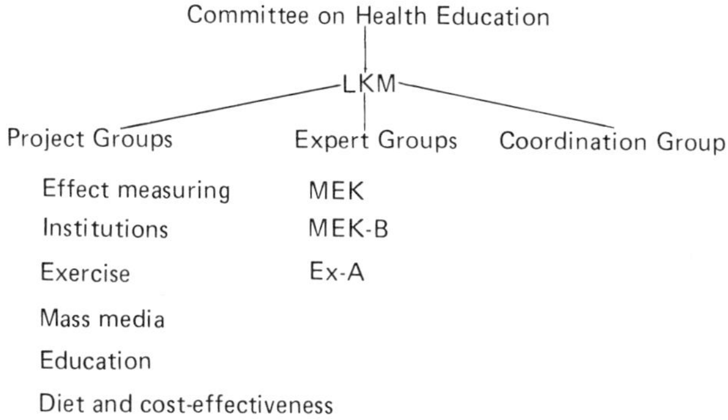

Fig. 4. The organization of the diet and exercise campaign

Monthly, they distributed posters with simple texts, partly intended for the staff (to be placed in the kitchen) and partly for the guests.

Another project group called Exercise cooperated with the sports movement, whose 200 000 leaders were expected to be able to function as communicators of the dietary principles, at the same time as they should motivate people to increase their physical activity. The National Sports Movement has a secretariat which produces and distributes a great number of pamphlets. They regularly arranged nation-wide exercise activities for different population groups, and then these activities also began to involve some sort of activity within the field of nutrition, such as competitions in diet knowledge.

At the beginning, the campaign organization also included the project group, Mass media. This group attempted to create cooperation with the various mass media but without success. There was also a project group, Education, which studied the extent of education in nutrition in the public schools and in adult education. Unfortunately, this type of education is very much neglected in Sweden, and this is considered one of the reasons for the present poor situation with respect to the dietary habits. This group worked out plans for improved education in schools, and the strategy by which to carry them out. The success has been limited and certain campaigns directed to the schoolchildren are, therefore, planned.

One inhibitory factor in all efforts to change food habits is food prices. It is common opinion among the public that nutritious food is more expensive than people can afford to buy. It was very easy for a special project group, Diet and Cost-effectiveness, to prove that it was possible to compose nutritionally well-balanced daily menus that satisfied all reasonable aspects of good food and still did not cost more than the traditional menus. This project group also presented the idea of a two-component menu, 'Base and supplement'. The basic diet included the cheap staple foods at defined quantities that cover the main part of the daily need of essential nutrients and energy. The supplementary foodstuffs cover the remaining need to make the menus varied, palatable, still inexpensive and within the framework of good nutrition.

An insufficient budget, however, reduced the activity plans so that they would by no means reach the public to the extent that they had been intended. It, therefore, became clear that it was necessary to try to seek cooperation within the industrial sector in order to achieve effective campaign. We were all rather surprised to learn that the small publication of the MEK group had been accepted as the official guide with respect to the product development of the food industry, and to an increasing extent also by other producers and by commercial organizations. In order to obtain direct support, a special coordination group was formed, later called the Advisory Committee on Industrial Questions, with representatives from the food industry and the retail trade organizations

Theme activities

It was soon apparent that the best form of cooperation with industry could be achieved within the framework of certain theme activities. The first example of this was the campaign 'Begin your day in a better way' which was directed towards the public. The background of the campaign was surveys which had shown that breakfast was the meal that people were most careless about in our country. Ten per cent of Swedes did not have breakfast at all in the morning. We also found that obese people usually had very poor breakfasts. Only a minority of Swedes consumed 25 per cent of the daily total energy and nutrients at breakfast, which was the recommendation of the MEK group. Recipes for some simple basic breakfasts and a programme for limbering up movements were worked out. All food industries which had a product that could be included in these or other good breakfasts were invited to participate in the campaign, provided that the product was marketed in its proper connection, in other words that the whole concept of breakfast and the importance of a good breakfast were emphasised. The retail trade contributed with window displays of suitable breakfast ingredients and by distributing centrally-produced pamphlets to the customers. These pamphlets were produced by the campaign office who also made available suitable texts to be used by the food industry in its advertising. In this way, the campaign was given increased coverage and made economically stronger.

In the spring of 1973, the campaign was tested in the Malmö region in southern Sweden. All of Sweden was reached during the following year.

A campaign, solely concentrated on products, took place during 1976, together with the Bread Institute, concerning our low bread consumption and the recommendations of MEK of a 25 per cent increase. This campaign was nation-wide and directly provocative as the public could read in all newspapers and on all advertising posters 'The National Board of Health and Welfare wants you to eat 6-8 slices of bread every day'.

The present program, operated via industry, takes place under the name 'Live well'. The object is to educate store clerks, both via the training programs of chain stores as well as by mechanized information. A brochure for the program has been worked out. This brochure is a unique document. First of all, it gives basic data in a simple manner about our dietary habits and the changes needed and, secondly, it contains text information which can be used by the individual store for its own campaign. Furthermore, it contains information on what would happen to profitability if the sales were changed in the direction desired. Finally, it gives examples on questions, which customers may-ask, and answers to such questions. As an example of this, I would like to mention a section on table fats, which is written and financed jointly by the dairy industry and the margarine manufacturers association and which contains a clear message to the consumer that he should reduce his consumption of table fats. As far as I know, the text writers are still employed by the respective organizations.

Unfortunately, the budget does not facilitate selective information to the extent required. The campaign must utilize information systems which already exist and now relies on four channels for this activity: provincial councils, schools, places of employment and large institutions. As much as possible is to be invested on the local level and the campaign organizers, therefore, cooperate with municipal authorities who arrange so-called health meetings where questions related to diet and exercise, and reduction in smoking are discussed simultaneously. However, many selective information campaigns have been planned but have never left the planning stage because of lack of money. This means that there are many persons in Sweden, especially among doctors, who still know nothing about the campaign.

Assessment

What can be said about the effects of the campaign? Unfortunately, we must admit that the scientific evidence supporting our opinion that the campaign has had some effect is rather small. A sociological study of a great number of variables in a representative sample of the population was carried out in 1971 by the project group, Effect Measuring, in order to define knowledge, attitudes, and habits of the population with regard to diet and exercise. The intention was that it should be repeated every fifth year but this has been impossible because of the lack of money. The most important instrument in the governing of the campaign is thus not yet available.

However, we can still justifiably maintain that there have been changes of attitudes in our country. People have become conscious of nutrition without knowledge of nutrition. The food industry has developed a number of new basic products which are in agreement with nutritional principles. Thus, the dairy industry has developed a low fat milk with only 0.5 per cent fat. There are types of lean cheese and table fats containing only 42 per cent fat. The composition of the margarines has been improved and leaner meat, pork, and sausages have been made available. Our bread assortment has changed towards more unsweetened bread and more whole wheat bread compared with the previously predominant sweet loaves, baked with flour of a low extraction degree.

From the Food Balance Sheets (Statens Jordbruksnämnd, 1977), it appears that no dramatic changes have occurred of the magnitude reported from the US, Walker, (1977) but the undesirable development of the dietary pattern during the sixties seems to have been broken. Consumption of potatoes (Fig. 5) continues to decrease regardless of the aim

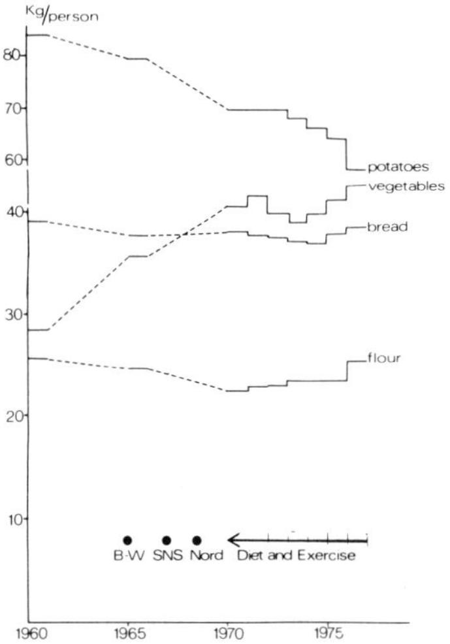

Fig. 5. Per capita consumption of potatoes, bread and cereals in Sweden during 1960-1976. BW = Blix-Wretlind's memorandum in 1965: SNS = Swedish nutrition society recommendations in 1967: Nord = collective recommendation on diet in the Scandinavian countries, 1968: diet and exercise = the campaign starting during 1970

of the campaign to increase it by 25 per cent. With regard to cereals and bread the declines have stopped and an increase was shown in 1976, the year the campaign was focused on bread. The bread campaign efficiency was higher than for any other campaign in our country with respect to observation (81 per cent), remembrance (70 per cent), and reading (36 per cent) of the adult population. As late as 8 months after the campaign, the number of Swedes who recalled the advertisement was as high as the number of Swedes who recall the colors of the Swedish flag. Bakeries all over the country reported an increase in sales which averaged 5 per cent for bread, at a time when price increases were expected to cause a considerable decrease in the consumption of bread. A decrease by 9 per cent was reported for pastries etc. In the campaign for better breakfast habits, there was participation by about 50 per cent of the stores in the country and 95 per cent of all daily newspapers reported on the campaign. A follow-up showed that people on average had improved their breakfast.

For sugar- and sugar-rich products (Fig. 6) the consumption of soft drinks and confectionary even decreased, while the consumption of candies and fruit syrups remained unchanged. Total consumption is on a high level, and it is a long way to the goal of a 25 per cent cut.

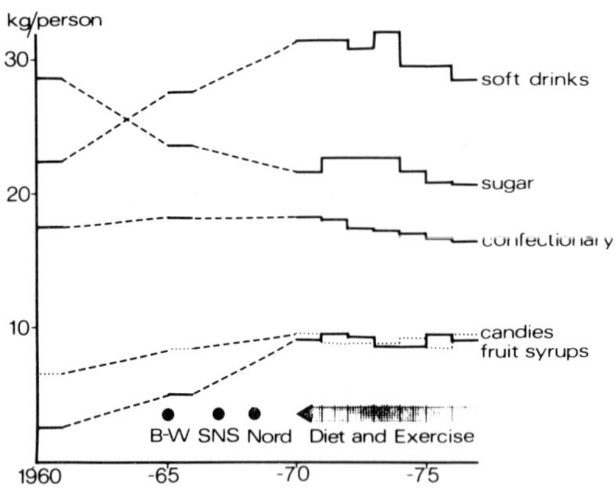

Fig. 6. Per capita consumption of sugar and sugar-rich products in Sweden 1960-76. Symbols, see Fig. 5

With regard to table fat (Fig. 7), during the sixties, a shift occurred in favour of margarine. Butter consumption increased again after 1973, when Sweden was the only OECD-land to decrease its total fat consumption significantly. The decrease in fat consumption also still has a long way to go.

The decrease in total milk consumption (Fig. 8) has changed to an increase due in part to the increase of low-fat milk, which covers a quarter of total consumption. On the other hand, the consumption of cream and other dairy products is increasing; the net result is probably the same fat intake from the dairy industry as during the sixties. It has not been possible to cope with the increase in pork consumption or meat consumption.

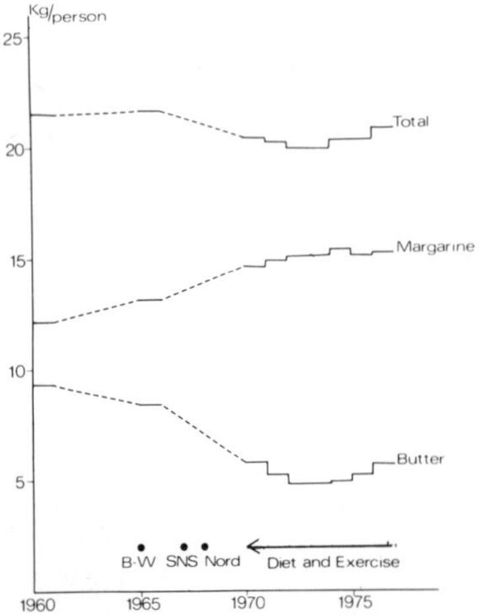

Fig. 7. Per capita consumption of margarine and butter in Sweden 1960-1976. Symbols, see Fig. 5

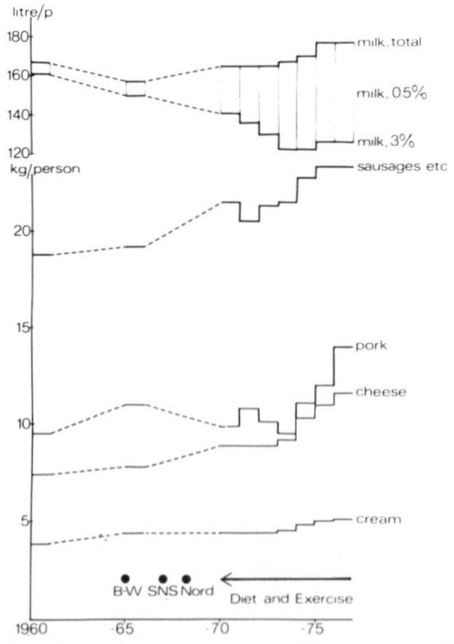

Fig. 8. Per capita consumption of milk, cheese and cream, sausages and pork in Sweden 1960-76. Symbols, see Fig. 5

The figures for per capita consumption should be compared to the results from some dietary surveys which show that people from higher social classes have changed their food habits and have considered the information supplied more than others. In reality, this would mean that in our society there are many people whose dietary habits continue to deteriorate.

Unfortunately, it is impossible at this stage to say whether the dietary changes have caused changes in the health of the public. The increase in death rate due to coronary heart disease seen during the sixties has levelled off, but not decreased as in the US (Walker, 1977). However, there are cardiologists who deny that our statistics allow us to draw any conclusions whatsoever on changes during the last decades (Tibblin *et al.*, 1970). For this congress, it would be of particular interest to know whether the dietary changes have involved changes in the incidence of obesity. In this connection, some data based on a population study performed on women in Gothenburg 1968/69 and reported on the same women in 1974/75 could be of interest. The increase in body fat with age expected from cross-sectional data failed to show up in this longitudinal study (Bruce, B., Bengtsson, B., Noppa, H. & Isaksson, B., unpublished data).

It must be established, however, that the campaign has not affected the agricultural policy in Sweden. The 1972 Swedish Governmental Planning Committee for the national farming policy has recently published its report (Jordbruksutredningen, 1977). Of the 420 pages, only about half a page is devoted to nutritional aspects with respect to production objectives. It was stated that the development as far as dietary habits are concerned is to be influenced primarily by means of information. At the same time, the committee recommends production changes and a subsidy of the foodstuffs which obviously must counteract the consumption changes required. Our new Minister of Health has expressed a desire to adhere to the World Health Organization resolution WHA 30.51 (WHO, 1977) which says that one should strive for a multi-sectorial, national nutrition policy program and that in this respect, the health sector should play a dominating role. Without participation of the agricultural, trade and food industries, the food stores, mass media, and the educational and health sectors, our diet and exercise campaign will not reach its goals.

References

Blix, G. (1965): *Acta Soc. Med. Upsal.* 70, 117.

Blix, G., Wretlind, A., Bergström, S. & Westin, S.I. (1965): *Vår Föda* 17:7, 1.

Jordbruksdepartementet (Department of Agriculture) (1977): Översyn av jordbrukspolitiken. Betänkande av 1972 års jordbruksutredning. Statens offentliga utredningar, 1977:17. Stockholm: LiberFörlag.

Keys, A. (1968): *Nutr. Rev.* 26, 259.

MEK (Medical Expert Group) (1975): *Kost och Motion,* h-fakta 1, Socialstyrelsens nämnd för hälsoupplysning, 2nd edn. Stockholm: LiberFörlag. (First edn 1971).

National Central Bureau of Statistics (1977): *Causes of death 1975.* Stockholm: LiberFörlag.

Statens Jordbruksnämnd (National Farming Council) (1977): Per capitakonsumtionen av livsmedel mm i Sverige 1960-1976. Mimeographed.

Tibblin, G., Vedin, A., Werkö, L. & Wilhelmsson, C. (1970): *Läkartidningen* 67, 4125.

Walker, W.J. (1977): *New Engl. J. Med.* 297, 163.

World Health Organization (1977): Thirtieth World Health Assembly, Geneva, 1977. Part I. Resolutions and Decisions, Annexes.

53
Obesity as a marketing problem. Can government use the solution?

J. HAUSER
Health Division, Statistics Canada, Ottawa, Ontario K1A 0T6, Canada.

Summary
Since obesity in North America is largely related to the choices individuals make about the food they eat or the exercise they take, it is possible, in order to reduce the incidence of obesity, to consider altering those choices as a marketing problem. Serious consideration has been given in recent years to applying marketing technology to social problems. Government and other public agencies with a mandate to reduce the prevalence of obesity can valuably use the concepts of marketing to meet their objectives.

This paper discusses the way in which marketing might facilitate social change and illustrates how, using the problem of obesity, it might be adapted for use by public service managers. The logical sequence of marketing activities are shown to be a common sense approach to achieving social change. The problems of using marketing technology in the public service are examined, and some of the ethical questions of the apparent manipulation of behavior and the potential limitation of individual freedoms, as a result of using marketing technology, are considered.

To the author's knowledge no large scale use has been made of a marketing oriented approach to change health related behavior used in North America. This paper suggests that such an approach to improving health should be seriously considered.

Introduction
Obesity is a widespread social phenomenon in North America which, although an integral part of our culture, can be considered a behavioral disorder of our own choosing. The choice to eat too much and exercise too little is taken by the majority of North American adults. Marketing is a technology whose purpose is to influence choice - the choice for one brand rather than another or, the choice for one life-style rather than another. Marketing, which in its purest form is applied behavioral science, can be used to influence the choice North Americans make to become and remain obese.

This paper will examine the concept of marketing and in particular assess the relevance of the proposed (Kotler & Zaltman, 1971) broadening of the concept to serve as a 'promising framework for planning and implementing social change'. If obesity can be adequately described as a social phenomenon, then social change is required to reduce its prevalence.

Public Health Agencies have increasingly expressed the concern that the only future improvements in national health will result from amelioration of life-styles detrimental to health (Lalonde, 1974). Notwithstanding the difficult decision of government to influence the life-style choice of its constituents, this article will suggest possible applications for marketing within the public sector.

**The opinions expressed in this paper are those of Dr. Hauser and in no way reflect upon present or proposed policies of Statistics Canada or the Canadian Government*

Marketing is popularly seen as a manipulative tool that has been widely used by profit-oriented industries to bring about a gradual dehumanization of the North American way of life. As will be seen, marketing technology is effective, but it only responds to consumer demand, and marketing does not reduce freedom of choice. Nevertheless, the ethics of directing social change, by whatever means, must be addressed.

After having described marketing and adapting it to the problem of obesity, having suggested how a marketing program might be managed, and finally considering the ethics of marketing, this paper will conclude by recommending that it be tried on both a small and large scale and that the results be evaluated against any other presently available technology to reduce the incidence and prevalence of obesity.

One word of warning, the author is not a marketing manager; all his knowledge of marketing is culled from the literature and from experts in the field. The description of marketing in this paper is solely for the purpose of illustrating the basic concepts of marketing. It is the application of those concepts to health problems that is the central thesis of this paper. For a more detailed discussion of marketing, the reader is encouraged to review the literature, to which some references are given at the end of this paper.

Marketing: a short description

The fundamental concept of marketing lies in the exchange process (Kotler, 1972*a*). Two parties exchange with each other something the other wants. Modern marketing management simply facilitates desired exchanges. The task of the marketing manager of a company with a product to exchange for money is to ensure that the product is known and available to persons willing to buy the product at the market price.

In other words, the task of marketing is to have the right product, at the right price, in the right place, with appropriate promotion. The four Ps of marketing - product, price, place (distribution) and promotion - illustrate that marketing is more than simply promotion. Advertising without a clearly defined and readily available product serves largely to promote the advertiser than effect any change. Promoting the advertiser is the unanticipated end result of many well-meaning public service advertising programs to 'educate' the public.

A marketing program may be initiated in response to a developed product that must be sold or, alternatively, by discovering unfilled needs and creating the goods or services to meet those needs. Whichever approach is used, the initial, and most important, function of the marketing manager is to define the market to be served. Analysis of the market (market research) plays a major role in all marketing programs. Markets are segmented by geographic location, by age or sex, by socioeconomic status. The wants, needs, desires, attitudes and behavior of potential markets are examined. Even if the product to be marketed already exists it may be 'packaged' by providing service, convenience, financing, etc. in order to meet the needs of the target market.

Essential to any successful marketing program is the distribution network. Having the product readily available, once the customer has decided to try it, is critical to the facilitation of the exchange process. Reaching, on the supermarket shelf, for a different brand advertised on television is a prime example of the importance of product availability. Too often, public advertising campaigns fail because the desired behavior change, such as trying a new brand, is not easy for an individual to make. Minimizing the incremental behavior change increases chances of a successful outcome to an advertising program.

Advertising campaigns are designed around the wants and attitudes of the target audience. Awareness, interest and knowledge of the product are important but a marketing campaign will fail unless knowledge leads to action - the desired exchange. A strategy of mass media communication, personal selling and sales promotion will lead the interested to buy. Often knowledge and acceptance of the product only follows buying the product and using it.

The more the desired behavior change can be a part of the daily activities of the target market and, the more it is apparently consistent with existing values and attitudes, the more likely is the behavior change to be made.

In summary, marketing serves to facilitate exchange guided by the wants and needs of the customer using a strategy that delicately balances the product, price, promotion and place to achieve the desired response (and maximum profit).

Social marketing

It has been suggested that the central concepts of marketing are universal and do not only apply to a market where goods are exchanged for money. Marketing concepts can apply to any situation in which items or ideas of value are exchanged (Kotler, 1972*b*). Anyone with a product or a service, an idea or a cause, to exchange in return for some valued behavior or attitude change can benefit from the technology of marketing.

For example, consider two components of an obesity program; the fact that obesity is unhealthy or, that a weight reducing service is available, are an item of information and a service respectively, both of which are willing to be exchanged by public service organizations in return for a valued attitude change or behavior change. This exchange of values can be stimulated and facilitated by the use of appropriate marketing management technology.

Marketing is independent of the institutions or persons using it, thus the tasks of social marketing are the same as those in commercial marketing. The analytical tasks are market research of the target population to aid in the choice of the appropriate presentation of the product. The planning tasks are the choice of appropriate price, promotion and distribution of the product (Liefeld, 1976).

Unfortunately, the word marketing is tainted with the specter of mass manipulation. One of the earliest suggestions that marketing technology can be used for things other than commercial products was in McGinnis' book 'The selling of the president, 1968', the theme of which is that you can sell a presidential candidate like you can sell soap.

Behavioral scientists may view the marketing of social causes with some distain knowing that entrenched human values, attitudes and behavior changes little throughout life. We are well protected from new ideas by our 'selective' perception. Marketing, it may be argued, simply directs the choice of one brand or another for a product the consumer has already decided to buy. This point is readily conceded and illustrated by the suggestion that marketing was simply used to influence the selection of a particular brand of president in an election, in which one or the other candidates would have to be chosen anyway.

However, such a criticism exemplifies the strength of marketing. Behavior change is rarely accomplished by challenging the fundamental values or the peer-supported life-style of an individual. A marketer only asks for a slight shift in preference, for the potential customer to try the product just once, often for free. It is the after-sales service, the face to face interaction, that slowly changes the attitudes and behavior of the customer towards the product. It is suggested later in this paper that in marketing obesity-control for example, a realistic objective would be to encourage the target population to attend, just once, a behavior modification type obesity program. Attendance would be the end point for marketing. By ensuring customer satisfaction with the results, it is then up to the program to achieve the true objective, ie weight loss.

In the marketplace, where very survival depends upon sales, the marketing orientation has shifted from a 'sales model', in which a preconceived product is sold by persuading an unsuspecting public that it meets their needs, to a 'marketing model', in which a product is designed to meet a perceived need after careful analysis of the potential market, in fact selling only to the interested. When transposing commercial marketing to social causes it can be argued that 'social marketing' must use an antiquated concept, the 'sales model'. One might ask how does one design a social cause to meet the wants, needs and values of the population? To use the 'marketing model' the social marketer does not change his underlying objective; he listens to the findings of market research and adapts by choosing intermediate 'products' that meet existing needs. A small change is more likely to be accepted than a large one. Public Health Officials have, for years, preached from the pulpit of 'truth' exhorting the masses to repent and give up their unhealthy life-styles. Such evangelistic selling is for the converted and is ignored by the unwashed masses. Social marketing advocates listening to those masses and adapting what is to be sold to their needs.

In reality, commercial marketing campaigns are a mixture of the sales and the marketing models. Companies must market existing products. Nevertheless, those products can be redesigned in line with the needs and attitudes of the target market. In the same way a social cause can be redesigned to reach one segment of the market. To quote Kotler (1971): 'The main point is that social marketing requires that thought be given to the manner in which manageable, desirable, gratifying, convenient solutions to a perceived need or problem are presented to potential buyers'.

An understanding of the central concept of marketing, ie *the exchange of value according to customer need,* is essential before it is possible to decide whether one's own concern for social change could benefit from the use of marketing technology.

Once having decided to use marketing technology, care must be taken to plan beyond product design and target market selection. The textbook suggestions for the establishment of the appropriate organization to co-ordinate the mix of product, price, place and promotion are simply good common sense management. In particular, marketing management places emphasis on the measurement of output and the modification of the original design in line with observed results.

There are real constraints in both government and public service organizations to the full implementation of a marketing program. Nevertheless, the public service can learn from marketing and apply its lessons judiciously.

The lessons of marketing: public service managers can learn from marketing

A study of marketing management would benefit most public service managers since it is simply good management. Once an objective is set based upon an assessment of the problem using research studies, it is followed by an orderly series of events which will achieve that objective, as measured by studies similar to those used to assess the problem.

Marketing performance is measured by the output, the achievement of the behavior change objective, rather than by the input which is the amount of promotion. The generation of posters, brochures, government funded projects and, the multitude of other government programs, unfortunately, are the usual measures of output in the public service.

Most public service managers, not only those concerned with health information and life-style change, can learn from both marketing as a concept and, marketing as a management process (Richie, 1973). How the ideas of marketing can be applied depends on the managers' own ingenuity and creativity. Marketing can be viewed, not as a set of answers, but more an orderly set of questions which will help you decide exactly what you are doing and for whom. A number of questions have been posed below, if you can answer them honestly, the answers may lead you in a market oriented direction. Hopefully, that direction will be more effective than most present government public information programs.

There are special problems with the use of marketing technology in the public sector. A number of recent articles, advocating a broader use of marketing principles in the public service, have drawn attention to the ethical, political and implementation problems. (Kotler, 1975; Liefeld, 1975; Hauser, 1976). The government budget cycle is a major roadblock. It requires detailed description and program justification before undertaking the market research studies that are needed to define the program. In addition, the presentation of full scale marketing proposals for social change to the public treasury will require a creative and persuasive agility with words as well as fundamental political support.

Other constraints to public service marketing will present themselves in answers to the questions below. Each question is asked and discussed from the perspective of a public service agency supported by government funds and dedicated to improving health by modifying life-style behavior detrimental to health. The comments made are in no way meant to be a comprehensive consideration of these important marketing questions.

Who are our customers?
Public agencies exist to serve the people. Therefore, a public servant has the responsibility to serve everyone. Yet, a marketing program directed diffusely to all is doomed to failure. Consider what different kinds of customers you have for the services you have to offer. How do they differ? Segment your market geographically, by age or sex, by attitudes, knowledge or behavior. The different target markets can be given priorities in terms of the extent to which they can benefit from the program and what the likely chances of success are. Unfortunately, the most needy are often the most resistant to change.

What are the needs of our customers?
Different target markets have different needs: obviously mothers with young children, overweight executives and adolescents eating 'junk foods', will have completely different needs for information and services. The needs should be measured using good survey methodology since the real needs may not be apparent. For example, a market segmentation study of female adolescents (Deitch & Watts, 1977) revealed that the perception of being overweight had little correlation with actual weight. Many normal weight girls had just as much desire to loose weight as overweight girls. The need of this group was not for more knowledge about dieting, since the level of knowledge regarding nutrition was high, but for a program designed to educate the girls about the 'right' weight. In a sense, more information about how to reduce weight might aggravate the struggle of normal weight girls to loose weight by semi-starvation, thus depriving themselves of essential nutrients. In summary, the knowledge we offer is not always the knowledge needed.

Who should be our target market?
Once having decided to direct the energy of the program at one segment of the market in order to achieve a measurable result, careful consideration should be given to who influences the behavior of the target market. The 'buying' role may be minor in relation to the 'user' role. The person who accepts the information may not be the person who can use the information to change behavior. Consider also the 'influencing' role of a third party which may be the critical factor in achieving a desired behavior change. The non-English speaking grandmother in ethnic neighborhoods is often the major determinant of family eating patterns. A marketing program aimed at second generation mothers who overfeed their children will have limited success if it ignores the grandmother's 'influencing' role.

Do we have a product?
As we have seen, the core idea of marketing is the exchange of things or ideas of value. Your product is that which you would like to exchange. A product can, for example, be information, a service, a grant, a community involvement center, a behavior modification program, an activity registration card. In short, a product is anything that, if accepted by the target market, achieves in some way the objectives of the agency. You have a 'product' when the buying or acceptance of it is an action that is measurable. Analysis of the potential market will aid in the process of defining a tangible product. Defining the product to be marketed is not easy but often it leads to a clearer definition of the agency's objectives.

In order to ensure that the product can be exchanged, it has to be presented in such a way that it is acceptable. A product is more than what is immediately visible. A product comprises a range of values, expectations and services. An automobile is more than mere transportation, it is dependability, status, comfort. The product should be designed to carry with it the values, expectations and services that are most likely to be accepted by the target market.

Careful consideration should be given to whether the target market is aware of the product; if aware, whether it is knowledgeable about it; and, if knowledgeable, whether it is interested in buying it. Often a market is willing to act and is just waiting for the product to become available.

If market research suggests good knowledge but little interest, design a product to stimulate interest, do not berate the public with more information. Sometimes action precedes knowledge, ie if the after-sales service is good the market can be taught more knowledge after the decision has been made, for whatever reason, to buy or accept the product.

Is price a factor?

Public Service Agencies rarely consider pricing policy as an integral part of their program. Their products are either free or at cost-plus. Yet, price is a component of the marketing program and can be varied. Obviously, in the private sector, products have to be competitive and make a profit. However, the same basic product can be sold at different levels of quality. Not all consumers want the top of the line model.

Another aspect of pricing policy to be considered in the public service is the psychic-cost of a product. The provision of free services are often ignored in favor of expensive, privately funded services. Presumably, the 'hidden' values attached to the product negatively influence its value to the target group. For example, it is often observed that the poor avoid free hospital clinics in favour of private medical practitioners. Apparently, there is a psychic-cost to waiting in hospital corridors and receiving impersonal service.

Does the distribution system work?

Many excellent products are viewed as imperfect by customers because the promotion promises a product which is unavailable when the customer is ready to 'buy'. A telephone nutrition information service may be an excellent 'product' but if demand is not anticipated, the busy signal may destroy the product's usefulness. The decision to lose weight may be made by potential customers in response to premature local promotion in a group weight loss program before the service is available. These are examples of common distributional problems which are critical to success or failure of a public program. There is often no second chance, failure of prospective customers to obtain the 'product' on the initial try tunes the market out to future promotion.

What is the anticipated demand?

Anticipating the demand is essential to marketing success. Philip Kotler has stated that the essence of marketing management is the regulation of the level, timing and character of demand for the products of an organization (Kotler, 1973). A marketer has as much responsibility to reduce demand when too high, as to increase demand when it is low. Kotler has classified demand into eight states, each requiring specific marketing strategies. The demand states range from negative demand, no demand, latent demand, faltering demand, irregular demand, full demand, overfull demand to unwholesome demand. The last two demand states mentioned require what he terms demarketing and countermarketing respectively, both worthy of further investigation by a social marketer, since many activities of public health officials are directed towards reducing interest in other organizations' products.

Should the marketing program be local or national?

The single most significant factor influencing the scope of a marketing program is the budget. National marketing programs with national advertising cost hundreds of million of dollars. In the private sector, any firm contemplating a national advertising campaign will also spend many millions of market research to aid product design for the appropriate target market. In addition, much of the resources of the company will be devoted to ensuring the distribution system is in place. In short, if you want a national marketing program it will cost many times the cost of the advertising. Since national problems are overwhelmingly local, public service agencies should perhaps devote their energies locally and ensure that the mix of marketing variables (the four Ps) are appropriate for the budget available. National governments usually feel some national responsibility for health education, with the result that their information budgets are lost in the daily cacophony of advertising with which we live.

How should our product be promoted?

This question has purposely been left until last because it is too often considered first. Social marketing is much more than social advertising. Social advertising (as distinct from socially responsible advertising practiced by some companies with a conscience) often promotes an idea but no tangible product. Slogans such as 'Speed kills', 'Eat less, live longer', allow for no measurement of their effect. The only measurement possible is the output, such as posters, brochures, TV spots, which are only the input to a marketing program. The public service manager may be able to measure his performance by considering this output but in reality his program often does little more than tell the public that his organization cares for them.

The promotional vehicles chosen should depend upon the needs of the target market. Do you need to make the market aware, make it knowledgeable or is the market ready to act and merely in need of being directed. Since personal selling is most effective for achieving attitude change, for most health promotions the advertising should be used to precipitate face-to-face contact. Advertising does not need to ask the customer to make a fundamental decision about his life-style, but simply to meet someone or attend a meeting. Marketing is aimed at small incremental changes in behavior. Publicity, unpaid promotion, should be carefully managed, since, it is both a goldmine of free advertising and often the cause of potential overfull demand, which strain the distribution services and, as a consequence, undermine the effectiveness of an otherwise good 'product'.

In summary, consideration of these questions should lead you in the direction of using a marketing approach to problem solving. At the very least their consideration should facilitate the planning by ensuring that most of the fundamental issues have been considered. If a formal marketing program is decided upon, the information presented thus far should allow adaptation of the technology to the particular social problem.

Marketing in the public service: a few ethical considerations

From a political perspective the use of marketing to influence behavior or bring about social change is unacceptable. No matter how lofty the objective, such as the improvement of national health, the politician who supports any program which has the appearance of reducing individual freedom runs a serious risk of not being re-elected. Marketing technology is often seen as a technology of manipulation. Although it has been argued in this paper that marketing does not reduce freedom of choice, a politician cannot afford such a debate. Nevertheless, if the word cannot be used, at least the principles of marketing, which are good common sense, can be applied in the design of programs to change life-style as a step towards improving health.

The essence of our democracy is that individual freedom of choice is to be preserved above all else. We choose how we live our lives, often blinded to the reality that the choice is largely ephemeral. Our choices are determined by our peers and constrained by the environment in which we live. We have the choice to opt out, although few of us really take it. Marketing, as applied behavioral science, recognizes how choice is determined and simply creates situations in which the results of choice or small behavior changes are maximized. A marketer does not challenge basic values and attitudes. He simply accepts existing values and attitudes and allows the choice to take place in a manner such that no major issues are at stake. Attitude change will take place once the product has been bought, and as this happens the potential customer simply moves into a different target market.

Some may feel that such claims for the effectiveness of marketing are exaggerated and that its role is to encourage the public to change brands. In fact, in the private sector, obtaining a 5 per cent share of the market with a new marketing program is considered a success. Thus, although the allegation may be true, it may be an argument in favour of the use of marketing by a responsible public service agency. If it does not change fundamental attitudes, then there is no harm in using it. It is apparent, however, that marketing can be a powerful technology if used appropriately. In fact, other than legislation and revolution, it is the single most effective technology of social change presently available.

Special consideration should be given to the ethics of marketing obesity control, using as a 'product' behavior modification programs. Behavior modification has been shown to be a particularly effective process of achieving weight loss. Yet, behavior modification has been condemned by some as manipulative and oppressive. To clarify the debate, separation of the two issues is in order. Marketing is used to inform the public of the availability of programs to help them lose weight. The marketing component of the program simply allows the public to make a free choice to attend the program. Once having attended the program, the public still has the choice of participating or not. Those that do participate will clearly see the behavior modification techniques as simple tools to enable themselves to have more control over their life and what they do with it.

Conclusion

Marketing has been presented as a technology worthy of investigation by those in the public health field. The application of the principles of marketing to social issues is clearly possible. Marketing has been presented, not as a science to be practised only by experts, but as an orderly set of questions that will allow a manager to decide if the marketing-oriented approach is appropriate to his problem. This approach to presenting the concepts does not suggest that a public service agency would not benefit from employing someone well trained in the art of marketing.

Marketing can be used to effectively transmit new ideas in nutrition, exercise and eating behavior to the public. Its use is recommended in controlled trials to confirm its apparent potential. If success, as measured by eating and exercise behavior change, is proved, its use should be recommended for national health education programs.

References

Deitch, P.K. & Watts, T.A. (1977): Segmentation of a social market by discriminant analysis of attitudes, presented at Canadian Public Health Association Conference, Vancouver.

Hauser, J. (1976): A bureaucrat learns from marketing, presented at Social Marketing Forum, University of Guelph.

Kotler, P. & Zaltman, G. (1971): *Journal of Marketing* 35, (July) 3.

Kotler, P. (1972*a*): *Marketing Management - analysis planning and control.* New Jersey: Prentice Hall.

Kotler, P. (1972*b*): *Journal of Marketing* 36, (April) 46.

Kotler, P. (1973): *Journal of Marketing* 37, (October) 42.

Kotler, P. (1975): Achieving social goals through social marketing. Proceedings of the *1st International social marketing congress,* Belgium.

Lalonde, M. (1974): *A new perspective on the health of Canadians.* Ottawa: Government of Canada.

Liefeld, J. (1975): Altering life-style risks through social marketing. In *Canadian marketing problems and prospects,* ed D. Thompson. Canada: Wiley (in press).

Liefeld, J.P. (1976): The concept of social marketing, presented at the Social Marketing Forum, University of Guelph.

McGinnis, J. (1969): *The selling of the president, 1968.* New York: Trident Press.

Richie, J.B. (1973): *Optimum* 4, 13.

54
Weight control and the food industry

J. SCALA
General Foods Corporation, Technical Center, 250 North Street, White Plains, New York 10625, USA.

Overweight is probably the most common problem of modern life. While its cause, elimination and subsequent control are simple in principle, they appear to be almost impossible in practice. Since the common denominator is calories - derived from food - it is fitting for the food industry to be part of a symposium on the subject.

In a consumer-oriented society the food industry offers options which, if viable, satisfy needs. Consequently, food options for weight control must satisfy needs and fill existing or emerging gaps in the marketplace. I will attempt to identify food product options which can be developed and the means by which they can be marketed.

Food product options for weight control must be designed with four issues in mind: does a need exist; what is the nature and origin of obesity and the eating habits of the obese; what are the points of intervention; and what does the consumer want? After these four issues have been considered, the means of marketing products within the context can be reviewed.

Need

Consumer need consists of two basic types; intrinsically 'real' and 'hedonic'. Health needs usually constitute the former, and pleasure and/or vanity, the latter.

'Real' need - an assumption

The need to achieve optimum weight has been documented on the subject of health by many experts, who have shown that overweight people lead shorter, more sickness prone, lives. (See Tables 1-3 for background). Indeed, I have concluded from the many papers and studies on the subject that more than 25 per cent of our population is significantly, if not seriously, overweight and the percentage is increasing. In the face of these observations I question why the achievement of individual optimum weight has not become a major national goal.

Table 1. Principal causes of death among people rated for overweight (Mayer, 1968)

Cause of death	Percentage of expected: Men	Women
Cardiovascular	149	177
Stroke	159	162
Cancer (all forms)	97	106
Cancer (liver and gall-bladder)	168	211
Cirrhosis of liver	249	147
Appendicitis	223	195
Gall-bladder disease	152	188
Suicide	78	73

Table 2. **Deviation from average weight - US** (Statistical Bulletin Jan 1960)

Age (decile)	Male 10%	Male 20%	Female 10%	Female 20%
2	21	7	21	10
3	19	6	25	12
4	21	5	27	12
5	21	5	26	10
6	21	6	27	9
7+	21	6	27	9

Table 3. Average weights (lb) corrected by age and height (US)

Age	25	35	45
		Men - Height 5′ 8″	
Year of study			
1912[a]	149	155	160
1940[b]	152	159	164
1959[c]	153	161	165
1960-62[d]	158	169	170
1971-74[e]	165	176	178
		Women - Height 5′4″	
Age	25	35	45
Year of study			
1912[a]	128	134	141
1940[b]	123	129	141
1959[c]	125	132	140
1960-62[d]	127	134	142
1971-74[e]	132	140	148

a - Medico - Actuarial Study 1912; b - Equitable Life Study; c - Build and blood pressure study, Society of Actuaries 1959; d - HES Survey 1960-1962; e - Hanes Survey 1971-1974

'Hedonic' need

Does a perceived need to maintain a 'lean look' exist without the fear of early death or disease as a driving force? The intangible standards on which our society judges personal appearance provide an affirmative answer.

Advertising

Although there appears to be a move towards using people who look 'real' in advertising (I refer mainly to facial structure), I cannot identify a tendency to use fat prople. Indeed, one would expect that, just as a proportion of various ethnic and racial groups are represented in advertising, some 30 per cent or more should be fat, but this is not the case. It is revealing to observe that even dresses for overweight (heavy) women are presented on slim models.

In conclusion, if we accept fat people as evidence of the fruits of the 'good life', advertising does not reflect this, since slim models are always used to show people happily pursuing everyday activities using various goods and services.

Public-elected officials

These people are characterized by a wide variety of qualifications, but very few state or national elected officials are genuinely fat. Some have a middle-age spread, some are large ex-athletes, but very few are fat.

Entertainers
Entertainers are usually slim and svelte; especially movie and theater actors. Some country and western singers are fat to obese, but those of national stature are very few. Opera stars are sometimes large (especially the women), but not necessarily obese.

From this brief look at the indices of how we wish to represent ourselves or be represented, it is significant that fatness is usually omitted or obscured. But, one needs only to watch people at a street corner, terminal or swimming pool to realize that there are a lot of fat people in the land. Is the stereotype of the fat, jovial, happy person a reality? On the contrary, purchase patterns suggest that they lead lives of quiet desperation, wishing that they were wrapped in a different body.

Diet literature
A viable business opportunity exists for anyone who can write a good diet book or article. In fact, every major women's magazine between January and June 1977 contained one or more complete articles in each issue on some aspect of weight control. Any bookstore clerk will point out that diet books are among the most viable of sellers. In short, a great deal of money, time and space is given to how to lose weight.

Weight programs
In addition to the purchase patterns of books and articles on weight loss, weight reduction programs meet in every town all across America with their various diet philosophies and plans; weight loss camps exist for the young and the old; devices can be purchased, all with one purpose, ie weight loss.

Fads
Fad foods - wafters, powders, drinks and additives - purport to offer short cuts to losing weight. In these products the consumer is often paying for no more than a crutch since he (she) is in reality reducing caloric intake.

There is thus a twofold need for weight loss: (1) from a health standpoint and (2) hedonically, because people wish to fit the image presented on TV, in the movies, on stage and in public life. Market researchers conclude that from 40 to 60 per cent of adults attempt some weight loss at one time or another during the course of a year. The sales of diet books and articles are a grim reminder that this estimate is probably correct.

Nature of overweight
'Of all human frailties, obesity is perhaps the most perverse. The penalties are so severe, the gratifications so limited, and the remedy so simple that obesity should be the most trivial of all aberrations to correct.' (Schachter & Rodin, 1974)

Thermodynamics - an assumption
Man has peered some 17 billion light years into our universe and found that the laws of thermodynamics apply; so I conclude that they prevail everywhere. In terms of food intake this means that a person consuming more calories than he expends will store the excess calories as fat. Conversely, if he expends more calories than he consumes, he will lose weight.

As Schachter's quote suggests, there is a simplicity to weight controls, ie calories. Experts from diverse backgrounds have shown that caloric manipulation can be employed to elevate or lower weight while maintaining a nutritionally balanced diet. Therefore, I assume that weight loss and weight control are governed by the manipulation of calories. I also recognize that the rates of change and final outcome are controlled by heredity and physiology.

Eating habits and behavior

Studies have shown that overweight people are not as active physically as their lean counterparts. Coupled with general inactivity is a tendency to eat more food.

Although there is no single eating habit which would clearly separate the obese from the remainder of the population, several characteristics appear to stand out. They seem to consume more food whether eating snacks or meals. The feeling of 'fullness' is either elusive to them or requires much greater intake than can be achieved in a short period of time. Eating appears to be important to overweight people and whether this results from the 'stresses' of living or is a 'habit' cannot be clarified. In addition, psychological studies have indicated that the behavioral origins of obesity are as frequently rooted in childhood as other stages in life and that no single event can be identified.

There appears to be a relationship between socioeconomic mobility and the desire to lose weight. If a potential for upward mobility exists, a desire to lose weight may emerge. Therefore, the desire to look lean is related in some way to social status.

In summary, it appears that we can make some generalizations about overweight people. They enjoy food and are less active, but do not focus as a group on any specific food or food category; consequently, as many become obese on 'meat and potatoes' as do those on 'candy and ice-cream'. Therefore, their problem cannot be solved with any single food product or group of products.

Understanding of the problem

Consumers in general do not appear to understand the relationship between calories and weight loss. This is inferred from the numerous fad diets and food gimmicks designed as adjuncts to weight loss. Indeed, in many weight loss programs, calories and general nutrition may not be discussed.

Coupled with a lack of knowledge about calories are the unrealistic expectations for rates of weight loss. Since positive reinforcement is essential to any weight loss program, realistic rates of loss, such as one pound per week, must be reinforced. Thus, some education is absolutely essential in the weight loss process and effective control of the new weight must be a primary goal.

Food options

Dietary trends

Dietary trends help to identify areas for potential food product intervention through the development of food options. They are also useful in the identification of points of need and general changes but cannot speak for specific foods or food products.

Figures 1 and 2, respectively, show the general trend in consumption of calories and

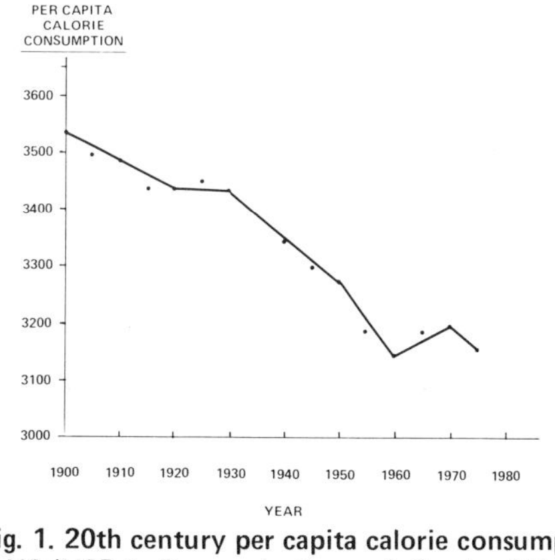

Fig. 1. 20th century per capita calorie consumption – US (USDA. Economic Research Service 31)

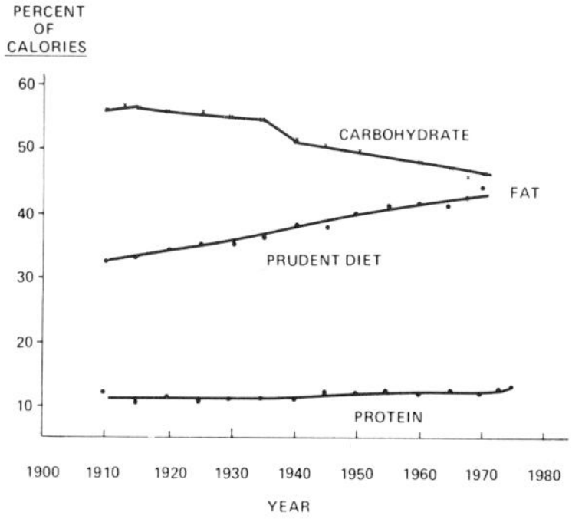

Fig. 2. 20th century calorie distribution – US (USDA. Economic Research Service 31)

their sources during this century. From them one can conclude that calorie consumption has declined, carbohydrate consumption has declined and fat consumption has increased. Since overweight is such a widespread problem it is reasonable to conclude that caloric expenditure has declined more rapidly than calorie consumption.

Table 4 shows the trend to derive more protein from animal sources while an increasing

Table 4. Sources of fat and protein in the 20th century - US (Friend, 1967).

Year	Protein		Fat	
	Animal	Vegetable	Animal	Vegetable
1909-1913	52%	48%	83%	17%
1933-1939	56%	44%	73%	27%
1965	68%	32%	66%	34%

Data rounded to nearest unit

percentage of fat has come from vegetable sources, especially since World War II. This reflects two trends, namely the consumption of more meat and the widespread use of vegetable oils and shortening in processed food and home preparations, explaining the dual nature of the increase in dietary fat. The data in Table 5 indicate that refined sugar has displaced starch as the chief source of carbohydrate while the discretionary use of sugar has declined markedly.

Table 5. Sources of carbohydrate in the 20th century - US (Page & Friend, 1974)

Year	Carbohydrate		Direct Consumer
	Starch	Sugar	Sugar
1909-1913	68%	32%	52 lb
1957-1959	50%	50%	
1973	47%	53%	25 lb*

* Data are for 1971

These trends should be used as background for Table 6 in which the last three decades are used to illustrate the increased use of processed foods. Based on this evidence, I conclude that the American diet has become more sweet, includes more processed foods (eg, 17 per cent of meat), contains less complex carbohydrate and has probably become more calorically dense.

Support for the concept of increased sweetness is based on the observation that total sugar in the diet has remained constant throughout most of this century, but that fraction as complex carbohydrate has declined. Therefore, one can argue that the sugar being used

Table 6. Annual per capita consumption of fresh and processed foods 1947-1976 US (Friend & Martson, 1977)

	1947-1949	1976
Meat, Fish, Poultry (lb)	176	233
Processed Meat Products (lb)	*	47[a]
Dairy Products (Milk Equiv.) (qt.)	236	222
Fruit, Fresh (lb)	164	106
Fruit, Processed (lb)	44	81
Vegetables, Fresh (lb)	184	145
Vegetables, Processed (lb)	47	69
Potatoes, Fresh (lb)	123	102
Flour and Cereal Products (lb)	171	140

* No data available

a - Includes all factory produced meat products such as sausage, luncheon meats (American Meat Institute, personal communication, unpublished data, 1977) is distributed among fewer total carbohydrates than previously. In addition, the use of artificial sweeteners has provided sweetness for soft drinks without sugar.

A question emerges from these patterns of consumption related to the human drive toward sweetness. If one assumes that trends in the marketplace represent a sort of natural selection and that product survival depends upon its appeal, then a drive toward sweetness appears inescapable. Since our diet is probably high in fat, the present level of sweetness is probably near its maximum.

The concept of increased caloric density in our diet is inferred from the observation that fat consumption increased. On a constant dry weight basis foods which are richer in fat will contain less water and more calories per unit weight since most of the calories are derived from the fat.

These conclusions are compatible with the drive towards sweetness and the increased use of convenience products. Both trends afford ample opportunity for food product options which are convenient but also provide adequate palatability at a reduced caloric density.

Possible modes of intervention (new food options)

Based on these dietary trends, one point of intervention is to reduce caloric density while maintaining food volume.

Diets which contain a larger percentage of calories from carbohydrate are, in general, more bulky. This comparison shown in the following table assumes that three 2500 calorie diets contain varying levels of fat and carbohydrate with constant protein. It also assumes that the reduction in fat is compensated for by carbohydrate which binds twice its weight in water and is calorically available.

	2500 calorie diets			
Fat percentage	42	35	30	20
Dry weight	479g	503g	521g	555g
Carbohydrate Index	1	1.14	1.25	1.45
Bulk Index	1	1.3	1.5	2.7

Although the above comparison is theoretical, it indicates that in order to eat a 2500 calorie diet as above the lower fat diets would be heavier and much more bulky. Thus, if people consume either a constant weight or a combination of weight and volume, the greater the amount of complex carbohydrate in the diet the less likely is overconsumption to occur. Indeed, at 20 per cent fat the diet is essentially 'vegetarian' and is bulky by any standard.

History indicates that a reduction in caloric density is most easily accomplished with beverages using artificial sweeteners (soft drinks) or removing fat (skim milk) and, with some difficulty, in fermented beverages (eg, light beer is a newcomer). However, reduced calorie versions of most other products are few and far between. For example, ice-milk and sherbet are really food products in their own right and alternatives to, but not low calorie versions of, ice-cream (see Table 7).

Cakes, pies and all sorts of sweet desserts and snacks could remain available with significantly fewer calories than their original counterparts, if proper diluents and artificial sweeteners are used.

The desire for sweetness and the reduction of discretionary dietary sugar provides a strong argument for the development of one or more artificial sweeteners. The introduction of sweeteners into solid food and snacks would permit more extensive caloric reduction than is now possible while satisfying the apparent drive toward sweetness. Table 7 also illustrates what could probably be accomplished with the availability of Aspartame or an artificial sweetener.

Another point for reduction of caloric density can be achieved by combining carbohydrate technology with meat processing technology and developing reduced calorie alterna-

Table 7. Ice-cream and alternatives

	Standard	Artificially* Sweetened
	kcal/serving	
Ice-cream	129	94
Ice-milk	100	65
Sherbet	88	33
Yogurt (Flavored)	260	175
Cookies (Butter)	115	80
Apple pie	156	111
Gelatin**	71	8
Pudding	166	112
Cake w/icing	365	255
Soda**	144	1
Lemonade	107	0

*Assuming suitable artificial sweetener and non-caloric carbohydrate
** Presently available

tives to processed meat products. The next extension of this concept would be to produce options that are new entrees in their own right, by making use of vegetable protein that reduces fat content or by the introduction of complex carbohydrate into meat entrees.

Table 8 illustrates the caloric reduction if 30 per cent of fat could be replaced with carbohydrate while maintaining palatability. Also shown in this tabulation are some products which are already on the market and widely used. Hamburger extenders illustrate the degree to which such changes are already available. It is important to note that, with one or two exceptions, hamburger extenders, which have been developed and have achieved caloric reduction, have not been marketed. This tabulation also includes consideration of some products if the carbohydrate is 50 per cent biologically available. These products could, in general, achieve a 25 per cent total caloric reduction with ease since the water content would probably increase markedly.

Table 8. Caloric reduction by replacement of fat with carbohydrate

Product	In the form presently available	Replacement of 30% fat with CHO	Replacement of 30% fat with CHO 50% calorically available
	kcal/serving	kcal/serving	kcal/serving
Hot dog	170	142	130
Lunch meat	195	169	157
Bologna	141	121	111
Sausage	152	133	123
Hamburger	243	193	–

I envisage the introduction of carbohydrate into processed meats as necessary if fat calories are to be reduced. These products would require some of the most sophisticated efforts of the food technologists, but are probably not beyond the reach of present capability.

Society is probably ready for such products, considering the widespread use of highly processed meats and fish available at fast food outlets. In fact, it is surprising that such variants have not already been introduced as new 'sensations'.

Alternatively, could we reverse the process and return to strict agriculture commodities with homemade snacks and desserts? In my treatise I have assumed that the relatively low percentage of disposable income directed to food in the US will continue and that our need to provide food at living centers far from farms will prevent this. More fundamentally, the convenience orientation of the American public would be incompatible with this reversion. Therefore, the use of technology to reduce caloric density in available food products and to provide alternatives with reduced caloric density to natural and some processed foods will, in my opinion, emerge. Indeed, the concept might be introduced as the *new horizon* in food science.

Products for weight loss

Since weight loss requires a calorie deficit, any products offering reduced caloric density become elements of a reducing regimen. Three types of products oriented specifically toward rapid weight loss (in excess of one pound per week) are readily available.

Protein supplements are used for fasting under a physician's supervision. These supplements are employed to maintain nitrogen balance.

Diet products based on providing one-fourth the RDA in vitamins and minerals per serving for four servings with an intake of 900 to 1200 calories have been used for over a decade. Basically, these products take the guess work out of dieting and result in rapid weight loss.

Although unbalanced protein (eg, gelatin) as part of a diet plan has been used for decades, there is no documentation of its effectiveness. In theory, these products elicit a specific dynamic action which in proper preloading results in greater satiation and less efficiency in caloric utilization. Surprisingly, unlike fasting or the use of complete dietary products, this approach provides the development of a modification in eating behavior which could be the basis for permanent weight control.

Other products are either combinations of the above or are simply 'gimmicks', not unlike a placebo which works because the consumer follows the low calorie diet which is usually provided with the product.

Serving size

A third approach to weight control is to make more extensive use of existing products presented in 'preselected' serving size. This would require packaging to produce servings of a preselected caloric size as opposed to a preselected serving weight. In this way the consumer could use the manufacturer's directions to develop his own diet or maintenance program.

The consumer

Would the consumer seek out foods which represent alternatives designed to help him lead a more healthful life? Three examples of products oriented towards health are low tar cigarettes, low fat milk and yogurt (Table 9). In the first, the consumer has recognized the risk of cancer inherent in smoking and desires to reduce his risk in the face of an inability to quit; in the second, fat and calorie reduction are desired for the purpose of minimizing perceived risk to the cardiovascular system or of reducing weight; yogurt represents the trend toward natural products based on the belief that they are more healthful.

Table 9. Consumption of health oriented products-US

Year	Low tar[a] cigarettes	Low fat[b] + skim milk (per capita)	Yogurt [b] (per capita)
	billions	fl oz	fl oz
1960	No figures	13	0.26
1965	13	15	0.32
1970	27	43	0.86
1975	65	61	1.64
1976	96	—	—

a - Historical Trends In the Tobacco Industry
b - Economic Research Service USDA

Each of the three issues exemplified by these products represents a consumer trend which should be analyzed for its potential as a vector of opportunity for food product options.

Risk reduction

Risk reduction through low tar and low nicotine cigarettes represents the translation of a rather complex statistical concept into an easily achieved behavioral pattern. Indeed, the consumer is sufficiently aware of the potential so that a company will publish the competitor's tar content while extolling the taste and pleasure which his product affords. Thus, choice probably includes flavor (a hedonistic factor) but focuses on health which is quasi-quantifiable through tar content.

Low calorie - low fat

Low fat milk is probably the 'classical' example of the low calorie alternative. Skim milk finds its place on just about every low calorie diet. Indeed, in the recent decade it has become an integral part of reduced fat diets designed for either cholesterol reduction or oriented towards those who are prone to cardiac disease. Its growth in the marketplace attests to the consumer's recognition of a need for milk and the clear understanding of its message.

The emergence of dietary alternatives to many soft drinks is testimony of the desire to remove calories from the diet while maintaining the pleasurable experience which these products provide.

Expanding this concept to a more sophisticated level we have the egg substitutes with the simple 'cholesterol free' message. Without belaboring the health value of such products, their message is clear and understandable by the user and their premium price, coupled with their widespread use, attests to the consumer's health orientation and desire for the products.

Natural

Yogurt, one of the oldest fermented foods, has emerged as a 'growth' food product in recent years. Indeed, it provides a natural food product which is convenient, moderate in calories, filling and 'seems' to have more fat than it does; in fact, it is a low fat dairy product. Thus, the consumer receives a convenient, healthy product, which is satiating and low in calories.

Addition of fiber to the diet through the introduction of high fiber cereals, breads and as a plain condiment shows that a 'healthful' dietary addition is not only welcome, but is very actively sought out. It indicates a willingness to add something for which one perceives a benefit. Since the use has occurred mainly in the ready-to-eat, high fiber, cereals, the consumer is clearly willing to use food products, indeed even presweetened products, to achieve his objective. It is important to note that the high fiber cereals promote bowel regularity which is obvious to the user and leaves no doubt in his mind that he is deriving a benefit from the use.

In conclusion, the search for health oriented products illustrates the consumer's desire to have good health and to reduce risk. If he understands the risk inherent in overweight, he will, in my opinion, seek risk-reducing alternatives.

Push-pull-education: the marketplace

This paper on weight control has examined the nature of overweight and the possible options for foods. It is now time to examine the marketplace. If products were made of reduced caloric density, would they be sought out by consumers? If so, would they use them properly? Will the food regulatory system permit them?

Conceptually, there is a 'technical push' potential for weight control foods. The concept of reduced caloric density is as apparent as comparing vegetables with beef, prepared in a wok, to the traditional steak, french fries and stringed beans. However, to place this concept before the consumer as meats processed along vegetarian lines, requires integration of carbohydrate, fat and protein technology utilizing meat, fish, fowl and biologically available complex carbohydrates. This three-way integration could bring to the fore a new horizon for food science and new food systems for the consumer. Since the products can be envisaged by the technician, their development becomes inevitable and they are being 'pushed' toward the marketplace.

Obviously, there must be a marketplace demand for any product or it will never survive, let alone thrive, in our economy. Therefore, the question of whether or not the consumer can understand how to use weight control food is critical.

This leads to the all important question of product use in a free-living, convenience-oriented society. Herein lies the second horizon which imposes on the producer the need to develop the product, conduct research to determine its best method of effective use and then explain this to the consumer. Clearly, the process is not simple, but experience proves that if the consumer can understand the need and the health value of his effort he will follow the plan.

An advantage in this effort is the widespread need for weight control. Indeed, controversy surrounds most health issues but the need to achieve and maintain optimum weight usually elicits little or no argument. In fact, it is the one consistency which pervades most health discussions. Educators and nutritionists agree on at least one continuing theme, ie energy balance.

Therefore, when a national nutrition policy is adopted, it should have optimum weight as its primary denominator and a consistent education program should be its objective. In this way the need for nutrition education can start on a common ground and be developed at every level. An understanding of calorie balance and its rewards will become commonplace. Therefore, all three elements of a successful marketplace system will be developed—technical push, realistic marketing concepts and consumer pull. The final outcome will be a reduction in health care delivery costs and better health for the American public.

References

Friend, B. (1967): *Am. J. Clin. Nutr.* 20, 910.

Friend, B. & Martson, R. (1977): Nutritional Review CFE (ADM - 299 - 11) 11.

Mayer, J. (1968): *Overweight: causes, cost and control,* p.103. Englewood Cliffs, NJ: Prentice Hall.

Page, L. & Friend, B. (1974): Level of use of sugars in the United States. In *Sugars in nutrition,* ed H.L. Sipple & K.W. McNutt, p. 97, 101. New York: Academic Press.

Schachter, S. & Rodin, J. (1974): *Obese humans and rats.* Washington DC: Erlbaum/Wiley.

Statistical Bulletin January 1960 and Current Population Reports, p. 25 No. 614 (Table 2 July 1, 1975).

United States Department of Agriculture. Economic Research 31. (1976): Nutrients available for consumption per capita per day, 1909-1975. In *Food consumption, prices, expenditure.* Supplement for 1975 to Agricultural Economic Report No. 138.

Author Index

Page numbers refer to this volume. 'A' indicates that an abstract is published in issue No. 3 or 4 of *International Journal of Obesity* (1978) 2.

Index

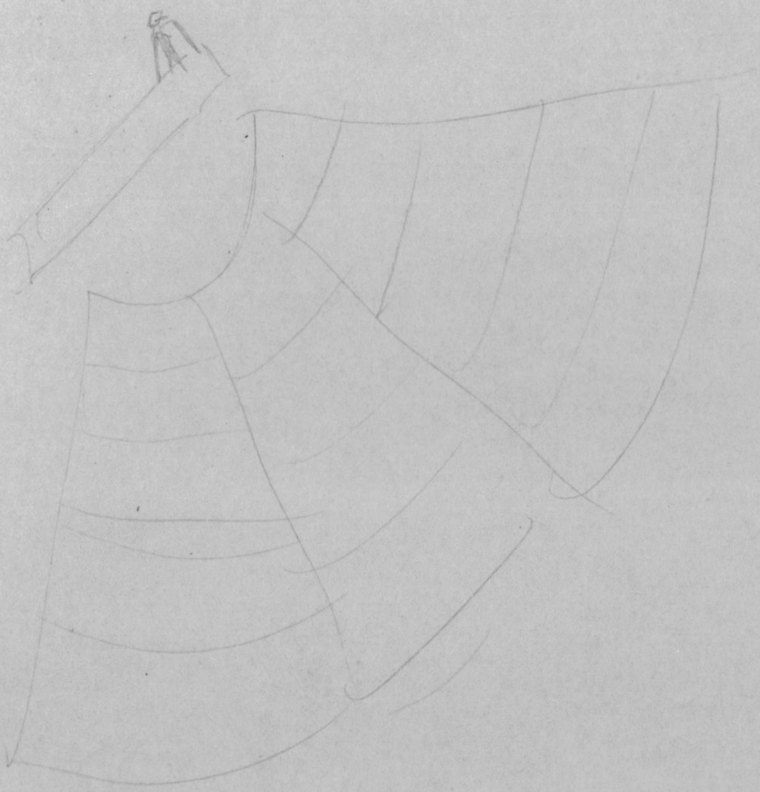